1979

Medical
and
Health Annual

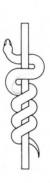

Encyclopædia Britannica, Inc.

CHICAGO · LONDON · TORONTO · GENEVA · SYDNEY · TOKYO · MANILA · SEOUL

1979 Medical and Health Annual

Editor	Ellen Bernstein
Associate Editor	Anita Wolff
Contributing Editors	Charles Cegielski, Robert Rauch, Christine Timmons, Linda Tomchuck
Medical Editor	Richard H. Kessler, M.D. Senior Vice-President for Professional and Academic Affairs Michael Reese Hospital and Medical Center; Professor of Medicine University of Chicago
Art Director	Cynthia Peterson
Design Supervisor	Ron Villani
Picture Editors	Barbara M. Epstein, Roberta J. Homan
Picture Staff	Kathryn Creech, Julie A. Kunkler
Layout Artist	Richard Batchelor
Illustrator	John L. Draves
Art Production	Richard Heinke
Art Staff	Paul Rios
Editorial Production Manager	J. Thomas Beatty
Production Supervisor	Barbara Whitney Cleary
Production Coordinator	Juanita L. Murphy
Production Staff	Mary Peterson Berry, Kathryn Blatt, James P. Carnes, Terry Geesken, Cheryl A. Johnson, Melinda Shepherd, James G. Stewart, Joyce P. Walker, Sylvia Wallace, Coleen Withgott
Copy Control	Mary C. Srodon, *Supervisor* Mayme Cussen
Computer Typesetting Manager	Robert Dehmer
Typesetting Staff	Ronald J. Laugeman, Arnell Reed, Melvin E. Stagner, Gilberto Valle, Elaine V. Yost
Index Manager	Frances E. Latham
Index Supervisor	Rosa E. Casas
Senior Indexer	Judith Anderson
Librarian	Terry Miller
Assistant Librarian	Shantha Channabasappa
Secretary	Marie H. Lawrence

Editorial Administration

Managing Editor, Encyclopædia Britannica, Inc.
Margaret Sutton

Director of Budgets and Control
Verne Pore

Encyclopædia Britannica, Inc.

Chairman of the Board	Robert P. Gwinn
President	Charles E. Swanson
Vice President, Editorial	Charles Van Doren

International Standard Book Number: 0-85229-345-3
International Standard Serial Number: 0363-0366
Copyright © 1978 by Encyclopædia Britannica, Inc.
All rights reserved for all countries.
Printed in U.S.A.

Foreword

Are modern life and advancing medical know-how turning us into hypochondriacs? Are many of the ailments, for which people today spend so much time undergoing costly tests, only imaginary? What are physicians to do when patients insist their common colds are really Legionnaires' disease or even cancer? Both the light and serious sides of this dilemma are presented in the 1979 *Medical and Health Annual*'s opening feature, "Hypochondria."

Consider the fact that 1.5 billion prescriptions are written for Americans each year. Another feature, "Therapeutic Drugs," addresses some of the complex issues surrounding the vast quantities of drugs people take, particularly the question of safety versus risk.

"Living with Leukemia," by Morris Abram, is a compelling personal story of a rare individual who has defied odds and lived for five years in remission from acute myelocytic leukemia. Abram is a New York City attorney whose achievements include winning a landmark decision before the U.S. Supreme Court in 1963, heralded for establishing one vote for every person. He tells of his battle to live, which began on the day of diagnosis. "The Acute Leukemias," by one of Abram's physicians, provides a more technical look at both the childhood and adult forms of leukemia. The pioneering treatment approaches presented in this article seem to signal great hope for the future of cancer therapy in general.

Also among the features in this volume: first-hand observations of mainland China's unique health care system; an inside look at the Mayo Clinic; and a study of the evolution of hospitals from early caring facilities to curing institutions of awesome technology to today's hospices, which symbolize a return to more humanistic care for the terminally ill.

The conquest of infectious disease is the subject of this year's symposium. In the United States one need only consider the case of polio to realize how great an impact the triumph over devastating infectious diseases has had. As little as 25 years ago parents panicked at the slightest sign of a cold or fever in their children, fearing the dreaded crippler. Today polio is a rare and totally preventable infection, but, ironically, Americans have become lax about having children immunized, so epidemics of the disease once again could threaten health. The symposium is comprised of four essays: "Epidemics and History," "Viruses: Drama Within the Cells," "Vaccines: Building Defenses Against Illness," and "Smallpox: Eradication of a Killer." The latter chronicles one of the most dramatic achievements in medical history—what has been called a "public health miracle." It is expected that in 1980 the World Health Organization will formally declare the eradication of smallpox from the face of the Earth.

The *World of Medicine* highlights recent advances in the major medical specialties, from alcoholism and drug abuse to world medical news. Fourteen special reports in this section cover such subjects as "Health Care for Teenagers," "Jogging Injuries," and "Recent Developments in Treating Obesity."

Twenty *Health Education Units* constitute the third section, which emphasizes the active and responsible role you must take in maintaining your own health. Some common concerns such as "Saving Money on Prescription Drugs," "Cosmetic Surgery," "Measles and German Measles," and "Fear" are covered with the intention of making you an informed patient or potential patient. Also in this section are challenging health quizzes that test your understanding of nutrition, exercise, the doctor-patient relationship, and sex.

Finally, the *First Aid Handbook* at the end of the volume was prepared in conjunction with the American College of Emergency Physicians. It offers up-to-date, lifesaving information that you should keep close at hand.

The third issue of the *Medical and Health Annual,* like the previous editions, is edited for laymen and contains topical articles by contributors who are among the most knowledgeable in their fields. The text is complemented by carefully selected illustrations. We emphasize that this book is not meant to be a guide for self-diagnosis or self-treatment and is not a substitute for the advice of your physician. We hope, rather, that it will help you to become more knowledgeable about how and when to seek professional care for you and your family.

Ellen Bernstein

EDITOR

Contents

Hypochondria

by Drummond Rennie, M.D.

In ordinary conversation we mean by a hypochondriac someone who has an unfounded belief that he is ill. We use the term in a condescending, mildly pitying, and derogatory fashion. We try to avoid meeting hypochondriacs because they are such terrible bores: when we greet them with a polite "How are you?" they are only too ready to tell us—at length.

A historical perspective

When Hippocrates used the term *hypochondrion* 2,400 years ago, it meant no more than the region below the chondral (rib) cartilages. Anatomically this part of the body contains the liver and gallbladder on the right and the spleen on the left. But as far back as 350 BC Diocles of Carystus and, later, Paul of Aegina blamed this region of the body in general and the spleen in particular for being the seat and origin of the humors of melancholia—our modern-day depression.

Splenetic and *hypochondriacal* came to be synonymous in ancient Greece. Indeed hypochondria was for many hundreds of years regarded as the male counterpart of hysteria. Hypochondria was due to vapors or humors from the spleen; hysteria (from the Greek *hystera*, meaning "womb") was due to vapors from the uterus. The question whether the spleen and uterus caused bizarre behavior in men and women, respectively, was argued up to the 20th century, despite what we would now call "hysterical" symptoms explicable in no rational anatomical or physiological terms in men and the inconvenient fact that women also had spleens.

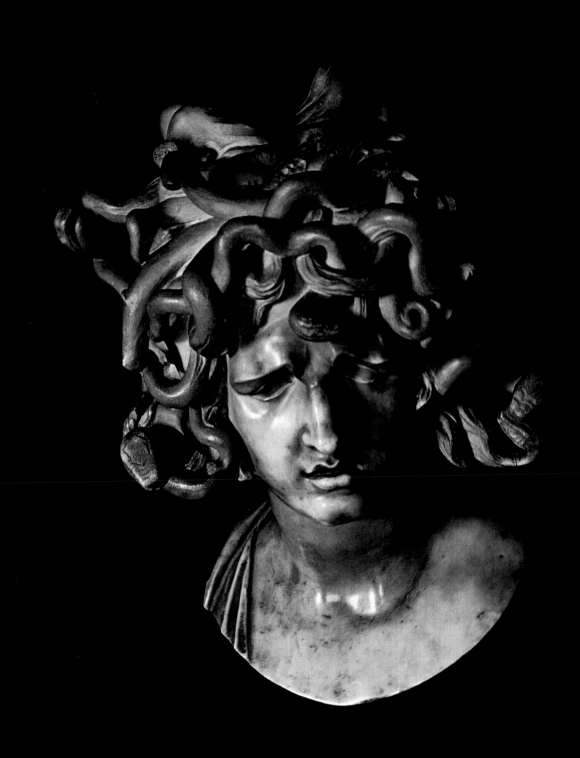

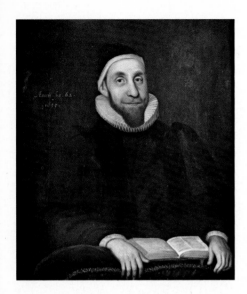

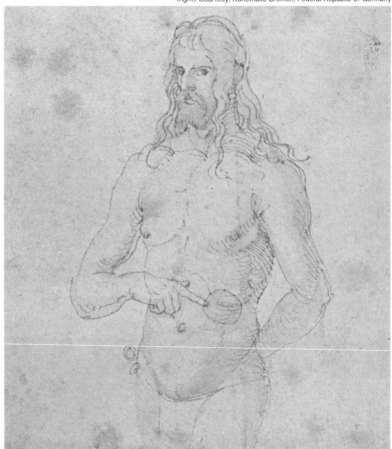

Robert Burton, an English clergyman, wrote *The Anatomy of Melancholy* in 1621. Burton himself was subject to "a sorrow without cause," explaining, "I writ of melancholy, by being busy to avoid melancholy." This long and complex book contains a classic description of hypochondria (melancholy), which had come to be associated with general malaise and unexplained gloom.

That which is but a flea-biting to one, causeth insufferable torment to another; and which one by his singular moderation and well-composed carriage can happily overcome, a second is no whit able to sustain; but upon every small occasion of misconceived abuse, injury, grief, disgrace, loss, cross, rumour, etc., (if solitary or idle) yields so far to passion, that his complexion is altered, his digestion hindered, his sleep gone, his spirits obscured, and his heart heavy, his hypochondries misaffected; wind, crudity, on a sudden overtake him, and he himself overcome with *Melancholy*.

Burton spelled out with elaborate charts all the features, causes, and cures of melancholy—his remedies including, sensibly enough, keeping merry company, dancing, kissing, and making love. The fact that *The Anatomy* was a best-seller, going through six editions in 30 years, meant that it struck a responsive chord in large numbers of people.

Burton's contemporary, the poet John Donne, also suffered from hypochondria. It is quite clear from *Biathanatos,* a theological justification of suicide, that Donne was subject to bouts of melancholia. Just as Burton's

Drummond Rennie, M.D., *is Deputy Editor of* The New England Journal of Medicine, *Boston, Massachusetts.*

(Overleaf) Head of Medusa by Gian Lorenzo Bernini (1598–1680), in the Palazzo dei Conservatori, Rome; photograph by Madeline Grimoldi Archives, Rome.

8

"torment" had produced an extraordinary literary work, so it was with the troubled Donne. His *Devotions upon Emergent Occasions* reflect his morbid preoccupation with his own health, though he always attempted to make useful generalizations from his personal predicament. Donne examined himself in a manner very reminiscent of Burton: "I have cut up mine own Anatomy, dissected myselfe. . . . how wanton and various a thing is *ruine* and *destruction!*" He complained about doctors: "The Masters of that *Art,* can scarce *number,* not *name* all sicknesses. . . . they cannot have names ynow, from what it *does,* nor *where it is,* but they must extort names from what *it is like* . . . the *Wolf,* and the *Canker,* and the *Polypus.*" Yet like so many hypochondriacs, pathetically he went on consulting those very doctors. "I am glad they know (I have hid nothing from them), glad they consult (they hide nothing from one another), glad that they write and prescribe *Physick,* that there are *remedies* for the present case."

Donne wrote with cynical insight, however. Though he acknowledged there was nothing wrong with his pulse, urine, or sweat, and there was no evidence of any dangerous sickness, and though his strength and appetite were good and his mind clear, he noted: "I feele, that insensibly the *disease* prevailes. The *disease* hath established a *Kingdome,* and *Empire,* in mee." In the most famous of his *Devotions* he expresses his own greatest fear—of death: "Therefore never send to know for whom the *bell* tolls; It tolls for *thee.*" He also presents the hypochondriac's ultimate vindication: "*Now, this Bell tolling softly for another, saies to me, Thou must die.*"

The 17th century was a time of great introspection about melancholy, and in 1673 the classic description in literature of a hypochondriac appeared in Molière's *Le Malade imaginaire.* The play has a jauntiness about it that is as hilarious as it is unexpected. Molière's dramas satirized every form of hypocrisy, miserliness, and pomposity. But he was at his best—and truest—when he turned his attack (as he did in six plays) on gullible physicians and their yet more credulous and fearful patients. In *Le Malade imaginaire* the rich hypochondriac Argan imagines he might ensure himself constant medical attention if he forces his daughter to marry a physician but is finally persuaded of a better solution: to become a physician himself. This he does in a farcical ceremony in which it is stated that he has, henceforth, a universal license to kill.

It is a peculiar irony that three years earlier Molière himself had been lampooned in a work called *Elomire hypocondre* as a hypochondriac for thinking his cough was due to consumption. Molière played the lead part in *Le Malade imaginaire,* that of Argan. Toward the end of the fourth performance, on stage, he suddenly suffered a massive bleeding from his tuberculous lungs and died minutes later.

Some hypochondriacs have bouts of illness; others are afflicted all their lives. In the 18th century James Boswell, friend and biographer of Samuel Johnson, wrote of Johnson's life-long hypochondria: "He felt himself overwhelmed with an horrible hypochondria, with perpetual irritation, fretfulness, and impatience; and with a dejection, gloom, and despair, which made existence misery." Meanwhile, Johnson himself wrote in his diary in 1777: "When I survey my past life I discover nothing but a barren waste of time

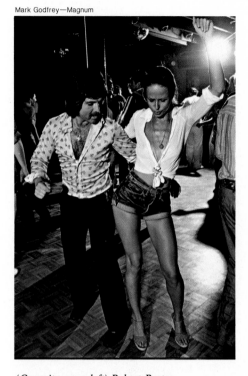

(Opposite page, left) Robert Burton, author of The Anatomy of Melancholy *(1621), the classic delineation of depression and hypochondria. (Above) Burton considered dancing to be a good remedy for melancholy. (Opposite right) Albrecht Dürer (1471–1528) drew this sketch of himself and sent it to his doctor with the notation "Where the yellow patch is with the finger pointing, that is where it hurts me." Dürer is pointing to his spleen. Hypochondria was once considered to be caused by "vapors from the spleen."*

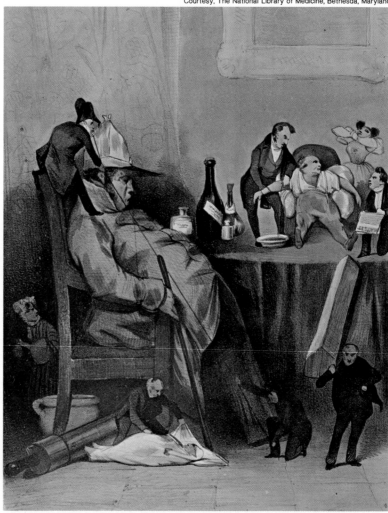

with some disorders of body, and disturbances of the mind very near to madness."

Mary Shelley records that her husband, the great poet Percy Bysshe Shelley, who went to Pisa to consult a famous Italian physician, was also a life-long hypochondriac. He was "a martyr to ill-health, and constant pain wound up his nerves to a pitch of susceptibility that rendered his views of life different from those of a man in the enjoyment of healthy sensations."

Throughout the 19th century hypochondriasis was a complex problem, replete with schools of thought. The Austrian neurologist and founder of psychoanalysis Sigmund Freud felt that hypochondria was an actual neurosis, meaning that the hypochondriac, in concentrating on the organ that was worrying him, withdrew his interest and especially his libido from the outside world. Freud himself had hypochondriacal symptoms. His biographer Ernest Jones wrote in 1958: "He was a chronic sufferer from an obscure abdominal complaint. . . . Increased discomfort, with various other symptoms of general malaise, always preceded Freud's best work." Freud recognized this: "I have long known that I can't be industrious when I am in good health; on the contrary, I need a degree of discomfort which I want to get rid of."

10

Hypochondriasis today

Over the years intense speculation based on little solid scientific evidence has brought us to the position Burton held over 350 years ago. Hypochondriasis is best seen as a manifestation of depression. Burton's melancholy, in its most severe form, was associated with severe slowing down of all functions, from pulse to bowels, from sexual performance to work. In the 1970s few doctors label patients solely with the diagnosis of hypochondriasis. Rather hypochondriasis is now thought to be a symptom.

The word merits only a few lines in modern textbooks of psychiatry, yet everybody thinks he knows what a hypochondriac is. Indeed, patients with severe organic problems sometimes delay seeing their physicians lest they be thought to be hypochondriacs.

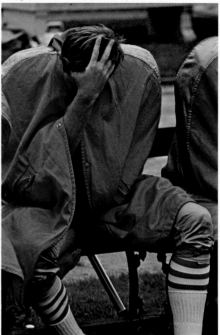

The symptom most commonly displayed by the hypochondriac is a morbid preoccupation with his bodily functions (bowels, heartbeat, body odor, sweating) together with exaggerated anxieties about ailments, real or imaginary, bodily or mental. Naturally, we all know a little of the terrors of this state of mind. We suddenly wonder if it's normal to hear our own heartbeats or imagine that our common cold is really pneumonia and quite possibly cancer. Even the fittest are not immune. Athletes, who have a tremendous spiritual and financial investment in health, are notorious worriers about minor symptoms. In their walk of life, the slightest ache assumes terrifying proportions, implying, as it does, a loss of form, of grace, of money, and of self-respect.

When, then, is a normally anxious person a hypochondriac? There is no clear line. Perhaps when the continuous series of unresolvable complaints exhausts the physician's reserves of reassurance or kindliness or when the doctor has used up his ability to think of new blood tests, urine examinations, X-rays, electrocardiograms, biopsies, and exploratory operations, all of them done in the fruitless attempt to convince the patient that there's nothing wrong, though there obviously is—in the patient's mind.

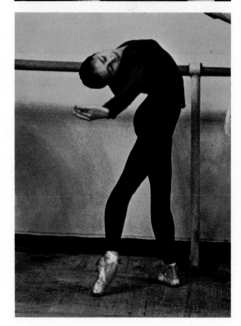

The hypochondriac presents a very special problem to the physician as diagnostician. Though the latter views the patient as a hypochondriac right from the start, his training and the horror stories he has heard of missed diagnoses—quite apart from obvious pressure from the patient and the unseen fear of the patient's attorneys—push him further and further to exclude more and more rare or untreatable conditions, though overinvestigation will, if anything, increase the hypochondriasis. Proof of normality having been repeatedly offered up to the impervious patient (who merely regards it as evidence that he has something yet more seriously wrong and beyond the powers of medicine to diagnose), patient and physician end up staring at each other in mutual frustration and, only too often, dislike. The doctor feels he has wasted valuable time and energy away from the really sick; the patient still has his complaints.

The true hypochondriacal patient has a conviction rather than a fear of disease or of malfunction of one of his systems, unlike the merely anxious patient who fears rather than believes. Bernard de Mandeville's witty book *A Treatise of the Hypochondriack and Hysterick Passions,* published in 1711, illuminated this conviction: "I have sent for you, doctor, to consult you

11

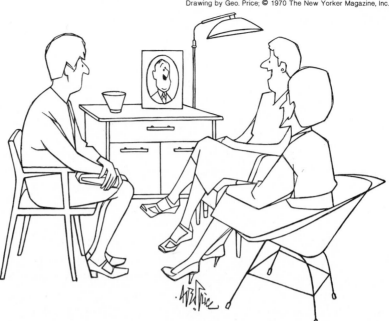

*"He didn't really die of anything.
He was a hypochondriac."*

about a distemper of which I am *well-assured* I shall *never* be cured." The patient may be disgruntled, discontented, and peevish, and he is usually convinced that his own symptoms are not merely of paramount interest to himself but should also be the only interest of his diminishing number of friends and of his increasing number of doctors. The patient may arrive with a meticulous list of dates, times, symptoms, and remedies taken. Frequently he seeks no sympathy, merely confirmation and applause. The symptoms are usually clearly bizarre and inappropriate. They do not hang together anatomically or physiologically and are often contradictory. "My whole body is flooding up; my catarrh is upsetting my nervous system. I scrape my tongue every day, and it's the wrong color. My gallbladder hurts. My eyes are yellow, and I see spots which make me feel faint. All my muscles are tight, I'm constipated all the time, my brain is melting away, and this affects my ascending colon and makes my flatulence worse. I've got diarrhea most days. My temperature is always low in the morning; my kidneys are blocked. I have a stench from my larynx. . . ." Frequently out of a brown paper bag spill 10 or 20 different bottles of tablets, capsules, suspensions, and fluids, which the physician reads glumly like a witch doctor scanning bones.

To complicate matters for the doctor, there are the varied ways hypochondriasis can present itself. The prejudice physicians themselves have toward these time wasters can interfere with diagnosis. The physician is also hampered by the knowledge that hypochondriacal symptoms may be superimposed on physical illness: he is only too aware that many diseases—chronic uremic poisoning due to kidney failure, long-continued drug abuse, diseases due to deranged metabolism such as porphyria or mercury poisoning, and generalized diseases such as diabetes, cancer of the lung, or syphilis—may produce such an enormously varied and peculiar combination of mental and physical symptoms and signs that he could be wrong. The doctor, listening to the long litany of woes of his demanding, manipulative patient, is certain

12

the patient's ills are imaginary, suspects the patient knows this, and yet he worries endlessly: when does the cry of "Wolf!" signal real danger? Most physicians have investigated a complainer, found nothing, and referred him or her to a psychiatrist, only to have the patient return a few months later with a now abnormal chest X-ray.

The problem of classification

There are numerous classifications of hypochondriasis; most are based on poorly understood, ill-defined, and inadequately investigated symptoms. The subspecialist in, say, kidney or cardiac diseases, who is used to arguments about minutiae but not about whether something exists, finds the attempts to classify hypochondria quaint and unscientific. Some authors divide it up by organ or complaint (nasal, abdominal, cardiac, and so on). While this is impractical, it has led to some glorious terms—*Schoenheitshypochondrie* is hypochondria about beauty ("Mirror, mirror on the wall, who is the fairest of them all?"), and *Haesslichkeitskummer,* preoccupation with ugliness. The trouble is that in some people the problem may always be the same, for example, an obsessive interest in chronic backache, while others have different complaints every week—or simply settle for total body malfunction from eyes to toes. Some hypochondrias are related to age; thus adolescents worry more about their genitalia or elderly people about hardening of their arteries.

Nose hypochondria is a particular oddity. It occurs only in male patients and is plausibly associated with a fear of castration. Freud's famous Wolf-man went through an episode of it. The great Russian author Nikolai Gogol wrote a short story, "The Nose," in which the hero finds on waking one morning that his nose is gone. He immediately thinks that he will never be able to marry. Later he meets his nose, now clad in the full dress of a privy councillor. It snubs him and then, just as he is about to approach it in church, a beautiful girl appears, and he feels unable to do so. Poor Gogol: he had a terrible complex about his own nose, a complex that he held up for the world to laugh at. One is of course reminded of the wretched Cyrano de Bergerac in Edmond Rostand's play: "No girl could ever love him because of his enormous nose." But the difference is that Gogol's nose looked entirely normal, despite his convictions.

Recognizing that depression, often heavily disguised, is the underlying theme of hypochondriasis, psychiatrist A. L. Lipsitt finds it unfortunate that the "familiar faces" in a clinic are frequently labeled "chronic complainers," "problem patients," or "crocks," with all their complaints or "organ recitals" (terms revealing of the doctors' frustrations, if not prejudices). Lipsitt describes these unfortunate patients as "hospital orphans," wandering on their own accord or by exasperated referral, from clinic to clinic.

The psychiatrist obviously sees a very different population from the internist, but to varying degrees most physicians agree on two general types. First, there is the hypochondriac whose symptoms are a sudden expression of some crisis or unresolved inner struggle and who at this stage may well be saved from a career of hypochondriasis by a sympathetic and thorough physician. Second, there is the chronic depressive who appears in many

13

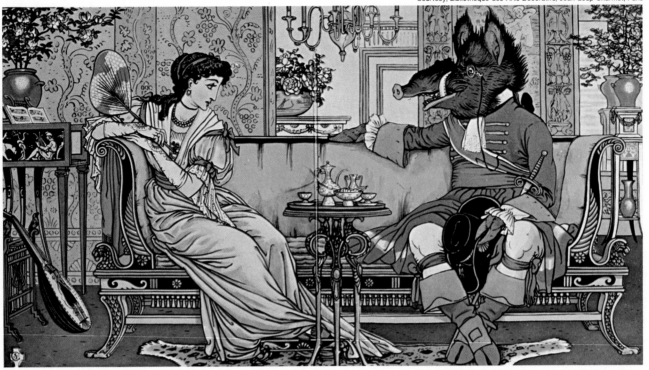

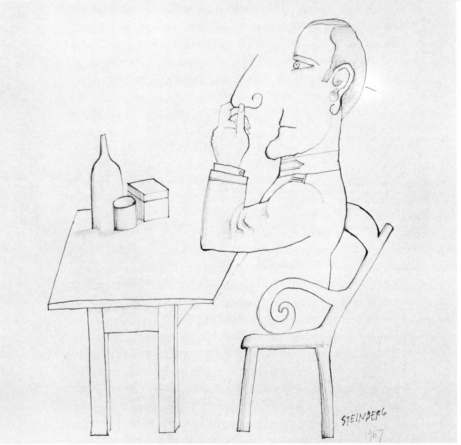

guises, often deriving smug satisfaction from a lengthy rehearsal of his or her innumerable illnesses and of sacrifices for others (perhaps in order to atone for guilt feelings reaching back into childhood). This patient is prepared to debate and do battle over treatment with as many physicians as he or she can find.

The first group is easier to understand because it is generally comprised of middle-aged people with middle-age problems, and they tend to respond more readily to therapy. The chronically depressed group, on the other hand, are dependent and clinging and rely on a doctor's office staff or clinic personnel for ceaseless sympathy. Without the ritual of chat, examination, and bottle of medicine, these patients fall apart.

Causes

Considerable advances have been made in detecting small chemical changes in the tissues of some people with gross psychiatric illness. Despite this, we know very little more about any biochemical causes of hypochondriasis than Robert Burton. Occasionally one may prove a biochemical cause, as is likely in the case of the prophet Job. He has been called a classic case of depression with hypochondriasis: "At night he scrapeth off my bones from me, but my veins do not rest." But it is far more likely that he simply had a deficiency of nicotinic acid, causing pellagra. Clearly, howev-

Hypochondriac fear may be generalized or may focus on one condition or part of the body. It may express itself in preoccupation with ugliness or beauty (opposite top), as in the French fable of Beauty and the Beast, 19th-century illustration by W. Crane. (Opposite bottom) Nose hypochondria is an exclusively male problem thought to be an expression of castration fears. (Below) Hypochondria is most often seen in middle-aged people, and men appear to be affected more frequently than women. It may be the physical mirror of unresolved internal turmoil. Painting by Francis Bacon, "Man in Blue Box" (1949), oil on canvas.

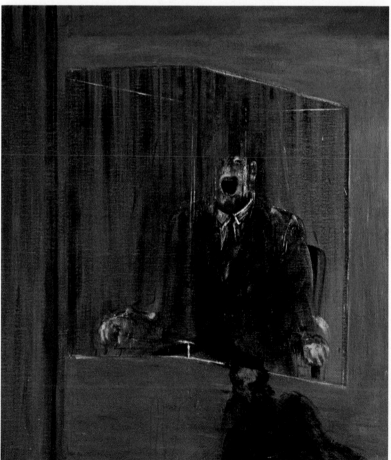

Courtesy, Museum of Contemporary Art, Chicago; gift of Mr. and Mrs. Joseph R. Shapiro

er, vitamin deficiencies do not account for most hypochondriasis today.

The presumed psychological causes vary with the type of hypochondria and are probably many, depending on the genetic make-up of the individual, *i.e.,* his *nature,* and the environment—his *nurture.* The problem here is that we lack facts. A great deal is known, for example, about the inheritance of schizophrenia, but as in the field of most neurotic illness, we are as yet unable to provide more than theories. One is left adrift on a sea of fascinating speculation. This is in part because most psychiatrists are not used to putting psychological theories rigorously to the test by using all the very considerable expertise that medicine, epidemiology, and statistics have accumulated in assessing, say, the causes of and therapies for disease. It is also due to the difficulty of definition (how hypochondriacal is hypochondriacal?), to the vagueness of the characteristics measured (on a scale of one to ten, how depressed are you?), and to the subjective nature of the psychiatrist's approach (one man's hypochondriac is another man's hysteric or misunderstood genius or henpecked husband or possible wronged patient). Indeed, so widespread is lay and professional knowledge—and misinformation—about psychological theories that the patient himself may have his own theory. For the physician it is always interesting to spin theories about each patient, but he must recognize them now for what they are—guesswork and a web of ideas—while he gives all his attention and sympathy to listening to that patient in order to help him come to terms with himself and to alleviate his depression and hence his suffering.

Incidence

There are almost no believable figures on the incidence of hypochondriasis, in part because different authors use different criteria for diagnosis, and all are subjective. G. A. Ladee, professor of psychiatry in The Netherlands, wrote a book on hypochondriacal syndromes in 1966. His 225 hypochondriacs, culled from psychiatric clinics, were all severe. (They made up 2.5% of the populations of these institutions.) They did not include the average, at home, chronic, boring complainer. Some general internists, on the other hand, might conclude that a quarter or half of their mildly depressed patients are hypochondriacal. The fact is we do not really know.

Ladee found hypochondriasis occurred more commonly in men, and the average age was the mid-forties, though those of retirement age also suffered. In general, people who tended to focus all their troubles onto their bodily organs in hypochondriacal complaints tended to be less educated. Such complaints are common in more primitive tribes, as has been shown by other authors, and there are other studies purporting to show that hypochondriasis is more prevalent in Orientals. Ladee observed that the incidence in Jews was four times higher than their percentage in his overall sample (15 Jewish patients, compared with an expected 4), but his population was far too small to allow generalizations. Studies in Israel have merely shown that hypochondriasis is four times commoner in Jewish immigrants from northern Africa than in those from Europe—a fact that remains unexplained.

None of this gives much support for our stock ideas about hypochondriasis. There is little question there are cultural differences that determine psychiatric symptoms, but who can say that the well-known hypochondriasis of the Germans or of the Jews is really excessive? The fact that of Ladee's 566 bibliographic references, 238 were in German, 231 in English, 72 in French, and 13 in Italian tells us much more about the state of the science of psychiatry in those European countries than it does about the relative incidence of hypochondriasis.

Treating hypochondria

The renowned hypochondriac Samuel Johnson once said to another hypochondriac: "Do not be like the spider man, and spin conversation incessantly out of thine own bowels." Well put, of course, but scarcely words for a physician to use, no matter what the provocation.

The doctor may not think much of his hypochondriac's *dis-ease,* but the patient does, so the fact remains it is the doctor's task to help him. The patient who suddenly appears with an excessive awareness of a normal bodily sensation and is morbidly oppressed by it can, after careful examination, usually be treated by encouraging him to discuss his inner conflicts and problems. This may prevent the problems from becoming intolerable and the hypochondriasis a fixed pattern. Sometimes tranquilizers are needed for agitation. When hypochondriasis is a symptom of a major depression, then the proper chemical treatment for depression (usually drugs of the tricyclic antidepressant family such as amitriptyline or imipramine) should be used.

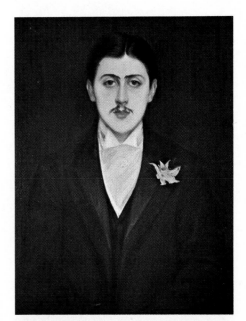

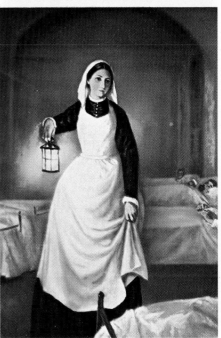

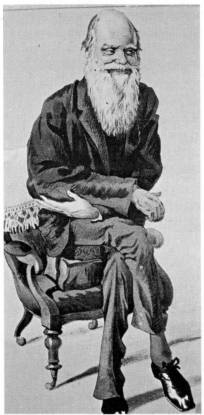

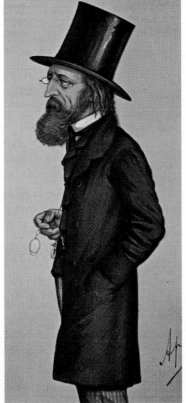

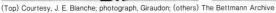

(Top) Courtesy, J. E. Blanche; photograph, Giraudon; (others) The Bettmann Archive

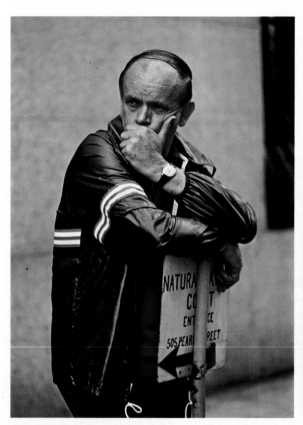

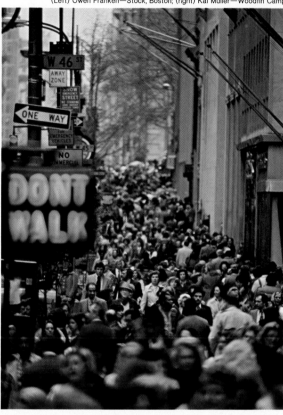

As 20th-century medicine becomes more successful in preventing and alleviating disease, there are, ironically, an ever increasing number of people who are worried and dissatisfied about the state of their health.

Electroconvulsive therapy (inducing convulsions in an anesthetized patient by electric shocks) somehow favorably shakes up the biochemistry of the brain and is still very much in use. In the far rarer cases where symptoms are utterly strange and extreme, a physician will suspect true psychosis.

There are many Argans of this world who are also depressed but are persistently, often aggressively, and, in a sense, triumphantly the bane of their physicians. The important rule for the doctor is to take their multiple complaints seriously while recognizing that these patients fundamentally do not want to get better. The patient suffers from the doctor's failure to cure him but at the same time gets sadistic pleasure out of causing this frustration. The doctor knows the hypochondriac cannot imagine a world in which his or her problems, failures, and conflicts are not excused by symptoms—so a truce must be struck. Indeed the patient may seek out doctors who do not try to cure him. It is no longer a matter of cure but of management, because to be cured would leave the patient stripped of all excuses, without his "crutches," and appalled at his psychological nakedness. The physician must resist the temptation to bounce this patient on to another doctor, compounding the problem for patient and for the profession, but accept and try to gain the patient's acquiescence while applauding his courage and, if necessary, provide him with a system of regular appointments as a workable substitute for the frantic calls about trivia at 2 o'clock in the morning.

Thus regular, appropriate examinations and minimal tests can be done and the patient gradually made to feel more secure as he comes to some sort of terms with his illness, while the physician, substituting the idea of "care" for "cure," no longer has to devote a totally disproportionate amount of his time to what are otherwise miserably frustrating problems. Lipsitt suggests the doctor has to be prepared to meet these patients at least halfway, and all his skill is needed to decide on the best mixture of discussion, explanation, investigation, drug therapy, and long-term support.

Three people who became famous largely because of the defense afforded them by their hypochondria illustrate some complexities of the issue of treatment. Several authors have suggested that the illness from which Charles Darwin began to suffer when he was 22, in 1831, before his famous voyage on HMS "Beagle" (1836), and which continued until he died in 1882, 51 years later, was Chagas' disease, or South American trypanosomiasis. This theory has been demolished by A. W. Woodruff, who proves Darwin's illness was psychological. Darwin was certainly a hypochondriac: he even kept a health diary, scoring days and nights for "goodness." Sir George Pickering has shed considerable light on Darwin's illness as well as that of Florence Nightingale, the founder of nursing as a profession and one of the most effective of health reformers, who was bedridden from the age of 37 until she died, aged 90. Lying on her couch year after year, she was totally devoted to her many pioneering activities—establishing schools of nursing, inaugurating training for midwives and nurses, reforming workhouses, even advising Indian viceroys. Both used their neuroses—their persistent hypochondriasis—as a defense and excuse to keep the world completely at bay so that there was never the least interruption to the full and exclusive pursuit of their life's work.

Marcel Proust is an example of a hypochondriac who also had a physical illness (bronchial asthma). As best man at his brother's wedding he was so padded beneath his three overcoats that he couldn't squeeze into his pew and had to stand in the aisle during the service. After his mother's death he became a recluse free to work out his obsession—himself—in his one vast novel. It was, in Pickering's words, another "creative malady." In each case one suspects the world would have lost hugely from an effective cure.

Prognosis

The English philosopher Thomas Hobbes was right when he said that the life of primitive man was "solitary, poor, nasty, brutish, and short." Yet it is our conceit to imagine that present-day life, which is by comparison ever so civilized, is full of many more stresses. It is a curious and tragic irony, however, that as medicine becomes more and more successful in preventing, detecting, and curing disease, people in general are bewildering doctors because they are less satisfied and worry more about their health. We feel that *any* depression, *any* worry, *any* anxiety, *any* ache is abnormal. For one thing, television ads say so. Indeed we have created a population of modern-day Argans, forever anxious, as was Molière's protagonist: "What I'm worrying about is all those ailments I've never heard of before." We must find some happy mean of serenity lest this hypochondria get out of hand. The right mixture of commitment, idealism, exercise, work, religion, and philosophy would surely help—a tall order, but necessary to prevent a whole world of worrywarts.

FOR ADDITIONAL READING:

Gogol, Nikolai Vasilevich. *The Overcoat and Other Tales of Good and Evil.* Translated by David Magarshack. New York: W. W. Norton and Co., 1965. Includes "The Nose."

Harris, Victor, and Husain, Itrat, eds. *English Prose, 1600–1660.* New York: Holt, Rinehart and Winston, 1965. Includes excerpts from *Devotions upon Emergent Occasions* and *The Anatomy of Melancholy.*

Idzorek, S. "A Functional Classification of Hypochondriasis with Specific Recommendations for Treatment." *Southern Medical Journal* 68 (1975):1326–32.

Jones, Ernest. *Sigmund Freud: Life and Work.* Vols. 1–3. London: The Hogarth Press, 1957.

Lipsitt, R. L. "The 'Rotating' Patient." *Journal of Geriatric Psychiatry* 2 (1968): 51–61.

Mandeville, Bernard de. *A Treatise of the Hypochondriack and Hysterick Passions.* 1711.

Pickering, Sir George White. *Creative Malady.* London: George Allen and Unwin, 1974.

Poquelin, Jean-Baptiste [Molière]. *The Misanthrope, and Other Plays.* Translated by John Wood. Baltimore: Penguin Books, 1959. Includes *Le Malade imaginaire.*

Sorsby, Arnold, ed. *Tenements of Clay: An Anthology of Medical Biographical Essays.* New York: Charles Scribner's Sons, 1975. Includes an essay on Job (C. J. Brim) and an essay on Charles Darwin (A. W. Woodruff).

Therapeutic Drugs

by Alexander M. Schmidt, M.D., and Timothy J. Larkin

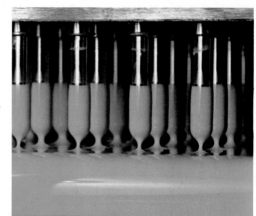

Since 1938, the year that the current U.S. law regulating drugs was passed, almost 1,000 new human drug entities have been approved by the Food and Drug Administration (FDA). Since each entity can be used in many individual products and combinations of products, patients and physicians are now confronted with a choice of over 100,000 prescription drugs, 90% of which did not exist before 1938. In addition, there are some 250,000 over-the-counter (nonprescription) drug formulations.

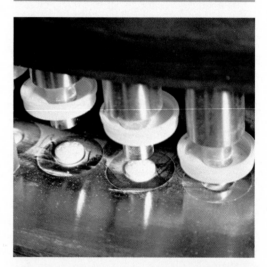

Americans now use more medicines than any other modern society. In 1976 physicians prescribed 1.5 billion drugs for their patients—*i.e.*, 5.7 prescriptions per person. And for Americans over age 65 the average per capita figure is much higher—13 prescriptions a year. Prescription drug sales have increased by 10% a year in the last decade to an estimated $7 billion in 1976. Americans also consume nonprescription drugs at an astounding rate—spending an average of $15 per capita in 1974 (the most recent figures available).

But such quantitative measures do not adequately reflect the impact of modern drugs on our lives. Drugs have contributed enormously to the improvement of public health and the quality of life. For example, it is difficult for most to understand the anguish felt by parents 50 years ago who learned that their children had diphtheria or polio or scarlet fever or tuberculosis since the death rates from these infectious diseases have declined so sharply in this century, largely because of modern medicines. The chemical compounds we call drugs are, therefore, capable of doing great good. But unless they are carefully screened there is a potential for doing great harm as well. It follows then that this dual character of drugs must be recognized and controlled.

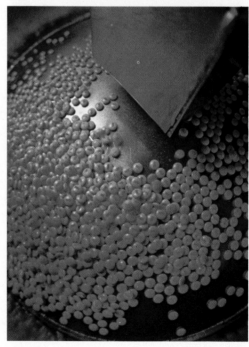

During recent years, how the United States regulates drugs for human use has become a matter of increasing controversy. That the controversy is complicated and arguments involved complex is illustrated by the contradictory nature of the charges made about the policies of the federal agency responsible for the task of regulating drugs, the FDA. The pharmaceutical industry complains that FDA regulations now make the discovery and testing of new drugs prohibitively expensive. Physicians see the FDA as inexcus-

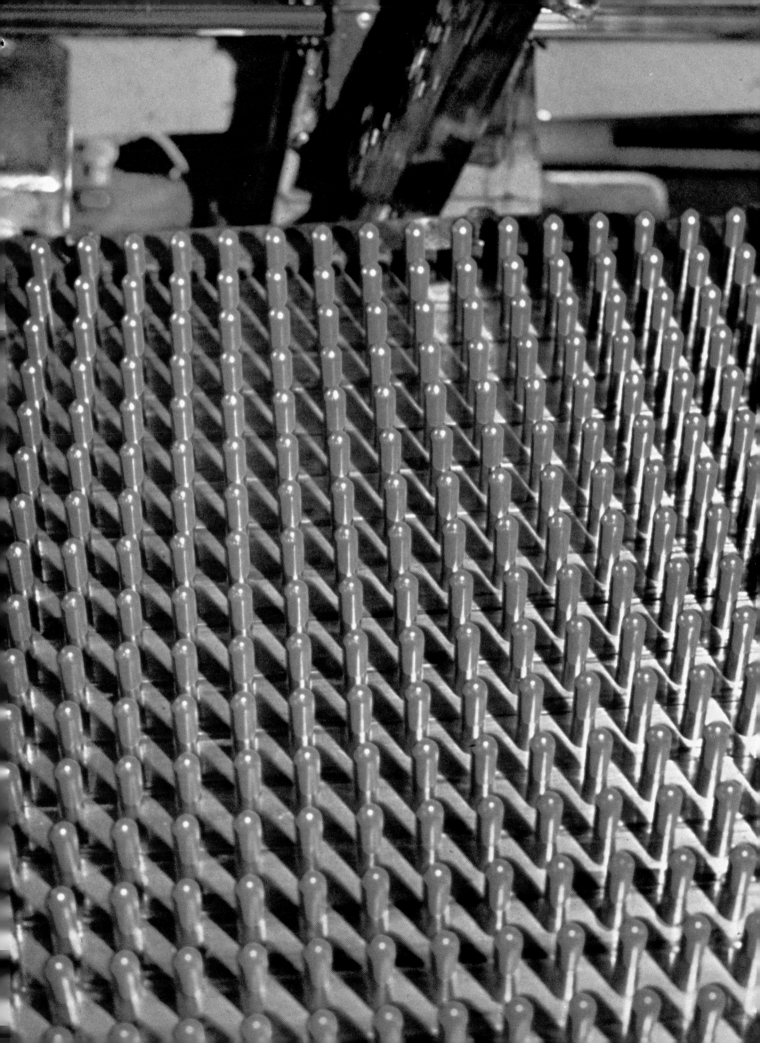

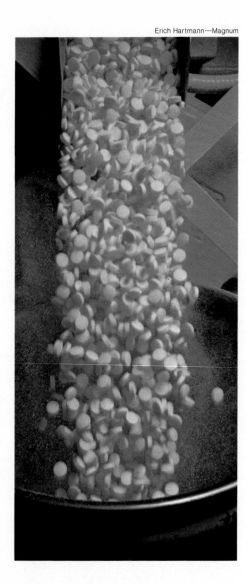

Alexander M. Schmidt, M.D., *is Vice Chancellor for Health Services, University of Illinois Medical Center, Chicago.*

Timothy J. Larkin *is Special Assistant to the Commissioner of the U.S. Food and Drug Administration, Rockville, Maryland.*

ably slow to approve promising new drugs. Consumer activists, along with articulate and powerful members of Congress, express great alarm over the danger of drugs already approved and call for even more stringent regulations. The result is that the general public is understandably becoming anxious about the drug regulatory process.

To deal with this anxiety in a constructive way, it is necessary to look at the dynamic, interacting, and sometimes conflicting forces that brought drug regulation into being, that produced subsequent changes in the law, and that now make certain elements of that law obsolete and in need of further change. It is also important to discard any idea that U.S. drug laws stem from clear, orderly, logical, or comprehensive policy deliberation. The historical reality is something quite different.

The first drug laws

When the first federal law regulating interstate drug marketing—the Food and Drugs Act—was passed in 1906, the goal was not to provide the nation with an ideal system of drug regulation but rather to deal with a specific and widespread problem: drugs that offered no medical benefit and were not intended to offer medical benefit. The new law was aimed at ridding the country of those drugs that sought to create a need through emotional and often fraudulent appeals, using every resource of the burgeoning art of advertising—*i.e.,* those drugs for which the prime motivation was not alleviating or curing or preventing illness but rather exploiting both illness and the credulity of those who were sick and wished to be well. Those drugs were, of course, the quack medicines that in a perversion of Jacksonian democracy made any American, no matter how ill-equipped in terms of education or ethics, into a potential drug creator and producer. As a mid-19th-century Ohio newspaper put it, "Any idle mechanic" could become a drug maker if he "by chance gets a dispensatory, or some old receipt book, and pouring over it, or having it read to him . . . he finds that mercury is good for the itch, and old ulcers; that opium will give ease; and that a glass of antimony will vomit. Down goes the hammer, or saw, razor, awl, or shuttle—and away to make electuaries, tinctures, elixirs, pills, and poultices."

Advertising for the thousands of varieties of mostly useless nostrums (by 1906 there were some 50,000) crammed newspapers and magazines, embellished handbills, billboards, and posters, and, eventually, sought out every conceivable flat surface—fences, sheds, rocks, bridges. The advertisements even leapfrogged ahead of America's advancing frontier, as indicated in 1876, when an editorial published in the *New York Tribune* complained that this visual pollution was "violating the beauty of mountain scenery and the seclusion of the remotest valleys. They have long since crossed the continent, and laid their unclean paws on the Rocky Mountains and the Sierra Nevada."

Muckraking journalists Samuel Hopkins Adams, Edward Bok, and others exposed the fact that many of these advertisements proclaimed the benefits of compounds that ranged from the useless to the deadly. Infants were narcotized into stupefaction with soothing syrups containing large amounts of opium. Potentially lethal coal-tar derivatives such as acetanilid were tout-

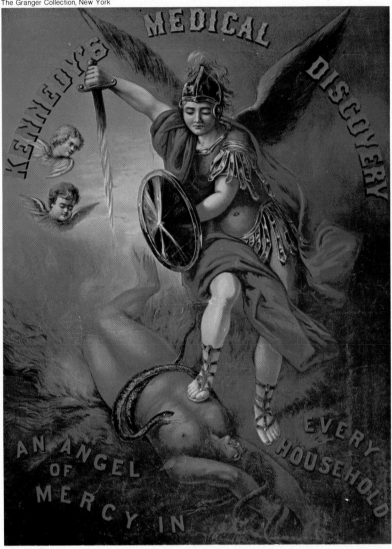

ed as effective, indeed wondrous, headache remedies. Medicines and potions claiming to eliminate afflictions from asthma to ulcer were submitted to chemical analysis. Many of these bogus panaceas turned out to be composed of up to 99% water, flavored with extracts of various herbs and tinctures of corrosive ácids. Other drugs were found to contain so much alcohol that the U.S. Office of Indian Affairs prohibited their sale on reservations, and states with prohibition laws banned them. One such drug, Dr. Hostetter's Celebrated Stomachic Bitters Tonic, which contained 32% alcohol, was served in shot glasses to frequenters of Sitka, Alaska, saloons, and this 64-proof potion was eventually declared a liquor for tax purposes by the Internal Revenue Service.

Despite the existence of such substances, when Congress finally passed food and drug legislation in 1906, the primary emphasis of the law was on food rather than drugs, for a number of reasons. The most obvious was that foods are universally consumed; drugs are not. Hence, food safety had a legitimate first claim on society's attention. And there was, by the end

Today there are some 250,000 over-the-counter drug formulations on which Americans spend an estimated $2.6 billion each year. Aspirin (opposite) is one of the most commonly consumed nonprescription medications. Before 1906 there were approximately 50,000 so-called patent medicines—drugs purported to cure every ill imaginable. Posters, such as the one for Kennedy's Medical Discovery (c. 1885), an angelic cure-all, seemed to fill every conceivable flat surface of America's advancing frontier.

23

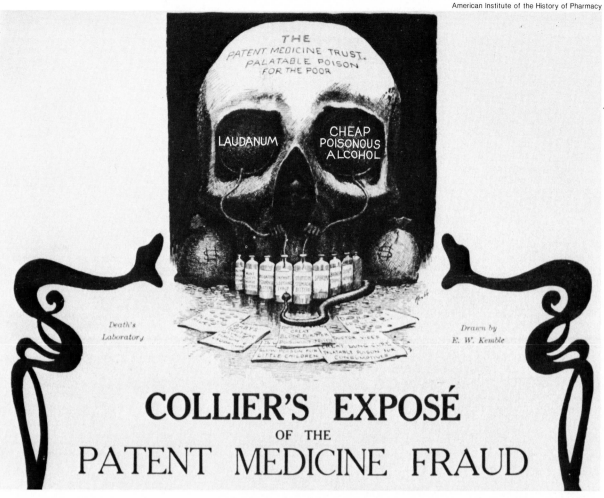

THE
PATENT MEDICINE TRUST.
PALATABLE POISON
FOR THE POOR

LAUDANUM CHEAP POISONOUS ALCOHOL

Death's Laboratory

Drawn by E. W. Kemble

COLLIER'S EXPOSÉ
OF THE
PATENT MEDICINE FRAUD

Detail of an advertisement (from Scientific American, *Dec. 16, 1905) for a series of articles in* Collier's *by Samuel Hopkins Adams, one of several muckraking journalists who exposed quack patent medicines. Adams attacked the manufacturers of 264 nostrums that ranged from the useless to the deadly.*

of the 19th century, a huge population that could not depend on the purity and quality of the food available to them. For a great many people, growing urbanization had broken the direct connection between food production and consumption. It became necessary to move, store, and market foods far from farm and feedlot, requiring the use of imperfect technology and a number of then novel processing and packaging methods, including chemical preservatives and other additives. The attention given to sanitation in manufacturing practices was regulated only by the sense of responsibility of the food manufacturer or processor.

The crusading leader of the demand for protection against flagrant abuses by food and drug manufacturers was Harvey Washington Wiley. Wiley, as head of the U.S. Department of Agriculture's Bureau of Chemistry, was the first director of what became, in 1931, the Food and Drug Administration. Because of his background and training, Wiley's professional orientation was understandably toward foods. Finally, and perhaps of greatest significance, a favorable emotional climate, which tipped the political scales in favor of enactment of a *food* and drug law, was created by Upton Sinclair's horrifying account of practices in the meatpacking industry in his book

24

The Jungle. Sinclair later looked upon the effects of his exposé somewhat ruefully: "I aimed at the public's heart, and by accident I hit it in the stomach."

Thus, federal authority to regulate drugs was, in a very real sense, a by-product of the need to regulate food production. The driving force for the law was moral outrage against deception and adulteration. This is particularly evident in regard to drugs, where the law essentially confined itself to matters of morality in the marketplace. Drug products were required by the new law to carry a label, and the label had to tell the truth. If a drug label claimed the presence of certain ingredients, those ingredients had to be present. If a label claimed that other ingredients were absent, those ingredients, in fact, had to be absent. In short, the manufacturer could not misinform. Yet, with the exception of requiring a label declaring the presence and amounts of a few obviously dangerous substances such as opiates, there was no requirement to tell the whole truth by informing the consumer about other ingredients, potential side effects, drug interactions, contraindications, or precise dosage recommendations. There was no requirement to test a drug for safety and, indeed, no stated restriction on what a drug might contain. It mattered less what was in the bottle than whether the label accurately described it.

The limited scope of the first drug law is surprising only from our present point of view. But the 1906 act was the product of a different period, a response to the major currents of political, social, and economic thought that characterized that period. Although Pres. Theodore Roosevelt's progressivism did attack certain business practices, the aim of that political movement was similar to that sought by the Food and Drugs Act—to eliminate the most egregious abuses. The idea was not to regulate business activity in any strict way but to facilitate laissez-faire policies by making shoddy competitive practices more difficult.

Less obvious, but equally responsible for the fact that the Food and Drugs Act did not outlaw quack remedies entirely, was the relatively immature status of drug science. Pharmacology and pharmaceutics were not as we know them today. Distinctions between quack remedies and legitimate drugs were fuzzy, and the scientific knowledge and tools needed to eliminate the fuzziness were not yet at hand. Though thousands of drugs were listed in official pharmacopoeias, many of them were useless and some actually injurious. For example, the fourth revision of the *U.S. Pharmacopeia,* issued in 1860, listed tobacco as a beneficial drug, along with other curious, even alarming, substances: silver nitrate, oatmeal, cadmium, charcoal, lead nitrate, potassium ferrocyanide, whiskey, Bay Rum, brandy, and tapioca. Tobacco was already known to contain nicotine, a stimulant, and was to be boiled, the resulting "infusum" then used as an enema for "twisted bowels" or hernias. Silver nitrate (or lunar caustic) was used to treat the insane ("lunatics"). The other substances were recommended as tonics, sedatives, soothants, antidiarrheals, etc. Many other commonly used drugs were based on speculative and bizarre beliefs such as the doctrine of signatures, which held that drugs signified their proper application through certain exterior signs. For example, nutmeg, with its brainlike, convoluted surface, was thought to be useful in treating brain diseases. Or because the leaves of the

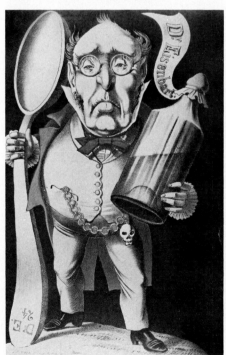

The terrible fact that in the mid-19th century anyone, no matter what his education or ethics, could be a drug maker—and thus a potential killer—is illustrated in this caricature of a quack.

25

Courtesy, Lederle Laboratories

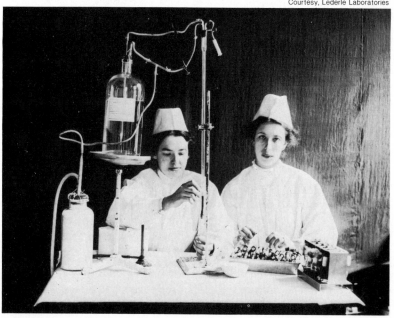

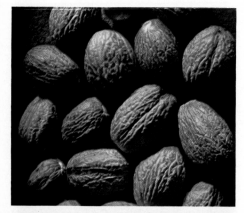

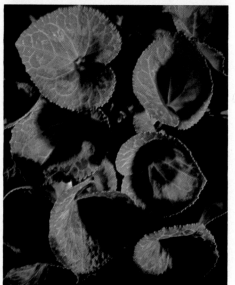

John H. Gerard

cyclamen plant were of an arrangement that resembled the human ear, this particular botanical was considered worthy in dealing with various disorders of the ear.

By the mid-19th century, the degree to which physicians held drugs in esteem was in inverse proportion to their enlightenment. One of the most enlightened, the physician, poet, and humorist Oliver Wendell Holmes, held a strong contempt for the growing numbers of medications that were being consumed by more and more Americans. In 1860 he expressed the new skepticism toward drugs when he wrote, "Throw out opium . . . throw out a few specifics . . . throw out wine, and the vapors which produce the miracle of anesthesia, and I firmly believe that if the whole materia medica, *as now used,* could be sunk to the bottom of the sea, it would be all the better for mankind—and all the worse for the fishes."

Alexander Pope once condemned apothecaries by charging them with being "bold in the practice of mistaken rules." The physicians who shared Holmes's conservative point of view demonstrated a different boldness by refusing to prescribe on the basis of mistaken rules. Instead, they relied on supportive therapy and a handful of drugs of proven effectiveness, such as quinine and digitalis. This therapeutic nihilism gradually eroded as new and truly useful drugs began to be available: amyl nitrate and nitroglycerine for anginal pain; chloral and codeine for sedation; ether, nitrous oxide, and chloroform to induce anesthesia; antipyrine and acetophenetidin for pain and fever; and a growing number of effective biologicals. Early in the 20th century, these were supplemented with the introduction of insulin to control diabetes, liver extract for pernicious anemia, and heparin as an anticoagulant. There was still, however, no magic chemotherapeutic bullet as Paul Ehrlich, the German bacteriologist and founder of drug therapy, had envisioned. No specific medicine capable of dealing with a number of intractable infections existed—that is until 1935, when sulfanilamide became available.

26

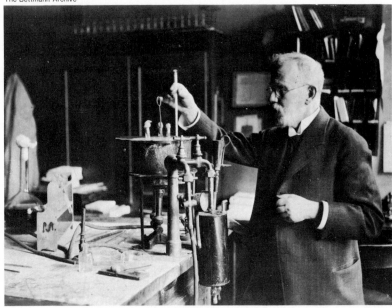

The sulfa drugs signaled a new era in chemotherapy. In 1924, when President Coolidge watched the red lines race up his son Calvin, Jr.'s, leg from a streptococcal infection, nothing could be done. A decade later, when President Roosevelt's son, Franklin, Jr., was suffering from the same kind of infection, it was swiftly eradicated with sulfanilamide.

The need for reform

With the increased reliance on drug therapy came problems not anticipated by the 1906 Food and Drugs Act, particularly the proliferation of unsafe medicines. These problems coincided with a political climate of reform, making it possible to contemplate eliminating the major weaknesses of the old law. A reform effort began in 1933 but lacked any true impetus.

Then, in 1937, there appeared the most compelling evidence of what could happen when the drug law permitted sale of an unsafe drug. A patent medicine manufacturer, seeking to exploit sulfanilamide's reputation as the first miracle drug, created a concoction called Elixir Sulfanilamide. To produce a liquid, nonprescription form of this drug, the company's chemist used a commercial solvent, diethylene glycol, normally employed to make such products as antifreeze and brake fluid. This concoction was tested for those features of primary importance when the goal is sales appeal—fragrance, appearance, flavor—but not safety. The company's lack of safety testing (entirely legal under the 1906 act) caused an FDA inspector to remark subsequently, "Apparently they just throw drugs together, and if they don't explode, they are placed on sale." While fewer than 2,000 pints of the Elixir were produced and only 93 were consumed, the death toll exceeded one per pint. The resultant uproar highlighted the weaknesses of the 1906 act. People learned that, with one exception, this lethal drug was entirely within the letter of the drug law. The exception—that all elixirs must contain alcohol, and Elixir Sulfanilamide did not—was the tiny opening that permitted

At the time of the first drug law the sciences of pharmaceutics and pharmacology were a far cry from their advanced states today. (Opposite page) The crudeness of the equipment (top) used by pharmaceutical technicians preparing diphtheria antitoxin in 1910 is apparent. At the time, many drugs were still based on folk ideas, such as the doctrine of signatures—a system employing natural products that signified their proper application through physical resemblance. Nutmeg (center), for example, was thought to be useful in treating diseases of the brain because of its brainlike surface. Cyclamen (bottom) was used for ear disorders owing to the design of its leaves. (Above) Paul Ehrlich (1854–1915) made many important contributions to developing the biomedical sciences and particularly to advancing drug therapy. Ehrlich envisioned a single magic chemotherapeutic bullet that would successfully treat a whole spectrum of diseases.

the FDA to track down and seize the undistributed supply. In short, only a technicality prevented a far greater toll of victims.

The public demand for action finally interrupted the seemingly interminable congressional debate on revising the law and, in June 1938, the new Federal Food, Drug, and Cosmetic Act was signed by Pres. Franklin D. Roosevelt. The act defined false labeling to include the omission of warnings when the potential for hazard was high. Also, common names of active ingredients were required on the label, as was a statement of quantity and proportion of hypnotic and narcotic substances. And drugs dangerous to health, dangerous even though taken as directed, were outlawed.

These were important and necessary actions. In a sense, they made drug laws conform more closely to the level of protection the American people mistakenly believed they had been receiving from their government right up to the moment when they read about Elixir Sulfanilamide.

But more important than the specific reforms were two basic principles established in regard to new drugs—principles that still stand. First, all new drugs must be tested for safety before marketing. Second, the manufacturer or whoever submits a New Drug Application to the FDA is responsible for conducting the tests necessary to prove the drug's safety. Together, these standards established for drugs what the Meat Inspection Act of 1906 had for meats—they created a measure for preventing injury.

The 1938 law came just as pharmacology began to harvest the fruits of a half-century of biomedical science. The role of living organisms—bacteria and viruses—in a great number of illnesses was being defined. Without this kind of *biotic* knowledge, medicine would not have been prepared for, indeed, would not have understood, the significance of the *antibiotics*. Certainly, the pharmaceutical companies would not have undertaken the

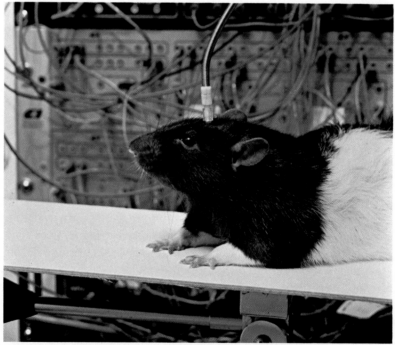

Pharmaceuticals must be tested for safety by the manufacturer before marketing. Every new drug must be tested on at least two species of mammals before it is given to humans. Laboratory rats are frequently used to test the effects of chemical compounds on behavior.

(Right) Courtesy, Warner-Lambert Company; photograph, Charles Harbutt—Magnum; (left) Jack Kath—Photo Trends

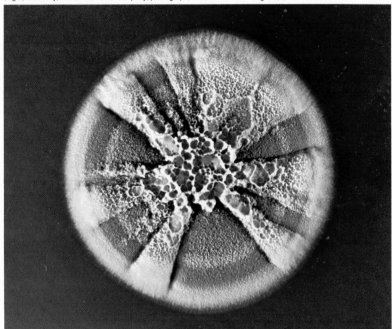

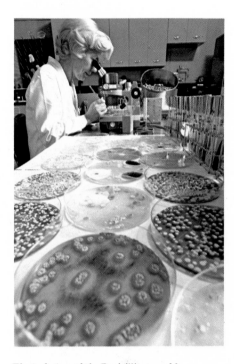

The isolation of the Penicillium *mold (left), from which the antibiotic penicillin is derived, meant physicians could cure illnesses once beyond the reach of medical intervention. Today new antibiotics are being sought for many specific purposes. A researcher (right) is searching for antibiotic agents to treat cancer.*

kind of research that realized the potential of penicillin and then moved on aggressively to discover streptomycins, tetracyclines, and a long list of other antibiotics. Thus, following hard on the footsteps of the first sulfa drugs, beginning almost simultaneously with the 1938 law, and picking up speed during and after the Second World War, biomedical science was arming physicians with powerful pharmaceutical agents that could actually cure illnesses that were once considered beyond the reach of effective medical intervention.

During the same period, there was a basic change in the development of new drugs. Most important drugs hitherto had been the subject of discovery; now they had become the product of purposeful invention. Where once new drugs had actually been substances familiar in other forms to the human species, now they often consisted of molecules never before encountered in the history of mankind.

But even as the availability of these new drugs was producing a kind of therapeutic euphoria, it was also inculcating a belief that there was, or soon would be, a drug for every ailment and every need. Even as pharmacology was exercising its new power to manipulate molecules to engineer new chemical entities, that power was, in almost classic fashion, silently corrupting the system by changing public attitudes toward drugs. Consumers began to take for granted that drugs could provide miracles in the form of chemical comforts. Modern advertising techniques echoed the newly powerful drugs themes that had been employed by nostrum manufacturers a century earlier. Illnesses were described that existed only in a copywriter's mind—tired blood, behavioral drift, tired mother syndrome, environmental depression— and then the advertising offered a prescription or an over-the-counter drug to deal with each new fancy. In one instance advertising created an entity called "imperceptible pain," for which a pain killer was offered designed with sufficient precision to block perception of the imperceptible.

During this period, the nation's use of drugs increased dramatically, signaling that many persons were overlooking the fact that drugs, because they *were* now effective, carried with them risks as well as benefits. In addition, pharmaceutical companies began manipulating molecules for the sake of novelty and sales, inundating the physician with a bewildering gallimaufry of new drugs.

As a result of this growing reliance on and the uncritical acceptance of drugs, all kinds of pathological symptoms began to appear—physicians prescribing at every turn; consumers adding numerous nonprescription capsules and tablets to already swollen and dangerous medicine cabinets; drug combinations that canceled or magnified the desired effect or that, interacting, produced wholly new effects; unanticipated adverse reactions; diagnoses skewed through high levels of various drugs in body fluids; and more.

Many of these drug excesses and abuses were exposed during the celebrated 1959 drug hearings of the Subcommittee on Antitrust and Monopoly, chaired by Sen. Estes Kefauver. And in response, once again, support began to grow for changes in the law governing the regulation of drugs. But, once again, it appeared that the matter would drag on until something sufficiently dramatic focused public attention on the deficiencies of the 1938 law. That something came in a form even more horrifying than Elixir Sulfanilamide.

The tragedy struck large numbers of European women who, while pregnant, had taken the sedative thalidomide and subsequently gave birth to seriously deformed children. Thalidomide was found to produce phocomelia ("seal limbs"), absence or malformation of the external ear, fusion defects of the eye, absence of the normal openings of the gastrointestinal tract, and other defects. Between 2,000 and 3,000 "thalidomide babies" were born in West Germany and 500 in Great Britain between 1959 and 1962. Only the insistence by an FDA scientist, Frances O. Kelsey, that the application to market this drug in the United States lacked sufficient evidence of safety kept thalidomide from being an American tragedy as well.

Preventing thalidomides

Once again the public demanded action, and Congress responded in 1962 by amending the Federal Food, Drug, and Cosmetic Act. The primary significance of the amendments was the addition of new general principles that furthered the concept of prevention of injury.

The 1962 revisions required drugs to be proved effective as well as safe before gaining access to the market. Evidence for effectiveness had to be of a certain, rigorous kind, "consisting of adequate and well-controlled investigations, . . . by experts qualified by scientific training and experience to evaluate the effectiveness of the drug involved, on the basis of which it could fairly and responsibly be concluded by such experts that the drug will have the effect it purports or is represented to have."

The goal of preventing drug-induced injury was greatly enhanced by the requirement that drug manufacturers make drugs in conformity with rigid "good manufacturing practices," as defined by FDA regulations that specified quality assurance techniques. In furtherance of this quality assurance

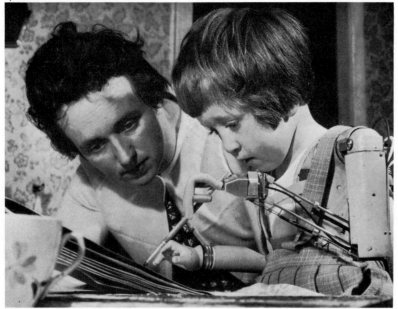

The problem of drug safety was highlighted in the 1960s when thousands of "thalidomide babies" were born with serious malformations to European mothers who had taken this sedative. during pregnancy. Here a Scottish victim of thalidomide shows her mother how she paints with her prosthetic arm and hand.

initiative, the FDA was given more extensive factory inspection authority and also required to conduct batch-by-batch testing of potency and safety of all biologicals for human use.

The FDA acquired the authority to regulate advertising of prescription drugs in professional journals. The amended law stated that drug ads had to contain information including the drug formula, a listing of side effects, warnings about when the drug should not be administered, and a statement about conditions for which the drug has been shown to be effective.

The 1962 amendments also addressed a significant human rights issue. Congress and the FDA were shocked to find that while the application for thalidomide was being considered, the manufacturer's sales representatives —"detail men"— had been actively distributing the drug to physicians in anticipation of approval. Instead of 50 or 100 clinical investigators who might have been expected to be supervising trials among human volunteers, there turned out to be many times that number of physicians possessing the drug. The FDA learned that 500,000 tablets of thalidomide had been given to 19,882 patients by 1,267 physicians. More than 3,700 of the patients were women of childbearing age. Despite the widespread publicity about thalidomide, over 400 of these so-called investigators failed to issue any warnings to patients given the drug. This was clearly a mockery of the "investigational use" provision of the 1938 act. Sen. Karl Mundt (Rep., S.D.) characterized the situation as "a loophole in the law through which you could drive a South Dakota wagonload of hay." As a result of these disclosures the 1962 Amendment reasserted in strong language that the FDA had authority to require consent of human test subjects, except in those rare instances where such knowledge might be harmful.

Finally, the law spelled out the ground rules governing removal of drugs from the market. Any prior drug approval could be withdrawn by the FDA after a hearing whenever tests or experience showed the drug to be unsafe

31

or whenever newly acquired evidence showed that the drug had not been proved safe or effective for its intended uses. Further, the 1962 amendments to the Federal Food, Drug, and Cosmetic Act also provided authority to the secretary of health, education, and welfare to order off the market a drug posing an imminent danger to public health.

These were important reforms, and they constitute the basic legal authority presently governing the way the FDA regulates human drugs. Despite the significance of the 1962 amendments, they do not and cannot be expected to represent the last legislative response to the challenge of modern drugs. The most productive way to respond to and accommodate the risks posed by the hundreds of powerful new drugs science has been making available is still being sought. While it is important to make the best possible response and accommodation, it is also necessary to recognize that the process involves a great number of controversial questions, some of which touch the very essence of the U.S. social and economic system. A number of these exceedingly difficult questions have emerged since 1962 and, to an extent, they serve to suggest the direction in which the most recent evolution of drug regulation is heading.

The growing debate over the law revolves around one central and basic issue: benefit versus risk. There are, as thalidomide so convincingly demonstrated, risks involved in letting drugs reach the marketplace without having been proved safe and effective. And even when there is scientific evidence of safety and effectiveness sufficient to satisfy our legal requirements, the risks are only mitigated or limited in number, not eliminated. There are other kinds of risks, less easily quantified, when potentially useful or even life-saving drugs are delayed from appearing on the U.S. market because of excessive concern or unnecessarily stringent regulations.

One of the charges made against the FDA is that the agency is overzealously protective, and this has resulted in an increase in the time taken to approve a new drug from two to seven years and an increase in cost from $1 million–$2 million per drug to $10 million. Some critics of U.S. drug regulation point out that as a result, there is a trend for the U.S. pharmaceutical industry to either stop new drug development or move it overseas to a more favorable regulatory climate.

New Drug Applications

The FDA is, by nature, predisposed to a conservative, cautious approach to New Drug Applications because once a drug is approved, unless there is a serious, proved danger—an "imminent hazard"—to the public health, the FDA cannot summarily remove the drug from the market. Without an imminent hazard to the public health, the FDA must first hold hearings, which in turn may lead to court appeals. This process can consume years, during which time the FDA can do nothing more than require appropriate changes in labeling, including warning statements. It is an either-or situation: either the data supporting the drug application are examined very carefully by the agency and must answer every question posed, or the agency may find itself having approved a drug that, while not an imminent hazard, is nonetheless too dangerous for unrestricted access to the marketplace.

32

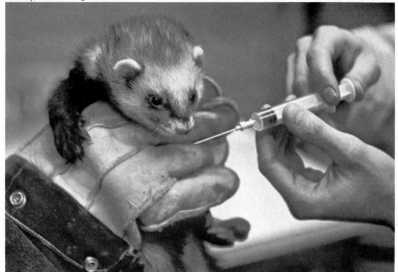

The FDA is required to conduct batch-by-batch testing of potency and safety of all biologicals for human use. Researchers (left) are preparing to place a virus in the nose of a ferret. Later the ferret's blood will be used to identify various strains of virus that are used in vaccines. As a result of the thalidomide tragedy, safety testing that involves the administration of new drugs to pregnant animals is standard procedure. A scientist (below) examines a fetal rabbit skeleton for abnormalities that may have been caused by a drug given to its mother.

There is an additional difficulty involved in securing the evidence needed to justify approving a new drug: the limitations imposed by clinical trials; *i.e.,* human experimentation. Ordinarily, only a few thousand volunteers at most can be included in such therapeutic trials, and the time during which the trials are conducted—generally a few weeks to a few months—is relatively short. But once a drug is approved for general sale tens of thousands, perhaps even millions, of persons will be exposed to it; and many individuals may take the drug for long periods of time. On a purely statistical basis, ignoring the fact that there are persons who may have an allergic or atypical reaction to the drug, serious unanticipated reactions not encountered during the clinical trial may very well appear among many of those taking the drug. The classic example of this phenomenon was the recognition of potentially fatal aplastic anemia following the widespread use of the antibiotic chloramphenicol in the 1950s. It has been estimated that about one case of aplastic anemia—a serious bone marrow toxicity—occurs for every 100,000 courses of therapy with chloramphenicol. In 1967 the Registry on Blood Dyscrasias, established by the American Medical Association, reported deaths to have occurred in 186 persons of a study group consisting of 408 individuals with chloramphenicol-associated bone marrow complications. A more recent example is the appearance of genital tract abnormalities including a unique cancer of the cervix or vagina in female offspring of women given diethylstilbestrol (DES) early in their pregnancies to prevent spontaneous abortion and certain other problems in pregnancy.

Imminent hazard provision

In those countries having national health programs with centralized health statistical services, particularly the United Kingdom and the Scandinavian countries, it is far easier to detect harmful drug reactions early and restrict use of the guilty drug or eliminate it entirely. The U.S. system is not centralized. Adverse reaction data do not automatically flow into some central federal agency empowered to make rapid decisions about the continued

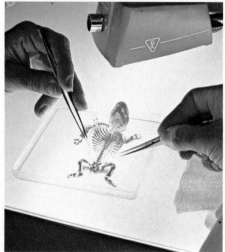

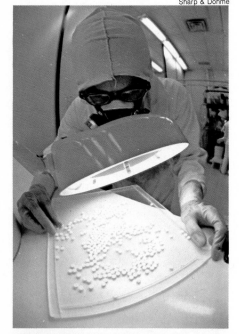

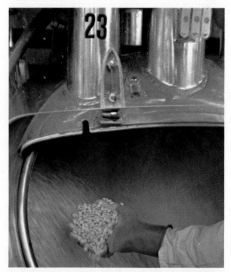

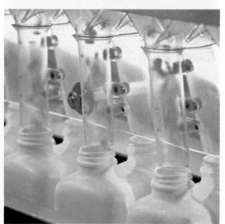

use of a drug. As we have seen, once the drug switch is thrown to "on," reversing to "off" is difficult. Indeed, only the secretary of health, education, and welfare can do so by invoking the imminent hazard provision. In fact, put bluntly, suspending a New Drug Application under this provision requires the demonstration of more than the potential for harm; it requires harm actualized—a "body count."

Therefore, it is not surprising that the imminent hazard provision has been invoked only once since 1962. On July 25, 1977, the secretary of health, education, and welfare ordered an end within 90 days to the general marketing of the oral hypoglycemic drug phenformin, used to lower blood sugar of diabetics, because of its unacceptably high risk of producing lactic acidosis, a buildup of lactic acid in the blood causing weakness, fast breathing, abdominal pain, and vomiting. The data supporting the secretary's decision were obtained slowly and with difficulty but eventually demonstrated that as many as 4 of each 1,000 persons taking phenformin during a one-year period developed lactic acidosis, with about half of such cases resulting in death. Since 336,000 persons, who could control their diabetes with other agents, were taking phenformin when the degree of hazard was appreciated, it was calculated that between 50 and 700 deaths per year could be attributed to the drug.

The infrequent use of the imminent hazard provision of the law illuminates how the American system has not been designed primarily for maximum speed but rather to assure, insofar as government can, that all citizens and every legitimate interest are accorded equitable treatment, often defined as due process of law. Thus, the 1962 drug law amendments, by carefully restricting the conditions under which a drug already marketed can be removed, take into consideration the fact that drug sponsors—usually the drug manufacturers—have invested large sums of money and scarce research resources to develop and market new drugs, and equity demands that this investment be accorded safeguards against arbitrary and capricious administrative action. By removing dangerous or ineffective drugs from the market the law also tries to provide equity for the public.

Drug lag

It is important to realize that in the United States, drug research, development, and production largely depend on private enterprise and commercial incentives. One of the reasons drug regulation has evolved in a halting fashion is that legislators see clearly that damaging the system of drug innovation can produce a net loss to society. As one illustration of this problem, safety and effectiveness data supporting New Drug Applications must now be kept confidential by the FDA because, the industry asserts, and the law tends to confirm, releasing such data would provide unfair competitive advantage to firms that did not invest in basic research. In the long run, this would serve as a disincentive to industry investment and innovation. On the other hand, those seeking legislation to remove this limitation of access to information in government files maintain that withholding safety and effectiveness data from the public domain requires duplication of expensive research—a practice that is deemed to be ethically unsound because it un-

34

necessarily exposes additional human subjects to experimental risks.

There are some who argue that the present drug laws and the FDA's interpretation of them already are serving as disincentives to new drug research and development, demonstrated by U.S. loss of leadership in new drug development and, more seriously, by the needless suffering and deaths from delayed introduction to the U.S. of new drugs. Those who contend there is a ''drug lag'' (by which is meant that the U.S. consistently falls behind others in drug innovation) marshall a number of arguments.

Unfortunately, not until recently has an objective assessment been made independently of the two parties involved—the pharmaceutical industry and the FDA. Two such assessments are now in hand, both contained in the *Final Report of the Special Panel on Drug Regulation.* The panel was formed by the secretary of health, education, and welfare to examine the entire U.S. drug regulatory process. One of the studies, ''Economic Effect of New Drug Regulation in the United States,'' concludes that economic analyses place undue emphasis on cost without considering benefits to society from the reduction of the number of ineffective drugs entering the market and better information about drug risk resulting from increased clinical testing.

The second study, ''Comment on Drug Regulation and Innovation in the Pharmaceutical Industry,'' prepared at the Massachusetts Institute of Technology Center for Policy Alternatives, points out that many factors are involved in differing international rates of drug innovation. The MIT study concludes that it is impossible to say whether there is a drug lag.

There is yet another study which, while compiled by the FDA, is based entirely on objective data published by Paul deHaen, Inc., the most authoritative source of statistics on international drug developments. The deHaen data reveal a fundamental deficiency in much of the evidence supporting a drug lag hypothesis. A more meaningful way to compare relative rates of innovation is to look at quality rather than quantity. The deHaen study does not include new drugs that are merely variations of existing drugs but, instead, focuses on important new chemical entities. Based on this distinction, the data tend to show that far from consistently lagging behind the rest of the world, the U.S. is ahead of some nations in the number of new drugs introduced and behind others.

While there does not appear to be any convincing evidence supporting the contention that the U.S. endemically and seriously lags behind the five other major drug innovating nations (France, West Germany, Great Britain, Italy, and Japan), it is nonetheless true that some important drugs are available in other countries and not in the U.S. It is also true that the cost in time and dollars to approve drugs in the U.S. has increased markedly during the past 15 years, so that it does take longer to approve drugs in the United States than in many other countries.

Some drugs are available in other countries prior to their introduction in the U.S. not because of regulatory inertia but because the decision to initiate or not to initiate a request for a New Drug Approval is made by private enterprise. The FDA must await initiation of an application before a drug can be considered for approval, and there is no way the FDA can force a drug

(Opposite) Techniques of drug manufacturing that meet the established standards for quality and purity: (top) inspecting tablets for imperfections under sterile conditions; (center) polishing and buffing tablets; (bottom) tablets being dropped automatically into sterile bottles.

35

Courtesy, Burroughs Wellcome Co., Research Triangle Park, North Carolina; photograph, Gail Shrader and Bob White

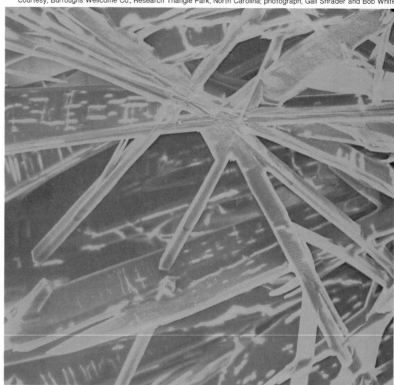

Sophisticated methods have been developed not only of synthesizing new drugs but also of examining their potential toxicity in animals and humans. A monkey (below) undergoes a blood pressure test in a trial with a hypertensive agent. (Right) A scanning electron micrograph of sodium allopurinol crystals (magnified 800 times). Allopurinol, introduced in the U.S. in 1966, was the first agent to block the formation of excess uric acid within the body, thus bringing about effective control of gout and hyperuricemia.

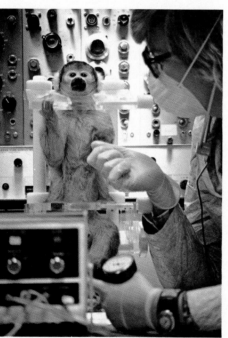

Courtesy, G. D. Searle & Co.

company to apply for permission to market a new drug. A recent illustration involves the drug valproate, reportedly used in Great Britain as an effective treatment for epilepsy in cases when other drugs have failed. As late as July 1977, no drug firm had taken the steps necessary to secure marketing approval in the U.S. In view of the potential benefit to epileptics, the FDA did as much as it could, under the law: the agency informed the American company that intended to market the drug in the U.S. (affiliated with the multinational firm marketing the drug abroad) that a prompt submission of a New Drug Application for valproate would be accorded priority attention. (On Feb. 28, 1978, valproate was approved for marketing and is currently available in the U.S. for the treatment of petit mal epilepsy.)

Too, as our scientific knowledge grows, we do tend to regulate more. The deHaen study pointed out that the fundamental reason why the drug approval process takes longer now than it used to has far more to do with science than government: "The real cause . . . is the progress of pharmaceutical and medical science . . . during the last 40 years. We are inclined to forget that during this time new drugs have been developed that are effective in minute quantities and permit therapy of diseases for which formerly no remedy was available. But these drugs also encompass great potential toxicity, and it is against this toxicity that we must guard the patient. New sophisticated scientific methods have been developed not only to synthesize these drugs, but also to examine their action in animals and man." The study then cites a fact that critics of regulation too often ignore: "Even if no regulations existed for the testing of the activity of drugs, scientific and corporate conscience would require a much longer testing period than in the past." In short, science has equipped society with the ability to ask far more piercing questions about risks and benefits, and it takes time and dollars to answer those questions. Thus, the fundamental problem, if it is a problem, does not result so much from some inherent lack of efficiency in regulation but rather from the growing efficiency of science.

Is safety enough?

The 1962 amendments added the requirement that drugs must be proved effective, and this provision has been a major target of critics of the law. Indeed, a bill to eliminate the effectiveness requirement is currently being considered by Congress. The stated reason for eliminating the effectiveness provision is that safety is primary, effectiveness secondary. Since proof of effectiveness is so onerous and time consuming, society is being exposed to unnecessary risk (by being denied promising new drugs) without gaining any significant benefit.

It is worthwhile, however, to recall that the effectiveness requirement resulted from the natural evolution of pharmacology and therapeutics. Previously, the therapeutic inventory consisted largely of useless drugs that sometimes seemed to work because a great many diseases are self-limiting or because of the placebo effect, which is that sometimes a medicine "works" because the recipient believes it will work. In prior times, there was little point in requiring proof of effectiveness—even if the needed scientific tools had been available. But as drugs appeared that had significant physiological effects, drugs that actually could work and did work, an ineffective drug was, by the very nature of its ineffectiveness, also unsafe. It was unsafe because it is dangerous to ingest physiologically active chemicals for no useful purpose. It was unsafe also because it would divert a patient from a drug that was effective—one of the strongest arguments against the purported anticancer drug laetrile. It is unfortunate that the law has created a distinction between safety and effectiveness, because the distinction can be supported neither by logic nor by science.

However one feels about the various controversies that continually surround the regulation of drugs, the evolutionary path along which further change will occur is now becoming clear. Society is asking whether there will be more benefits than risks accruing from making the requirements of law less inflexible, by allowing greater disclosure of safety and effectiveness data, by instituting mechanisms to get certain drugs of high therapeutic potential to patients earlier, and by arranging for patients to be more fully informed about drugs prescribed for them. These questions are soon to be answered, and they must be answered carefully, on the basis of the best science available, and with an eye to the practicalities of administering the law. The questions must also be answered in such a way that the great benefits to be derived from drugs are not diminished, and the equally great risks are not increased. The public welfare must be protected, but scientific innovation and discovery ought not to be repressed. Finding the balance presents one of the greatest challenges facing our government, and the public, today.

FOR ADDITIONAL READING:

Dowling, Harry F. *Medicines for Man: The Development, Regulation, and Use of Prescription Drugs.* New York: Alfred A. Knopf, 1970.

How Safe Is Safe?: The Design of Policy on Drugs and Food Additives. Washington, D.C.: National Academy of Sciences, 1974.

Ross, Walter S. *The Life/Death Ratio: Benefits and Risks in Modern Medicines.* New York: Reader's Digest Press, 1977.

U.S. House of Representatives. Committee on Interstate and Foreign Commerce. Subcommittee on Public Health and Environment. *A Brief Legislative History of the Food, Drug, and Cosmetic Act.* Washington, D.C.: U.S. Government Printing Office, 1974. LC card 74–600990.

Young, James Harvey. *The Medical Messiahs.* Princeton, N.J.: Princeton University Press, 1967.

———. *The Toadstool Millionaires.* Princeton, N.J.: Princeton University Press, 1961.

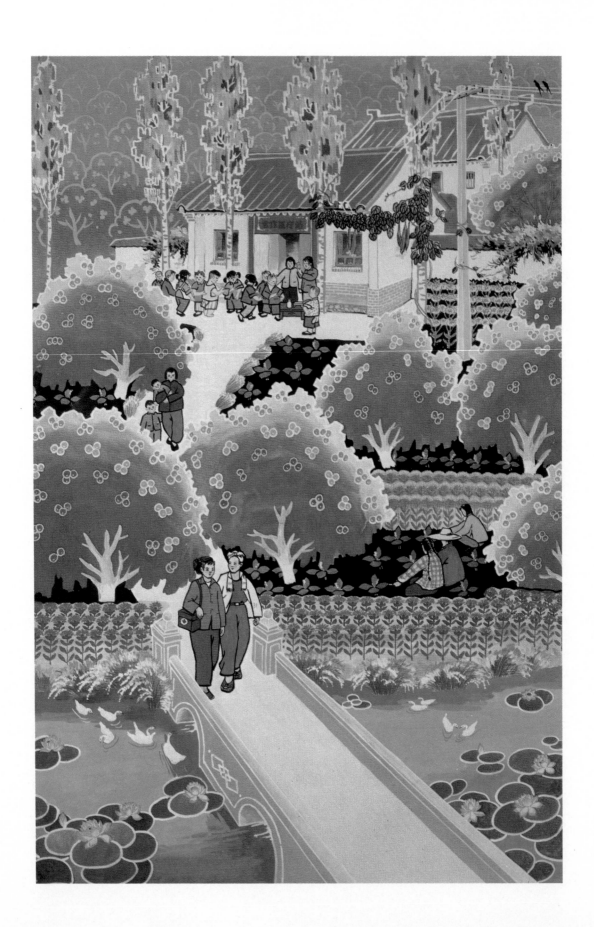

Health in China Today

by Marian S. Kessler
and Richard H. Kessler, M.D.

It was in August 1976 that we were informed our application to visit mainland China had been approved. The trip was scheduled for the following January, which gave us a full five months lead time to turn our attention, scholarly and otherwise, toward the Orient. We were to visit the People's Republic with a group of 22, mainly from the Evanston and Chicago campuses of Northwestern University—a group diverse in interests and disciplines: medicine, sociology, mathematics, computer science, engineering, management, law, education, political science, languages, and health administration. Like the other members of our group, we read widely and avidly. As a result, many of the facts and, to a lesser extent, the opinions we are about to present about health care and medicine in China were realized prior to the visit. However, any amount of study carried out in anticipation of the trip proved to be totally inadequate preparation for the stunning experience we had.

For example, the fact that most of the Chinese people live in rural areas is widely known. One can read about this but is not likely to understand its critical implications until, having traveled thousands of miles through the countryside, it ceases to be an abstraction that no landscape, however remote, is free of inhabitants. This fact has monumental significance for the system of health care in China, as we shall see.

Because of the heavily rural quality of China, early revolutionary leaders made the rural peasants, rather than the urban-based proletariat, the focus of their political strategy. The frequently quoted statement of Chairman Mao, "Stress the rural areas," which owes its origin to political pragmatism, ultimately led to dramatic improvements in the nation's health.

39

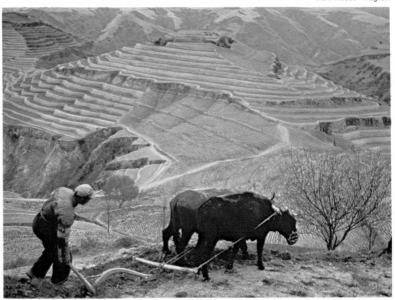

The late Chairman Mao's decision to "stress the rural areas," where 76.5% of the Chinese population lives, ultimately led to dramatic improvements in the nation's health.

Marian S. Kessler *is Director of the Department of Health Systems Studies for the American Hospital Association, Chicago.*

Richard H. Kessler, M.D., *is Senior Vice-President of Michael Reese Hospital and Medical Center in Chicago and Medical Editor of the* Medical and Health Annual.

(Overleaf) "A Production Brigade Clinic" (1973), by Li Cheng-hsuan, part of an exhibition of peasant paintings from Huhsien County of the People's Republic of China.

But many of the achievements in Chinese medicine are elusive. It is difficult to obtain good public health statistics on pre- and, frequently, on postrevolutionary China. Where older records are available, they relate to small and often unrepresentative segments of the population. Most pre-revolution investigations were carried out by Western-trained health workers who studied urban rather than rural groups. Moreover, even contemporary Chinese health authorities seem uncomfortable with current epidemiological reporting methods. In some cases they do not have good record-keeping systems; this may explain an apparent reluctance to publish. But most notably, Chinese priorities lie in grappling with present needs, not in studying past experience.

There are good reasons for the lack of comprehensive and systematic statistics on national health. Effective centralized government is new to China. Historically, the Chinese social-political structure stressed regional rather than national organization, a phenomenon that continues to be characteristic of China. Although major political and economic policies may issue from Peking, local organizations (communes, residential groups, or factory committees) enjoy considerable freedom to modify or interpret those policies to fit local needs. Health statistics are available from these smaller units of government—any deficiencies or signs of unwillingness to share this information appear strongest at the national level—but in all cases the data that are forthcoming may not be consistently reliable. Much health care is provided by sanitation workers, "barefoot doctors," and other minimally trained practitioners who, appropriately in many cases, are not pressed to make and record definitive diagnoses. If a respiratory illness fades in time, helped by herbs or occasionally an antibiotic, the prevailing sentiment argues against expending scarce and costly resources to identify the causative agent of the self-limited disease. Many pneumonias are probably never pinpointed by X-ray or cultures and, we suspect, numerous other common diseases share such anonymity.

However, one doesn't need hard epidemiological facts to know that through the first half of this century health in China was at best fragile. In some regions the death rate exceeded the rate of live births. The inferior status accorded women, which often meant indifference to the health of mothers and infant daughters, was in large part responsible for exceptionally high mortality rates. Too, periods of turmoil—wars, droughts, and epidemics—decimated whole communities. In short, poverty and malnutrition were endemic, ill health the norm, life expectancy poor.

Health care before the revolution

The few Western medical facilities predating the Communist takeover in 1949 were almost exclusively in cities. And even there Western medicine never really gained popular support. The centuries-old insularity of the Chinese was reflected in their medical care customs. For example, local medicine men and herb doctors were compassionate, familiar to the people, and in harmony with Oriental folk beliefs in ill winds, noxious spirits, and imbalances of yin and yang as causes of disease.

But herbs, moxibustion—a form of cautery involving the burning of herbs upon the skin—and other forms of therapy had questionable value, particu-

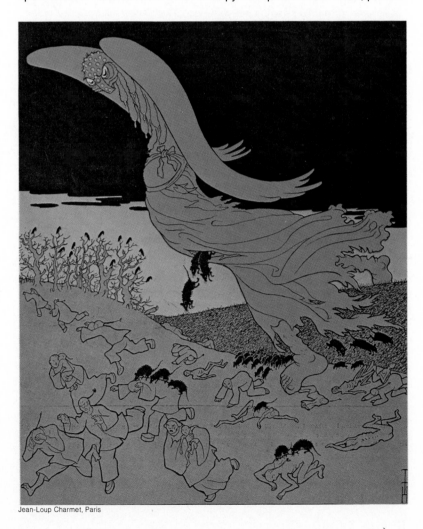

Jean-Loup Charmet, Paris

During the first half of this century China was ravaged by wars, droughts, and epidemics of infectious disease that decimated whole communities. The engraving by Simplicissimus (1911) depicts "The Plague of Manchuria."

larly in the treatment of infectious diseases, which until quite recently constituted a substantial health problem in China. Syphilis, smallpox, tuberculosis, malaria, and the parasitic disease schistosomiasis ravaged the people. Little in the venerated medical practice of China could favorably affect these scourges. In major cities, where the occasional medical schools and hospitals patterned after the Western model were clustered, even the privileged classes utilized Western medicine only as a last resort, so strong was the preference for their own cultural traditions.

The few Western institutions that existed in urban centers were never intended to assume delivery of care as their primary responsibility but rather were organized to affect the course of health in China through education of the public and professionals in sanitation, hygiene, and nutrition. The Kuomintang government, established in 1928 by Chiang Kai-shek, was enthusiastic about the potential offered by Western sanitation methods and created an elaborate public health administration in its capital at Nanking. Few programs were implemented, however, and little thought or budget went toward translating policy into action.

Reports from a few studies undertaken in the 1920s suggest the magnitude of problems that literally plagued the country. In Peking from 1926 to 1932 there were 2,055 deaths per year per 100,000 population. The comparable figure for New York City in 1930 was slightly more than half that rate—1,130 per 100,000. Similar contrasts are evident in the following table:

Causes of Death, rate/100,000

	Peking, 1926–32	New York, 1930
Tuberculosis	303	66
Pneumonias	260	108
Gastrointestinal diseases	244	21
Cardiac diseases	166	480

As mentioned earlier, not all attributions of death were made by trained people, nor were standards uniform within the professional groups. Compounding the problem, ancestor worship in China essentially precluded definitive diagnosis by postmortem examination. Nevertheless, the data are reliable enough to reveal a sharp difference in incidence between the principal killers in the U.S. in 1930—heart disease (as well as cancer and stroke)—and those of China—infectious diseases.

At the turn of the century, well before the advent of antibiotics, improvements in sanitation and general living conditions in New York had mitigated the threat of infectious diseases. The Chinese, on the other hand, faced devastating health problems as a legacy of poverty, a lack of public health technology, deficient medical care facilities, and a medical tradition unsuited to solve the nation's major health problems.

Poverty was so widespread that at no time in prerevolutionary history had the Chinese been free of the anguish of starvation. Malnutrition, chronic and pervasive, was periodically exacerbated by catastrophic famines from crop failures, wars, and epidemics. Diseases of childhood such as measles and mumps, relatively benign in Western nations, were often fatal to malnourished children in China. Malnutrition took its toll in other ways, too, affecting intellectual capacity over a lifetime. Not only does hunger preempt human intellectual endeavor but lack of proper diet in mothers impedes fetal brain development. How many humans were thus denied their full mental, creative, and spiritual potential we will never know.

Poverty also led to the selling of children into prostitution, which fostered an incidence of venereal disease said to exceed 25% in certain urban centers. Overcrowding in housing and worksites provided an environment ripe for transmission of respiratory disease. Tuberculosis not only killed from 15 to 20% of the population, it also severely debilitated uncounted numbers of the living. Smallpox, diphtheria, and influenza were common. Inadequate living conditions, coupled with the use of untreated human feces as fertilizer, also favored transmission of intestinal diseases. Typhoid, bacillary dysentery, and cholera took great tolls in lives and human productiveness. Neonatal tetanus (caused by fecal contamination of birthing sites) contributed in large measure to high maternal and infant mortality.

Parasitic diseases of the gastrointestinal tract, primarily hookworm and schistosomiasis (marked by fever, allergic symptoms, diarrhea, and often severe and chronic infection of the liver, lungs, and nervous system) pervaded the south of China. In a limited study of vegetable farmers during the 1930s over 60% were found to be infected. Contamination of drinking and irrigation water in the heavily populated Chekiang Province resulted in a 55% incidence of schistosomiasis among rice farmers there. Insect-borne diseases such as malaria, plague, typhus, and kala-azar (an infection with a high fatality rate, often called "black fever") were endemic because of the failure to treat sewage, to control the quality of drinking water, and to educate the peasants in simple hygienic measures.

The revolution: new focus on health

At the time of the revolution in 1949, conditions remained deplorably poor. The following year the First National Health Conference was organized to confront China's major health problems. Prevention was the keynote. Four major areas were identified for immediate action: smallpox vaccination, control of syphilis, midwife training, and public sanitation. Mao Tse-tung set the tone of the conference with three widely quoted slogans: "In medicine and health put prevention first," "Stress the rural areas," and "Combine Chinese with Western methods."

At that time the incidence of venereal disease in urban areas approached 25%. Syphilis in particular constituted a major national health problem for both living and future generations since it is transmitted not only to sexual partners but also from the mother to the fetus. The wholesale attack on syphilis and its subsequent control became the prototype for alleviating other infectious diseases, both in rural and urban areas. The strategy devised illustrates the unique and effective methods applied in the People's Republic to achieve dramatic improvements in health in less than three decades.

The organization of the population into multifunctional units is a critical element in the extraordinary progress the Chinese have made since the

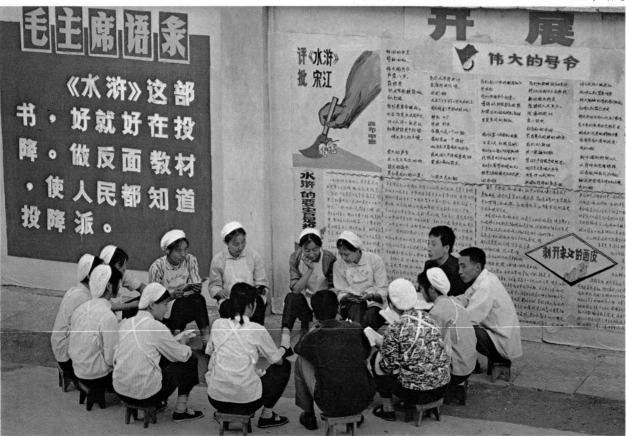

The organization of both urban and rural populations into communes has facilitated education about public health matters. With the aid of those trained in detection of the disease, the masses ultimately assumed responsibility for the dramatic decline of syphilis and other infectious diseases. After the revolution employment opportunities for women increased measurably; women's improved status had a great impact on the general state of health in China.

revolution, specifically in medical care. In both urban and rural areas the commune is the basic living and working unit. Rural communes are centered around farms, urban communes around factories, places of business, or neighborhoods, and both encompass essentially all the major interdependent elements of daily life—housing, schools, health care, employment, recreation, and, of course, politics.

Such collective living and working arrangements facilitate public education about health matters; after the First National Health Conference syphilis became a prime target of discussion at regular group meetings in urban communes throughout the People's Republic, fostering an awareness among neighbors and fellow laborers about the course of the disease. Poverty, the low status of women, lack of employment opportunities for women, and prostitution were identified as key factors in the rapid spread of syphilis, one of the most virulent forms of venereal disease.

The problem and its genesis were clear to the revolutionary leadership. By redistributing land, closing houses of prostitution, and creating job opportunities for women some reduction in the number of syphilis cases was obtained. The cure, penicillin, already proven abroad, was available in China. But identifying the diseased population remained an obstacle. It was necessary to screen high-risk groups by blood test before treatment could be initiated, and that issue aroused much political conflict.

Professional health workers proposed to institute screening programs.

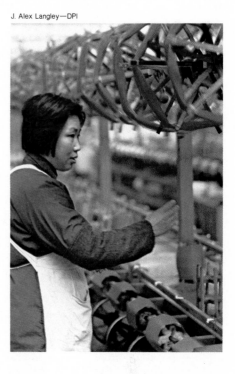

Although qualified for the task, these practitioners were few in number and to the masses represented an intellectual elite. In keeping with the revolutionary doctrine to be self-reliant, the people rejected the efforts of health workers because, if the revolution as conceived by the early leadership was to succeed, the laboring class had to be the major implementer of policy. Accordingly, amateur health workers, driven by an intense spirit of social responsibility, offered their own screening system for syphilis.

They were assisted by professional health workers in designing a ten-item questionnaire that could identify high-risk individuals in a test population. Some 3,000 volunteers, who were provided an intensive one-week course in the use of the questionnaire, were also instructed in a simple blood-screening method to detect syphilis. More than 80% of these amateurs passed the qualifying exam, and within two months of working amid a select-ed population of about 300,000 they had found over 10,000 cases. Retesting of a sample of this same population by professional health workers demon-strated that the novices had successfully detected about 90% of the active cases in that population.

In addition to effective screening, the control of syphilis was in large part abetted by stringent measures to eliminate sexual promiscuity. The strict self-discipline of the masses has contributed enormously to the extremely low incidence of venereal disease in China in the last few decades.

From this example, it was clear that health and political needs in China could be served simultaneously, and a curable disease like syphilis could be successfully contained by the use of highly motivated, minimally trained amateurs. With the aid of those schooled specifically in detection and pre-vention of disease, the masses could assume responsibility for their own health. Accordingly, other public health problems, including most infectious and nutritional diseases, were successfully conquered in a similar manner—through a combination of group efforts, resourcefulness, and discipline.

Clearly, the organization of commune members into intensively structured units and the suffusion of politics into every phase of life have greatly in-fluenced the status of contemporary health in China. Indeed, the self-con-tained commune organization represents a public health worker's dream: the population is accessible, limited in size, encompassed within a definable territory, and presents no problems of compliance. What the central commit-tee dictates as health policy for the common good is accepted virtually without question.

If the postrevolutionary Chinese had followed a Western mode of over-coming disease, at least by U.S. standards, it would have entailed training one million physicians and building hospitals with a total capacity of five million beds. But China's leaders adopted a far more expedient approach. Our trip provided the opportunity to observe firsthand in many areas the results of such pragmatism.

A commune clinic

At the Evergreen commune outside Peking, on a gray, bitterly cold day in January, we were warmly welcomed by the vice-chairman of the local revolu-tionary committee, the "Responsible Person." During the not-so-brief "Brief

45

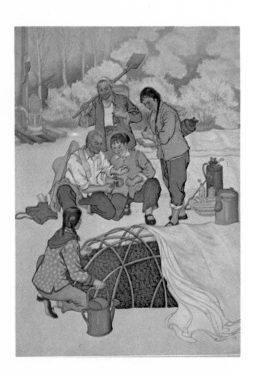

"Nursing Sprouts" (1974), by Lui Chih-teh, from the peasant paintings from Huhsien County.

Introduction" we were served green tea, Golden Deer cigarettes, and a great deal of political rhetoric. (Smoking is a source of some embarrassment to the Chinese; they denied the association of tobacco with lung cancer or heart disease. Cigarettes are a luxury in the same way that candy is, and they are used as a gesture of friendship, particularly between host and guest. Cigarettes were offered to us with great frequency.) We learned that the 42,000 citizens at Evergreen were engaged in vegetable farming and in maintaining minor acreage in grain and fodder. Nonfarming assets included a small factory that produced land-grading machinery, a chemical plant to purify phosphate for fertilizer, and, because Peking's winter climate requires hothouse horticulture, a glass factory to support the many acres of green-houses. Schools, housing, shops, and some cottage industries, along with health care and recreational facilities, completed the inventory.

The commune supports 14 medical clinics, each staffed by about ten health personnel. The clinic we inspected consisted of four rooms, none heated or supplied with plumbing. One room, devoted to storing and dispensing herbs, was dominated by a 70-drawer cabinet containing carefully labeled specimens of dried leaves, roots, berries, bark, seeds, petals, and blossoms of both cultivated and wild plants. Each was reported to have proved its value by generations of trial-and-error experimentation. (We would hasten to add that as many as 48 herb teas of 36 botanical varieties are said to be effective for 13 specific therapeutic purposes, according to one of the standard reference works in U.S. medical schools, *Stedman's Medical Dictionary*. Moreover, many drugs in common use in Western medicine are either purified extracts or synthetic analogues of botanical products. Examples include digitalis, adrenaline, belladonna, quinidine, colchicine, caffeine, and penicillin.)

The second room was also a pharmacy, but one supplying Western drugs in both pill and injectable forms. All are made in China—a source of great national pride. These two adjacent pharmacies stand as concrete evidence of Mao's dictum to "Combine Chinese with Western methods."

The third room was for the examination of patients. It was simply equipped, with a table, chairs, blood pressure machine, stethoscope, and other basic diagnostic tools. But imagine undergoing a physical examination at an ambient temperature well below freezing!

The last room, largest of all, was used for general treatment and was modestly supplied with necessities for performing minor surgery, first aid, and acupuncture therapy. A familiar portrait of Chairman Mao hung side by side with one of his successor, Chairman Hua. Posters illustrating acupuncture sites and birth control instructions filled much of the remaining wall space. (The Chinese are so concerned about containing the growth of their population that birth control advice and materials are readily available. Pills, mechanical devices, and surgical procedures are commonly employed. We suspect that the Pill is most frequently used.)

This clinic serves a population of approximately 3,000 peasants at a daily rate of about 20 outpatient visits and 5 house calls. The bedridden and the elderly are cared for in the commune's nursing home, while the children get treatment at their schools.

46

The cost of operating this particular unit is largely borne by the commune through an annual tax. The patient is charged an amount equivalent to about 5% of his monthly discretionary income per visit. In other locations the patient may be charged a direct fee for service. Whether supported by the group or paid for wholly or partially by individual recipients, medical care in China is inexpensive but not free.

The clinic described above provides inoculations against tuberculosis, poliomyelitis, diphtheria, measles, pertussis, tetanus, smallpox, encephalitis, and meningitis (meningococcus A and B). This kind of preventive program is said to be carried out throughout China. Evidence of success is apparent in the following data from the Chinese Medical Association:

Incidence of Infectious Disease
rate/100,000, Peking

	1951	1971
Diphtheria	13.4	0.1
Pertussis	103.0	16.1
Measles	598.0	46.4
Poliomyelitis	5.3	0.7

In addition to providing mass immunizations, the local clinic is the focus of other infectious disease programs: insect and animal vector control, sewage processing, and controlling the quality of drinking water. At the local clinic we visited, the Chinese penchant for numbers was evident: three slogans emphasize the "two controls" (water and sewage), "four pests" (rats, bedbugs, flies, and mosquitoes), and "five improvements" (wells, latrines, pigsties, stoves, and hygiene).

Barefoot doctors

But none of the progress we observed at the Evergreen commune—or elsewhere in China—could have been achieved without "barefoot doctors,"

At a typical commune clinic both Western drugs and herbal medicines are dispensed. Wild plants as well as carefully cultivated specimens of dried leaves, roots, berries, bark, seeds, petals, and blossoms are used and have proved their value over generations of experimentation. It is interesting to note that many Western drugs are purified extracts or synthetic analogues of botanical products.

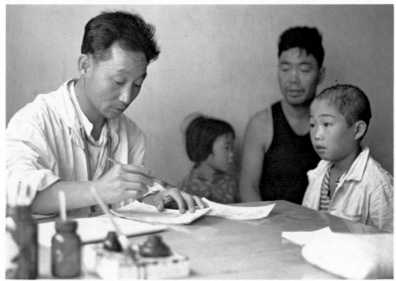

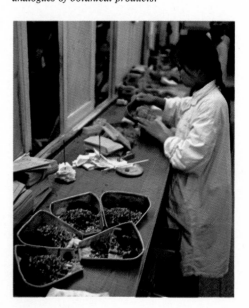

(Left) Richard Balzer—Stock, Boston; (right) Bruno Barbey—Magnum

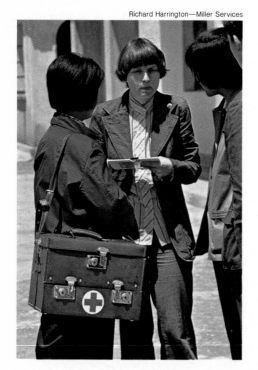

"Barefoot doctors" *have had a major* *impact on health improvement in China.* *The title applies to most nonphysician* *health workers, who are involved in acute* *care, sanitation, cultivation of herbs,* *midwifery, birth control, and* *infectious disease programs.*

a generic title that applies to most nonphysician health workers. Their activities vary with the setting and with the availability and skill level of their associated health practitioners. In addition to maintaining the infectious disease programs, they may have sole or collaborative responsibility for acute care, sanitation, cultivation and collection of herbs, midwifery, pre- and postnatal care, birth control advice, and, when the problem at hand seems beyond their competence, referral to higher echelons of medical care. Their training appears as eclectic as their tasks. We spoke to some barefoot doctors who had received two years of university education and to others whose training was exclusively on the job. Occasionally a clinic will have a physician or surgeon assigned both for help in patient care and for the continuing education of the barefoot doctors.

In their last year of secondary education students are allowed to indicate their future work preferences. (If not assigned to a task of their choice, all seem quite willing to do what is best for the group, the revolution, and society.) Barefoot doctoring is a popular occupation, and the number of students and older commune residents who wish to become candidates often exceeds commune needs—a familiar situation to those involved in selecting applicants to U.S. medical schools. In China, however, members of the commune elect from the group of aspirants those they believe will best satisfy their needs.

A Shanghai infirmary

It is difficult to estimate the extent to which the widely distributed clinics are successful in solving health problems, but certain observations lead us to conclude that they carry the major burden. The best evidence rests on the fact that there are few facilities beyond the local clinics.

The next link in the Chinese medical care system—infirmaries for the bedridden ill who do not require highly sophisticated care—has no modern Western counterpart. A 30-bed infirmary that we visited on the outskirts of Shanghai was said to be typical of this second level of medical care in China. Adjacent to a modern apartment complex housing factory workers, the two-story building contained many of the same facilities as a local clinic plus a small surgical suite, a dental chair, and 15 two-bed rooms. Patients from about 14 clinics scattered through the suburb are referred here for "secondary" care. It was reported that during the winter respiratory ailments are seen most often, while intestinal problems predominate in the summer.

At the infirmary approximately half of the professional staff are barefoot doctors; the remainder are "physicians" and "surgeons." Overall, women on the staff outnumber men by about two to one. But, typical of the difficulty in getting hard facts, essentially everyone we asked gave different answers about staff size and composition. This should not necessarily be interpreted as deliberate deception but more probably is an indication of the underplaying of job titles and credentials. It should also be noted that significant numbers of practitioners rotate at irregular intervals through this infirmary from hospitals in Shanghai.

It was equally difficult to obtain estimates of the numbers of patients seen. We can attest only to the fact that on the day of our visit business was

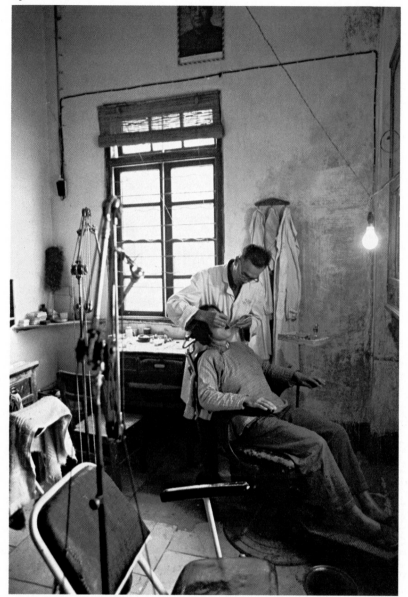

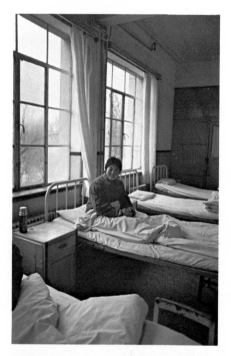

While there has been stunning progress in health care, some of the medical facilities, such as the dental clinic (left), are distressingly dirty, drab, poorly lighted, and often unheated. Hospitals are few in number and are often underutilized. The Friendship Hospital in Peking (above) contains 650 beds but here is only about half occupied.

minimal: neither the two barefoot doctors nor the dentist was seeing patients; the operating room was empty; and only 4 of the 30 beds were occupied. Half a dozen ambulatory patients were undergoing acupuncture, moxibustion, or cupping treatments—the application of a cup-shaped glass to the skin to induce a flow of blood to the area—for such complaints as infected jaws or muscle spasms.

This infirmary was probably the most unattractive of the numerous medical facilities we visited. In the rural commune clinic one expects rustic, somewhat crude firstline facilities and services, but in an infirmary in the suburbs of Shanghai we assumed conditions would be better. However, the rooms were drab, poorly lighted, minimally furnished, and distressingly dirty. While antibourgeois sentiment might discourage decorative trappings, it was surprising from the standpoint of hygiene to see soiled walls, dirt-spotted floors,

49

and chipped and peeling paint. Independent of political attitudes, most visitors to China soon become ambitious for the Chinese to succeed with their social welfare goals. This was quite evident in our own group. Observing the earnestness of the Chinese, who are justifiably proud of their many recent achievements in nutrition, housing, education, medical care, and public health, visitors readily become enthusiastic advocates for their continued success. So we were perplexed by the fact that our hosts selected to show us this dismal, underutilized, probably unsanitary infirmary. That visit forced us to agree with their frequent admission, "We have a long way to go."

A Peking hospital

It should be obvious from the foregoing description that institutional care is not high on the list of medical priorities in China. Hospitals are few in number, underutilized, and bear a significant primary care responsibility. Peking, with a population of close to ten million, has 11 general hospitals. The Friendship Hospital, one of the largest, contains 650 beds. A casual walk through on one cold January day revealed an occupancy rate of about 50%. We were particularly interested in the cardiac intensive care units here. Two units consisted of four beds each, serviced by electronic monitors of heart rate, a single electrocardiograph, and a defibrillator (a device used to restore erratic heart rhythm to normal). Seven of the eight beds were empty. But unfortunately that statistic probably does not reflect a city of healthy hearts. With infectious and nutritional diseases largely under control today, even meager statistics reveal that the major killers of the adult population in China are the same as in the West—heart disease, cancer, and stroke. In a metropolis the size of Peking one could therefore predict heart disease sufferers by the tens of thousands, many hundreds of whom would benefit from specialized intensive care. Where were the victims of heart attacks being treated? We don't know the answer, but it is certain that this eight-bed facility in the prime teaching hospital of Peking does not reach many cardiac sufferers of that city.

Friendship Hospital is organized along traditional Western lines, with clinical services arranged by discipline—medicine, neurology, pediatrics, surgery, and so on. Although the staff of approximately 800 is said to be composed of about equal numbers of doctors, nurses, and technicians, it is difficult to compare these figures with typical hospital staffing patterns in the U.S., since not only do the professional titles differ but so do the tasks. For example, at any given time one-third of Friendship Hospital's staff is engaged in medical care outside of the hospital. Teams of 15 to 20 health workers do tours of duty in urban and rural clinics, some as distant as Tibet. Each member of the professional staff is obliged to spend one-third of his or her time in "grass roots" work. Maintaining contact with the peasantry is considered one means of counteracting the elitism that is thought to result from specialized hospital activities.

We have made reference to "doctors" and "nurses," and some elaboration of that terminology is in order since these expressions do not necessarily convey the same meaning in China as in Western society. Uniform criteria do not exist for conferring these titles. A consequence of the Cultural Revo-

50

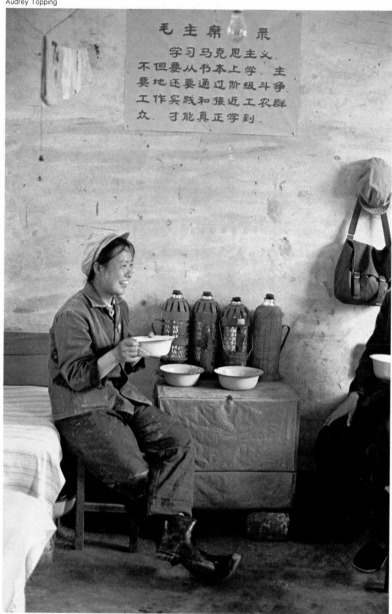

lution has been the blurring of the line between the intellectuals and the peasants, and nowhere is this politically motivated step toward a classless society more evident than in medicine.

The lack of uniform educational standards also helps to dispel the mystique prevalent in other cultures surrounding the title "Doctor." What better way to keep doctors humble than to give them the same title as "barefoot" workers, to minimize the pay differential, and to permit communities to confer the "degree" as they see fit? In the United States there is universal recognition that a "doctor" has graduated from a college and a medical school, has passed a licensure examination, and has worked for at least three years under close supervision as a resident physician before beginning independent clinical practice. In China there is an accommodation both to

All professional health workers are required to spend one-third of their time in so-called grass roots work. The Chinese consider maintaining contact with the peasants a means of counteracting elitism.

51

Photographs, Bruno Barbey—Magnum

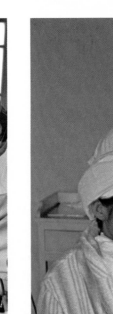

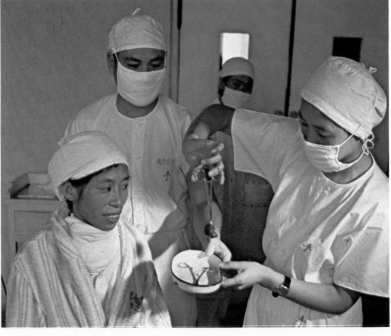

Acupuncture is used by the Chinese for two purposes: to relieve pain and to cure disease. As an anesthesia it has proved to be remarkably effective. The patient above underwent a thyroidectomy after receiving acupuncture to numb the throat area, was conscious throughout the surgery, experienced little pain, and was free of the postoperative complications that can arise from drug anesthesia. Future generations in China (opposite) and the United States would benefit from cooperative efforts to solve mutual health problems, in particular, cancer, heart disease, and stroke.

the vagaries of local health needs and to the mandates of national political purposes. Each school of medicine or nursing establishes its own curriculum and promotion standards. What is more, no paper credentials attest to satisfactory completion of a particular course of study.

Acupuncture: an effective anesthesia

Later in our travels a visit to the Honan Provincial Hospital in Cheng-chou reaffirmed our earlier impressions. What enthralled us here was a spectacular demonstration of acupuncture anesthesia.

In recent years there have been many reports out of China on this technique; however, it is essential to note that the Chinese employ acupuncture for two different purposes—relief of pain and cure of disease. For the former, acupuncture is undeniably successful in certain circumstances; for the latter, it not only defies clinical rationale but borders on the occult.

To witness acupuncture's remarkable effectiveness, our entire group, physicians and nonphysicians alike, were dressed in clean white caps, gowns, and masks. Accompanied by our equally awed translators, we were given free access to five separate operating rooms. During our two-hour stay we were encouraged to inspect, photograph, and talk with the patients who were undergoing the surgical procedures.

A 55-year-old patient harboring an ovarian cyst received most of our attention. She was spirited, confident, and obviously pleased to be the object of attention. After preoperative medication consisting of a mild tranquilizer, anesthesia was induced by insertion of four needles placed symmetrically under the skin of her lower back, plus one in the sacral canal (just below the base of the spinal cord). Each needle was connected to a source of alternating current of 120 hertz (cycles per second) at a voltage of from five to ten volts. After about 15 minutes she could no longer feel a pinprick over the

52

skin of her abdomen. The surgery lasted about 30 minutes, during which she continued a dialogue with us, wincing only at the moment when a grapefruit-sized tumor was delivered through a nine-inch abdominal incision. On completion of the procedure she moved unaided from the operating table to the wheeled stretcher for return to the ward. It was clear that pain was minimal and that she would be free of complications of inhalation anesthesia.

China and the U.S.: toward an information exchange

We returned to the U.S. from our month's sojourn in the People's Republic of China convinced that there would be many benefits for both countries if the Chinese experience in health care could be integrated with ours. The five physicians in our group who witnessed the operations in Cheng-chou feel sure that acupuncture anesthesia could play a vital role in American medicine. It holds an appeal because it is simple in application and avoids the administration of drugs in surgery that in themselves may be injurious. Certain problems are apparent that may limit the use of acupuncture anesthesia, but in selected cases its efficacy, safety, and simplicity confirm it as a major technical advance. Yet as long as the mode of action of acupuncture remains mysterious, the reluctance of Western physicians to accept it will persist. The limited trials in this country have yielded disappointing results despite the fact that the Chinese claim success in 40 to 50% of preselected cases. They have obtained best anesthesia in procedures of the head and neck regions, although acupuncture is also employed in chest and abdominal surgery. Many have observed that acupuncture is a function of hypnosis-suggestion, but the Chinese utilize acupuncture extensively for surgical anesthesia in farm animals, and its use in veterinary surgery would indicate a physiologic basis for its effectiveness.

From here on, the rate of progress in the People's Republic will undoubtedly slacken, because as the population ages, having survived the ancient killers of children and young adults, the Chinese will fall—in fact are falling—prey to the same diseases as Westerners. Thus we find that in 1972 the primary causes of death in Shanghai were, in order, cancer, stroke, and heart disease. Currently the U.S. reports the same three leading causes, although the order differs—heart disease, cancer, and stroke. There is growing evidence that the top three killers are significantly influenced by life-style—diet, physical activity, stress, etc. Many cross-cultural clues may exist that would help uncover the etiology of diseases currently seen in both populations.

A new administration in the People's Republic is striving to bring many advances. Though we lack full diplomatic relations, an increasing number of U.S. physicians and health care professionals have visited China in recent years and have observed, as we did, the strides in medicine and health. The cordial relations American and Chinese health care specialists have enjoyed should be allowed to develop so that we can study effects of environment, social structure, work habits, and ethnic backgrounds on patterns of disease, since we share not only similar problems but, more importantly, the desire to solve them.

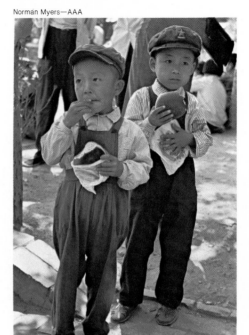

FOR ADDITIONAL READING:

Comparative Study of Traditional and Modern Medicine in Chinese Societies. *Medicine in Chinese Cultures: Comparative Studies of Health Care in Chinese and Other Societies.* Edited by Arthur Kleinman et al. Washington, D.C.: U.S. Government Printing Office, DHEW publication, no. (NIH) 75-653; S/N 017-053-00036-1, 1975.

Hogness, J. R., et al. *Report of the Medical Delegation to the People's Republic of China.* Washington, D.C.: National Academy of Sciences, Institute of Medicine, 1973.

Medicine and Society in China. Edited by John Z. Bowers and Elizabeth F. Purcell. New York: Josiah Macy, Jr. Foundation, 1974.

Sidel, Victor W., and Sidel, Ruth. *Serve the People: Observations on Medicine in the People's Republic of China.* New York: Josiah Macy, Jr. Foundation, 1973.

Caring and Curing
The evolution of hospital design

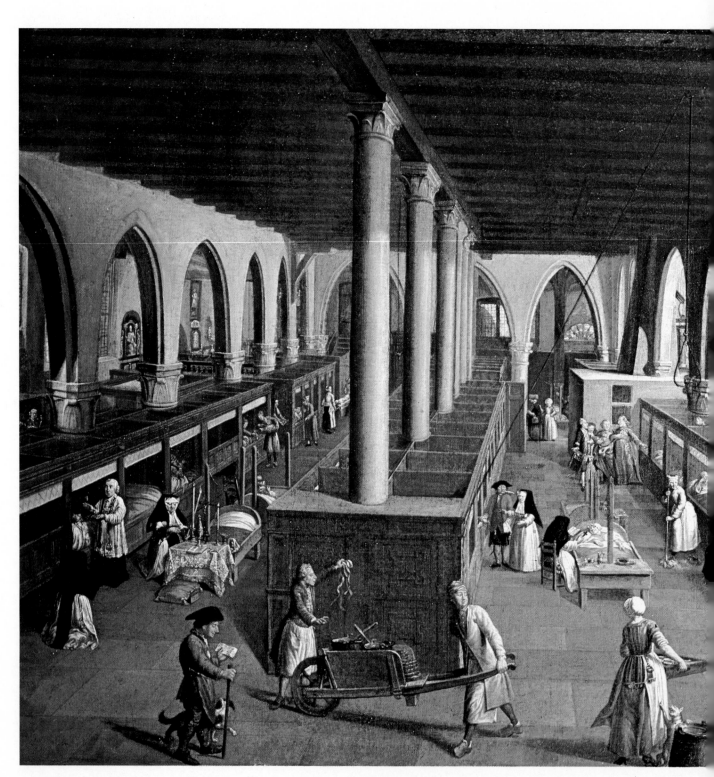

by John D. Thompson

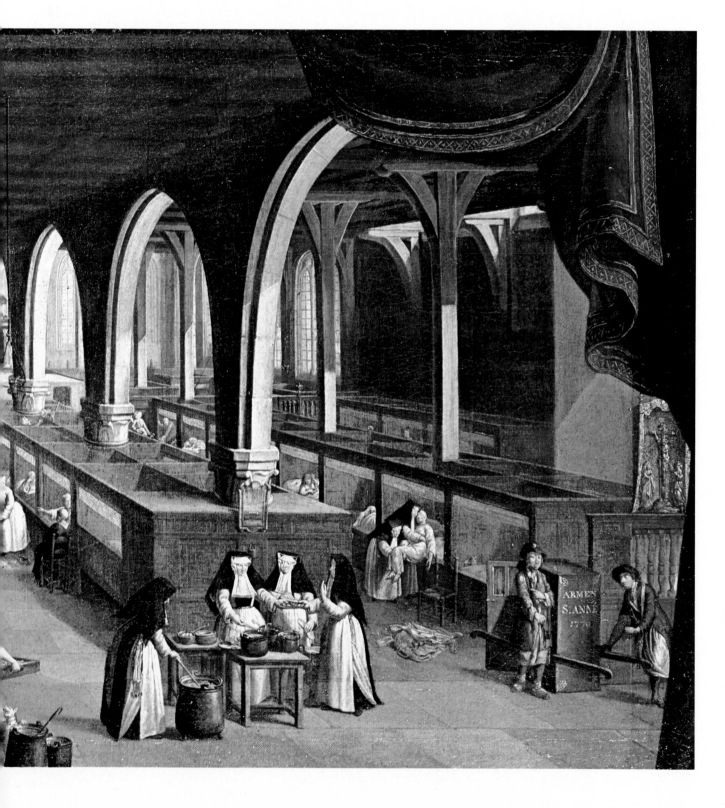

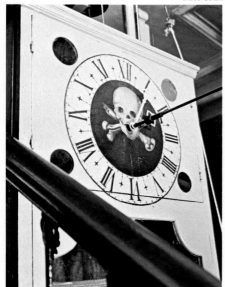

While the driving forces in the previous periods were social, it was progress of medicine and surgery which now called for a new type of hospital. . . . the character of the hospital changed fundamentally. It was no longer a hospice to provide shelter for the indigent, no longer an institution in which charity service was given to the sick poor exclusively. From the dreaded place where poor people went to die, the hospital became a medical center to which patients of all classes go to seek recovery, a place in which new life is brought to light.

—Henry E. Sigerist

A study of the design of hospitals provides not only insights into the development of a particular kind of building but also a framework for the examination of the history of medicine as an art and a science. Until a little over 100 years ago, hospitals were not specific places for the treatment of disease. They were institutions for social rather than medical care. Anyone who had a home where he or she could be cared for without danger to himself or others was treated there. Hospitals sheltered travelers, pilgrims, the poor, the insane, or those who were considered harmful to the community, such as lepers. They were multipurpose institutions, derived from inns and poorhouses, though special facilities for the mentally ill and for those considered carriers of disease had appeared as early as the 1st century AD as separate institutions. The buildings that housed patients tended to reflect the characteristics of the social sponsor of the hospital, such as the church, local government, or a lord. The structures themselves were adapted from monasteries, palaces, estates, prisons, and barracks.

During the 19th century a transformation of the hospital from a social to a medical care institution took place. Development of the hospital as a medical institution involved first assuring the basic safety of the patient; later its adaptation into a positive therapeutic force could be accomplished when the medical sciences began to develop. This meant that hospitals no longer sheltered just the sick poor. The middle classes and the wealthy who previously were cared for at home when they were sick since the home could provide more comfort, a greater number of amenities, and a more sanitary environment now began to go to hospitals for therapeutic treatment. In fact, as facilities and services developed that truly could aid the ill, *most* beds were occupied by the affluent. This key shift in the hospital's population had an important effect on the physical features of these healing institutions. Beginning around 1860, then, medical factors, as they were perceived at the time, became important influences in the design of hospitals. Hospitals took on their own recognizable architectural characteristics; they no longer looked like churches, palaces, or civic buildings. Each hospital began to resemble other hospitals regardless of sponsorship or even location. After 1860 hospitals were specifically designed to care for the ill, and in the past several decades they have become healing machines of awesome technology, devoted to curing or prolonging the lives of patients of every age and social class.

The history of modern hospital architecture is often considered in terms of three periods: before Nightingale (1860), from 1860 to 1950, and from 1950 to the present. However, these periods do not in any way conform to a dominant architectural style; there are examples of Romanesque, Gothic, Renaissance, baroque, neoclassical, and modern hospitals.

John D. Thompson *is Professor of Public Health and Chief of the Division of Health Services Administration at Yale University School of Medicine, New Haven, Connecticut.*

(Overleaf) "View of the Sick Ward of St. John's Hospital" by Johannes Beerblock, 1778. In St. John's Hospital, Bruges, Belgium. Reproduced with permission of St. John's Hospital, O.C.M.W., Bruges.

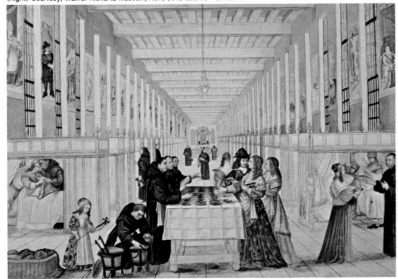

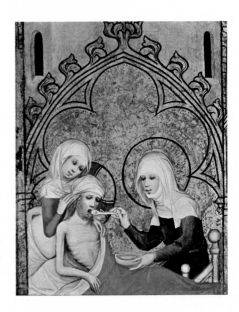

Early history

The hospital in the Western world began as a Christian institution. With the emergence of Christianity the ill, crippled, and maimed assumed a special, blessed place in the community. This was indeed a radical change in society's view of the diseased: the Greco-Roman view idealized the *perfect* human body. This new regard for the sick was two-sided. Not only were the ill viewed as being specially marked by God but they were the instruments of salvation for the other members of the church. The "seven works of mercy" focused on caring for the ill and the poor and were considered the way to eternal life. Six of the works were stated in Matthew 25:35–36: "For I was hungry and you gave me food, I was thirsty and you gave me drink, I was a stranger and you welcomed me, I was naked and you clothed me, I was sick and you visited me, I was in prison and you came to me." Burying the dead is the seventh work of mercy. In early Christian history, then, the hospital, or hospice, was the institution in which Christians carried out the words of Jesus. For the next thousand years hospitals in the Western world were shaped by the seven works.

It is not surprising to find that the architecture of these early caring institutions was ecclesiastical, whether monastic or urban. Unfortunately there are no examples of the early Christian hospices, most of which were inns for pilgrims, although we know these institutions existed from the writings of the early church fathers, both in Rome and Constantinople. Inns served those who were considered more or less sick, having made long journeys as penance. Foot travel was both painful and hazardous, and illnesses were often contracted along the way. Food was inadequate. Provisions for those who died of illness were necessary. In all likelihood many of these buildings were converted from some other use, just as the early churches were converted temples. For example, the recreated pandochaeion (hospitality inn) at the monastery of Turmanin (Syria) is typical of buildings in Syria of the Roman period, with its columned porticos on all sides.

The Middle Ages. It is almost accidental that we know as much as we

Hospitals in the Western world began as Christian institutions. Until a little over 100 years ago they were not specific places for the treatment of disease; rather they provided shelter for travelers, pilgrims, and the poor. (Opposite) The clock above the entrance staircase in St. Nikolaus-Spital, a nursing hospital at Kues, West Germany, founded in 1458 for aged priests, noblemen, and paupers. A 17th-century engraving by Abraham Bosse (left) shows Anne of Austria with monks who cared for the sick at the Hôpital de la Charité in Paris. Detail of a late-14th-century altarpiece (right) by the Master of Cologne depicts St. Elizabeth of Hungary, who devoted most of her life to caring for the sick, at a hospice that she founded in the 13th century.

do about the development of the hospital's early monastic form in Europe. A single piece of parchment contains a copy of the recommended plans for a monastic community worked out in two synods on ecclesiastic reform held in Aachen in the years 816 and 817. This copy was made for the abbot of the monastery of St. Gall, in Switzerland, to be used as a guide for rebuilding his monastery. The monastery typified the manner in which monks looked after the sick, which later became a model for the laity. At St. Gall there were structures labeled as a hospice for pilgrims and paupers, a physicians' house with two rooms for the seriously ill, an herb garden, and a house for distinguished visitors. There was also a separate infirmary for the monks and a blood-letting house. It is now believed that these outbuildings, as opposed to the church and cloister, were probably built in some form of vernacular architecture rather than in a formal design of the period. They may well have looked more like barns than churches. We do know from the recreation of the monastery at Cluny, in France, two centuries later, that these various forms of monastic hospices expanded and probably became more devoted to the treatment of the sick as the monasteries themselves grew.

Another reason for the close link between hospital and ecclesiastic architecture was that many of the hospitals built in the Middle Ages contained altars within them or churches alongside them. Faith and prayer were the primary therapies available at the time. At the same time, sponsorship of hospitals was broadened within the church by the council at Aachen to include bishops and specific religious orders such as the Hospitallers and the Order of the Holy Ghost and even extended outside of the church to royalty who were anxious to demonstrate their piety. This transition from religious to secular auspices was primarily a shift in the assumption of responsibility for the care of the poor and ill, but the hospitals were still staffed by religious orders.

Fortunately a few examples of these hospitals remain, among them the infirmary of the abbey at Ourscamp, France (1210), and the Hôpital Notre Dame des Fontenilles (1293) in Tonnerre, France—probably the most outstanding surviving example of the early "open ward" architectural style; *i.e.*, a patient ward that opened into a chapel. The hall at Tonnerre measures 88 meters (288 feet) by 19 meters (61 feet) and is covered by a wooden barrel vault. There are differences in the architectural details in the chapel at the end of the ward and the patient spaces within the ward, including "sacred and profane" windows. Large open wards that were adjacent to chapels predominated not only because religion was the key therapy but also because religious feelings were intense among the ill or those about to die.

St. John's Hospital at Bruges, in Belgium, started out at the end of the 12th century with a relatively small ward constructed alongside a church. As that beautiful city grew in the high period of Flemish prosperity, two additions to the original ward were constructed in the 13th century, and another enlargement was added during the first half of the 14th century. Though we do not know how the hospital functioned during those times, there is a marvelous painting, Johannes Beerblock's *View of the Sick Ward of St. John's Hospital* (see pages 54 and 55), that depicts the interior, indicating the different architectural styles employed for these additions. All of the activities carried

In the Middle Ages monks cared for the sick. Monastic hospices expanded and probably became more devoted to treating the ill as the monasteries themselves grew. The monastery at Cluny, France, about 1157, as restored by Kenneth J. Conant, shows the great infirmary hall built by Peter the Venerable (c. 1135), in the left foreground; adjoining it, middle foreground, is the infirmary built by St. Hugh (c. 1082).

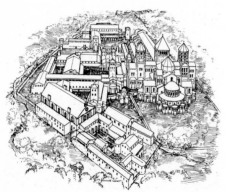

Courtesy, Mediaeval Academy of America

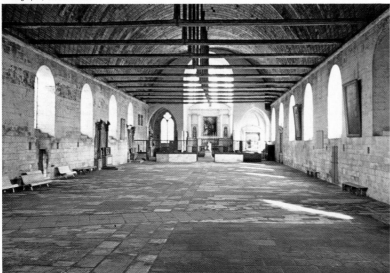

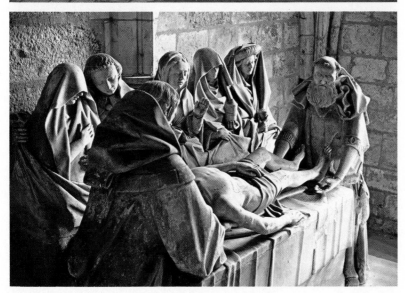

on within the hospital are represented—from the admission of a new patient brought in on a sedan chair ambulance, to the care of a dying patient, to the preparation for the last rite of extreme unction to another patient. Sisters are shown nursing, feeding, and making rounds with a physician or apothecary; clergy are visiting patients; the patients are searching their heads for lice or chasing cats between their bedded cubicles.

The reason few examples of these hospitals remain is that many of them were situated in front of cathedrals so the communicants, on their way to mass, could contribute to the hospital's upkeep. It was a sort of "poor box" near the church door. During the 19th-century Gothic revival the architect Viollet-le-Duc and others had the hospitals razed in order to obtain a better view of the cathedrals.

The Renaissance. Growth and prosperity of European cities characterized the Renaissance and influenced architecture, including the design of hospitals. One hospital, Brunelleschi's Ospedale degli Innocenti (1419), in

The Hôpital Notre Dame des Fontenilles (1293) in Tonnerre, France, is probably the most outstanding surviving example of "open ward" design—a patient ward that opened into a chapel (top). Religious feelings among the sick were usually quite intense. This design meant patients could see mass from their beds. (Below) A deposition in the hospital at Tonnerre by Jean Michiel and Georges de la Sonecte. The 15th-century sculpture depicts the laying out of Christ's body for anointment.

59

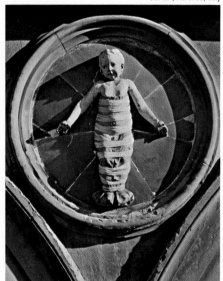

A foundling in swaddling clothes, one of the terra-cotta medallions by Andrea Della Robbia adorning the facade of the Ospedale degli Innocenti in Florence. Della Robbia's sculptures of children have been replicated in children's hospitals throughout the world.

Florence, is considered by many to be the first important institution constructed in Renaissance style. The glazed blue and white terra-cotta plaques portraying children which embellish the spandrels were sculpted by Andrea Della Robbia. These have been replicated in children's hospitals throughout the world.

Filarete's (Antonio Averlino's) Ospedale Maggiore in Milan was the best known of the Renaissance hospitals. Its outstanding feature was the cross-shaped ward with an altar at the juncture of the two arms of the cross. While the cross was a Christian symbol, it was also used in many hospitals as an architectural solution to the problem of increasing capacity. When a medieval hospital had grown too large, rather than double the length of the open ward that adjoined a chapel so that patients at the far end would no longer be able to see or hear mass, logic led to a new design: a cross with four wards and an altar in the middle.

Filarete described his original plan for the Ospedale Maggiore in some detail in his *Treatise on Architecture,* written during 1460–64. The hospital was intended for the care of the "needs of the infirm, both men and women, and of children born out of wedlock." The Ospedale Maggiore was a grand hospital in every respect. Set in a rectangle 235 meters (770 feet) long and 94 meters (308 feet) wide, the hospital consisted of two crosses, eight courts formed by the arms of the crosses, and a large central court with a chapel in the rear. Although it had been designed to hold 300–350 patients, often more than 2,000 were cared for at one time, using all the space available. The auxiliary wards and the service departments were in the inscribing buildings. The staff also lived in these buildings. The cross-ward altars were used for livestock until they were slaughtered. There were vaults for the dead with "parallel iron bars, like a grating, where the bodies [were] laid." However, the smell of dead bodies that wafted upward was a great problem. Sponsored by the Sforzas, the nobility of Milan, the hospital was begun in 1457 by Filarete and not finished until 300 years later. Filarete resigned from the project in 1465, but his original plan, including a most complex internal drainage system for the latrines in the exterior walls with entrances between each two beds, was followed by a series of subsequent architects. Thereafter, the cross ward assumed predominance as a desired form for hospitals. The Ospedale Maggiore was in active use until part of it was bombed during World War II. It now serves as a library for the University of Milan.

Pre-Nightingale England. The history of hospitals in England differed from that on the Continent. Though it is estimated that more than 750 multipurpose hospitals, apart from actual monasteries and friaries, were established in that country from the 12th to the 15th century, most were, as in Europe, under various church auspices. When Henry VIII dissolved and expropriated the monasteries during the Reformation in the mid-1500s, the hospital system in England was destroyed. From 1536 to 1544 the crippled, maimed, and sick crawled through the streets. The situation was so bad in London that the people had to petition the king to reopen some hospitals. In the latter part of his reign St. Bartholomew's—founded in 1123—was reopened. However, since Henry considered Thomas Becket a traitor, the hospital established in *his* honor—St. Thomas's (founded around 1173)—

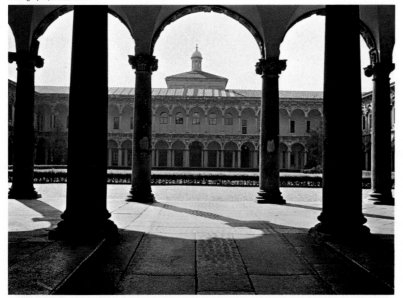

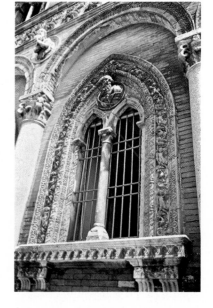

was not reopened until Henry's son, Edward VI, on his deathbed in 1553, gave the royal assent. At that time London had three other hospitals supported by the crown, called "royal" hospitals: Christ's Hospital, a combination foundling hospital and school for orphans; St. Mary's of Bethlehem (Bedlam), a mental hospital; and Bridewell, a prison hospital.

St. Thomas's, as rebuilt in 1693–1709, was a rectangular building that consisted of three large adjoining quadrangles. The first court (three stories high) was for women. The ground floor wards were dark and narrow. Every other window was bricked up to avoid a tax on windows, levied in 1695. The second court included the service areas, the treasurer's house, the parish church, the chapel, the chaplain's quarters, the counting house, and the great hall. The third court comprised the wards for men. In 1819 there were half as many beds for women as men (114 to 226) because "the habits and ways of the latter expose them to a greater number of casualties and diseases than women." Off the men's wards there were "foul wards" for syphilitics, who were regarded as "victims of a disease so degrading to humanity" that they were not admitted to most other hospitals.

While some condemned the quadrangle plan of St. Thomas's as fatal for the free circulation of pure air, others, including Francis Bacon, praised it as an outstanding institution. Benjamin Golding, a physician, wrote in his *Historical Account of the Origin and Progress of St. Thomas's Hospital*:

The whole design of the building gives it a bold and commanding appearance. It is constructed upon a magnificent scale. . . . The white stone pilasters in every square afford a pleasing contrast to the red brick body of the building, and relieve, with a peculiar lightness. . . . Instead of that heavy sombre appearance, which is so frequently complained of as making an hospital resemble a prison or place of punishment, and striking a repulsive awe in the sufferers who apply for relief, it bears a striking similitude to an agreeable private mansion.

The real renaissance of hospitals in England did not occur until early in the 18th century with the rise of "voluntary" hospitals—hospitals no longer

The Ospedale Maggiore in Milan was the best known of the Renaissance hospitals. Begun in 1457 by the architect Filarete, the construction was completed in the 18th century. The large central court and chapel (left) and the ornate terra-cotta window (right) still stand; the building now serves as a library for the University of Milan.

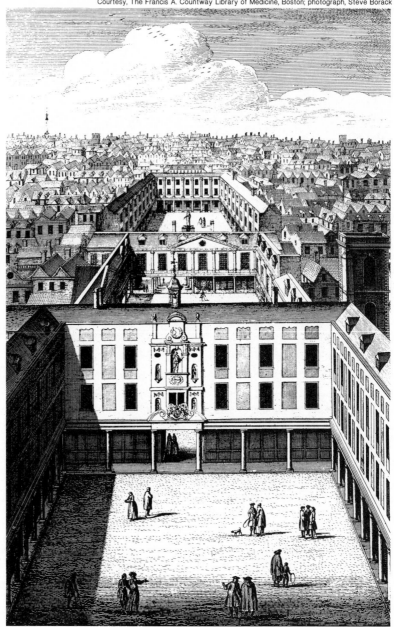

under church or royal auspices but supported by voluntary action. In 1719 laymen and physicians in London organized the Charitable Society in West-minster to build a hospital and provide care for the sick poor. Within 25 years four more such voluntary general hospitals had been established in London under similar auspices. This permitted England to follow the lead of the University of Leiden in The Netherlands and undertake bedside teaching of medical students on the wards. During the 18th century, owing to the growth of the cities, many patients were crowded into the urban hospitals, which permitted physicians, particularly the French anatomists, to relate the ob-served illnesses of a great many patients to autopsy findings and begin to build a science of medicine.

Hospitalism. The crowding of the sick poor into institutions took its toll. Sanitary conditions in many hospitals were abominable, and social reformers such as John Howard, who turned his attention from prison reform to hospital reform, began to lay the groundwork for the sanitary revolution in the 19th century. Criticism of hospital architecture and of unsanitary hospital environments was leveled by a physician disciple of Howard, John Aikin:

The architect considers it his business to manage his room and materials in such a manner as to accommodate the greatest number of people in the least possible space. The physician on the contrary would leave as much vacant space, occupied by fresh air alone circulating freely, as was in any degree compatible with use and convenience. It is to the prevalence of [the architect] above [the physician] that all our complaints are owing. . . . It does not belong to my profession to lay down an architectural plan for one of these buildings . . . but by pointing out what to avoid, we in effect give rules what to aim at.

The disease that swept through the crowded institutions—more often than not there were two patients to a bed—was called "hospitalism." Probably an erysipeloid streptococcal or a staphylococcal infection or both, the contagious illness affected patients by the hundreds and was often fatal. Indeed, the situation was so unhealthful that a recommendation was made toward the end of the century to relocate the Hôtel-Dieu of Paris (the largest hospital in France at the time). Louis XVI appointed an eminent committee from the Royal Academy of Sciences to examine the hospitalism problem. So-called healthy hospitals were inspected, among them the Naval Hospital at Plymouth, which was similar in structure to the design concept the committee ultimately chose for a new Hôtel-Dieu: the patient accommodations consisted of 14 separate three-story buildings connected by a one-story corridor with a flat roof, which could be used for airing patients. The committee devised their own plan for the new Hôtel-Dieu from many sources and called the separate buildings "pavilions," a term that may be derived from the arrangement of Louis XIV's retreat at Marly. Pavilion describes an open ward of limited extent, ventilated on both sides by windows and on both ends by doors; it is connected to a corridor that serves similar pavilions but is self-contained with its own service areas. The French Revolution delayed the application of the plans, but a new hospital, the Lariboisière, based on the committee's report, was built in 1846, just in time to be regarded as a model by the English during the next wave of hospital sanitary reform.

Florence Nightingale's contribution to hospital design

It was impossible to ignore Florence Nightingale's chronicle of sanitary conditions in hospitals during the Crimean War:

It may seem a strange principle to enunciate as the very first requirement in a hospital that it should do the sick no harm. It is quite necessary, nevertheless, to lay down such a principle, because the actual mortality in hospitals, especially in those of large crowded cities, is very much higher than any calculation founded on the mortality of the same class of diseases among patients treated out of hospital would lead us to expect.

General anesthesia was used successfully in the 19th century, but sanitary conditions of the hospitals were so primitive that many patients

The courtyards of St. Thomas's Hospital, London, in the early 18th century. Every other window was bricked closed to avoid a window tax. St. Thomas's was first established near London Bridge in honor of Thomas Becket in 1173 and rebuilt in Long Southwark 1693–1709. Constructed under the supervision of Florence Nightingale, it was reopened in 1871 across from the Houses of Parliament. St. Thomas's was largely destroyed during World War II; parts are being rebuilt.

63

At no time in its long history did the Hôtel-Dieu have adequate space. More than one patient to a bed was not unusual. Thus, contagion, or "hospitalism," a disease that swept through this and other crowded institutions, was always a great concern. Miniature from the 15th century in the Book of the very active life of the nuns of the Hôtel-Dieu of Paris.

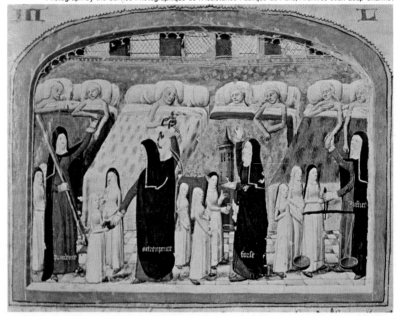

died of postoperative infections instead of shock or hemorrhage. The cleansing of the hospitals in the mid-1800s was really just one extension of a far broader phenomenon known as the Sanitary Revolution. The sanitary reformers of the 19th century differed from those of the previous century in four important respects: they knew enough about statistics to identify the problems; they had adopted a theory to explain why the problems existed; the theory proposed a solution; and when the solution was applied, it worked. The theory held that disease was caused by "miasmas" arising from rotting material in the ground. The fact that it was a misguided conception was beside the point. In fact, the cleansing efforts employed to combat the so-called miasmas were also somewhat effective against bacteria. "We are very clean," said James Lind, the naval surgeon and pioneer in naval sanitation, who also discovered preventive measures for scurvy. In fact, the miasma theory was so strongly believed, and its application achieved such dramatic results, that it delayed the acceptance of Lord Lister's experiments in antisepsis, first published in 1867, which were an extension of Louis Pasteur's research on germs.

In her *Notes on Hospitals* Nightingale was not as retiring as Aikin was in the previous century about "laying out a plan" for a hospital. In fact, her instructions to architects were most specific about the pavilion's length (128 feet), width (30 feet), ceiling height (16–17 feet), number of square feet per bed (96), cubic feet of air (1,600 per bed), number of stories (2), type of floor (polished oak), and paint color (pure white or the palest possible pink). Under her supervision were built the Herbert Hospital in Woolwich and the relocated St. Thomas's across the Thames from the Houses of Parliament. In both, the neo-Gothic facades almost, but not quite, disguised the fact that the pavilion ward was an adapted barrack. The pavilion design soon became the standard plan for hospitals throughout Europe and even in Europe's colonies in America.

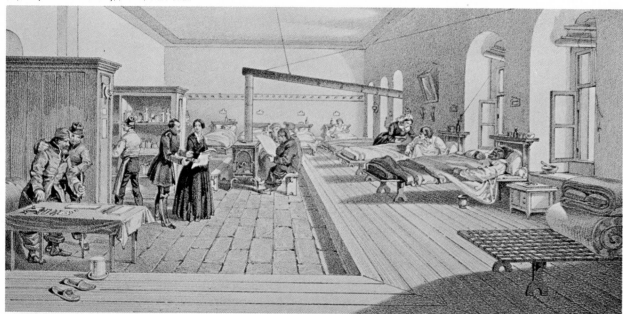

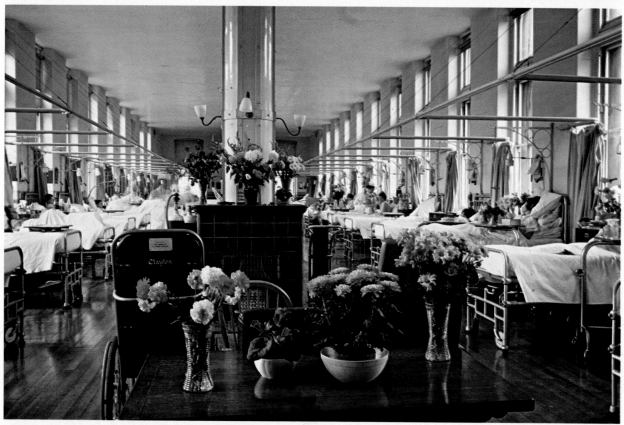

Florence Nightingale was active in hospital sanitary reform during and after the Crimean War. Her instructions for the design and upkeep of patient wards were most explicit. She is pictured in a ward in the military hospital at Scutari (now Uskudar), Turkey (top), where she was responsible for greatly improving conditions. The 19th-century lithograph is by E. Walker from a drawing by W. Simpson. (Bottom) A ward at St. Thomas's in London as it appears today with its polished oak floors, soft white walls, radiators down the center, and, everywhere, brightly colored flowers—precisely as Nightingale prescribed.

Hospital architecture in America

The three earliest hospitals in American colonies were Pennsylvania Hospital in Philadelphia, New York Hospital in New York City, and Massachusetts General Hospital in Boston. They followed the charitable organization type of sponsorship recently introduced in England. Benjamin Franklin was president of the board of Pennsylvania Hospital, which was constructed in three stages: the east wing opened in 1755, the west wing in 1796, and the center in 1804. It is a fine example of colonial architecture (it can be termed that since the plans were drawn before the Revolution).

Massachusetts General Hospital admitted its first patients in 1821. Before this could happen the hospital had to be justified as an institution. Two physicians who proposed the original plans for the hospital pointed out that some lying-in women and most mental patients had no other recourse. Almshouses took in the community's least desirable members. As a result, respectable but poor members of society often chose to die rather than enter an almshouse. Massachusetts General began then as a place that cared for the sick poor: working men who lived in garrets were taken in when they were sick because their homes were cold and they were without proper food or attendance; ill women abandoned by intemperate husbands stayed there; and young apprentices who had accidents or illnesses healed or recovered in the new hospital.

As urban hospitals became crowded, the problem of hospitalism appeared in the U.S. When Massachusetts General had to transfer all of its patients to private homes in 1827 because of the presence of an erysipelatous infection, physicians wrote that "behind the ambitious front, foul air breeds disease." One claimed, "There is but one remedy possible for a pyemia [pus-forming bacteria] ridden hospital, the pick axe."

The Nightingale Crimean War experience was first applied in the U.S. during the Civil War. An attempt was made to duplicate the activities of the British Sanitary Commission through the organization of a voluntary association of physicians, clergy, and interested women led by Frederick Law Olmsted, the landscape architect responsible for Central Park in New York City.

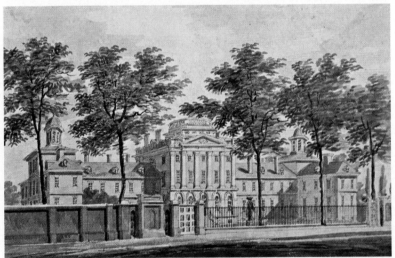

The Pennsylvania Hospital in Philadelphia, built 1755–1804, was one of the three earliest hospitals in the American colonies; watercolor by Pavel Petrovich Svinin.

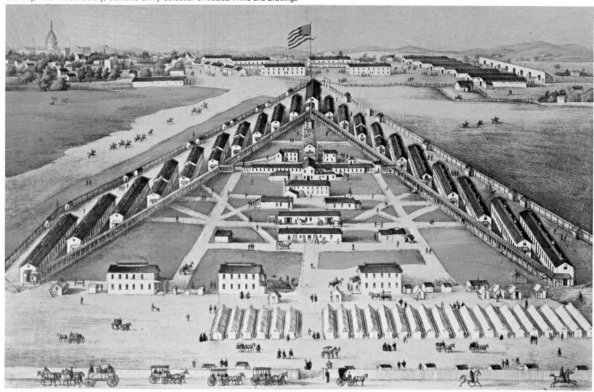

After the debacle of the First Battle of Bull Run, the commission was set up and, as an autonomous body working with the Army, recommended "barracks hospitals" and other sanitary reforms throughout the war. Even when the Army took over existing hospitals, as in New Haven, Connecticut, the main building served as the administrative center, and the Army built barracks hospitals with proper ventilation for the sick and wounded soldiers. At the end of the war the commission stated, "Our sick and wounded were better cared for in military hospitals than ever before and the rate of mortality in them was far lower than had been observed in the experience of any army since the world began."

This experience greatly affected the design and construction of the Johns Hopkins Hospital, which has been called the Ospedale Maggiore of the U.S. Johns Hopkins was the ultimate in pavilion hospitals. It was laid out to prevent the spread of "contaminated air," closely following the dictates of the miasma theory. A series of elevated, two-story pavilions were separated by open walkways. Elevators were not included in hopes of preventing foul air from passing between levels. Patients had to be carried up the stairs to the wards. All service buildings were separate from the wards, connected by the same passageway.

Later the conquest of infectious diseases led to the construction of multi-story buildings at Johns Hopkins. At the close of the 19th century the need for the pavilion system was subordinated to land cost (Mr. Hopkins had purchased 13 acres on Loudenschlager's hill for his hospital) and efficiency of operation. The elevator was then considered safe for patients, and the

Lincoln Hospital, Washington, D.C., 1864, an American Civil War "barracks hospital." Its pavilions, in the shape of a triangle, emphasized proper ventilation. Quarters for medical officers were in the two-story houses along the base. The tents in the right foreground were used for infectious cases. The buildings in the center housed the kitchens, dining rooms, and nurses' dormitories.

67

The Johns Hopkins Hospital, Baltimore, Maryland, begun in 1877, represents the ultimate in early pavilion design; it was laid out to prevent the spread of "contaminated air."

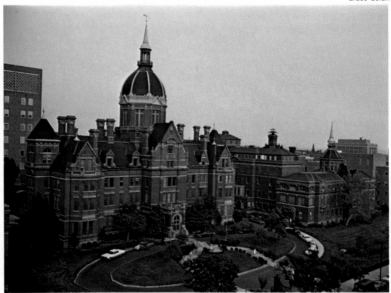

"skyscraper" hospital was developed. More importantly, new developments in medicine required operating rooms, radiology departments, and clinical laboratories. Most of the advances were in the field of surgery and in the prevention of communicable diseases.

During the Great Depression hospital architecture, like the economy, was in the doldrums. One notable exception appeared in the 1930s: Paul Nelson, an American expatriate architect living in Paris, created two studies that examined the best features of modern architecture with an attempt to articulate some of the newest medical services, such as the oval operating room and special emergency entrances. These were later included in his American Memorial Hospital at St.-Lô, France, built following World War II.

Modern influences

The modern era of hospital function and design coincides with two remarkable medical advances: the discovery of antibiotics and the development of psychotropic drugs. The first changed forever the kinds of treatments given as well as the types of patients seen in the general hospital, while the second had an even more dramatic effect on mental hospitals. As important as these innovations were, they were but the first indications of a scientific and technological revolution every bit as important as the sanitary revolution that preceded it.

Antibiotics shifted the place of treatment for certain diseases, such as tuberculosis, streptococcal throat infections, and bacterial pneumonias, from the hospital to the home. They also prevented complications of these diseases from developing, such as rheumatic fever, bone infections, and lung abcesses.

The psychotropic drugs added a new group of patients to the general hospital, the mentally ill, many of whom could now be treated effectively and safely without the trauma of admission to a state mental hospital. Psychiatric patients had previously been housed in long-stay institutions, formerly called

68

asylums. An important social change occurred when the preferential site of treatment of the mentally ill shifted: it was now thought they should be as close as possible to the community to which they would return.

While hospitals were attempting to adapt to these new demands, there arose the practical necessity of rebuilding the hospital system, which in the U.S. had been neglected during the Depression and World War II. The Hill-Burton Act, which matched federal moneys with those raised in communities for hospital construction, stimulated (many believe, overly so) the construction of hospitals. In spite of this criticism, the Hill-Burton Act did make a positive contribution to hospital architecture in that it required the states to develop and maintain statewide hospital plans, which introduced institutional health planning. The architects on Hill-Burton's federal staff also began issuing a series of design and equipment manuals for the various elements of the hospital, including setting minimum standards for safety.

As valuable as these guidelines were in preventing costly errors in the design process, there were two problems with this approach: it could not keep up with the new technology, and little or no attention was paid to assembling these elements into a smoothly functioning and aesthetically pleasing structure. Consequently, innovative designs were rare. Most hospitals of this period could be categorized as being in the style of late PWA (Public Works Administration) functional.

Current concepts of hospital design

In the meantime, hospital based technology has increased at a dizzying pace. Cobalt "bombs" have been replaced by linear accelerators; the intensive care unit has multiplied and evolved into coronary care units, neonatal intensive care units, shock units, and specialized burn centers. Laminar flow rooms that assure relatively germ-free air and hyperbaric chambers for treating tetanus, among other conditions, have become necessary adjuncts to certain hospitals. Computerized axial tomography units have begun to scan the entire body. Organ transplants require redesigned operating rooms. Coronary bypass surgery and total hip replacements have become daily procedures in large medical centers. Life-support systems can maintain a patient long after some of his vital centers have ceased to function. As many people now come to the hospital for ambulatory care in the emergency rooms and outpatient departments as are admitted as inpatients. Day surgery is being performed without formal admission to the hospital altogether.

All of this has changed the design requirements for the hospital in dramatic ways. Most of the growth and change is occurring in the diagnostic and therapeutic support departments such as the operating rooms, special care units, radiology, and laboratories; today the relatively unchanging section is the nursing unit on which most of the previous concern was focused. Patients stay in the hospital for shorter periods of time, so a restful view is less important. Traffic in and out of the hospital has become a complex problem because both bed patients and ambulatory patients are being routed to the same support facilities. Above all, hospital costs have risen so fast that deconstruction programs are being recommended with Luddite frenzy, which may be a reflection of society's ever increasing concern with the too

Prentice Women's Hospital and Maternity Center and the Institute of Psychiatry at Northwestern Memorial Hospital, Chicago, designed by Bertrand Goldberg and dedicated in 1976. The four-story rectangular base is topped by a seven-story cloverleaf bedtower.

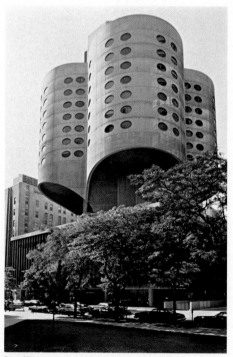

Peter Kiar

rapid advance and consequent depersonalization of the various medical sciences.

It is difficult to predict the future of hospital architecture particularly in light of this lack of balance between society's willingness to support advances and medical science's natural desire to extend itself as far as possible. So much disease has been eradicated; yet so much more remains to be understood about cancer, the process of aging, and debilitating chronic diseases. Hospitals that are part of major university medical centers are the places at which many of these answers will be found.

But even without a clearer definition of the future role of a hospital system, three important architectural implications *can* be projected: many hospitals will become larger, fewer new hospitals will be constructed, and other types of caring institutions and programs will be developed as hospital adjuncts.

These projections are based on a hospital system that differentiates among various levels of care. Clearly not every hospital should have a linear accelerator, heart pumps for cardiac surgery, or a laminar flow room. In fact, not many patients require these facilities, and they are extremely expensive to install and maintain. They should be available in tertiary care institutions, specializing in complicated cases. Primary and secondary hospitals can treat the large majority of patients and transfer those who require specialized technology to those hospitals equipped to care for those kinds of diseases.

An application of hospital design that synthesizes many aspects of traditional architecture and newer building technology has emerged in the past decade and has been employed extensively in the U.S. by architect Bertrand Goldberg, though derived in part from Paul Nelson, James Moore, and others. Among Goldberg's endeavors in the health field are the Affiliated Hospitals Center at Harvard University; the Health Sciences Center at the State University of New York, Stony Brook; Prentice Women's Hospital and the Institute of Psychiatry at Northwestern Memorial Hospital, Chicago; and St. Joseph Hospital, Tacoma, Washington. Goldberg's designs take advantage of technology that has enabled the building of nonrectilinear shapes. In most hospitals traditional design has dictated that patient rooms must be

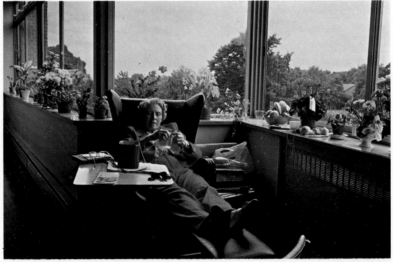

A patient at St. Christopher's Hospice in Sydenham, south London, where institutional care provides comfort and cheerful surroundings for the dying.

Grace Goldin

arranged basically in straight lines. But Goldberg has carefully balanced countervailing forces with exterior structures and has managed to eliminate the need for load-bearing columns. His exteriors are self-supporting; his interiors are larger and more adaptable because no columns take up space.

The building that houses Prentice Women's Hospital and Maternity Center in Chicago is representative of this style. A four-story rectangular base is topped by a seven-story cloverleaf bedtower. The curvilinear hospital is composed of sets of patient rooms arranged in clusters, or pods. The design provides privacy while allowing for optimal patient care. On maternity floors at Prentice, nurseries are centered among clusters of private and semiprivate rooms so that infants are close to mothers at all times. Nursing stations are located at a minimal distance from every patient so that professional staff can respond quickly and efficiently to patient needs, and the patient never fears she is all alone at the end of a corridor.

Since the number of new hospitals will be limited, a complex architectural problem is raised, namely the modernization of existing hospitals. The designer in such projects must become intimately familiar with the operation of the hospital because he must identify what is to be renovated or replaced, consider the precise effect the modernization will have on all existing elements of the hospital, and at the same time determine the pattern for future expansion. Another complication in renovation is the fact that hospitals cannot shut down during such programs, and the architect must carefully and safely stage his modernization. A good example of such a plan was that carried out by architect Bruce Arneill at Lakes Region General Hospital in Laconia, New Hampshire. Previously combined facilities were separated; these included support, ambulatory, ancillary, and bed patient services. This was achieved by constructing a new connecting patient tower on the edge of a cliff, permitting support services to penetrate the hospital three stories below the existing inpatient beds and two levels below the emergency and ambulatory patient facilities.

The trend toward shorter patient stays in the general hospital, due in part to soaring costs, means that nonacute institutions and programs providing care in the home must be planned as hospital-affiliated institutions. Unfortunately, nursing homes in the U.S., which house 5% of the older population, in many cases provide little more than basic custodial care; half of all nursing homes do not even meet basic sanitation and fire standards.

A notable exception is the hospice movement, adapted from St. Christopher's Hospice in Sydenham, south London, where both home care and institutional care are dedicated to the needs of the dying patient and his or her family. The St. Christopher's environment is cheerful and optimistic, generated, among other things, by physical characteristics—a tasteful architectural style, gardens, a nondenominational chapel, and so forth. General hospitals are inappropriate both in scale and milieu for death with dignity. There are now several hospices in the United States as well as special units within hospitals for the care of the terminally ill. It will be most interesting to see if architect Lo-Yi Chan's small, exquisite hospice for the terminally ill now under construction in Branford, Connecticut, can bring the human values back to a hospital system.

FOR ADDITIONAL READING:

Filarete [Antonio Averlino]. *Treatise on Architecture.* Translated by John R. Spencer. New Haven: Yale University Press, 1965.

Foucault, Michel. *The Birth of the Clinic.* Translated by A. M. Sheridan Smith. New York: Pantheon Books, 1973.

Hospital Plans: Five Essays. New York: William Wood, 1875.

Leistikow, Dankwart. *Ten Centuries of European Hospital Architecture.* Ingelheim am Rhein: C. H. Boehringer Sohn, 1967.

Nightingale, Florence. *Notes on Hospitals.* 3rd ed., rev. London: Longman, Green, Longman, Roberts, and Green, 1863.

Rosen, George. *A History of Public Health.* New York: MD Publications, 1958.

Thompson, John D., and Goldin, Grace. *The Hospital: A Social and Architectural History.* New Haven: Yale University Press, 1975.

The Mayo Clinic
by Peter R. Stoler

Photographs by Michael Marienthal

Rising out of the Minnesota prairie 80 miles south of Minneapolis, Rochester is an unquestionably attractive city, a checkerboard of neatly laid out streets just off the interstate highway, a cluster of modern concrete-and-glass buildings and tasteful shops. To the west of the city, cornfields stretch off for seemingly endless miles; to the east lies a range of low, wooded hills that marks the edge of the Mississippi River Valley. Rochester has museums, a symphony orchestra, good restaurants, and a modern, all-weather airport into which major airlines make 50 scheduled flights every day.

Taken together, Rochester's amenities might attract a few thousand tourists each year. Why, then, do more than a quarter of a million travel to the city each year, coming from all 50 U.S. states and a few coming, quite literally, from the ends of the earth? "For my health," explains a tanned, rawboned man who had driven 125 miles to Rochester from his farm outside Waterloo, Iowa. "For the same reason," says a well-coiffed, fur-coated matron who has flown to the city from New York City.

A unique medical institution

Their answers are not flippant but factual. Health—or the absence of it—is exactly what attracts people to Rochester. The city does not possess mineral springs like Badgastein or Marienbad. It does not have the dry, salubrious air of New Mexico or Arizona. What it does have is the Mayo Clinic, a world-renowned medical mecca that has become—with some justification—not merely the symbol of what doctors can do when they put the needs of the patient before all other considerations but the standard against which other polyclinics, which have taken the Mayo as their model, are judged. The Mayo Clinic has been decribed as a "secular Lourdes"—not unlike the town in southwestern France that in 1858 became a pilgrimage center for the sick and disabled after a 14-year-old girl had visions in the nearby grotto, which were later declared authentic by the pope. The underground spring in the grotto is said to have miraculous qualities and attracts hundreds of thousands to Lourdes every year.

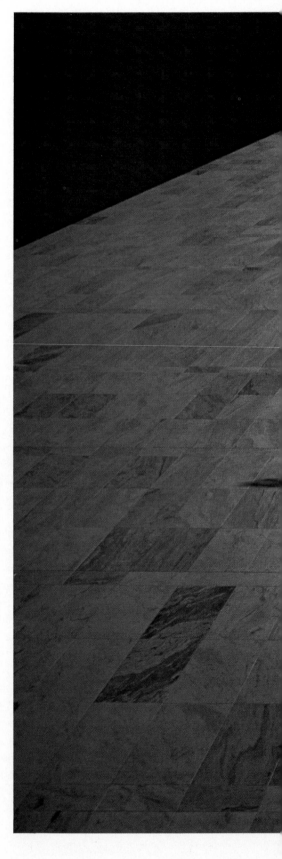

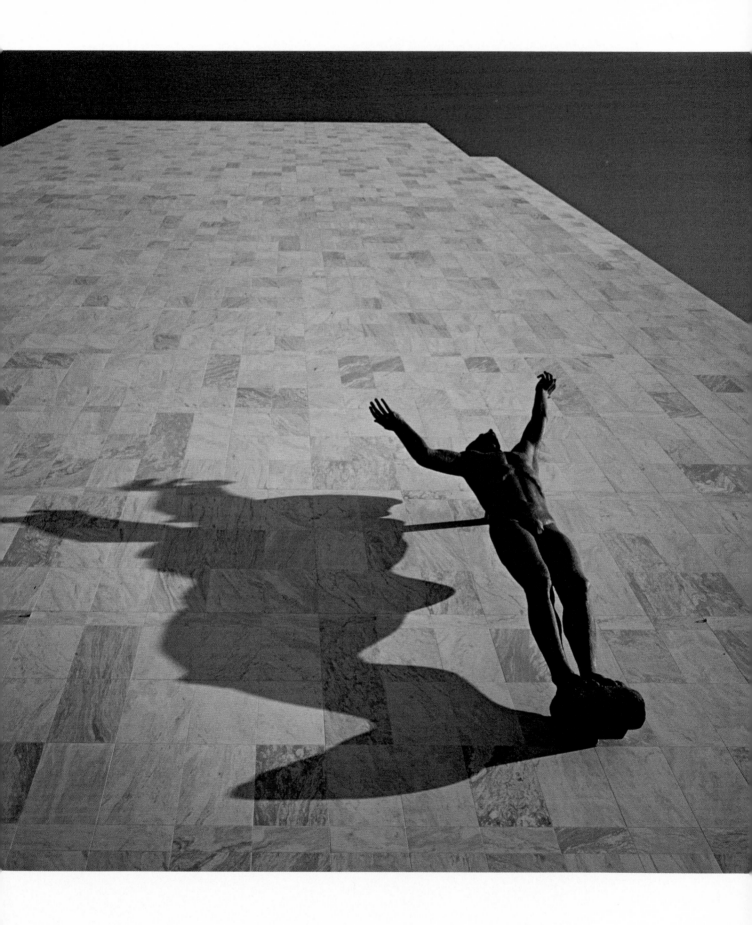

Others avoid religious allusions when describing Mayo. But they do not refrain from hyperbole. "There is no place like it," says a New York City physician who has himself been a patient in Rochester, Minnesota. He explains, "Some institutions educate. Some treat specialized diseases. Some treat patients. The Mayo Clinic treats people. It is, quite simply, the world's greatest medical practice."

The term *clinic* suggests a small, often inadequately equipped facility in which a handful of people attempt to provide basic medical care. The sobriquet "clinic in a cornfield" is often used to describe the Mayo. But far from a shoestring or storefront operation, the Mayo Clinic is a $111 million complex of a dozen buildings, most of them strikingly modern and crammed with the most technically sophisticated equipment. Together with the two private, independent hospitals affiliated with it, the Mayo Clinic is part of a medical center that includes 1,800 examining rooms, 1,700 beds, and 62 operating rooms. Among the clinic and the hospitals Rochester has nearly 11,000 people involved in medical care. Of these, the Mayo Clinic alone accounts for 6,000, including over 600 physicians and medical scientists and some 4,000 administrative and paramedical personnel.

The location has its advantages. Big city hospitals must try to operate and maintain everything from diagnostic to surgical services, from well-baby clinics to emergency rooms. As a result, they often find themselves overwhelmed as patients begin using their emergency and outpatient departments instead of family doctors, or bogged down trying to train physicians in too wide a variety of specialties. The Mayo Clinic maintains neither an emergency room nor surgical services. Nor does it find itself functioning as the American equivalent of a Chinese-style "barefoot doctor" or community hospital. Freed of these functions by local hospitals and its own organization, it is better able to concentrate on diagnostic and rehabilitative medicine and to keep the quality of such services at a level that many urban medical centers—even those connected with major teaching institutions—can only envy and dream of achieving.

However, Mayo has not always enjoyed this uniqueness. In fact, were it not for a fortuitous set of circumstances involving such disparate elements as a pioneering medical family and a tornado, the shrine to healing known as the Mayo Clinic might never have come into being at all.

The contributions of the Mayo family

The Mayo Clinic, says the official history, owes its existence to the remarkable doctors Mayo, three men whose place in medical history is as secure as the places held by such giants as Galen, Jenner, and Osler. The first of these unusual men was William Worrall Mayo, who was born near Manchester, England, in 1819 and came to the United States 25 years later. Like many immigrants to the new land Mayo worked his way westward, ending up, 15 years after his arrival, in Le Sueur, Minnesota, where he practiced as the kind of country doctor Americans wish still existed. He did not remain there long. In 1863, following his appointment as an examining surgeon for the Union Army Enrollment Board, Mayo moved to Rochester. When the Civil War ended, he stayed there.

Peter R. Stoler *is an Associate Editor for* Time *magazine, New York City, who specializes in science writing.*

Michael Marienthal *is a Chicago-based photographer. His work has appeared in numerous magazines, books, and corporate publications.*

(Overleaf) The north facade of the Mayo Building, with Ivan Mestrovic's bronze sculpture symbolizing man and freedom.

74

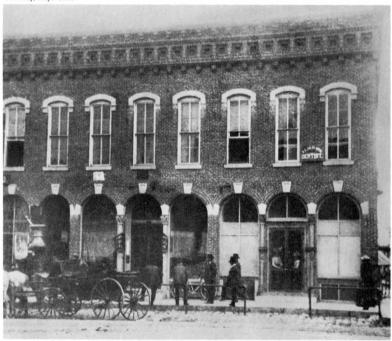

Mayo might have remained a simple country doctor, but circumstances dictated otherwise. In 1883 a tornado swept through the area, killing 20 people and injuring scores of others. Mayo responded to the emergency by asking the Sisters of Saint Francis to provide nursing care for the injured. The sisters did, and after a short while Mother Mary Alfred Moes proposed that her order build a hospital in Rochester with Mayo in charge of planning. Mayo agreed. The result of their collaboration was Saint Marys Hospital, a 27-bed facility that opened its doors in 1889.

The creation of the hospital, however, was only one of the steps that led to the creation of the Mayo Clinic. The other—and more important—factor in the establishment of this unique house of healing was the combination of talent and compassion that characterized the Mayo brothers.

Mayo's two sons, William James and Charles Horace, were born in 1861 and 1865, respectively, and learned medicine, quite literally, at their father's knee. During their boyhood years the brothers assisted their busy father in his medical practice, doing everything from assisting at childbirths to scrubbing in while father Mayo performed surgery. "My brother and I came along in medicine like farm boys do on farms," William recalled many years later. "We learned as we went along. And as we got older, we could do more and more things."

Given such a background, it is hardly surprising that the brothers decided to formalize their medical training. William went to medical school at the University of Michigan and graduated in 1883. Charles attended Chicago Medical College, later part of Northwestern University Medical School, and graduated in 1888. What was surprising was that the brothers both decided to return to Rochester, joining their father in the medical practice then housed above a drugstore in the center of town.

The Mayo brothers joined their father's medical practice on their graduation from medical school in the 1880s. In the first years their office was located over a drugstore in downtown Rochester.

75

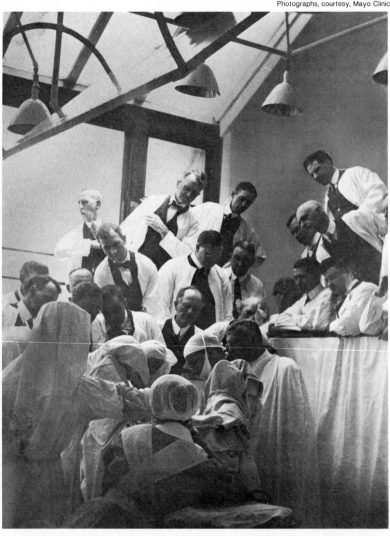

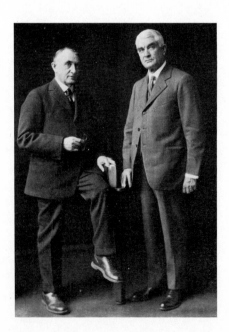

The practice thrived. One reason for its success was the skill of the three Mayo doctors, all of whom were voracious readers of the medical literature and ardent innovators of new techniques for treating their patients. But the major reason for the practice's acceptance and growth was the attitude of this talented trio toward medicine: from the very beginning the three made it clear by their actions rather than their words that what motivated them was not money, not prestige, not power, but the welfare of their patients. Dr. Will and Dr. Charlie, as the brothers were called, exuded an aura of competence that made their patients feel completely secure. But beyond their competence, the pair was surrounded as well by an air of concern that made their patients feel—and rightly so—that the doctors were genuinely interested in them and their problems. Indeed, as one of the Mayos' admirers has commented: "Dr. Charlie could walk into some little old lady's room, say, 'Hi, I'm Charlie Mayo,' and the next day she would be cured."

The tale is a tall one; the Mayos were not faith healers and never attempted to treat disease by mere laying on of hands. Both, in fact, were men of science. William specialized in abdominal surgery; Charles concentrated on

76

surgery of the head and neck area. Both were also keen observers who learned from every experience, seemed to forget nothing, and shared their knowledge freely with their colleagues in the medical profession. Some prolific modern researchers manage, in part by attaching their names to work done by their subordinates, to publish 500 papers in the course of a career. The Mayo brothers contributed more than 2,000 papers, reports, and articles to the medical literature.

Patients began seeking out the Mayos in increasing numbers. Soon the load became too much for the three doctors to handle themselves. In 1892 the Mayos invited A. W. Stinchfield, an experienced physician, to join the practice; two years later Christopher Graham joined them. The result: what may well be the first true group practice in the United States or, for that matter, in the world.

By word of mouth, by citations in the medical literature, the reputation of the growing Rochester practice spread quickly beyond the borders of Minnesota. The Mayos' group approach to medicine initially drew the disapproval of the American Medical Association, which believed that doctors should be their own entrepreneurs and charge individual fees for their services, and not be salaried members of a medical group. Eventually, however, each brother was elected president of the association. The group idea won the immediate approval of patients, who began flocking to Rochester by horse-and-buggy to see the doctors about their problems. By the 1890s physicians had begun referring their patients to Rochester or traveling there themselves to observe the Mayos and learn from them. By the end of the century people were referring to the unique practice as the "Mayo Clinic." By the early 1900s the name had come into general use.

The appellation proved appropriate. From 1883 until 1914 the rapidly expanding practice was housed in local buildings. But then the brothers formed a clinic in fact as well as in name, moving their practice into a five-story red brick structure designed especially for their group approach to medical care. Over the years, as the practice continued to expand, the single building evolved into the complex of eight buildings that now dominates Rochester's downtown.

The facilities, however, were not the only things that evolved. The Mayos had long regarded themselves as the "custodians of the sick man's dollar," considering themselves morally bound to turn all but their own modest salaries back into the development of their practice. In 1915 they decided to formalize this belief by establishing a school for graduate medical education. With a gift of $1.5 million from their personal resources, the Mayo brothers set up the Mayo Foundation for Medical Education and Research affiliated with the University of Minnesota. Four years later the brothers established the Mayo Properties Association (now known as the Mayo Foundation). They transferred to this nonprofit charitable corporation the ownership of all the properties and facilities of the Mayo Clinic. They also assigned to the foundation the right to receive all future earnings of the Mayo Clinic and gave it the obligation of spending any "profits," or funds left over after the clinic's running expenses had been met, on education and research. "The people's money, of which we have been the moral custodians, is being

(Opposite left) Charles (left) and William Mayo. (Opposite right) A rapt audience of physicians observe surgery in the clinic's operating theater, circa 1900. By the late 1890s visiting physicians had begun to gather to observe the Mayos' surgical techniques. In 1915 a school for graduate medical education was established; today it is the world's largest graduate medical education program.

77

irrevocably returned to the people from whom it came,'' said William Mayo.

The Mayo brothers died within a few months of each other in 1939. But their innovative approach to medical care has not only survived but thrived, and their attitudes still inform and guide the clinic that bears their name today. The clinic has grown, of course, and changed from a small, simple partnership to a more complex arrangement. The basic unit of the present-day medical center is the Mayo Clinic, a so-called voluntary association of physicians whose revenues are derived mainly from patients' fees. Funds in excess of those needed to run the clinic, which has an annual budget for staff alone of more than $100 million, are, in keeping with the arrangement developed by the Mayo brothers, turned over to the Mayo Foundation for education and research.

Mayo today

The Mayos, of course, no longer control the clinic and have not since the brothers themselves died (although Dr. Charlie's son was on the staff until 1963). Instead, administration of the clinic is the responsibility of a board of governors consisting of nine doctors and two professional administrators. Much of the day-to-day decision making is handled by a plethora of committees appointed by the institution's board of governors.

The institution's finances are complex. A large chunk, in fact some 65%, of the Mayo's more than $27 million annual research budget comes, as does most medical research money today, from the federal government, the rest from private gifts and Mayo Clinic funds. But the lion's share of the clinic's costs is paid by the patients themselves—or by their governmental and private insurers.

In its early days the Mayo Clinic had a sliding fee scale for its services; the business office would ask each patient how much he could afford to pay and would charge accordingly. As a result, the clinic quickly got a reputation for overcharging the wealthy and subsidizing the poor, a reputation that was enhanced when the Mayo brothers would, on occasion, dig down into their own pockets to give a destitute patient the price of a train ticket back to his home.

Today things are different. The clinic has a fixed scale of fees under which all patients are charged the same amounts for the same services. But in keeping with the philosophy expounded by the institution's founders, patients are always treated, without regard to economic status.

Another thing that remains unchanged is the relationship of the Mayo Clinic and its doctors. Physicians at most American hospitals and medical centers are individual entrepreneurs who make their own financial arrangements with the patients they treat. The Mayo Clinic's doctors are not private practitioners but salaried professionals. These doctors do not seem to regard money as a major concern. Indeed the work ethic is alive and well in the community of Rochester, Minnesota.

So, apparently, are the Mayo brothers' standards of excellence. Doctors do not come to the Mayo Clinic looking for jobs; the clinic neither solicits nor entertains applications. Instead it ''invites'' physicians to join its staff, seeking out the best and most highly recommended people it can find to fill the

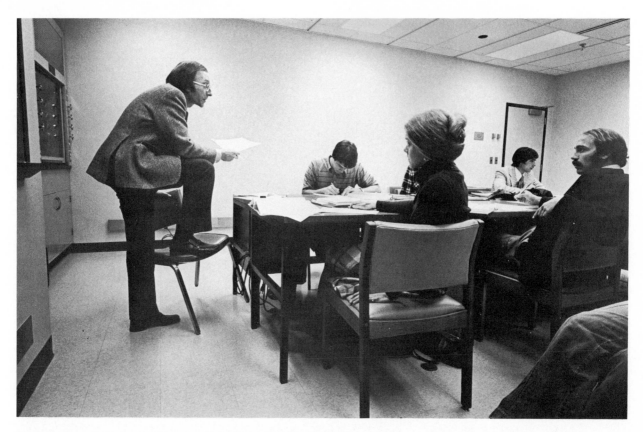

few openings that occur each year. Only 20 to 30 Mayo physicians resign or retire each year; dismissals are so rare that most doctors on the staff cannot remember one.

Many, indeed most, Mayo Clinic physicians are themselves products of the institution. The clinic usually has some 700 postgraduate residents undergoing training. The Mayo Clinic also has an undergraduate school of medicine. Established in 1972, the Mayo Medical School has an enrollment of 160 students and admits a class of 40 new students each year. Of this number, at least 35 are from Minnesota. The competition for acceptance is stiff: at least 2,000 apply for entrance every year. By the time students have completed their training, most are imbued with the Mayo Clinic spirit, and many eventually return.

Medical educators rate the Mayo Medical School's undergraduate programs as excellent, although they generally agree that the programs at such schools as Harvard, Yale, Cornell, and Stanford are better. Medical educators do, however, rate the Mayo's postgraduate medical education programs (*i.e.,* internships and residencies) as outstanding and consider them equal to the best offered by the endowed or major state-supported institutions.

The medical specialties at Mayo run the gamut. There are psychiatrists on the clinic staff, but psychiatric treatment is not one of the institution's specialties. Doctors in the Midwest who refer patients with organic illness to the Mayo are, according to our Mayo Clinic sources, just as likely to refer those with psychiatric problems to another Midwestern institution, the Menninger Clinic in Topeka, Kansas.

Today the clinic is part of a major medical center that also includes two hospitals and the Mayo Medical School, an undergraduate facility, which was established in 1972. Each year more than 2,000 students apply to fill the 40 openings in each class.

79

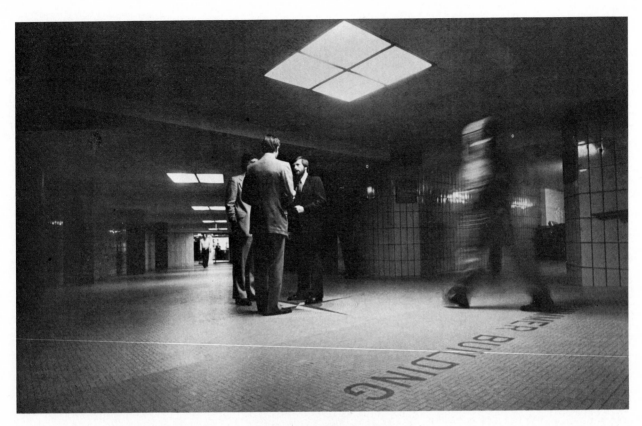

The patient who arrives in Rochester for treatment or diagnosis discovers an atmosphere of total involvement in the healing arts; the interaction of the best in medical technology and human skills makes Mayo the standard against which all other clinics are judged. An underground pedestrian walkway (above) joins all of the buildings in the Mayo complex, providing protected access to offices, hospital rooms, and technical services (opposite), as well as to hotel accommodations.

Emphasizing the patient

Rochester, which has grown up around the clinic (the only other major employer in the area is an IBM installation), has gone out of its way to make the patients who come there feel welcome. The city has ramps at every curb so that people in wheelchairs can move freely in the streets. In addition, some hotels have extra-wide doors to accommodate wheelchairs, not to mention dining rooms that serve special salt-free or other specially prepared meals, plus staff nurses who are available to help patient-guests get ready for examinations. "Where else can you call room service and order an enema?" asks an official at Rochester's Kahler Hotel, the city's major hostelry, located right across the street from the clinic.

All this attention is appreciated by the Mayo Clinic's patients, who have numbered over three million since the beginning of the century. Many come because, among other reasons, they appreciate the clinic's policy of protecting its patients' privacy. Patients come to Mayo at a rate of nearly 1,000 a day (in 1977, the last year for which complete figures are available, the clinic saw 245,000 patients). Of these, about half have been referred to the clinic by physicians when the latter have been unable to help them because their illnesses defy treatment, diagnosis, or rehabilitative therapy. A Midwestern doctor who is baffled by a patient's condition, or who has found himself unable to do anything about what he, at least, thinks this condition to be, is, according to Mayo officials, their chief referral source. The rest come on their own—and for a variety of reasons. "I haven't had a good, complete physical examination in my life," said one Minneapolis woman as

80

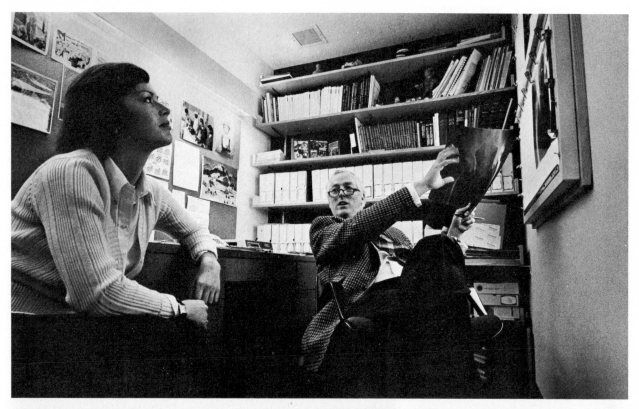

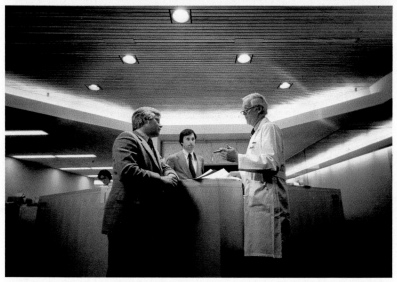

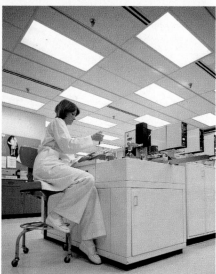

she sat in a waiting room. "If I can't get it here, then I can't get it anyplace." Many come to Mayo as a last resort: they've been going from one doctor to another for years, and nobody's found out what's wrong, let alone helped them. Indeed some come because they are desperate.

A visit to the institution begins in the street level waiting area of the 19-story Mayo Building, which opens its doors around the time many neighboring farmers are beginning their days. There the arriving patients are assigned numbers, and there they remain until their numbers are called.

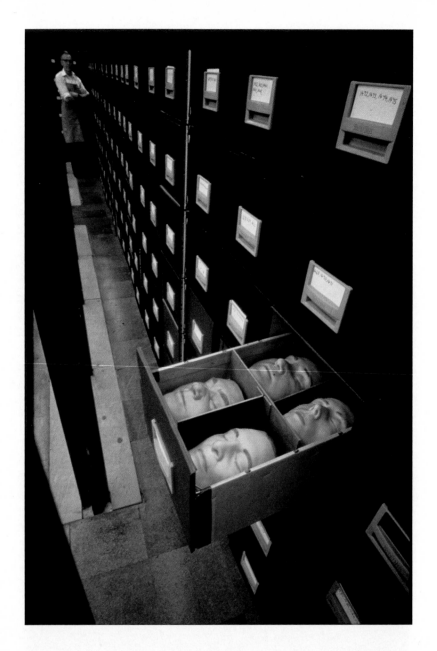

Martin Roessler, a medical sculptor, displays a cabinet filled with models of faces; other drawers contain models of limbs and organs, all with medical significance. The models were designed as educational tools to illustrate specific diseases or conditions.

The wait can be a long one, and many patients find the delays distressing. Patients who come to the clinic by prearrangement may wait several hours. Patients who come to the clinic without appointments may wait even longer. The clinic attempts to work patients with urgent medical problems into its schedule as quickly as possible and will, for example, push a woman who has shown up with a lump in her breast into the schedule ahead of, say, a patient referred by his doctor for a general physical examination.

The Mayo Clinic has yet to find a way to relieve the tedium of waiting. But once a patient's name is called, the institution does handle him expeditiously. The patient is first sent to an examining room where a doctor takes his personal medical history and gives him a general medical examination, a process that takes about an hour and a half and begins the assembly of the medical record that will follow a patient throughout his visits to the clinic and go into the institution's massive permanent storage systems when he dies.

The physician who conducts the examination, usually a specialist in internal medicine, will remain in charge of the patient's case, becoming, in effect, his personal doctor for as long as he remains under the care of the clinic. The main reason for this practice is simple. Specialists, according to the Mayo Clinic philosophy, treat specialized diseases; the Mayo is interested in treating the whole patient. "The definition of a specialist as one who 'knows more and more about less and less' is good and true," wrote Charles Mayo in 1938. "Its truth makes it essential that the specialist, to do efficient work, must have some association with others who, taken altogether, represent the whole of which the specialty is only a part."

But there is another reason for this practice; it places one individual in overall charge of each patient and leaves no question where responsibility for his care lies. Also, placing one physician in charge helps to develop the doctor-patient rapport that is essential to communication, and this in turn is essential to effective diagnosis and treatment.

After the initial examination, diagnostic tests are scheduled according to the patient's needs. Depending upon the patient's specific complaints, various medical and surgical specialists may be called in to consult. The close working relationships of such specialists and their ready availability under one roof constitute one of the main strengths of the clinic.

Doctors at the Mayo Clinic can make appointments in such a way as to allow ample time not just to examine patients but to talk to them as well. The result is improved communication and, according to physicians, better medicine. "I don't have to be concerned with the patient's finances or with keeping my waiting room filled," said a Mayo Clinic cancer specialist. "All I have to do is see patients. You can practice good medicine when you're not in a hurry." Mayo Clinic physicians, who know nothing of a patient's financial condition, can order all the tests they feel are necessary without the temptation to skimp in ways that ultimately might not be in the patient's best interest.

Generally, people who go to the Mayo as a last resort do find the kind of help they need. The Mayo has a good record for diagnosing difficult problems, at least in part because of its thorough work-up of each patient. There are no figures that would show how many patients the Mayo fails to diagnose, but that number appears to be minuscule. With its cadre of specialists the clinic can probably find out what is wrong with anyone who comes there. It cannot, of course, cure everyone; medicine has not advanced that far.

A complete Mayo Clinic physical, which can cost anywhere from $300 to $600 or more depending upon the tests and examinations performed, takes around three days, though it can occasionally run even longer. When it is completed, the results of the examinations and tests are sent to the patient's primary Mayo physician, who first evaluates them, then sits down for a long, leisurely talk in which he explains them to the patient. The explanation is complete. Patients are told, in language that they can understand, exactly what the examinations and tests have shown and what the results mean. If the news is good, a patient is told that he is in good health and told what

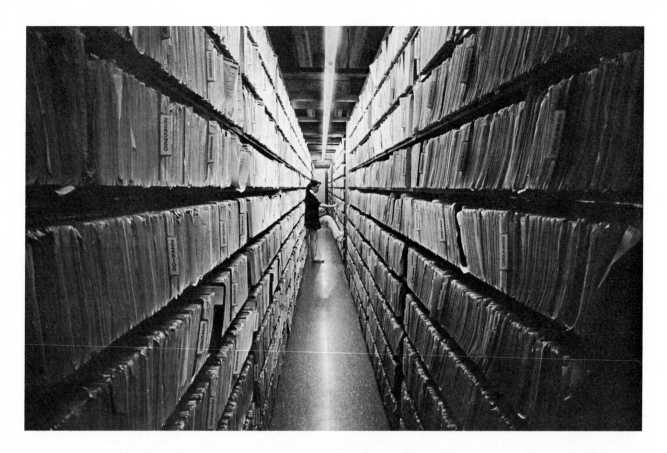

A medical librarian files information in the medical records storage room. Nearly a thousand patients a day come to Mayo Clinic, totaling millions of people treated since the turn of the century.

he must do to stay that way—lose weight, stop smoking, drink less, exercise more, or whatever else is necessary. But not even if the news is bad is a patient ever told anything but the truth. A patient who has a serious or terminal illness will be told just how dire his situation is and advised as to what he can or must do in order to cure, control, or adjust to his condition. The Mayo philosophy is that patients have a right to know, and they must know if they are to help themselves and make intelligent decisions about treatment and care.

Most patients wind up their examinations with a session in which they are told what the doctors have found and are referred to their own physicians, to whom the clinic will send the examination results and the recommendations that were made to the patient. Some patients are sent on their way with a friendly handshake and the knowledge that what may be the world's most complete physical examination has uncovered no serious problems. But some require treatment, which can be provided in the clinic or the affiliated hospitals if the patient prefers to be treated in Rochester rather than his hometown. Many are treated as outpatients, visiting the clinic periodically over several days or weeks, but about one out of every five requires hospitalization for medical treatment or surgery. The Mayo Clinic does not own or operate a hospital; it does, however, staff both St. Marys and Rochester Methodist hospitals, which have facilities for all types of care ranging from minor emergency room problems to open-heart surgery and every kind of cancer treatment.

For those for whom care is provided in the clinic's outpatient facilities, treatment is efficient, effective, and, most important, humane. Everyone, from physicians and therapists to the aides that change the linens in the examination and treatment rooms, exudes compassion, and everything at the clinic, from the records rooms with their bustling staffs of blue-smocked workers to the tasteful, nonthreatening decor seems designed to increase efficiency and put the patient at ease.

On just about every count the Mayo Clinic seems to pass this test. When a patient is shown into a treatment room, for example, a light outside the door signals that he is ready for the doctor. If the doctor does not show up within a few minutes to turn off the light, it begins to flash, alerting aides who can monitor the corridors from central stations and page the physicians to get them there. Other aides stand ready to help patients in and out of whirlpool baths, on and off tables, or merely to show their interest.

A physical therapist not only instructs but empathetically encourages a man with a badly scarred arm as he slowly claws his way up a ridged board on the wall with his fingertips, trying to exercise the injured limb back to normal. "I know it's uncomfortable," she says, "but you're doing so much better than you were last week." Her compassion is rewarded a moment later when the man, with an effort made as much for her as for himself, manages to crawl a few inches up the wall before dropping the arm down to his side.

The staff's concern is evident in other areas, too. The Mayo Clinic maintains close contact with its patients, many of whom return regularly for additional examinations or continuing treatment. "I always felt that I was just another sick body as far as my doctors back in New York were concerned," said a Manhattan woman as she took her place in the Mayo Building waiting room. "Here, I'm treated like a human being who happens to be sick."

Continuing standards of excellence

Such treatment seems likely to continue. The Mayo Clinic has no plans to change a system that has worked so well for it and its patients and no intention of "franchising" its operations or licensing miniclinics around the country as some have suggested. Nor do clinic officials see any reason why it should. A national health insurance plan is likely to increase the demand for the type of services Mayo provides, and the clinic may require some moderate expansion to meet these needs. The clinic is cautious of getting too big to retain the personal touch considered crucial to good medicine.

Mayo Clinic colleagues, physicians throughout the United States and around the world, and the thousands of patients who make their pilgrimages to Rochester each year in search of the kinds of miracles earlier generations expected only from saints can only hope that the clinic succeeds in staying the same. Every profession has its paragons, every area of human endeavor its meter sticks against which the accomplishments of others are measured. Medicine has its giants, too, but none stands taller than the Mayo doctors and the clinic they founded. The Mayo Clinic is such a world medical treasure that if it did not exist, it would be necessary to invent it—and today, at least, that would probably be impossible.

FOR ADDITIONAL READING:

Clapesattle, Helen B. *The Doctors Mayo.* New York: Pocket Books, Inc., 1956.

————. *The Mayo Brothers.* Boston: Houghton Mifflin Co., 1962.

Cohn, Victor. "The Marvelous Mayos." *The Saturday Evening Post*; three-part article in issues dated 26 November 1960, 3 December 1960, and 10 December 1960.

Mayo, Charles William. *Mayo: The Story of My Family and My Career.* New York: Doubleday, 1968.

A Symposium

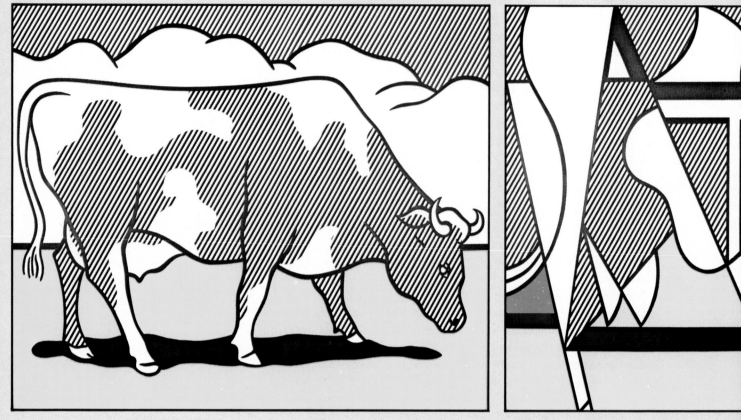

The Conquest
of Infectious
Disease

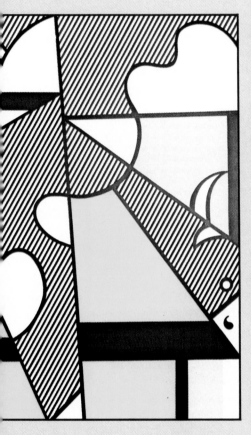
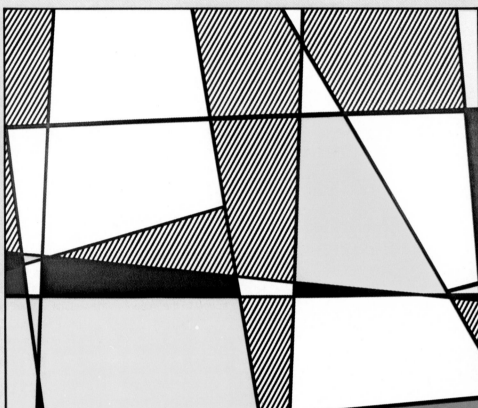

Epidemics
Viruses
Vaccines
Smallpox

Epidemics and History

by David M. Ozonoff, M.D., M.P.H.

At the end of an indecisive year of war between Athens and Sparta, early in the summer of 430 BC, the Athenian general Pericles encouraged refugees from the countryside to retire within the walls of Athens as part of his defensive strategy. The result was severe overcrowding and the overtaxing of the city's resources. Athens was soon struck by a devastating outbreak of plague that took the lives of a quarter of the population. It has come to be known as the Great Pestilence.

The plague apparently had come from Ethiopia by way of Egypt, appearing suddenly in the overcrowded harbor district of the Greek city. At first it was thought that the enemy had poisoned the local reservoir, but soon deaths were also occurring in the upper city. People were suddenly stricken with burning pain in the head, reddening and swelling of the eyes, and bleeding of the throat and tongue. Next came hoarseness, sneezing, chest pain, cough, stomachache, vomiting of bile, and an ineffectual retching. There was little fever and no pallor; the skin was flushed and later broke out into small pustules. Insomnia, unquenchable thirst, and a fierce restlessness added to the misery of the victims. If death did not come by the seventh or eighth day, the disease descended to the bowels. There it produced ulceration and uncontrollable diarrhea, killing a great many of those who had survived the first ravages of the affliction. Not even habitual scavengers, it was claimed, would eat the abundant human carrion that littered the city, and those few animals and birds that did partake of the flesh died soon afterward. Those victims of the Great Pestilence who survived suffered lasting scars, some losing portions of fingers, toes, or genitals and others going blind.

The displaced rural population, crowded together in badly ventilated huts, were particularly hard-hit, and they died like flies. The historian Thucydides, an eyewitness, recorded the event:

The bodies of the dying were heaped one on top of the other, and half-dead creatures could be seen staggering about in the streets or flocking around the fountains in their desire for water. . . . [The] catastrophe was so overwhelming that men, not knowing what would happen next to them, became indifferent to every rule of religion or of law. . . . As for the gods, it seemed to be the same thing whether one worshipped them or not, when one saw the good and the bad dying indiscriminately. As for offences against human law, no one expected to live long enough to be brought to trial and punished.

We shall probably never know the exact identity of this ancient Greek plague, although this has not stopped medical historians from arguing at length and with passion for their favorite scourges. Thucydides' description, however, makes it clear that a great epidemic is not only a biological event but a social one as well. The saga of epidemic infectious disease has shown that neither established conventions nor hallowed traditions can survive the calamity of a major pestilence.

David M. Ozonoff, M.D., M.P.H., *is Assistant Professor of Public Health at Boston University School of Medicine, Boston, Massachusetts.*

88

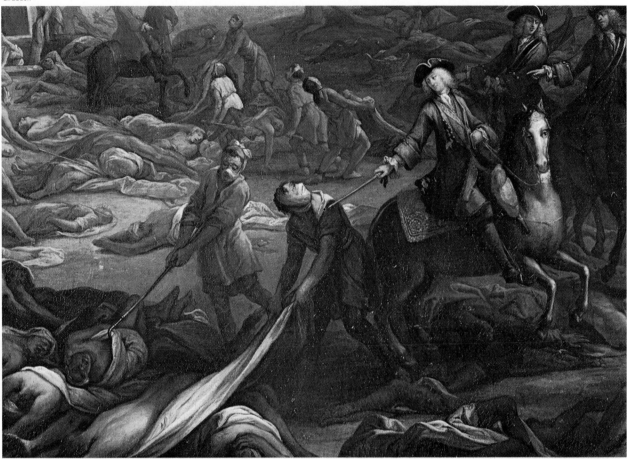

The host-parasite relationship

Man's body is always open to attack by minute specks of living matter. While the skin is generally resistant, if it is broken, organisms can penetrate it, causing boils, abscesses, or blood poisoning; and germs, such as those that cause tetanus or rabies, can be carried through the skin when it is bitten or cut. Mucous membranes lining the nose, mouth, and upper respiratory tract are open to attack by influenza and other viruses. Infective agents can also be swallowed with food or drink, causing intestinal diseases. Microorganisms can enter the body through the delicate membranes of the genital tract, the eyes, and even through the placenta before birth.

The relationship between human beings and lower organisms is not always (or even usually) antagonistic, of course. Humans often live intimately with viruses, bacteria, and other microorganisms in the mutually profitable fashion known as *symbiosis*. For example, normal intestinal bacteria synthesize nutrient substances essential to the human host. Microorganisms may also establish a totally indifferent relationship with a host, one organism living harmlessly within an environment produced by another. Consider the abundant variety of bacterial life on human skin. Only in the special kind of relationship called *parasitism,* where one organism lives at the expense of another, is there the possibility of what we call "disease."

Detail of La Peste à Marseille en 1720, *an 18th-century painting depicting the calamity of a major epidemic, from the collection of the Musée Atger–Faculté de Médecine, Montpellier.*

89

The symbiotic and indifferent relationships are the most gainful to both the microorganism and the host. The parasite is dependent on the host for its own nourishment and reproduction; ultimately, destroying the host offers little advantage. It is likely, in fact, that in the course of centuries or millenia, adaptation and evolution have tempered many previously antagonistic relationships, and in the process diseases have disappeared. However, when organisms invade new hosts or come into new relationships with old ones, new or unusual forms of parasitism may appear. *Virulence,* the property of being especially harmful or dangerous, then, does not belong solely to an infectious organism but is a property of the host-parasite relationship.

Defenses against disease

As important as the host-parasite relationship is to disease epidemics, we are largely in the dark about the adaptive and evolutionary aspects of the history of infectious disease. Because modern microbiological methods were unavailable until the 19th century, we can never be sure of the identity of many major historical epidemics, even those as well documented as the great plague of Athens. We presume, however, that many epidemic infectious diseases have been with us for some time.

In addition to natural immunity—the body's sensitive mechanisms that react quickly and specifically against disease organisms when they attack—there are also acquired defenses. In the cases of measles, smallpox, and mumps, for instance, it is clear that the body defends itself by manufacturing

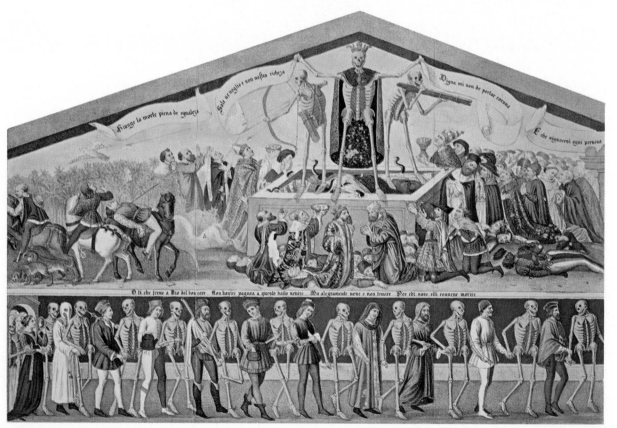

Bibliothèque des Arts Decoratifs; photograph, Jean-Loup Charmet, Paris

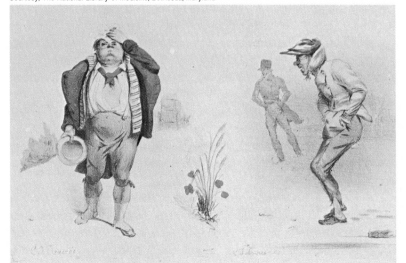

Hippocrates made the impressive connection between weather and the kinds of diseases prevalent—respiratory in winter and intestinal and malarial in summer. But the notion of contagion—the transmission of disease from one person to another—eluded Hippocrates and most physicians for the next two millenia. Lithograph, Les Contrastes—le chaud, le froid, *by Charles Joseph Traviés, 1804–59.*

antibodies against the offending organism; if the victim survives, there is immunity to further attack. For the responsible viruses to propagate, therefore, they must have available to them an *unexposed* population of human hosts—"susceptibles." Since a population of a certain size is necessary for this susceptibility, it has been speculated that epidemic infectious diseases first became possible at the time of the first agricultural revolution (about 10,000 years ago), when an increase in food supplies allowed human settlements to become large enough to support disease infestations.

Human beings have developed other ways to ward off the personal and social destruction caused by epidemic disease; *i.e.,* "cultural" defenses. Often these responses are so spontaneous as to appear instinctive, as when the scene of an epidemic is deserted by a fleeing populace (ironically this often spreads the disease even more widely).

Cultural defenses frequently take a magico-religious form, an apparently timeless and universal phenomenon. In the earliest surviving Greek writings, the Homeric poems, we find an offended Apollo smiting the Achaeans with divine arrows, causing a plague that was halted only when the wrong against Apollo's priest was rectified and suitable sacrifices were made to placate him. The Greek myth is not so different from the contemporary phenomenon of church congregations setting aside prayer or fast days in times of such unexplained or unstoppable pestilences as influenza or polio. The Greeks created the magico-religious cult of Aesculapius, whose symbol, a staff entwined with a snake, remains the emblem of the medical profession today.

Hippocrates' contribution to epidemiology

But, characteristically, it was the Greek world that also launched one of the most impressive scientific-rational traditions in medicine, appealing to a special combination of theory, observation, and experience. Hippocrates (5th century BC), the Greek physician who is traditionally regarded as the father of medicine, put forth a set of theories in this tradition in what is called the Hippocratic Collection (the Hippocratic writings were, however, the product of several hands).

(Opposite) The Dance of Death, *a 19th-century lithograph. The dance of death, or* dance macabre, *was a form of medieval allegory representing the equalizing power of death—a concept that gained momentum in the late Middle Ages, when obsession with death was inspired by an epidemic of plague. All ranks of living and dead figures are pictured—the living being led to the grave by the dead.*

91

Among the works are two remarkable examples of what we would today call *epidemiology*, the modern discipline that studies the types and patterns of disease present in a population. The first of these Hippocratic treatises, *Airs, Waters, and Places,* includes an examination of the powerful effect of cultural habit, geographic location, and prevailing climate on the kinds of diseases prevalent in a given area. Among the impressive observations in this work is that respiratory diseases prevail in the winter, intestinal and malarial ones in the summer, while stagnant, marshy areas (often polluted and now known to be infested with disease-bearing mosquitoes) are sites of summer epidemics of "dysentery, diarrhea, and long quartan fever" (probably malaria).

The second Hippocratic work, *Epidemics,* essentially a doctor's case-book, makes an important attempt to correlate weather conditions and atmospheric states with prevalent diseases. Since breathing the air was one of the few things that appeared to be common to the many victims of a widespread epidemic, this was thought to be a plausible explanation for transmission of disease. This theory lasted well into the 19th century, when the new science of bacteriology shifted everyone's attention from malign influences in the atmosphere to germs.

The notion of contagion

The Hippocratic writings, and indeed most of the medical writings that followed them in the next two millenia, were also remarkable in another way: they seem to contain no idea of contagion—the transmission of disease from person to person. Curiously the reticence of the medical authorities on this point is not matched by the lay or religious sources of either antiquity or the Middle Ages. In these nonmedical writings an idea of contagion was present, and rational measures to protect against it were sometimes proposed. Thucydides' account of the plague at Athens, for example, recognized that those who cared for the sick were more likely to contract the disease than others. And a disease that is usually identified as leprosy, although its relationship with what we now know as Hansen's disease is uncertain, is the subject of some famous passages in the Old Testament, Leviticus, chapters 13–15, where instructions are given for the diagnosis and isolation of confirmed cases. Many other nonmedical writers of antiquity, among them the poets Virgil, Ovid, and Lucretius, also understood that some diseases could be transmitted from one victim to another, and in that respect they were ahead of the medical authorities by many centuries. The *Georgics* of Virgil, for example, contains a clear description of a terrible epidemic of malignant anthrax that killed off the herds of northern Italy and Austria in the 1st century BC. The herder was advised to eliminate sick sheep to avoid ultimate disaster:

> When you see a sheep drift off to the gentle shade
> Too often, tug the grasstops idly, lag,
> Or stretch out prone mid-pasture, or retire
> Alone and last as deepening night draws on,
> Check the guilt with steel, before contagion
> Winds its way through all the careless herd.

In 1347 Europe was hit by the infamous Black Death, which killed from a third to a half of the population in a few years. (Opposite top) Goya's A Procession of Flagellants *(c. 1793) depicts the ritual whippings and floggings that were common as people sought by prayers and physical sacrifice to escape imminent death from the plague. An 18th-century print (bottom) shows a plague doctor wearing strange protective clothing and a long beak filled with antiseptic substances. He is carrying a rod used to take pulses.*

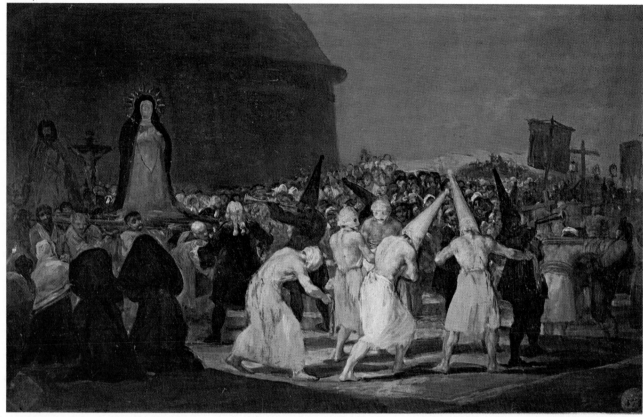

It is through the notoriety of three diseases of the Middle Ages, however—bubonic plague, leprosy, and syphilis—that the image of contagion was burned into the popular mind.

Bubonic plague. Bubonic plague was probably responsible for a number of epidemics in antiquity. The characteristic swellings, or "buboes," of the lymph glands in the groin, armpits, and neck are well described by several early sources. But it was only with the so-called Plague of Justinian in the 6th century AD that the disease first came into clear focus.

The eastern Roman Empire was rising in Byzantium when the emperor Justinian, crowned in AD 527, embarked on a program of reconquest of the territories that had fallen away when the old empire, centered at Rome, began to disintegrate. The initial years of Justinian's reign were a time of splendor and military achievement, and the future looked bright. But in AD 542 the empire was visited by a devastating plague that returned again and again in successive waves for over half a century and left Byzantium in a state of wrack and ruin. The emperor's secretary, Procopius, left a chilling account of the onslaught, noting that the epidemic had started on the coast and then had moved inward, proceeding inexorably from place to place and "always moving forward and traveling at times favorable to it." The death toll was so frightful that timely burial was impossible; instead, the towers of fortifications were crammed with corpses.

Descriptions make it clear that the plague of Justinian started as bubonic plague. Bubonic plague is a disease of rats and rat fleas. Under suitable

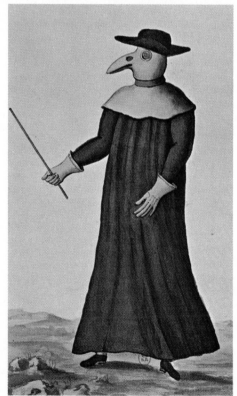

93

conditions fleas can pass the infection on to humans, but the rat–flea–human route of transmission is slow and inefficient, and therefore the bubonic form of the plague usually occurs sporadically rather than in massive epidemics. Sometimes, however, under conditions poorly understood but perhaps involving generally lowered resistance in the human host population, the plague causes not buboes but a sudden, severe, rapidly fatal pneumonia, which spreads from person to person by coughing and sneezing. It is plague in this form that is propagated in widespread epidemics, although it is often still called "bubonic" plague.

Whatever the reasons for the lethal transformation of the plague infection from bubonic to pneumonic form—perhaps a crop failure and malnutrition combined with an unusual number of infected rats—a plague similar to the Plague of Justinian hit some 600 years later. (Though there are no records of plague between the 8th and the 14th centuries, this does not necessarily mean that it was absent.) When it did definitely return to Europe in 1347, it was in the form of a colossal, unimaginable disaster: the infamous Black Death, which caused the destruction of from a third to a half of the European population in the space of a few years. The poet Petrarch, witnessing the events from Avignon, wrote: "Has one ever seen anything like this, ever heard reports of similar occurrence? In what annals has one ever read that the houses were empty, the cities deserted, the farms untended, the fields full of corpses, and that everywhere a horrible loneliness prevailed."

A Franciscan monk, Michele Piazza, describing how Venetian galleys brought the plague to the harbour city of Messina, wrote of the symptoms:

Because of an infection of the breath passed around among them as they talked, one so infected another that all were seen as if racked with pain, and, in a measure, severely shaken; as a result of the pain, the shaking, and the infection of the breath, pustules appeared on the thigh or arm in the manner of *lenticulae,* which thus infected and penetrated the body, wherefore they violently spat forth blood; after spitting for three days incessantly without any cure for the dreaded disease, they departed from life; and not only did whoever talked to them die, but indeed whoever bought, touched, or seized anything belonging to them.

During the Black Death complete social disorganization was the rule, and the extremes of utter lawlessness and licentiousness coexisted with the harshest self-abnegation and mass self-flagellation—the practice of beating, flogging, and whipping oneself. Organized efforts to halt the spread of the disease were difficult under the circumstances, but several maritime cities did try to place restrictions on incoming ships to ensure that new cases were not being imported. In 1377, for example, the Italian town of Ragusa required that passengers on ships from infected places be detained a month before being given the liberty of the city. Later this interval was increased to 40 days (*quaranti giorni*), giving us our word *quarantine.*

Plague continued to smoulder for the next several centuries with regular flare-ups, the most prominent occurring in England in 1664–65. Major cities were almost deserted. The famous diarist Samuel Pepys recorded that in London there was "little noise heard day or night but tolling of bells." For unknown reasons, not long after this episode plague largely died out in Europe. A recrudescence at the end of the 19th century was but a pale

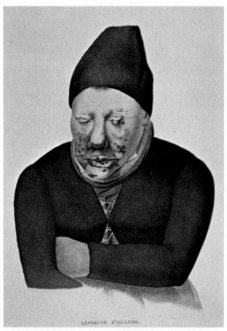

The terror inspired by leprosy, a disfiguring skin disease that was epidemic in the Middle Ages, generally was out of all proportion to its actual medical effects. Engraving by L. Bevalet from Voyage en Islande et au Groenlande, *1838.*

94

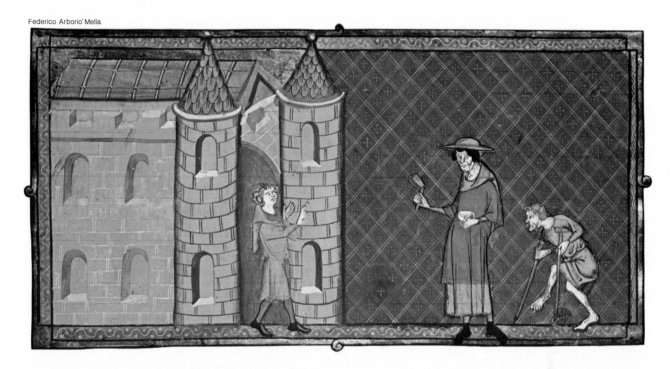

shadow of its earlier manifestations in Europe but killed some ten million people over a period of 20 years in Asia.

Leprosy. A medieval scourge of a very different kind was leprosy. This name was probably used for a number of chronic disfiguring diseases of the skin that had been known since biblical times. But coinciding with the Crusades, in the 12th and 13th centuries, the prevalence of disease or diseases called leprosy suddenly increased dramatically. The terror the affliction inspired was out of all proportion to its actual medical effects.

A strict Old Testament tradition identified the disease with moral and physical uncleanliness. Victims were stigmatized because of the deformed features, open sores, and gangrenous digits. Incredibly stringent laws had the effect of declaring the victim dead as far as society was concerned. The biblical tradition had earlier identified contact as the mode of spread and prescribed isolation of the victims as a protective measure. But true leprosy is a chronic, indolent disease that mimics many others, and its diagnosis is anything but easy. It is not surprising that few voluntarily stepped forward to suffer forced isolation in a leper house, exclusion from all normal human contact, life as itinerant beggars, and even summary execution in a few places. Instead the diagnosis was often suggested by suspicious neighbors and "certified" by a panel of medical and ecclesiastical experts. The similarity to the epidemic of witch-hunting some centuries later in Western Europe is probably more than coincidental, since similar social forces and tensions were at work in both cases.

The epidemic of leprosy reached its peak in the same century as the Black Death, and it has been suggested that the plague eliminated leprosy by killing off its weakened victims, who were conveniently crowded together in leprosaria—leper colonies. Whatever the reason, leprosy disappeared as suddenly as it appeared, and while its image is indelibly stamped on Western

Lepers were stigmatized because of the deformed features, open sores, and gangrenous fingers and toes; many led lives as itinerant beggars, sounding clappers, horns, or bells to warn of their approach, as seen in this miniature from the British Museum, London.

95

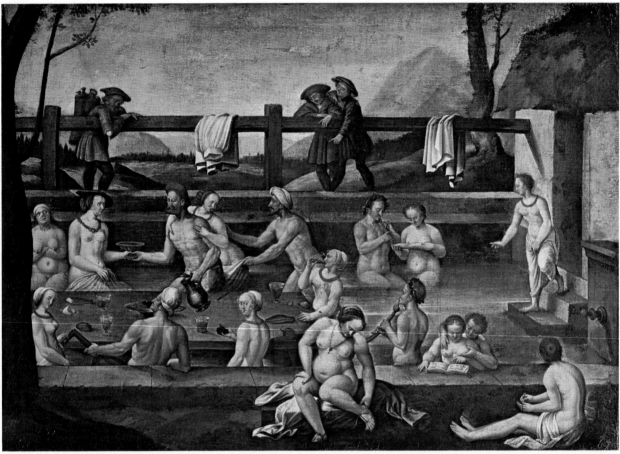

Syphilis reached epidemic proportions in Europe in the late Middle Ages and Renaissance. Mixed bathing in public baths had been a popular treatment for many ills, sometimes accompanied by other procedures such as bloodletting and by feasting and drinking. But as knowledge of contagion grew and syphilis was recognized as a disease spread by sexual contact, the practice of bathing in common tanks died out. Das Bad zu Leuk, *oil painting by Hans Bock, 1597.*

culture, the disease had ceased to be a major factor in the health of the population by the 15th century. Its place was taken by another morally stigmatizing affliction: syphilis.

Syphilis. The disease we know today as syphilis is a mild illness compared with the virulent form that struck in the first years after Columbus' first voyage to America. The conjunction of its appearance with the opening of the New World immediately suggests that it was an imported disease. This theory has been at the center of what one historian has called "the most controversial subject in all medical historiography" ever since. We would note only that if syphilis existed in the Old World prior to 1493, it was in a form quite unlike the one it assumed after that time. The following description makes clear that this was a particularly horrible malady:

There were boils, sharp, and standing out, having the similitude and quantity of acorns, from which came so foul humours and so great stench, that who so ever smelled it, thought himself to be infected. The color of these pustules was dark green, and the sight thereof was more grievous to the patient than the pain itself; and yet their pains were as though they had lain in fire.

Early-16th-century writers knew that the disease sometimes occurred after sexual intercourse, but other causes, including unfavorable astrological conjunctions, were also thought to be important. It received the designation "venereal" from a 1527 work of Jacques de Bethencourt of Rouen, France,

96

who noted the special influence of Venus, the Roman goddess of love. Indeed, until the science of bacteriology would identify the causative organisms, in 1905, there was continued debate as to the possibility of contacting venereal disease (including gonorrhea) from a variety of inanimate sources such as horse saddles, bicycle seats, or toilet seats. We know that the organisms involved are too fragile to survive for very long outside the human organs that are their natural habitat, yet little else demonstrates the large social component of our ideas about disease as well as the fact that it still seems terribly important to us whether a disease—whose strict definition is merely that it is an infection by a particular organism—should have been caught from a toilet seat or from another human being.

It is odd that such an unpoetic disease should derive its modern name from the title of a work written in Latin hexameters, but such is the case. Girolamo Fracastoro, a Veronese gentleman who was a true Renaissance man, accomplished in philosophy, poetry, music, astronomy, and geography as well as medicine, wrote a poem entitled "Syphilis, or the French Disease" (1530). (Syphilis was called the French disease, by the Italians, at any rate, since it was first recorded in the French campaign against Naples in 1495. The French, naturally enough, preferred to call it the Neapolitan disease.) Fracastoro fancifully traced the new sickness to blasphemous idolatry committed by an ancient herdsman and his country people. As punishment for this sacrilege Apollo sent a scourge through Syphilus, the herdsman. (The name, in good Renaissance fashion, was that of a herdsman in a poem by Ovid.)

Fracastoro first held the common medical view that syphilis was not contagious, but by 1546, in a renowned work called *On Contagion and Contagious Diseases,* he had registered his growing perception that a number of diseases were by nature transmissible. It was a perception probably widely shared by the many who lived in those centuries when plague, leprosy, and syphilis were ever present realities. It seems all the more remarkable that the mainstream of medical writings adhered much more closely to the ancient Hippocratic tradition, which declared disease to be the result of atmospheric corruptions or personal predispositions rather than contact with existing cases. It should be remembered, however, that most of the observed phenomena were compatible with either viewpoint and that ancient medical tradition weighed heavily against contagion.

In his second book Fracastoro made the additional observation that over the preceding 20 years syphilis had become noticeably less virulent, tending to run a milder, longer course. This was just 50 years after its first appearance. Syphilis is a prime example of the accommodation between host and parasite mentioned earlier. It is sobering to realize then that the three principal scourges of the Middle Ages and early modern period—plague, leprosy, and syphilis—all disappeared or reverted to milder forms on their own.

Personal and environmental factors blamed for the transmission of disease

Well into the 17th century the bulk of illnesses continued to be placed within the Hippocratic framework, which regarded them as systemic imbalances resulting from personal indiscretion or malign environmental influence, although by the 18th century some members of the medical profession had accepted a few diseases as contagious.

Smallpox was one such malady that was beginning to be understood as capable of transmission by personal contact. It was recognized, too, that a single attack brought immunity from the disease. Therefore, when reports began to circulate of the Eastern folk practice of inoculating susceptible individuals with matter from pox pustules to produce a mild case of the disease, the ground for what became smallpox vaccination had been, in a sense, prepared. The practice of artificially immunizing a population, initiated in Boston in 1721, occurred at a time when smallpox was becoming a major hazard for the rapidly growing urban populations that accompanied the Industrial Revolution. The general principle of prophylactic inoculation is still one of the most effective defenses we have against certain epidemic infectious diseases.

The doctrine of disease contagion was not yet the order of the day, however. It is a historical irony that in the 75 years immediately preceding the triumph of the germ theory, the idea of contagion reached its low point in popularity. Instead, personal and environmental factors were deemed to be the obvious and irrefutable elements in the production of epidemic illnesses.

The same forces of urbanization and industrialization that provided such luxuriant opportunities for the smallpox virus to spread also produced physical and intellectual conditions that obscured the transmissible character of most infectious epidemic disease. The crowding, poor drainage, inadequate waste disposal, and insufficient and unclean drinking water in the major cities were ideal grounds for pestilence. In the 19th century devastating epidemics of yellow fever and cholera spotlighted these conditions and drove home the connection of disease with the poverty and squalor of the urban slums. At the same time, classical liberalism and its philosophy of free trade resisted any public health practices that restricted commerce. Chief among its targets was quarantine, which rested squarely on a contagionist conception. Adopted instead was a strategy of moral education and environmental sanitation, tracing disease to individual defects or corrupted habitats.

The notion that disease was connected with individual uncleanliness and sloth surfaced first in an ideology that blamed the victims of disease for their own misfortunes. Whether the fault lay in deep-seated moral defects, ignorance of "laws of health," or irresponsible and self-indulgent vices (intemperance, for example), the responsibility was clearly the victim's. One result was the beginning of social service and visiting nurse associations whose aim was to go into the homes of slum dwellers to reeducate them by precept and example. It also produced a convenient attitude under the cover of which major social evils could be ignored.

Sanitary reforms

Sometimes, however, it was seen that the alleged irresponsibility of the so-called lowest segments of society endangered all. Epidemics did not always stay safely confined to the poorest parts of town but threatened all

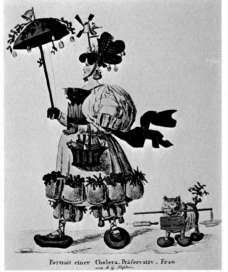

Portrait einer Cholera-Präfervativ-Frau
von H. G. Sophie.

The Bettmann Archive

98

orders. Thus in the wake of massive yellow fever and cholera epidemics in the 19th century attempts were made to enact sanitary reforms. We now know that foul odors emanating from overflowing cesspools, uncleaned streets, and stagnant pools in undrained alleys do not cause disease. But the piped-water supplies and sewer systems developed to eliminate these odors had a major beneficial impact on the health of the population.

The provision of public water supplies, for example, was especially important in eliminating such water-borne diseases as typhoid, cholera, and the dysenteries, although the motive behind these supplies was, first, to provide a copious source of flushing water to clean the streets and, second, to fight fires. The efficient distribution of drinking water, however, if the water was obtained from a polluted source, produced dangers of its own. The preoccupation with the foulness of the air, encouraged no doubt by the appearance and odors of the 19th-century industrial city, made the recognition of the connection between disease and dirty water surprisingly long in coming.

The credit for this discovery is given to John Snow, although in truth his achievements are not as clear-cut as admiring 20th-century sanitarians portray them. Snow was a London physician best known to his contemporaries as the doctor who administered chloroform, an anesthetic, to Queen Victoria in childbirth. But he is known to public health specialists today as the author of a remarkable series of investigations into the cause of epidemic cholera in London in the 1850s.

The water of the city at that time was provided by several competing private companies who drew their supplies from the heavily polluted Thames River. Since his youth Snow had been an ardent temperance advocate, and it is likely that his belief in the poisonous nature of alcohol also stimulated his interest in toxicology and directed his attention to poisons possibly present in the water supply. Using this "drinking-water theory" as a working hypothesis, he was able to show that in the epidemic of 1849 cholera deaths were especially high in the south district of London. This district was supplied by two companies that drew their water from a portion of the river downstream from the city's main sewer outflow. Between the 1849 outbreak and another in 1854 one of these companies had moved its intake upstream of

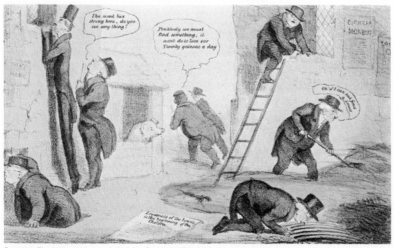

Courtesy, The National Library of Medicine, Bethesda, Maryland

Before the sanitary reforms of the 19th century, cholera epidemics were associated with foul odors, corrupted habits, and moral defects, among other things. Frantic citizens wore bizarre costumes to ward off the disease: (opposite) a 19th-century Austrian engraving, Portrait of a Cholera-Protected Woman. *(Left) A cartoon (no. 27, by Robert Seymour) from "McLean's Monthly Sheet of Caricatures," depicts* A London Board of Health Hunting After Cases like Cholera.

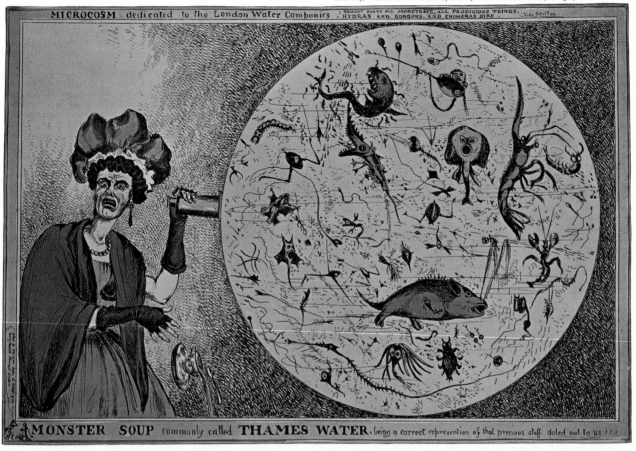

MICROCOSM dedicated to the London Water Companies

BROUGHT FORTH ALL MONSTROUS, ALL PRODIGIOUS THINGS, HYDRAS AND GORGONS, AND CHIMERAS DIRE. Vide Milton.

MONSTER SOUP commonly called THAMES WATER, being a correct representation of that precious stuff doled out to us!!!

John Snow, known as the "father of epidemiology," showed that cholera deaths were related to sewage-polluted water from the Thames. The anonymous 19th-century caricature above portrays a woman dropping her tea cup when she sees the poisonous creatures contained in Thames water, or Monster Soup, when it is magnified. But several decades passed before the substances in polluted water were identified as pathogenic microorganisms. This discovery was possible in part because of improvements in the microscope. (Opposite page) Microscopes from the 17th century (bottom right), 18th century (top right), and an electron microscope today.

the sewer outflow, while the other had not. In a detailed investigation of deaths in the area where the two companies competed on a house-to-house basis, Snow showed that deaths from cholera were relatively frequent in households supplied by the sewage-polluted source and infrequent in neighboring, otherwise identical households supplied with water that had come from the cleaner area.

For this pioneering work Snow is given the title "father of epidemiology." Unfortunately, the elegance and force of his argument did not bring immediate acceptance of his views. Several decades were to pass before the drinking-water theory won universal recognition, and this came only after independent work in the new science of bacteriology had successfully identified the poisonous substance present in polluted drinking water as being composed of pathogenic microorganisms.

Microbiology and other developments

The triumph of the germ theory in the last quarter of the 19th century was the most profound advance yet in our knowledge of the etiology of epidemic disease. The explosive development of the science of bacteriology was the result of the convergence of several separate lines of work. Louis Pasteur made fundamental contributions to microbiology while working with the cultivation of French grapes. Pasteur adamantly rejected the materialistic doctrine of the time that living organisms could arise from nonliving material. He

100

had noticed that previously virulent bacterial cultures would produce milder diseases if incubated in a culture medium slightly warmer than the optimum growth temperature. Using these attenuated cultures Pasteur successfully demonstrated the principle of prophylactic inoculation in anthrax, swine erysipelas, and rabies.

Meanwhile, other developments made possible the identification and isolation of the causative organisms of a large number of diseases. Improvements in the microscope, the availability of new stains from Germany's infant aniline dye industry, and the introduction of solid culture medium by Robert Koch contributed to the incredible speed with which discoveries were made once the new techniques were mastered. The use of bacteriological diagnosis and the development of preventative immunizations were great achievements and are often given credit for the virtual elimination of epidemic infectious disease in our own century.

The addition of the antibiotics to our therapeutic armamentarium in the 1930s and '40s is considered by many to be the final and decisive accomplishment in the conquest of infectious disease. This view, however, should not be accepted as offhandedly as it sometimes is.

For many deadly diseases of the 19th century, among them tuberculosis (the greatest killer), scarlet fever, diphtheria, measles, and whooping cough, the greatest part of the decline in incidence took place *before* the time when we could do anything about them. Just as the incidence of leprosy and plague decreased for unknown reasons, so have tuberculosis and other infections. Scarlet fever has been significantly reduced and has reverted to a milder form, as syphilis did earlier. Undoubtedly, better living conditions and improved nutrition have played their part. It is also true that for some diseases the use of antibiotics has made possible the treatment of those sporadic cases that do occur. And the use of prophylactic immunization, while coming *after* the major decline of such diseases as diphtheria and whooping cough, may be preventing a recrudescence. But the evidence as

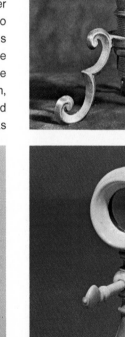

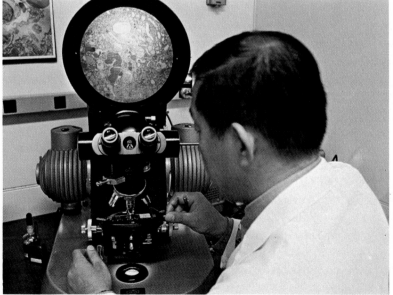

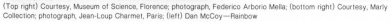
(Top right) Courtesy, Museum of Science, Florence; photograph, Federico Arborio Mella; (bottom right) Courtesy, Marly Collection; photograph, Jean-Loup Charmet, Paris; (left) Dan McCoy—Rainbow

FOR ADDITIONAL READING:

Burnet, Sir Frank Macfarlane, and White, David O. *Natural History of Infectious Disease.* 4th ed. Cambridge, England: Cambridge University Press, 1972.

Cartwright, Frederick Fox, and Biddiss, Michael D. *Disease and History.* New York: Thomas Y. Crowell Co., 1972.

Dubos, René Jules. *Mirage of Health: Utopias, Progress, and Biological Change.* New York: Harper and Row, 1959.

Rosebury, Theodore. *Microbes and Morals: The Strange Story of Venereal Disease.* New York: Bantam Books, 1973.

Rosenberg, Charles E. *The Cholera Years: The United States in 1832, 1849, and 1866.* Chicago: University of Chicago Press, 1962.

Sigerist, Henry E. *Civilization and Disease.* Chicago: University of Chicago Press, Phoenix Books, 1962.

Winslow, Charles Edward Amory. *The Conquest of Epidemic Disease: A Chapter in the History of Ideas.* Princeton, N.J.: Princeton University Press, 1943.

Zinsser, Hans. *Rats, Lice and History.* Boston: Little Brown & Co., 1935. Reprint. New York: Bantam Books, 1965.

it now stands seems to indicate that conscious human efforts were not the decisive factor in the overall decline that has taken place in many infectious diseases.

Nor have epidemic infectious disease outbreaks been entirely eradicated. The devastating 1918 influenza pandemic is reputed to have killed more human beings than any other disease in human history within a comparable period of time. Known as the "Spanish flu," this acute respiratory malady spread throughout the world. During the two-year period it was rampant more than 21 million people died—1% of the world's population. It was known for killing an unprecedented number of healthy young adults. We still do not know why this happened, and the recent swine-flu scare suggests we are not sure it could not happen again.

The future

While advances in standards of living have generally aided in the fight against infectious disease, in some cases, notably poliomyelitis, those very advances have been responsible for transforming a sporadically occurring disease into an epidemic one. Prior to the end of the 19th century sanitation was so universally bad that most people had been naturally immunized to this intestinal virus in early infancy by exposure at an age when they still possessed some protective immunity from maternal antibodies. As sanitation improved, however, entire generations of unexposed populations appeared, with the result that huge epidemics of polio occurred. They were not halted until the introduction of mass immunization in the 1950s eliminated the huge reservoir of susceptible hosts.

Other aspects of our modern world have also created new conditions for epidemic spread of infectious disease. Air transport has made it possible to fly virtually anywhere on earth within the incubation period of every known infectious disease. A less exotic example of the wonders of modern transportation is reflected in a diary kept by a prostitute with venereal disease that reveals that she had had sexual contact with individuals (all long-distance truck drivers) from 37 states, Canada, and Mexico.

These are not the only, or even the major, issues of contemporary epidemiological concern, of course. One could add the current rapid spread of antibiotic resistance in many kinds of bacteria, especially the causative agents of lobar pneumonia and gonorrhea. There is also the fear that radically new types of biological technologies such as recombinant DNA experimentation might introduce new and unknown kinds of organisms into the general population. (This last question has already sparked a thorough review of genetic research and the safety of the laboratories that carry it on.) The list could go on.

If our luck holds, some epidemic diseases, like the dramatic example of smallpox, may soon become historical curiosities. But we cannot rest secure in the knowledge that infectious diseases no longer pose a threat of epidemic outbreak. The recent example of Legionnaires' disease suggests the possibility that previously unknown organisms might have been and continue to be unrecognized threats to the population. In this respect we have not yet reason to suppose the future too different from the past.

102

Viruses: Drama Within the Cells

by H. Sherwood Lawrence, M.D.

Viruses are unique among all infectious agents that plague mankind. This uniqueness derives from the fact that viruses are infectious nucleic acids, genetic messengers either naked or lightly disguised in an envelope of protein, and, unlike free-living bacteria, they exist in a state of suspended animation until they can broach the defenses of their host and penetrate deep into the intimate corridors of his cells. Once nestled snugly inside such cell membranes, the infective virus sheds the protein topcoat, seeks out and inserts itself into the components of a related nucleic acid in the cell, and borrows the host's cellular copying machinery to reproduce itself over and over again.

This wild need of the virus to ensure its survival continues unabated even though it causes the cell that harbors and nourishes it to grow sluggish and sicken and often burst in consequence—a process that can cause visible abnormalities such as skin blisters (pox), red spots (measles), or intrinsic liver damage (hepatitis).

The hard reality of the matter is that a virus can assume living properties and reproduce itself only while inside other living cells. The fact that the virus causes disease, devastation, or even death in the process is a chance outcome of evolutionary pressures it has responded to in its own battle for survival. The same pressures caused some viral families to take refuge in plants or insects or bacteria, rather than in humans. The virus has no other particular commitment but that of self-reproduction and thereby passing on its genetic information to its progeny, which then does the same. Viruses are not driven to cause disease, nor is there any spirited inclination on their part to do so. The latter event from our viewpoint is the unfortunate and, ironically, the chance outcome of our capacity to provide temporary or sometimes permanent lodging while satisfying the evolutionary pressures that compel the virus to reproduce itself packaged in such a form that upon leaving the afflicted host it may set up housekeeping in another victim and begin the cycle again.

In the discussion to follow we shall consider the natural events surrounding viral infections: what it is about the virus that causes human disease and how the disease is transmitted, how we develop immunity and resistance to repeated infections by the same virus, how some viruses manage to evade this rule of the game, how certain viral infections gone awry can produce so-called autoimmune disease, and how several newer strategies of immunologic intervention may be employed to rescue the patient afflicted with an infectious viral disease from an otherwise bleak outcome.

H. Sherwood Lawrence, M.D., *is Professor of Medicine and Head of the Infectious Disease and Immunology Division at New York University School of Medicine, New York City.*

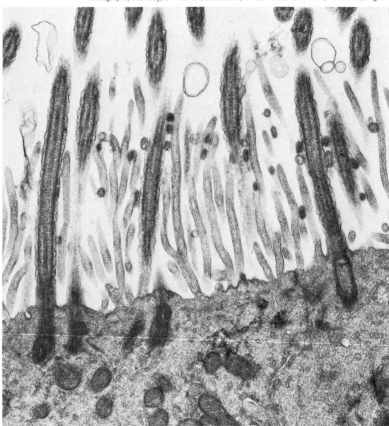

Influenza viruses in action. A cross section of a windpipe, magnified 35,910 times, shows flu viruses—the small dark particles—invading the respiratory tract. The long, waving fronds are cilia, hairlike extensions of cells. When a flu virus reaches the cell surface (opposite, magnified 70,000 times), the membrane of the cell forms a pocket in an attempt to swallow the intruder. But once inside, the virus easily works its way into the interior of the cell, where it multiplies and eventually causes the cell's death.

The viral odyssey

The most common way for viral particles to get into the interior of the cells of a human host is via infected secretions and bodily products. The most common vehicles of transmission are air inhaled into the respiratory tract (*e.g.,* influenza, common cold), food and water ingested into the digestive tract (hepatitis, poliomyelitis), or breaks in the skin or mucous membranes directly accessible to the bloodstream (rabies, mosquito-borne encephalitis). These methods of transmission are usually and most efficiently accomplished directly from person to person but may occur indirectly via contamination of objects (food, hands, linen) or infection of bloodsucking insects (mosquitoes, ticks).

There are two types of viral infection: one in which the virus comes into direct contact with its target cell (common cold, influenza), and the other, in which access to the bloodstream must be gained before delivery to the target cell can occur. In the latter circumstance the viral particles have a bit of an uphill journey, like salmon swimming upstream to their original spawning grounds, to arrive intact and operative at their destination contiguous with the appropriate target cells.

Thus, both hepatitis and poliomyelitis viruses upon ingestion share the same portal of entry, and each must traverse the cells of the intestine to gain access to the bloodstream but then have widely divergent journeys. Hepatitis viruses seek out the liver cells, attach to the cell membrane, penetrate,

104

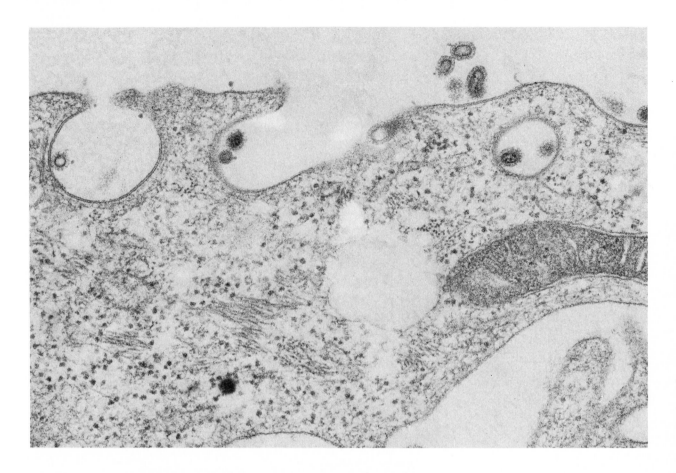

and take over the cell metabolism, producing sickness in the patient, accompanied by fever, jaundice, nausea, and vomiting. In contrast, poliomyelitis viruses seek out the particular nerve cells in the anterior horns of the spinal cord to result in sickness or death of the nerves while producing headache, fever, muscle aches, and finally weakness and wasting or complete paralysis of a limb.

It is this type of behavior that has fostered the notion that viruses have a homing instinct or predilection for residence and multiplication in specific tissues or organs. However, it is more likely that many, if not all cells, are infected with a particular virus, yet this generalized infection is overshadowed by the critical tissue damage that is reflected in the malfunction of a *single* organ system such as the brain or liver or a single cell type in the spinal cord.

Yet cells must have a specific receptor for the particular virus, and the initial attachment of the virus to the cell must have the symmetry and congruence of a key fitting into its proper lock before passage into the cell can occur and the replicative goal of the virus can be realized.

Immunologic deterrents to viral invasion

We all produce antibodies that circulate in our blood and protect us against certain diseases; this is called humoral immunity. The exact repertoire of such protective antibodies varies from individual to individual and is largely

105

Humoral Immunity

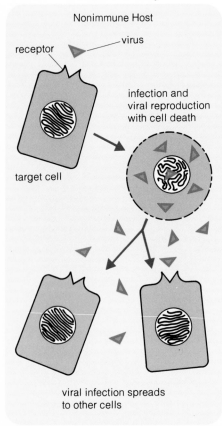

Nonimmune Host

receptor

virus

target cell

infection and viral reproduction with cell death

viral infection spreads to other cells

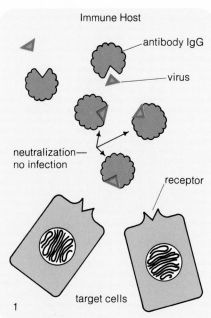

Immune Host

antibody IgG

virus

neutralization— no infection

receptor

target cells

1

a matter of chance confrontation in nature with a vast array of infectious agents, including viruses, or deliberate encounters via active immunization.

Antibodies are proteins that usually circulate in our blood as a second line of defense or are excreted to line the mucous membranes of our respiratory and intestinal tracts as a first line of defense against microbial or viral invasion. Antibodies are called immunoglobulins (Ig) and are of several classes, such as Immunoglobulin G (IgG) in our blood serum and Immunoglobulin A (IgA) in the mucous secretions of our digestive and respiratory tracts, where our cells are in direct contact with an exterior, hostile environment.

Specificity is the key to all our immune responses and the touchstone of survival when we are confronted with viral infections. For example, those of us who have had measles in childhood harbor a highly specific memory of that event in our antibody-producing cells. The antibody we carry as a result of that encounter will neutralize and inactivate the measles virus and protect us upon exposure to our children when they acquire measles, but it will not protect us against chickenpox or poliomyelitis. If we possess the antimeasles virus antibody (IgA) in the mucous secretions lining our respiratory passages and inhale that virus disseminated in droplets coughed or sneezed by another, it is promptly enveloped by our antibody and its infectivity neutralized. Should we lack IgA in our respiratory tract, and the measles virus gains access to the bloodstream, the IgG antibody will neutralize it there (*see* Figure 1).

If these two arenas of confrontation are evaded, and the virus makes the perilous journey to the target cell and even inserts itself into the cell membrane, it can still be neutralized and infection prevented by specific IgG in the neighborhood. Yet once through the membrane and divested of its protein coat, the virus is safe and the host now in danger, since antibody cannot cross the cell membrane and penetrate our cells. This fact is important to the timetable for administration of passive immunity to nonimmune children or adults following exposure to a patient with measles. An instant loan of immunity to a susceptible individual can be accomplished by injecting purified IgG antibody prepared from the blood serum of patients who have recovered from measles. Yet to be effective in preventing the infection the IgG has to be administered as early as possible in the incubation period of the disease—usually within five to six days after exposure—during which time the virus is making its voyage from the respiratory epithelium (a thin layer of tissue lining) to the target cells via the bloodstream. If administered later, after the virus has penetrated the cell membrane, the infection may be ameliorated but not prevented.

The specific example of measles applies with equal force to all viral infections acquired via the respiratory route. With minor alterations the model is adaptable to viruses that infect via the intestinal tract.

An invitation to repeated infection

Fortunately, many natural viral infections provoke an indelible immunological memory of their presence and, having recovered from an illness, the patient possesses a lifelong immunity that prevents reinfection by the same virus.

106

Notable examples of this protective remembrance of the past include such diseases as smallpox, chickenpox, measles, German measles, and yellow fever. There are also families of viruses that seem to cause the same disease two or three times, but this is due to the inherent individual antigenic or immune provoking difference of one virus from other members of the family. For example, hepatitis virus A differs from hepatitis virus B in this important respect despite the fact that infection with either virus produces an almost identical disease of the liver, distinguishable only by the type of antibody provoked or by isolation of the virus itself. At the most practical level recovery from hepatitis A infection protects the individual from reinfection by hepatitis A but does not protect against hepatitis B.

This state of affairs is quite different from the case of influenza A virus infections, which threaten highly developed as well as less developed countries annually on a global scale. Most people have experienced influenza more than once, and the disease produced is generally indistinguishable from the last bout. Yet, although each manifestation of disease produced is immutable and seemingly identical to the last, the cause is fundamentally different. The reason lies in the capacity of the influenza virus to switch its genetic composition and with it the protein outer envelope during its passage through large numbers of victims.

This evasion of the "rules of the game" probably has great significance for the overall survival of the virus but not necessarily for infected individuals, since it leads to recurrent episodes of the same illness in the same individual and widespread dissemination of the disease in uniformly susceptible populations. In switching its protein envelope the virus alters the identifying mask by which the immune system remembers it. Last year's antibody cannot recognize and hence cannot neutralize this year's virus, and a new infection is the result, independent of prior recovery from infections with earlier versions of the same strain of virus.

Moreover, it is this genetic mutability of the virus and resultant acquisition of an unlimited repertoire of viral protein disguises that subvert influenza vaccination programs. It is not that influenza vaccines are ineffective; they are most effective immunizing agents, which protect the patient and prevent or ameliorate the disease. Carefully controlled studies have shown that in addition to preventing actual infection in most people vaccinated, if such infection does occur the patient sheds much less virus in respiratory secretions. Thus, vaccination programs reduce disease transmission to nonimmune individuals by at least two mechanisms: fewer susceptible people and reduced transmission of disease by immune people who become infected.

Hence, the subversion of flu vaccination programs is just another expression of the subversion of man's acquired immunity following infection. It is not the vaccine that is at fault any more than the patient's immune response but rather the evasive tactics employed by the influenza virus itself. This year's vaccines can contain only influenza viruses isolated from prior epidemics, and they cannot be expected to contain predictions of which labyrinthine turn in the protein coat the next genetic mutation of the virus will produce. And even if the virus had an intelligence, which is sometimes intimated by such wily behavior, it is doubtful that it could predict what the

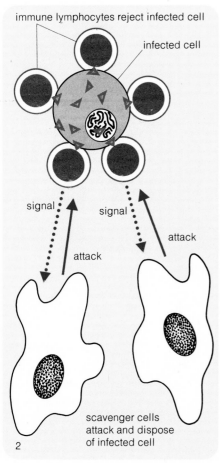

Cell–Mediated Immunity

immune lymphocytes reject infected cell

infected cell

signal

signal

attack

attack

attack

scavenger cells
attack and dispose
of infected cell

2

next turn would be since each turn is fraught with unpredictable circumstance.

In sharp contrast, the story of the global eradication of smallpox by vaccination is an illustrious example of the stunning success that can be achieved when the virus exhibits genetic stability and the game is played according to *man's* rules, which do not always coincide with those of nature.

Cell-mediated immunity

We have considered the interactions of viruses and target cell membranes and the role of the antibodies of humoral immunity in either preventing access of the virus to the bloodstream (IgA) or intrusion into the main arena of viral activity, within the cell itself (IgG). We have also emphasized that humoral antibody cannot penetrate cells. Once the virus has reached this sanctuary, another type of immune response is called into play.

This other arm of the immune response is called cell-mediated immunity (CMI), and its prime vehicle is a lymphocyte or white blood cell, called the T cell since its unique functions are under the influence of the thymus, a small gland in the neck. We become most aware of thymic influence and T cell functions that are critical for our survival when we see children born without a thymus or with defects in T cell function. These children can die from an overwhelming viral infection or from a smallpox vaccination, both of which in normal children will produce only mild indisposition.

The critical role of cell-mediated immunity in recovery from viral infections is highlighted in congenital immunodeficiency diseases involving defective T cell function such as the Wiskott-Aldrich syndrome. Individuals with this condition, which is characterized by chronic eczema, deafness, anemia, and hemorrhages, can succumb to viral infections despite relatively normal humoral antibody responses. In contrast, children born with congenital agammaglobulinemia, who have extremely low levels of gamma globulin in their blood and lack the capacity to produce antibody, have functional cell-mediated immunity and are easily infected but nevertheless are able to deal with and recover from viral infections much as normal children do.

The behavior of viral infections in such children with birth defects of immune function has underlined the distinctive and different functions of the two arms of the immune response: humoral antibody is most effective in the prevention of infection or in dealing with the extracellular life cycle of the virus, and cell-mediated immunity works by eradicating the virus-laden cell once an intracellular residence has been established (*see* Figure 2).

Autoimmune disease

Powerful evolutionary pressures for survival must have been placed on an infective virus spawned in the primeval ooze countless eons ago to make the long odyssey from the cells of one individual to those of another in an unbroken chain to the present. The opportunities for termination of this chain of descent through chance mishaps, abortive infections, or the precipitous and untimely death of the infected individual are incalculable.

Confronted with such evolutionary pressures for survival, certain viruses probably responded by evolving a more amicable intracellular accommodation. This would allow viral reproduction within the cell without killing it outright while the virus acquires host cell camouflage and refrains from calling excessive immunological attention to itself.

Whatever the explanation, there appear to be certain viruses that have a predilection to cause what are termed slow viral or persistent viral infections. Slow viral infections are characterized by their tendency to persist in the cell over prolonged periods. This is in contrast to the usual viral infection, where the duration of illness is short and the eradication of the virus is generally an integral part of the recovery process.

The persistence of a virus inside or at the surface of a cell has several important consequences that result from the alterations produced in the face of the cell, which make it look foreign to our own lymphocytes. Lymphocytes are versatile memory banks equipped to react promptly against foreign cells or tissues while sending out distress signals to other cells to join the fray. This delicately poised espionage system is engaged in constant immunologic surveillance, and the lymphocytes function to police our internal milieu against alien intruders.

Thus the viral alterations on the face of our cells inadvertently fool our lymphocytes into thinking our own tissues are foreign, such as someone else's cells in a transplanted kidney might appear, and provoke aggressive behavior that attempts to reject promptly all cells bearing such an altered appearance. This event serves as the invitation to trigger unfriendly "autoimmune" responses when host lymphocytes attack altered self-tissues in the mistaken belief that they are overtly foreign. Thus, depending upon which tissue or organ is involved in such alteration of cell surface antigens, a different type of disease pattern is expressed, which forms the basis for the autoimmune diseases. Two classical examples of this outcome are seen in the persistent inflammatory involvement of the liver cells in chronic active hepatitis and in the brain cells following a measles viral infection that results in a devastating brain disorder called subacute sclerosing panencephalitis (see Figure 3).

There is also evidence accumulating to support the notion that infection of our pancreatic cells with coxsackieviruses, which resemble poliomyelitis viruses, can cause juvenile diabetes through a similar mechanism. In this instance it appears that instead of inheriting diabetes, a child inherits the highly individualized arrangement of glycoprotein molecules on the face of his cells—called histocompatibility antigens and comprised of proteins and carbohydrates—which have a relationship with the infecting viruses that favors a persistent or slow viral infection with all the autoimmune overtones discussed above.

This congruence of host cells and infecting virus may be at the root of subacute sclerosing panencephalitis—a chronic destructive, generally fatal, disease of the brain that arises in certain children as a consequence of an ordinary childhood measles infection gone awry. There is also the suspicion that multiple sclerosis, another chronic devastating neurological disease of young adults, may also be caused by a commonplace viral infection gone wrong and converted to a slow viral infection of the brain in certain individuals who have inherited a particular histocompatibility type.

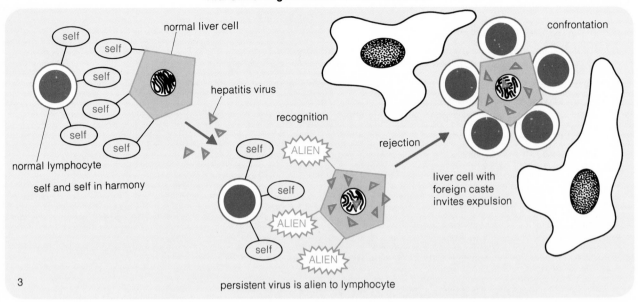

self
self
self
self
self
self

normal liver cell

normal lymphocyte

self and self in harmony

hepatitis virus

recognition

self
self
ALIEN
self
ALIEN
ALIEN

persistent virus is alien to lymphocyte

rejection

confrontation

liver cell with
foreign caste
invites expulsion

3

New strategies for treatment of viral infections: chemotherapy and immunotherapy

The search for effective agents for the treatment of viral infections has quickened consequent to recent research findings illuminating our understanding of the precise nature of viral organisms, their relation to the intricate machinery of the infected cell, and the cascade of immunologic responses triggered by infections. The contributions of epidemiology, sanitation, and vaccination to the eradication or subjugation of viral infections have been vast. The role of humoral antibody in preventing, aborting, or ameliorating viral infections during their extracellular phase is important. But the rules of the game can change for viruses once they are inside our cells. There are two approaches to this phase of the problem: to disable the virus directly without hampering the cell that harbors it and to bolster the host's capacity to dislodge the virus. A great deal of research is being done with antiviral drugs, and in 1977 adenine arabinoside (ara-A) was found to be effective in treating herpesvirus encephalitis—a serious and generally fatal inflammation of the brain. Ara-A is currently being investigated for treatment of other viral infections.

For many scientists, however, immunologic intervention designed to augment the host's capacity to eradicate the virus is seen as an equally promising method of attacking the problem. While this discussion will be restricted to immunological approaches, in the future it is anticipated that both chemotherapy and immunotherapy will be employed to accomplish a common goal.

It will be recalled that humoral antibody directed against an infecting virus can function to prevent it from reaching the bloodstream or, having reached the bloodstream, prevent it from invading our cells. Yet, having penetrated the cell, the virus is protected against the neutralizing effects of humoral antibody, and the host is dependent upon cell-mediated immunity, negotiat-

110

ed by lymphocytes (T cells) and macrophages (scavenger cells), to eradicate the virus along with the cells that give it asylum (*see* Figure 2).

Fortunately, most of the time the host achieves this feat with his own immunologic apparatus. Recovery and, in its wake, staunch immunity generally ensue unaided. However, this is not always the outcome, particularly in patients with inborn or acquired defects of cell-mediated immunity; such individuals need some help to restore this arm of defense to full vigor and efficiency, hence the current application of immunologic reagents that can achieve prompt restoration of cell-mediated immunity.

Transfer factor. Transfer factor is a tiny, nontoxic material that can be extracted from the white blood cells of individuals with cell-mediated immunity. It has the capacity to confer that type of immunity on nonimmune individuals very promptly. Transfer factor also has the capacity to boost and augment cell-mediated immune responses that are latent or depressed due to an infection. In this way it has been shown to boost cell-mediated immunity when administered to patients suffering from intracellular infectious diseases caused by fungi and bacteria as well as those caused by viruses. Following the administration of transfer factor there is a generalized spurt in cell-mediated immunity, and the patient's clinical state usually improves. There is also evidence of eradication of the infectious agent.

There are several chronic viral diseases that have responded to transfer factor administration. These include chronic active hepatitis, subacute sclerosing panencephalitis, and cytomegalovirus infections. The acute viral diseases that have responded to transfer factor include herpes zoster, generalized vaccinia—a systemic infection often following smallpox vaccination —herpes simplex, and measles pneumonia.

The response to transfer factor in the case of herpes zoster will serve to illustrate the point. A patient suffering from Hodgkin's disease, a tumor of lymphatic organs, which resulted in depressed cell-mediated immunity, developed a herpes zoster viral infection, so-called shingles. The skin blisters caused by the infection spread over his body despite treatment with antiviral chemotherapy (ara-A), and culture of the blister fluid revealed herpes zoster virus. At this time the patient exhibited a generalized absence of cell-mediated immunity, and his lymphocytes did not respond when confronted with the zoster virus in a test tube. Transfer factor was prepared from the lymphocytes of another individual who was immune to herpes zoster virus and injected into the patient. Following several injections, the patient's lymphocytes acquired cell-mediated immunity to zoster virus; the skin blisters dried up and healed; the virus could no longer be isolated from the patient; and clinical improvement ensued.

This immunologic type of treatment is still in its infancy and highly experimental since so much more needs to be learned about transfer factor, namely its chemical composition, the optimum dosage needed, and precisely how it selectively boosts cell-mediated immunity. Additionally, as is true of any new therapeutic agent, the results of carefully controlled clinical trials will decide the effectiveness of this new type of therapy. Such clinical trials are currently in progress to determine the value of transfer factor therapy in recalcitrant viral infections such as chronic active hepatitis, subacute

FOR ADDITIONAL READING:

Ascher, M. S.; Gottlieb, A. A.; and Kirkpatrick, C. H. *Transfer Factor—Basic Properties and Clinical Applications.* New York: Academic Press, 1976.

Lawrence, H. S. "Transfer Factor in Cellular Immunity." Harvey Lectures, series 68. New York: Academic Press (1974): 239–350.

Mims, C. A. *The Pathogenesis of Infectious Disease.* New York: Academic Press, 1976.

Talal, N., ed. *Autoimmunity.* New York: Academic Press, 1977.

Youmans, G. P.; Paterson, P. Y.; and Sommers, H. M. *The Biological and Clinical Basis of Infectious Diseases.* Philadelphia: W. B. Saunders, 1975.

sclerosing panencephalitis, and congenital cytomegalovirus infections.

Interferon. Human cells in tissue culture infected with live influenza virus are stimulated to secrete a substance that protects other cells from infection. This substance is called interferon. Interferons are composed of a family of molecules whose production and export are stimulated not only by viral infections but by other intracellular microbial infections such as those caused by fungi and bacteria. Unlike the requirement of specificity for antibody discussed above, the interferons triggered by one viral infection have activity against any other viruses. Despite this immunologic nonspecificity, however, interferon produced by human cells will protect human cells only and not those of other mammals, and vice versa.

It is of interest that among the many cells that can produce interferon upon viral infection are immune lymphocytes. Indeed, upon administration of transfer factor to a patient with subacute sclerosing panencephalitis large amounts of interferon were produced, presumably from viral interaction with immunologically rehabilitated lymphocytes.

Interferon may have been responsible for aborting the common cold when instilled in the nasal passages of volunteers at the time of or shortly after exposure to the cold virus. It is also being explored as therapy for herpes zoster and chickenpox infections, and initial results are promising enough to warrant further exploration. The clinical application of interferon therapy is on the verge of getting under way, and future developments are awaited with interest.

The adaptation of new immunologic and biologic reagents to rescue the patient from the consequences of intracellular viral parasitism is currently an area of intensive investigation. At best the results of such investigations hold promise for amelioration and perhaps even cure of life-threatening diseases; at the very least we can confidently anticipate a clearer understanding of the immunological plight of the afflicted patient. In the best of all possible worlds such information can be tailored and adapted to suit specific situations, and a combination of such reagents may be employed to bolster host defenses and limit propagation of the virus while chemical reagents distract or otherwise engage or cripple the intracellular viral parasite directly.

One may justifiably view the promise afforded by such new developments with a degree of circumspect optimism, if only since man is unique among all species in his capacity to think, and to plan, and to remember. This capacity has allowed his own direct intervention to tip the scales in his favor when a conflict of evolutionary pressures for survival arises, such as happens in infectious diseases. The challenge presented by the virus to propagate its own genetic heritage in the nucleic acids it imparts to our cells was originally met by the evolution of natural immune responses adapted to ensure man's propagation of his own genetic message in an unbroken line. For most of us, most of the time, the capacity for immune responses that we have inherited is adequate, and we surmount viral assaults—although sometimes at great bodily cost. By studying the composition and life-style of viruses as well as our own responses to their presence and behavior in order to devise means to survive the challenge and thwart the invader, man is contributing in a spectacular way to his own evolution.

Vaccines:
Building Defenses Against Illness
by Lawrence K. Altman, M.D.

In the early part of this century, thousands of infants choked to death each year from diphtheria; a toxin from the diphtheria bacillus produced wax plugs that cut off air in the children's windpipes. Other children were struck with severe paroxysms of whooping cough; as they gasped for breath, air sucked through their windpipes produced the characteristic whoop that gives the disease its name. Some children became brain damaged from encephalitis, a complication of measles. Athletic, vigorous teenagers suddenly were paralyzed, unable to walk or write, because the virus that causes poliomyelitis destroyed a section of their spinal cords. Many other polio victims could not breathe outside an iron lung. Men or women who pricked a hand with shears while gardening or cut themselves while doing handywork at home developed tetanus; a few days after the tetanus bacterium entered the body through an innocuous wound, a toxin was produced that injured a nerve and "locked" their jaws. Today we so seldom hear about these and other infections that we have lost perspective on the problems posed by infectious diseases. Only a few decades ago there were so many cases of highly contagious diseases that entire hospitals existed just to treat them, and they were among the leading causes of death in the United States.

Today such preventable infectious diseases remain very common in the less developed countries of the third world, where they are the leading killers. However, in the United States and other developed countries they have been wiped out or reduced to a near-zero level. Today when a case of diphtheria or tetanus or polio is diagnosed in a U.S. hospital, doctors and medical students from miles around gather to discuss what has become a medical oddity—an exotic disease. Two factors have been primarily responsible for wiping out these killers and threats to the quality of life: better hygienic and living standards, and the development of vaccines and immunizations to prevent infections.

While improved sanitation, nutrition, clean water, and population control certainly have been a major force in reducing the toll of infectious diseases on society, it is unlikely that the death and sickness rates would have fallen to zero or near-zero levels on the basis of improved hygienic and nutritional standards alone. Because polio, diphtheria, tetanus, and the other infectious diseases still can strike well-nourished, "clean-living" people, even today an individual has no assurance that he or she may not be the next victim.

The development of vaccines and immunizations is clearly among the most impressive achievements of medical science. Ironically, modern medi-

Lawrence K. Altman, M.D., *is a medical correspondent for the* New York Times.

(Top) Jean-Loup Charmet, Paris; (bottom) courtesy, The National Library of Medicine, Bethesda, Maryland

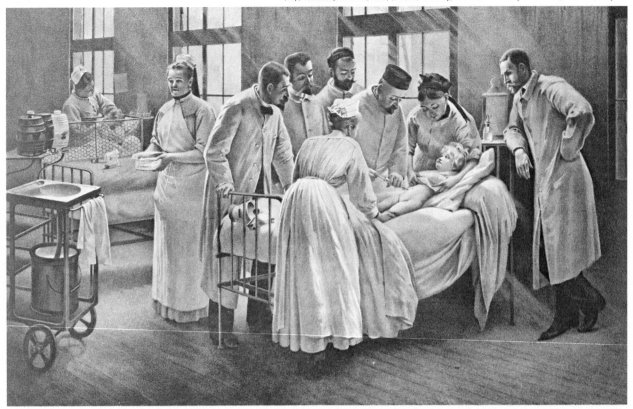

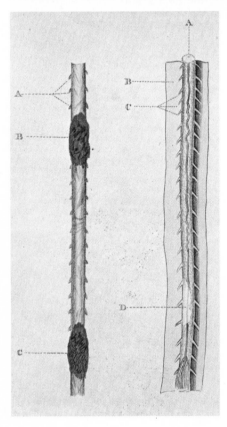

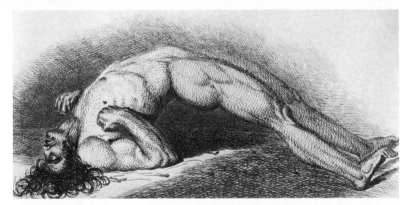

cine probably does a better job of preventing diseases than it does of curing them. Immunization offers an excellent chance of protection against many noncurable diseases. In fact, most immunizations offer more than a 90% chance of protection, although some, such as those against cholera and influenza, are considered about 60% effective. However, polio vaccine is more than 90% effective. Mothers whose children are adequately immunized no longer feel compelled, as they did in the 1940s and '50s, to keep them from crowded swimming pools on sweltering summer days because of the fear that they might contract the paralyzing illness. The fears of polio have been so reduced that many children do not know what the word polio means, except perhaps that it is one of the vaccines they swallowed in a sugary liquid solution at a young age.

114

But immunization is not an absolute guarantee of protection for everyone who receives an inoculation. Even in a protected population there are a small number of cases of disease attributed to vaccine failure, often for biological reasons that doctors do not fully understand. And vaccines can lull an individual into a false sense of security. An individual who has been immunized against cholera or typhoid, for example, can still succumb to these infections if he or she drinks or eats contaminated foods. The risk of getting the infections is substantially lessened, but it is not reduced to zero. And for this reason health experts advise individuals traveling to cholera- or typhoid-infected areas not to consider immunization a substitute for proper hygienic standards.

The history of vaccines

The concept of immunization is as old as mythology. Mithradates VI Eupator, king of Pontus from 120 to 63 BC, protected himself against poisons by drinking ducks' blood that had been mixed with the poisons. Crude forms of smallpox vaccination were performed by the ancient Chinese and the Turks long before Edward Jenner developed the first smallpox vaccination in 1796. It is known that *variolation* (inoculating directly with the human smallpox virus) was practiced in the 17th century in Africa and Asia.

Louis Pasteur carried the science of immunization forward with the development of vaccines against chicken cholera, anthrax, and rabies. Pasteur described the notion of specificity, which underscores the concept of im-

The development of vaccines and the widespread practice of immunization have made the scenes on these pages history. (Opposite top) Pierre-Paul-Émile Roux, at extreme right, an associate of Louis Pasteur, supervises the administration of diphtheria antitoxin to a child at the Paris Children's Hospital; lithograph from the Musée Carnavalet, Paris. (Opposite center) Scottish physician and anatomist Sir Charles Bell sketched the rigors of the spasms of tetanus in a soldier on the battlefield at Waterloo. (Opposite left) The spinal lesions caused by the tetanus bacterium are clearly seen in this illustration, the frontispiece from Robert Reid's On the Nature and Treatment of Tetanus and Hydrophobia, *Dublin, 1817. (Below) A nurse attempts to cheer a child with polio whose breathing must be sustained by an iron lung. Such scenes were common in the terrifying epidemics of "infantile paralysis" of the early 1950s, before the development of the polio vaccine. The quarantine warning (bottom) dates from about 1910, evidence of a futile attempt to contain smallpox when it was epidemic in the United States.*

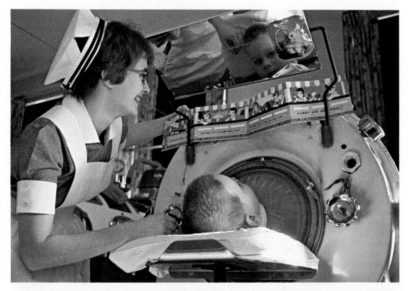

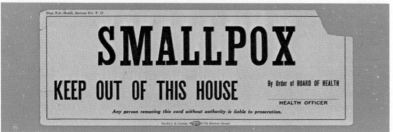

(Top) Courtesy, The Children's Hospital Medical Center, Boston; (bottom) courtesy, The National Library of Medicine, Bethesda, Maryland

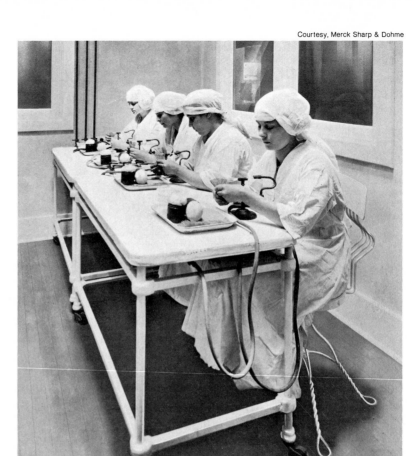

The technology of vaccine manufacturing struggled to keep pace with the snowballing scientific advances. In this early photograph technicians seal test tube points over gas flames.

munology, by showing that chickens protected against cholera remained defenseless against anthrax.

The special merit of protection against further attack after surviving one bout of an infectious disease probably was recognized from observations going back to ancient times. But it was not until the late 19th century that Emil von Behring, a Prussian Army surgeon, and Shibasaburo Kitasato, a Japanese bacteriologist, first recognized that acquired immunity to tetanus and to diphtheria was due to a factor in the blood plasma; animals that had been injected weeks earlier with small doses of tetanus and diphtheria toxins had produced the factor. They recognized that animals built their own immunity, and they showed that animals susceptible to tetanus acquired immunity if they were injected with blood plasma from an immune animal. This was the first demonstration of passive immunity. Following the animal experiments, Behring tested antitoxins in man. Finding his human tests successful, he began producing the antitoxins on a mass scale as the specific treatment for diphtheria, which led to immunizations against tetanus and other bacterial infections.

Behring was the first recipient of the Nobel Prize for Physiology or Medicine, in 1901, and others were awarded Nobel Prizes later for developing vaccines against other diseases. For example, Max Theiler won the Nobel Prize for Physiology or Medicine in 1951 for developing a vaccine against yellow fever, a viral disease. But success in developing vaccines

116

against viral diseases was limited until John F. Enders, Thomas Weller, and Frederick Robbins began developing a Nobel Prize-winning technique for growing viruses on cells in test tubes in 1946. It was this step that proved crucial in allowing other scientists to develop vaccines against poliomyelitis, measles, and rubella (German measles).

The vaccination principle

The word *vaccination* is derived from vaccinia, the cowpox virus that is scratched into the skin to protect against smallpox. Literally, there is only one vaccination—that against smallpox. But the word *vaccination* has come to be used generically to cover virtually any immunization.

Now both *immunization* and *vaccination* are used to describe a technique of modifying an infectious agent or its product such as a toxin to the point that when artificially introduced into the body it does not cause the infection yet still is potent enough to stimulate the body to develop immunity to the infectious agent. In general, immunizations are made against infectious agents. But the principle has been used to protect against at least one noninfectious disease, the potentially fatal anemia called erythroblastosis fetalis that can develop in a baby born to an Rh-negative mother and an Rh-positive father. When a pregnancy results from parents with such a combination of blood groups, the baby's blood can be Rh-positive. In the first pregnancy of such a combination, the baby's Rh-positive cells have little chance of entering the mother's body to stimulate her to form antibodies to the baby's Rh-positive red cells. However, at birth both the mother and the baby bleed—the mother from the uterus and the baby through the placenta, or afterbirth. If some of the baby's Rh-positive red cells enter the mother's veins (and there is a good chance this will happen during delivery), the mother forms antibodies against the baby's red cells. She becomes immunized against the Rh-positive cells, and if she has another Rh-positive baby, the antibodies in her blood can pass through the placenta and damage the baby's red blood cells, producing erythroblastosis fetalis.

Due to an immunization process erythroblastosis fetalis has become much rarer. It can be prevented by injection of a gamma globulin solution that is rich in Rh antibodies within 72 hours after delivery. The immunization must be given after each pregnancy because it does not stimulate the mother to make her own antibodies, and the injected antibodies are destroyed over a six-month period.

Against infectious diseases there are two main types of immunization agents—active and passive—and the distinction is based on the way in which the protection is gained. Both types work by stimulating the body to produce antibodies, the proteins that the body forms in response to the invasion of an antigen, a foreign substance such as an infectious microorganism. Antigens are proteins that differ from the body's own proteins. When an antigen enters the body, antibodies combine with the antigen in an effort to thwart its dangers. Antibodies are specific; they fight only the particular antigen that led to the antibody's formation.

Passive immunity. Passive immunity involves injecting an antiserum that contains specific protective antibodies against a specific condition. Such

Jonas Salk injects a child with polio vaccine. Statistics reflect the drama of the success of polio immunization: in one state alone, Massachusetts, there were 3,950 cases of polio in 1955; in 1956 there were 100 cases, and deaths dropped from 175 to 6.

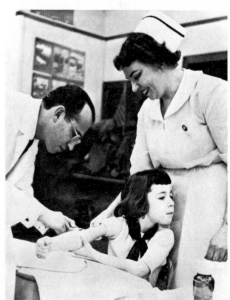

Courtesy, The National Library of Medicine, Bethesda, Maryland

117

antisera are prepared by injecting toxoids into animals and harvesting the resulting antitoxin. Another form of passive immunity is injection of gamma globulin strained from the blood of people who already have protective antibodies against such infections as hepatitis and chickenpox. Because the biological materials used in passive transfer do not stimulate the recipient's body to produce antibodies, technically they are not vaccines. Rather, they are immune serums. Passive immunity takes effect immediately after injection. But the immunity continues only as long as the injected material is sustained in the body, usually a period of just several weeks. Its protection then is temporary.

Active immunity. In contrast, active immunity takes several days to weeks to become effective. But when it does, it provides longer-lasting protection, usually for many months or years. Active immunity can be provided by injection or by a solution taken by mouth. It results from the stimulation of the body's own natural disease-fighting mechanism by the injection of the causative organisms of the living disease, which have been modified so as not to cause a damaging case of the infection. Examples of such vaccines are live measles, oral polio (developed by Albert Sabin in 1955), smallpox, and the bacille Calmette-Guérin (BCG), sometimes used to protect against tuberculosis. When scientists cannot attenuate an organism, they often make vaccines from killed organisms. Examples are whooping cough, tetanus, injected polio (developed by Jonas Salk in 1954), and injected measles vaccines.

In general, scientists say that live vaccines are theoretically more effective than killed vaccines but that live vaccines pose risks that do not exist with killed immunizations. Killed vaccines can lead to production of antibodies, but not all antibodies are fully protective. In order to ensure full protection against certain infections, cell-mediated immunity must be produced. This type of immunity follows vaccination or infection with an organism that replicates in the body. Tuberculosis, for example, is caused by the presence of *Mycobacterium tuberculosis*. Injection of killed tuberculosis bacteria leads only to some antibody production, not to protective immunity. For immunity to develop, live *Mycobacterium tuberculosis* in the form of the BCG vaccine must be injected. There is, however, a potential danger in live virus vaccines: the attenuated, or weakened, strain might unpredictably revert to a more dangerous form, thus causing rather than preventing infection.

The immunizations against tetanus and diphtheria contain no bacteria. For their action they rely on the presence of toxoid, which is a toxin in the bacteria rendered harmless by treatment with formalin or another chemical.

Current use

The U.S. government currently licenses vaccines for general use against at least 13 major infections: cholera, diphtheria, influenza, measles, meningococcal infections, mumps, pneumococcal pneumonia, poliomyelitis, rabies, rubella (German measles), tetanus, whooping cough (pertussis), and yellow fever. (There are also a few vaccines for limited use against special conditions.)

Because antibiotics, with rare exceptions, are not effective against viral

A Chronology of Immunizations

Date	Disease	Researchers	Type of Immunity and Vaccine	Expected Duration of Immunity	Similar Vaccine in Current Use
1796	smallpox (viral)	Edward Jenner	active immunity/live virus vaccine	3–10 years	yes, in a few countries
1885	rabies (viral)	Louis Pasteur	active/attenuated	[1]	yes, to a limited extent by the French
1890	diphtheria (bacterial)	Emil Adolf von Behring Shibasaburo Kitasato	passive/antitoxin	3–4 weeks	yes
1892	cholera (bacterial)	Waldemar M. W. Haffkine	active/attenuated	[1]	no
1892	tetanus (bacterial)	Emil Adolf von Behring Shibasaburo Kitasato	passive/antitoxin	10 days	rarely
1895	plague (bacterial)	Alexandre Yersin Albert L. Calmette Amédée Borrel	passive / active/killed	[1] [1]	[1] [1]
1896	cholera (bacterial)	Wilhelm Kolle	active/killed	unknown	yes
c. 1896	plague (bacterial)	Waldemar M. W. Haffkine	active/killed	6–12 months	yes, for lab workers only
1896	typhoid (bacterial)	Almroth E. Wright; Richard Pfeiffer and Wilhelm Kolle	active/killed	2–3 years	yes
c. 1904	diphtheria (bacterial)	Alexander T. Glenny	active/killed	[2]	[2]
1906	pertussis (bacterial)	Jules Bordet[3] Octave Gengou[3]	active/killed	several years	yes
1912–13	diphtheria (bacterial)	Emil Adolf von Behring	active/live	[1]	no
c. 1917	Rocky Mountain spotted fever (rickettsial)	Roscoe R. Spencer Ralph R. Parker	active/killed	unknown	no
1921	tuberculosis (bacterial)	Albert Calmette Camille Guérin	active/attenuated	unknown	yes, but not in U.S.
1923	diphtheria (bacterial)	Gaston Ramon	active/killed	7–10 years	yes
c. 1927	tetanus (bacterial)	Gaston Ramon Christian Zoeller	active/killed[5]	5–10 years	yes
1930	diphtheria (bacterial)	Alexander T. Glenny	active/killed	[1]	[1]
1930–33	epidemic typhus (rickettsial)	Rudolf Weigl	active/killed	6 months	no
1935	yellow fever (viral)	Max Theiler	active/attenuated	10 years	yes
1937	influenza (viral)	Thomas Francis, Jr.	active/inactivated	several months to one year	yes
1941	Rocky Mountain spotted fever (rickettsial)	[1]	active/killed	unknown	yes, for lab workers only
1945	pneumonia—pneumococcal types 1, 2, 5, 7 (bacterial)	C. M. MacLeod R. Hodges M. Heidelberger	active/polysaccharide	6 months	no
1948	mumps (viral)	Thomas H. Weller John F. Enders	active/killed[5]	3–10 years	yes[4]
1954	poliomyelitis (viral)	Jonas E. Salk	active/killed	2–3 years	yes, but not in U.S.
1955	poliomyelitis (viral)	Albert B. Sabin	active/live	5–6 years	yes
1957	rabies (viral)	[1]	active/killed	2–3 years	yes
1960	measles (viral)	John F. Enders	active/attenuated	6–10 years	yes
1966	rubella—German measles (viral)	Harry M. Meyer, Jr. Paul D. Parkman	active/attenuated	3–5½ years	yes
1969	meningococcal infection (bacterial)	Emil C. Gotschlich Malcolm S. Artenstein I. Goldschneider	active/polysaccharide	unknown	yes
1969	rabies (viral)	R. Keith Sikes W. G. Winkler R. C. Schmidt	passive	3 weeks	yes
1977	meningococcal infection (bacterial)	H. Peltola[6] P. Helena Mäkelä[6]	active/chemical	unknown	yes
1977	pneumonia—pneumococcal types 1, 2, 3, 4, 6, 8, 9, 12, 14, 19, 23, 25, 51, 56 (bacterial)	Robert Austrian Researchers at Merck Sharp & Dohme	active/chemical	estimated at 3–5 years	yes

[1] information not available
[2] not applicable
[3] cultivated the causal bacillus; vaccine developed simultaneously in several countries later
[4] attenuated vaccine
[5] immune globulins conferring short-term passive immunity are also available
[6] demonstrated efficacy of group A vaccine for children 3 months to 5 years of age

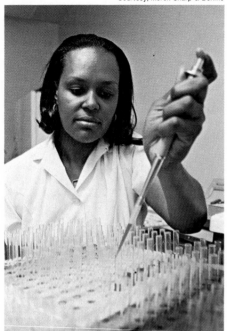

The testing of a vaccine for safe and effective use on human patients is rigorous and time-consuming. It may take a decade to ready a vaccine for use. The many steps in the manufacturing process must then be tightly controlled so that quality is maintained.

diseases and can cure bacterial, fungal, and parasitic diseases only after they occur, most experts regard vaccines as the chief prospect for preventing the myriad of infections that still threaten human life. Researchers are now trying to develop vaccines for hepatitis, chickenpox, respiratory syncytial virus (a principal cause of acute bronchiolitis, a serious lung infection among infants), gonorrhea, malaria, and several other parasitic diseases. The U.S. military spends millions of dollars trying to develop vaccines against exotic infectious diseases such as Bolivian hemorrhagic fever, chikungunya, and Rift Valley fever, which American troops have encountered in battle in the past or are likely to encounter in the future. It was military research that played an important role in producing the recently licensed vaccine against the meningococcal bacterium, which can cause meningitis.

Producing vaccines

Making a vaccine is easy in principle. In simplified terms: first, the causative germ is grown in eggs or cells in test tubes; then the organism is weakened or killed; and finally a preparation is extracted that produces immunity by stimulating the body to produce protective antibodies against the antigens in the vaccine. But in reality developing vaccines is very costly and time-consuming; the applied research that produced the meningococcal vaccine cost U.S. taxpayers at least $11 million. However, even if money is available, scientists must carry out basic research before any vaccine can be made. They must isolate not only the organism that causes the disease but also each antigenic type. Then the vaccine derived from an attenuated or dead germ must be tested separately for safety and for ability to produce antibodies. Finally, efficacy against the disease must be proved in field trials. Generally the process takes at least ten years.

Once scientists believe they have been successful in making a vaccine in test tubes in the laboratory and in experiments on animals, they must then tackle other problems—particularly whether the vaccine is safe and effective in humans. The vaccine must be tested in man; the first volunteers often include the scientists who developed the vaccine. Thereafter, the human tests move slowly on to increasingly larger groups in what are called field trials. In these series of tests data are collected to answer a wide variety of questions. How safe is the vaccine for different age groups? What types of adverse reactions, if any, occur? How often? How rapidly and to what extent does the body produce antibodies? Do these antibodies provide protection, or are they just artifacts in the research? How effective is the vaccine when the presumed immune volunteer is exposed to the causative organism? What is the most effective means of giving the vaccine: by injection into a muscle or under the skin, by swallowing, or by spraying into the nose? Which groups should receive it? At what age? Will there be a difference in protection if the vaccine is given too early in life? What is the overall benefit-to-risk ratio?

The answers to some of these questions depend on the reported incidence of a disease and its nature. If the incidence of an infectious disease is low but the risk of death (case fatality rate) is high, it may be necessary to immunize hundreds of people to prevent a single death. If the incidence

Photographs, courtesy, Merck Sharp & Dohme

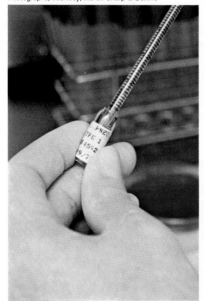
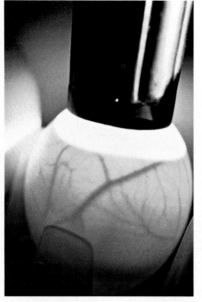
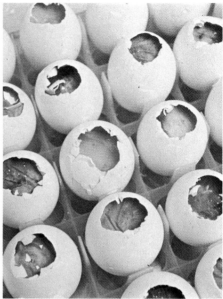
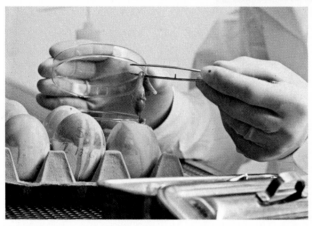
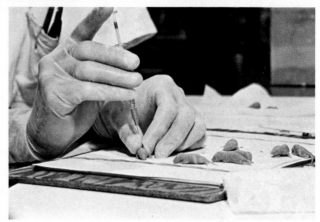

is high but the case fatality rate low, immunization of the same number of individuals could prevent the same number of deaths. Deaths from a disease may be rare, but the manifestations of the infection can be troublesome enough to cause significant time lost from school or work. In such a case the aim of prevention is to reduce the amount of temporary illness.

Because the incidence of preventable infectious diseases remains so high in the third world, the World Health Organization (WHO) has called for an expanded immunization program to reduce the death and sickness toll in less developed countries. But since health services are frequently rudimentary, one of the practical problems is the difficulty in giving the immunizations on a frequent, repeat (booster) basis, as is done in the industrialized countries. Accordingly, one research priority is to develop combinations of vaccines that can be given at one time.

Once a vaccine is approved for marketing, drug companies develop elaborate procedures for making as pure a product as possible; rigid quality controls are built in to each step of the process. The steps vary according to the specific vaccine. To produce a vaccine against most viral diseases,

Manufacture of a vaccine begins with the disease-causing virus or bacterium. The vial at top left contains pneumonia bacteria. Some killed viral vaccines are grown in fertile eggs. Red veins seen in the candling process (top center) indicate the egg contains a live embryo. (Top right) After the seed virus is allowed to grow in the eggs for a precise period of time, the tops of the eggs are sheared off, and the vaccine material—in this case, influenza virus—is separated, the virus killed, and the vaccine purified. (Bottom left) A duck embryo is removed from its egg. It will be processed into a growth medium for rubella virus. (Bottom right) A technician injects a vaccine into mouse fetuses in a standard test of vaccine safety. Animal tests of a vaccine must be successful before human trials can begin.

121

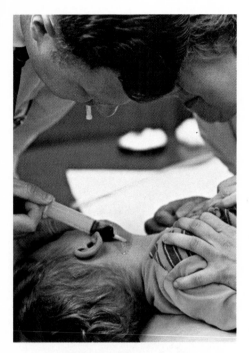

Once a vaccine has given satisfactory results in laboratory tests, the next step is a field trial for effectiveness in a varied population. A vaccine's ability to produce antibodies can be determined by taking blood samples before and after inoculation. The photograph above shows an unusual case—blood samples are usually taken from an arm vein. In February 1978 a new vaccine, Pneumovax (below), was made available for protection against pneumonia for high-risk patients who are most threatened by the disease. Five years of field trials preceded the release of the vaccine.

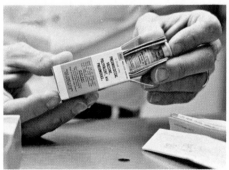

Courtesy, Merck Sharp & Dohme

for example, rows of bottles are stacked on their sides on mechanical rotators. In each bottle living cells are grown in a thin layer, a process called tissue culture. The cells are nourished in a fluid that bathes them as the bottles are turned. In vaccine manufacturing a seed virus is added to some tubes, which become breeding places for the viruses. As the virus grows inside the cells, it is discharged into the nutrient fluid. The unseeded bottles are used as scientific and quality controls.

Some killed vaccines are made by injecting the seed virus into duck or chicken eggs that contain live embryos and that are obtained from special breeds from hatcheries. Machines punch tiny holes in the top of each egg, and then precise amounts of seed virus are injected into each egg. The virus is allowed to grow for a specified period, for example, 48 hours. Then a hole about the size of a dime is sheared off the egg, and the fluid, which is removed or "harvested," contains the raw, impure vaccine and the chicken cells in which the virus grew. In a several step process the vaccine material is separated from the chicken cells through filter papers and by a high speed centrifuge. The chemical formaldehyde then is added to the resulting vaccine to kill the virus. After safety tests are made, the vaccine is sealed in vials, ready for distribution.

Contemporary problems

Just as there is a risk in taking any drug, so too is there a risk in "taking" a vaccine. The frequency and type of adverse reactions vary widely according to the vaccine, and the degree of possible complications permitted is related largely to an immunization's potential benefit. For instance, the risk of death from rabies is so great that doctors and patients in weighing the potential risks and benefits have long accepted the risk of nerve damage that could follow inoculations for this acute viral infection with the Pasteuric-type rabies vaccine. Newer rabies vaccines, however, are considered safer.

Nevertheless, any vaccine can, in unusual circumstances, cause death from allergic reactions. Anaphylactic shock, an induced sensitivity, or allergy, characterized by rapid distress in breathing and sudden fall in blood pressure, is one of the most severe possible side effects. People who are allergic to eggs are warned not to receive injections of vaccine prepared in eggs. Measles and mumps vaccines are currently made in chick fibroblast cell cultures, while German measles vaccine is made in duck fibroblast cultures. (Fibroblasts are connective tissue cells.) A vaccine prepared from such cell cultures is usually devoid of potentially allergenic substances, in contrast to vaccines prepared from viruses grown in whole eggs. More than 90 million live measles vaccines doses have been given in the U.S., but there has not been a single report of anaphylactic reaction.

Encephalitis (inflammation of the brain) is a rare complication of vaccinations. An often temporary form of paralysis called Guillain-Barré was discovered to follow swine influenza immunizations in 1977. Impurities and errors in the vaccine production process have led to serious allergic and paralyzing reactions. However, the most common adverse effects are the mild fever, headache, and redness of the skin at the injection site that follow some immunizations. But it should be emphasized that adverse reactions are rare.

122

Although existing vaccines have more than proved their value, and medical leaders point to the need for developing new ones, a wide variety of scientific, economic, and legal problems have been cited as hampering further progress. Additionally, the very successes of vaccines create the need from time to time to call into question the policy of continued immunization. The dilemma for public health officials is determining at what point a therapy that has proved effective in the past and that carries with it a certain rate of adverse reactions becomes more dangerous than the disease it is designed to prevent. In other words, the risk of the vaccine may have been acceptable when thousands of cases occurred each year, but when the incidence drops to near-zero levels, the risks of the vaccine might outweigh those of acquiring the disease. However, the danger of discontinuing vaccination against infections is that the organisms that cause the diseases and that lurk in the environment will strike unexpectedly and cause epidemic outbreaks. Unfortunately, the exact point when stopping a certain vaccination is more beneficial than continuing it cannot be precisely determined.

Improving existing marketed vaccines is a major scientific concern. The whooping cough vaccine, for example, has been credited with dramatically reducing the incidence of that childhood scourge. But the vaccine preparation is considered crude. Critics in Great Britain argue that the vaccine causes severe brain damage in enough cases to make its dangers outweigh its benefits. This line of reasoning is disputed by infectious disease experts who at the same time urge more research to develop a purer whooping cough vaccine, possibly through new genetic engineering techniques.

The steady attrition of pharmaceutical manufacturers from the vaccine field is also a current problem. Relatively low profit margins, high production risks, rising costs of research and development, difficulties in clinical testing, and increasingly stringent governmental standards of safety and efficacy were cited by a federally sponsored National Immunization Work Group in 1977 as formidable constraints to private investment in vaccine development. The National Immunization Work Group also found that the need for planning and coordination is impeded because no single government agency has the authority to formulate, implement, or evaluate immunization policy, thus hampering the use of beneficial vaccines. Merck Sharp and Dohme of West Point, Pennsylvania, has become the dominant vaccine-producing firm in the United States. A number of other companies have cut back on vaccine manufacture or pulled out of the field entirely.

Declining immunization of U.S. children

Recent surveys have found that the immunization levels of a large percentage of American children are inadequate. Just 65% of American children under the age of 14 are adequately protected against polio, diphtheria, and other infections. The lag has been attributed to apathy among the public, health professionals, and government aides. Immunization programs have been so successful that many Americans have all but forgotten the widespread panic polio caused 25 years ago. And when health officials, trying to motivate parents to immunize their children, speak of an outbreak of two or three cases of an infectious disease as an epidemic, some people regard it as overstatement, thus creating a credibility gap. The call for a program to immunize every American against a strain of influenza that affected 13 soldiers at Fort Dix, New Jersey, accentuated the problem. But the threat of outbreaks will remain as long as a sizable percentage of the population is not protected against an infection. Many health officials say that only smallpox can be totally eradicated, and only the need for smallpox vaccinations can be eliminated in the future. Because the organisms that cause the other infections are present in the environment, ready to strike without warning when they come in contact with a susceptible individual or group of individuals, immunizations must be continued. For that reason the current administration has begun an immunization program designed to lift the lagging immunization level of children above 90%. Health officials have begun a crackdown on enforcing laws that require children to be immunized before attending school. Yet because of the effort to have each individual (or his parent or guardian) sign an informed consent form before being vaccinated, conflicts are arising. Informed consent clearly gives the individual the right to refuse treatment. Most laws have waiver clauses for people who object to vaccinations on religious grounds. Though few laws provide waivers if the individual objects on the basis of informed consent procedures, if substantial numbers of individuals decline immunization, then the goal of immunization levels of more than 90% might not be reached.

Legal issues

Immunization program workers have said that their efforts to raise the immunization levels were being hindered by the costs and problems involved in protecting against professional liability. Vaccine experts agree that the combination of laws, regulations, and liability factors have made it very difficult to do the tests that were necessary to improve available vaccines against whooping cough and other infections. The national study group recognized the seriousness of the problem. It called the area of vaccine development the most threatened of any clinical research field by the problems of liability, informed consent, and other proposed limitations on the use of human subjects in nontherapeutic research.

Legal problems, particularly the potential liability of manufacturers, have confronted vaccine trials and mass immunization programs since the first large-scale polio immunization programs were begun in the 1950s. Drug companies that manufactured the Salk and Sabin polio vaccines were sued. But the legal issues were not regarded as real impediments until the government's ill-fated swine influenza immunization program in 1976.

Few disagree with a report that contended that an adequate diet is the best immunization against common infectious diseases. But common infections will still be health hazards. Federal officials in charge of vaccine development programs contend that the potential for immunization has not yet been fully realized. Application of basic research into genetics of humans and organisms could lead to new and improved vaccines. But these experts warn that in the final analysis, the development of new and improved immunizations may be hampered more by legal factors than by a lack of scientific know-how.

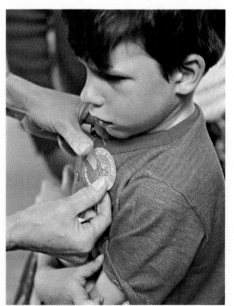

In recent years apathy has led to declining immunization among American children. The threat of outbreaks of diphtheria, whooping cough, polio, and other infections remains unless a sufficient proportion of each generation is immunized. Current efforts are geared to raising levels to 90%.

Courtesy, Merck Sharp & Dohme

Smallpox: Eradication of a Killer

by Donald A. Henderson, M.D., M.P.H.

Smallpox—preeminent among the great pestilential diseases and once prevalent throughout the world—is all but a chapter of history. The world's last known case occurred on Oct. 26, 1977, in eastern Africa. The patient, a 23-year-old man, Ali Maow Maalin, was a resident of the seaport town of Merka, Somalia.

Since then, tens of thousands of national health workers assisted by World Health Organization (WHO) staff have searched village by village throughout Somalia, the adjacent countries of Ethiopia, Kenya, and Djibouti, and in other countries where smallpox has been present within the past decade. Cash rewards have been offered for the discovery of a case: village residents and health staff have reported thousands of different types of illness involving a skin rash. Specimens obtained from patients have been examined in WHO-collaborating laboratories in Atlanta, Georgia, at the Center for Disease Control (CDC) and in Moscow at the Institute of Virus Preparations. All, however, have proved to be cases of chickenpox, scabies, and other types of infection. Final confirmation that the disease is extinct must wait until two full years of such active search in each previously infected country have been completed. In addition, an independent WHO global commission, comprised of recognized experts, must conduct field inspections of each country's program to satisfy itself that the work has been sufficiently thorough to detect cases if they were present. A final declaration that smallpox has been eliminated from the face of the Earth awaits only this

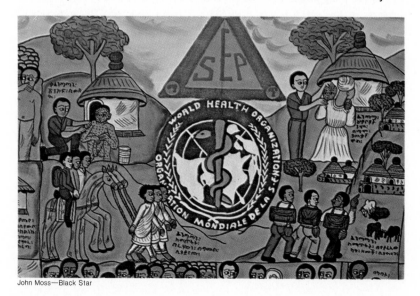

John Moss—Black Star

Donald A. Henderson, M.D., M.P.H., *is Dean of the School of Hygiene and Public Health at The Johns Hopkins University, Baltimore, Maryland; he was formerly Chief of the World Health Organization's Smallpox Eradication Program.*

Smallpox Eradication Program (SEP) poster painted in traditional Ethiopian style by a native artist.

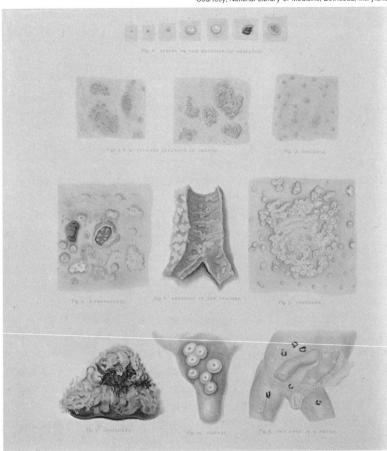

final phase of confirmation; the declaration will mark the first instance in which man has succeeded in the global eradication of a disease.

A devastating viral disease

In 1934 the eminent pathologist Theobald Smith of the Rockefeller Institute for Medical Research in New York City wrote of smallpox: "There is perhaps no disease next to leprosy so loathsome as this, none which has played so important a part in human life everywhere in the world." Smallpox is a disease caused by a virus. It is transmitted directly from person to person in minute droplets expelled from the mouth and nose. There is no known animal or insect reservoir. The susceptible person inhales the virus particles and after a period of about 10 to 12 days experiences high fever and aching pains, similar to the symptoms of severe influenza. In the typical case a rash appears on the face after two to four days and rapidly spreads over the rest of the body, the lesions being most dense on the face, arms, and legs. Small red pimplelike papules become filled with fluid. During the succeeding days they gradually form blisterlike vesicles. Gradually these become larger, and the fluid becomes pustular. In severe cases the pustules are so dense that they merge, forming a confluent mass. Swelling of the face also occurs, and the acutely ill patient is often unrecognizable. Subsequently scabs form and eventually separate during the third or fourth week of rash. Of those afflicted

Smallpox, along with leprosy, has been considered one of the most loathsome diseases known to mankind. The lithograph showing the smallpox rash was drawn by Byrom Bramwell for An Atlas of Clinical Medicine, *1896.*

126

with variola major, the most severe form of the disease, from 20 to 40% die. Death usually occurs during the first two weeks of the illness and is caused by an overwhelming virus infection. Of those who survive smallpox, two-thirds bear permanent pitting scars over the face and body, and some are blind.

During the past decade variola major has been confined principally to Asia. However, cases periodically were imported into Europe. There, despite the greater availability of medical care, the disease proved no less severe because there is no effective treatment. As recently as 1972 a pilgrim returning from Iraq introduced smallpox into Yugoslavia; 175 cases occurred, and 34 victims died.

Historical accounts suggest that until the late 19th century variola major was the only form of smallpox in the world. In the late 1800s, however, a mild form, called amaas (later termed variola minor or alastrim), was described in South Africa. The disease was less severe, and the mortality rate was only 1%. About the turn of the century this form of smallpox appears to have been introduced into the Caribbean and from there spread to North and South America and subsequently to Europe. Gradually, in these areas, it replaced the more severe form of smallpox. Though little is known of the history of smallpox in Africa, during the past two decades a form of intermediate severity has been present there, which causes death in 5 to 15% of its victims.

A 3,000-year history

The origin of smallpox predates written history. It was described as early as 1122 BC in China and is referred to in the ancient Sanskrit texts of India. The mummified head of the Egyptian pharaoh Ramses V, who died about 1156 BC, bears lesions that resemble those of smallpox. Insofar as historical records show, the disease appears to have changed little in character over the centuries. Since it can be maintained only by a continuing chain of human transmission, the virus passing from one infected person to another, population concentrations had to be large enough to permit the infection to persist. Thus, the first cases probably occurred within the past 4,000 to 5,000 years in populated areas of northern China, India, or the Middle East. One can only speculate that the virus strain that first infected humans originated as a result of mutation of one of many related poxviruses in lower mammals.

Although the disease existed in ancient India and China and probably for at least a brief period in the Nile Valley, there is no mention of smallpox-like disease in either Hebrew or Christian biblical writings. A disease of this severity, to which all were susceptible and which spread readily, would almost certainly have been mentioned had it been prevalent. A plausible explanation for its apparent absence relates to an epidemiological characteristic of smallpox—a characteristic critical to its eradication: the smallpox victim can transmit infection only from the time the rash first appears until the scabs separate. Subsequently he is immune to reinfection. Since there are no known animal or insect reservoirs, an unbroken chain of infection is necessary if the virus is to persist. In isolated villages and among populations of low density, there comes a time when there are so few susceptible persons that the disease dies out. It does not recur unless it is reintroduced. This phenomenon was repeatedly observed during the recent global eradication campaign.

In ancient times continuing smallpox transmission would have been possible only in the few densely populated areas of the world. The slow pace of travel and the tenuous contact between the more heavily populated areas may have largely confined smallpox to Asia in the pre-Christian era. With increasing trade and travel and rising population densities in Europe and Africa, smallpox became a more frequent occurrence and eventually became endemic. In 1520 the Spanish conquistadors brought it to the Americas.

A killer of millions

Historically smallpox has wrought unprecedented havoc. Since there is no natural immunity, virtually all persons in endemic areas eventually contracted infection. Cases varied in their degree of severity, but even the least seriously afflicted developed a rash and a prostrating illness, and death occurred in at least 20 to 40%. Beginning in AD 165, then again in AD 251, "plagues," which may have been smallpox, spread throughout the Roman Empire over 15-year periods and killed between one-quarter and one-third of the population. Large urban and rural populations quickly died off, which precipitated economic and civil disruption and eventually led to the collapse of the Mediterranean civilization.

Latter-day parallels are the downfall of the Aztec and Mayan civilizations following the introduction of smallpox in 1520 by the relief expedition that joined Cortés. Fully 3.5 million Indians are estimated to have died. The decimation by smallpox of North American Indian tribes paved the way for European settlement.

In Europe the problem was no less severe. Thomas Macaulay in his *History of England* wrote: "This disease was one of the most terrible of all ministers of death. The havoc of the plague had been far more rapid, but the plague visited our shores only once or twice within living memory; but the smallpox was always present, filling our churchyards with corpses."

Inoculating against smallpox

The earliest form of protection against smallpox was achieved through variolation. This technique, recorded as early as the 6th century BC in China, consisted of taking material from the pustules of a patient and scratching it into the skin of the susceptible recipient. Infection by inoculation, in contrast to infection by the natural respiratory route, resulted in a milder form of smallpox, usually with fewer pustules and less fever. The death rate was about one-tenth as great as that from natural infection. However, the variolated individual represented a risk to those in contact with him since he could readily transmit infection to others by the respiratory route. Variolation spread from Asia into Europe as a folk practice and in the early 18th century was introduced into western Europe, where it was extensively practiced, especially in England. Variolation, however, was utilized to a varying extent in many parts of the world. Even during the past decade large numbers were

128

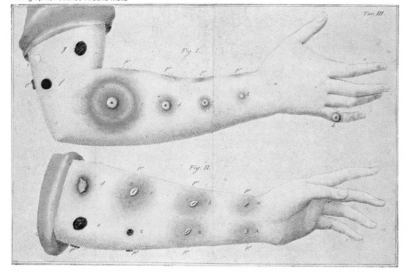

Edward Jenner performed his famous vaccination experiment in 1796 by taking the material from a cowpox lesion on the hand of a dairymaid and inoculating it into an eight-year-old boy. He later showed that the boy was immune to smallpox infection. (Left) Engraving from Treatise on Vaccination, *by Luigi Sacco, Milan, 1809. (Below) Marble sculpture of Jenner vaccinating a child, completed in 1873 by Giulio Monteverde, Genoa.*

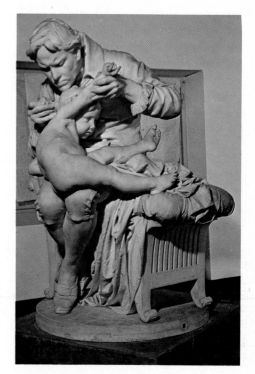

still being variolated in Afghanistan, Ethiopia, and Dahomey, and occasional practitioners were found in Brazil and Pakistan.

Jenner's vaccination. In the course of widespread variolation in England, it became common knowledge that dairymaids who had been infected with an illness called cowpox would not "take the smallpox" when they were variolated. They also were observed to be immune to the natural infection. Basing his work on these observations, Edward Jenner, an English country physician, performed his well-known vaccination experiment in 1796. He took material from a pustular cowpox lesion on the hand of a dairymaid, Sarah Nelms, and inoculated it into the arm of an eight-year-old boy, James Phipps. He showed subsequently that the boy was immune to smallpox infection. Jenner also showed that protection was afforded to others inoculated with cowpox material passed from the arm of one individual to another. Just five years after performing the first successful vaccination, Jenner prophetically announced: "The annihilation of the Smallpox, the most dreadful scourge of the human species, must be the result of this practice."

Within a few years cowpox material was being distributed around the world. Sometimes it was dried on a thread or a glass slide and later reconstituted with water for inoculation. Dispatched in this form, the virus all too frequently died in transit. An alternate approach was to recruit a group of susceptible children who were successively vaccinated by arm to arm passage of the virus during the course of a journey.

Difficulties in providing an assured and adequate supply of cowpox virus curtailed the number of vaccinations during the 19th century. When arm to arm vaccination was used, the not infrequent failure to obtain a successful vaccination resulted in the need to seek fresh cowpox material. Since cowpox-like lesions were sometimes caused by other microorganisms, this sometimes proved difficult. Moreover, in the process of arm to arm vaccination the syphilis spirochete, hepatitis virus, and staphylococcus bacillus were sometimes transferred simultaneously. An important advance was the discovery that large amounts of vaccine could be obtained by scarifying and

129

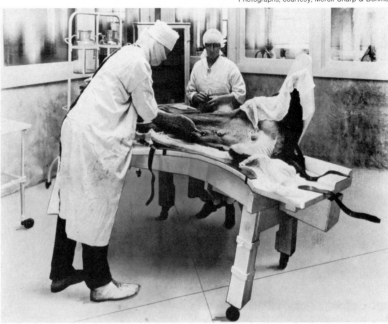

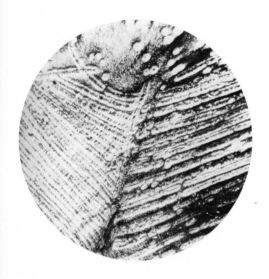

Large amounts of vaccine were obtainable from pustular material on the shaved flanks of inoculated calves.

inoculating the shaved flank of a calf—a technique for vaccine production that is still in use. For many years the pustular material scraped from the flank of a calf was simply suspended in a 50% solution of glycerol and distributed in glass capillaries. Preservation of the virus, however, remained a troublesome problem, especially in tropical areas.

In Europe and North America, use of vaccine prepared in this manner led to a marked reduction in smallpox incidence. On both continents, however, smallpox persisted until World War II, the United States alone recording almost 10,000 cases as recently as 1939. More rigid enforcement of compulsory vaccination and the increasing availability of the electric refrigerator for vaccine storage eventually terminated smallpox transmission. But in the tropical and less developed countries the disease was essentially uncontrolled.

Improving smallpox vaccines. Although Jenner himself had noted that the vaccinia (or cowpox) virus survived longer in a dried than in a pustular form, practical methods for drying large quantities of vaccine of assured potency were slow to evolve. Much of the early research was conducted in France and Germany, countries confronted with the problem of sending vaccine to tropical colonies. Progress in the chemical and physical sciences led to the use of desiccators, then to the drying of vaccine by exposure to sulfuric acid vapor, and eventually to freeze-drying. However, not until the 1950s was an effective, simple, commercially feasible technique developed for large-scale production of freeze-dried vaccine. Leslie Collier of the Lister Institute in London perfected a technique that employed differential centrifugation to partially purify the crude pulp suspension and that added peptone. The material was then freeze-dried in ampules for distribution and the vaccine subsequently reconstituted for use with a glycerol solution. Batches of Collier's vaccine were found to be still potent after storage for two years at 45° C (113° F). In contrast, the effective life of the glycerolated liquid vaccine

130

at this temperature was only a few days. This technological development was a key step in the eventual realization of smallpox eradication.

The monumental problems of eradication

Not until after World War II was smallpox recognized as a disease requiring formal quarantine regulations. A Swiss delegate to the 1926 International Sanitary Conference summed up the problem: "Smallpox has, in reality, no place in an international convention. It is not a pestilential disease in the proper sense of the term; it is, in effect, a disease that exists everywhere. There is probably not a single country of which it can be said that there are no cases of smallpox."

When WHO was established in 1948 as a specialized agency of the United Nations, it approached the problem of smallpox control cautiously. Its interim commission in 1946 had stated, in fact, that it was "impracticable as yet" even to standardize smallpox vaccines.

A primary impetus for smallpox eradication came from Fred Soper, director of the Pan American Sanitary Bureau (later known as the WHO Regional Office for the Americas). Soper had previously directed a remarkably successful program to eradicate yellow fever from the Americas. Although this effort was thwarted by the unexpected discovery of a mammalian jungle reservoir of the virus, yellow fever was successfully eliminated from urban areas. Persuaded of the virtues of eradication as the ultimate, most cost-effective means for prevention, Soper in 1950 proposed a program for smallpox eradication in Central and South America. The feasibility of such an approach had already been shown in the elimination of smallpox from Europe and North America as well as some countries, such as the Philippines, that had less highly developed health services.

This program, undertaken with technical assistance from the Pan American Health Organization, began in 1950. By 1959 smallpox had been effectively eliminated from all countries of the Americas except Argentina, Brazil, Colombia, Ecuador, and Bolivia. That year, at the instigation of the U.S.S.R., the World Health Assembly called for worldwide smallpox eradication. It proposed that all countries where the disease was endemic should undertake programs of vaccination and that countries free of the disease should provide voluntary contributions in support of the effort. WHO and UNICEF were asked to assist countries in developing vaccine-production institutes. In the meantime, donations of vaccine were offered by several countries, and a number of those with endemic smallpox began mass vaccination.

Progress, however, was slow. The interest and energies of many governments were tied up in a WHO global program to eradicate malaria. But the program was costly and required large numbers of health workers. Many countries were reluctant to consider a second eradication program. Moreover, increasing difficulties were experienced with the malaria program, and it became clear that for numerous reasons it was doomed to failure. Not surprisingly, government officials and public health experts alike questioned the possibility of eradicating *any* disease.

Most countries that did undertake mass programs of smallpox vaccination soon experienced difficulties. Vaccine quality was frequently in doubt. There was no mechanism for systematically monitoring quality, and because of production problems or improper preservation vaccination failures were common. Vaccine donations were far too limited to meet the need; voluntary contributions of all forms rarely exceeded $100,000 in value per year. Smaller countries, which experienced some success in their programs, were beset by importation of smallpox across open borders from still-infected neighboring countries. By 1966 little progress had been made, and some countries, such as India, profoundly discouraged by what had been achieved, contemplated reversion to so-called perpetual control programs.

The ten-year WHO campaign

At the 1966 World Health Assembly it was proposed that a special allocation of $2.5 million per year be provided through WHO's regular budget to develop a fully coordinated, intensified global eradication program. It was suggested that this be confined within a ten-year period. Many delegates and scientists had misgivings, doubting that any disease could ever be successfully eradicated. Their reservations were not unrealistic, given the practical problems that could be foreseen of coordinating an activity extending over some 50 countries, the remote areas that would need to be penetrated, and the reluctance of countries to participate in and to support the eradication program over the preceding eight years. Although ultimately agreeing to embark on the intensified eradication program, most delegates privately expressed the hope that better control of smallpox might be achieved, but few expected more than that.

However, the program commenced on Jan. 1, 1967, with the objective of stopping smallpox transmission by Dec. 31, 1976. From the start two major problems were apparent: (1) the need for adequate supplies of full-strength, stable vaccine and suitable vaccination devices, and (2) the selection of a suitable strategy, since mass vaccination alone had proved to be of doubtful value.

Supply of vaccine. In 1967 the endemic countries were all conducting some type of vaccination program to control smallpox. Vaccine was being obtained from diverse sources. Two laboratories, one in Canada (Connaught Laboratories) and one in The Netherlands (Rijksinstituut voor de Volksgezondheid), agreed to collaborate with WHO and to routinely test batches of vaccine being employed in the infected countries. The initial results revealed that not more than 10% of the vaccine then in use met accepted standards. Some batches of vaccine, in fact, were found to contain no detectable virus whatsoever. The total need for vaccine was estimated to be approximately 250 million doses each year. At a cost of one cent per dose, this was equivalent to the total WHO budget provided for all activities in the program. The only practical solution was to encourage the development of vaccine production in the endemic countries and, in the interim, to solicit vaccine contributions from countries already producing it.

Improved vaccine quality was essential. A group of consultants was convened, and a simplified step-by-step manual of production and testing procedures was developed. Selected consultants traveled from laboratory to laboratory in the endemic areas to assess their potential for vaccine production, to determine their needs for equipment, and to participate in the training of local staff. As these laboratories commenced production, each batch was tested by one of the international testing laboratories. Eventually the quality of vaccine improved, and smaller proportions were tested. Throughout the program, however, efforts were made to test at least three batches of vaccine from each laboratory every three months.

During the first years the U.S.S.R. contributed some 140 million doses of vaccine a year and the U.S. some 40 million doses for countries in western and central Africa. Smaller amounts of vaccine were eventually donated by 20 other countries. Increasing quantities of high-quality vaccine gradually became available. By 1970 essentially all vaccine met the accepted rigorous standards. Among other requirements, freeze-dried vaccine had to meet potency standards after incubation at 37° C (98° F) for 30 days. By 1973, 80% of the vaccine being used was produced in the less developed countries, and several of these countries were contributing vaccine for the use of others.

Vaccination technique. Since Jenner's time, vaccine had been applied by some sort of scratch technique in most parts of the world. In the U.S. a better method for vaccination—the multiple pressure technique—had been developed, which produced a higher proportion of successful takes. Unfortunately it proved difficult to teach to lay vaccinators.

A better approach for vaccination appeared to be the jet injector, which had been developed by the U.S. Army Research and Development Command and field-tested for use in smallpox vaccination by the CDC. With this gun, vaccine is expelled under high pressure through a very small opening into the superficial layers of the skin. By 1967 field testing of the gun had been completed, and it was introduced for use in Brazil and countries of central and western Africa. Although theoretically as many as 1,000 persons per hour could be vaccinated with this device, logistically it was impossible to realize this potential: most teams in western and central Africa averaged no more than 1,000 to 2,000 vaccinations per day. With dispersed populations, difficulties of travel, and problems in organization, greater numbers simply could not be vaccinated. Moreover, there was a continuing need for maintenance and repair of the jet injector. In the less developed countries these proved to be formidable tasks.

An optimal approach to vaccination proved to be the very simple bifurcated needle, which was developed by Wyeth Laboratories in Philadelphia, Pennsylvania. The needle, approximately two inches long, has two small sharpened tines at one end. In 1967 it was being tested for possible application for multiple pressure vaccination. But it was reasoned that the needle might be equally effective if held at right angles to the skin and multiple punctures made. The design of the needle was such that only superficial penetration of the skin was possible, a desirable attribute since the vaccinia virus multiplies only in surface layers. Tests of the technique revealed that it was as effective as vaccination with the jet injector or the multiple pressure method. Using the new needle and the multiple puncture method, a vaccinator could be trained in minutes. Another important advantage was that much less vaccine was required for vaccination. When the needle was dipped into

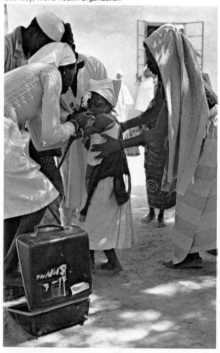

Field testing of the jet injector method of vaccination—an improvement over previous methods—was completed by 1967, and the device was used in Brazil and central and western Africa. But the continuing need for maintenance and repairs made the injector method less than optimal.

133

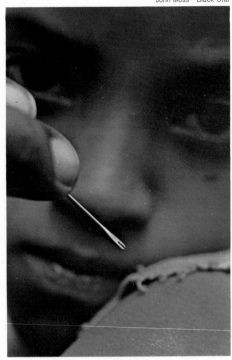

The bifurcated needle—an extremely simple device—proved to be the best method for mass vaccination. (Below) A worker in Delhi, India, carries all the equipment he needs for a day of vaccinating.

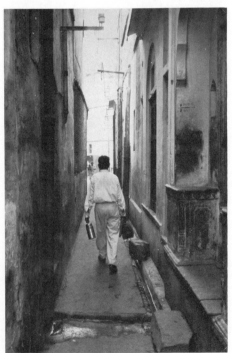

a vaccine vial, only a small amount of solution adhered between the two tines, but an amount sufficient for effective inoculation. Previously a drop of vaccine had been applied to the skin and a scratch made through this drop. A vial that previously was sufficient for vaccinating 25 persons could now be used for nearly 100 persons. Wyeth Laboratories had envisaged that the needle would be used once and discarded, but with the limited budget available, it was stipulated that needles be made of a hard steel alloy that would permit them to be repeatedly sterilized and reused many times.

A further refinement involved "sterilizing" the skin. Earlier studies had shown that use of a 70% alcohol solution achieved little in cleansing arms of those to be vaccinated. Accordingly, studies were conducted comparing two groups of children, one vaccinated without cleansing the skin and one to whom alcohol was applied. There was no difference in the frequency of septic complications. Vaccinators were thus instructed to dispense with cleansing the skin unless the vaccination site was caked with dirt, in which case they removed what they could with a moist cloth. The savings in alcohol, soap, and cotton sponges was significant enough to pay a substantial proportion of the travel costs for vaccinators to get from one area to another.

Finally, a special container for vaccination needles—a simple thermo-resistant plastic receptacle—was developed, which permitted one needle at a time to be dispensed. A vaccinator was issued two such plastic containers, one containing approximately 100 needles and the other empty. As each needle was used, it was placed in the originally empty container. At the end of the day, the container holding used needles could be boiled for 20 minutes, shaken once or twice, and used again the next day. Thus, the vaccinator's equipment consisted only of these two containers plus a few vials of vaccine, all of which could be placed in a shirt pocket. Since the dried vaccine remained potent for a period of one month at 98° F (37° C), a vaccinator could work in tropical areas over long periods far from a source of supplies.

Strategy. Before 1967 progress in national smallpox campaigns had been measured in numbers of vaccinations performed. Unquestionably, a program of vaccination was important, but the real objective was "zero" cases of smallpox. Thus, a two-pronged strategy was developed: vaccination and surveillance. In most of the endemic countries vaccination immunity was low. Thus, systematic campaigns were planned with the objective of reaching 80% of the population—a feasible operational goal—tailored to the particular needs of the country, depending on the health structure as well as social, economic, and other considerations.

The program in Afghanistan illustrates the methodology. The starting point in the campaign was the securing of a map that showed villages and roads. When the program began there, available maps were obsolete and often erroneous. Over the years new villages had been built, and old ones had disappeared. In many parts of the country vaccination was unknown, and there was active resistance to the new procedures. Accordingly, each vaccination team was assigned an "advance man" whose responsibilities included preparation of an updated map that showed each village, school, and

134

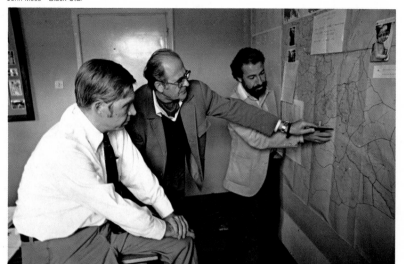

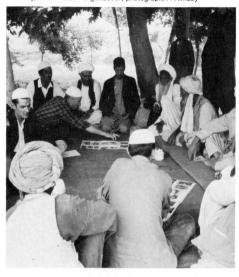

Maps of each target area provided a starting point for eradication efforts. The author (left, in white shirt) and other WHO leaders look at maps of Ethiopia in the program headquarters in the capital, Addis Ababa. In Afghanistan (above), eradication teams explained the nature of the smallpox program to village leaders and solicited their help.

health facility. To do this he traveled ahead of the team to a known village and inquired there about other villages in the area. Each of these was specifically identified on the map and was visited, and information in regard to other villages was sought. The nature of the eradication program was explained to village leaders, and their support was solicited. Later a team performed vaccinations house by house in each village. The team kept no records of individuals vaccinated; rather, when work in a village had been completed, they counted the number of needles that had been used and recorded this number. Few records were thus required, and the teams were able to move rapidly. Ten to 14 days later an assessment team visited a 10 to 20% sample of the villages. If on inspection the assessment team found that less than 80% of those under five years of age bore marks of recent or past vaccination, the vaccination team was required to return to the area *without daily compensation* to revaccinate the area. This technique served admirably to motivate the vaccination teams to reach a high proportion of the villagers.

Regular reporting of all known cases was essential if outbreaks were to be identified and contained. In 1967, however, the reporting of smallpox cases was in ruins. By international convention, smallpox cases were required to be reported weekly to WHO. However, some countries submitted no reports, some reported only sporadically, and some suppressed reports of smallpox altogether. Reporting from national levels was actively encouraged through frequent telegraphic messages and personal contact with government authorities. Concerted efforts were made to persuade governments that it was better to acknowledge known cases and to indicate that action was being taken than to suppress such reports. Eventually weekly telegraphic reports were received from all endemic countries, although the problem of suppression of reports recurred occasionally throughout the course of the program.

The problems at state, district, and local levels were no less serious. Frequently, for example, it was found that some 200 cases would be known at a local level, but owing to casual recording practices or sometimes delib-

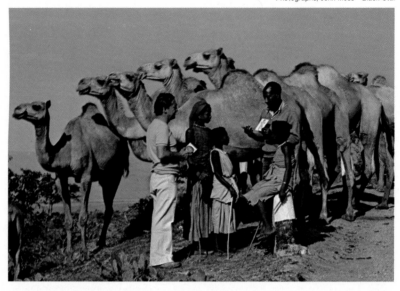

erate suppression of information, no more than 100 cases would be reported to the district level. The same process was often repeated at the district level, so that only 20 cases out of the original 200 would eventually be reported to national authorities.

Various approaches were employed to improve reporting. One of the most effective was to assign a mobile team of two to four persons for each population numbering from two million to five million. The team would visit each health unit on a regular basis to encourage them to report each week the name, age, sex, village, date of onset of rash, and vaccination status of each case discovered that week. Following discovery of cases, the team participated with local health staff in the containment of the outbreak. By repeated visits and by working with the local health staff in containment of outbreaks, reporting steadily improved.

The initial strategy in 1967 called for a two- to three-year mass vaccination program during which the reporting and surveillance system would be developed. It was thought that if 80% of the population were vaccinated, smallpox incidence would be so reduced that with improved surveillance the remaining foci of infection could be rapidly identified and eliminated.

Early in the campaign it became evident that sufficiently effective reporting procedures could be developed more rapidly than had been thought and, moreover, that even in densely populated areas transmission could be interrupted when less than 80% of the population had been vaccinated. William Foege, senior adviser of the eradication effort in eastern Nigeria, discovered that smallpox transmission could be interrupted in less than six months simply by intensive search for cases, isolation of patients, and vaccination of the infected village. The last cases of smallpox in eastern Nigeria occurred when less than half of the population bore marks of previous vaccination. Similar observations were subsequently made in Indonesia and in Brazil. These results led to a shift in the program's strategy to a new emphasis on "surveillance-containment" as the primary goal and mass vaccination as a secondary objective. So-called firefighting teams actively checked rumors of

Reporting suspected cases was an important part of the eradication strategy. (Top) A native worker and a WHO consultant show pictures of people with smallpox to children in Ethiopia. When cases were reported, "firefighting" teams checked rumors, isolated cases, and vaccinated all contacts in the area. (Opposite) An Ethiopian child is vaccinated.

136

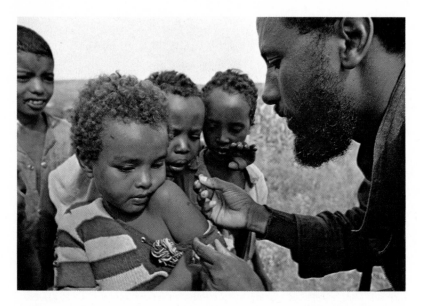

outbreaks, isolated cases, and vaccinated all contacts in the village or area where the infected person resided.

During the surveillance-containment effort it was discovered that smallpox is less easily transmitted from one person to another than had previously been thought; a given patient rarely infected more than two to five others. Since there is a two- to three-week interval between each generation of cases, outbreaks developed slowly. Transmission almost always occurred as a result of close face-to-face contact between the patient and susceptible contacts within a household. As a result, subsequent cases usually occurred among family and friends and tended to concentrate in one part of a town or a portion of a district. Thus, relatively small teams could concentrate their efforts in localized areas and quickly interrupt transmission.

Rapid progress was made, especially in the smaller, less populous countries. In 1967, when the program began, 34 countries were considered to be endemic—*i.e.,* experiencing smallpox continuously among the native population—and 11 others experienced importations. By 1970 the number of endemic countries had decreased to 17 and by 1973 to 6. However, these included India, Pakistan, Bangladesh, and Nepal, which together had a total population of more than 700 million. Techniques employed in Africa were far less successful in these Asian countries. Traditional vaccination programs had been in progress for many years but were poorly supervised. Despite efforts to improve the reporting of cases, many outbreaks remained undetected, and reports were suppressed by local health offices. Containment efforts were less than optimal, and in more densely populated areas, the disease spread more rapidly. Overall, profound pessimism prevailed.

Eradication in India. In June 1973 a plan was developed in India and later extended to the other countries to utilize for one week each month all health workers in a village-by-village, later house-by-house, search for cases. Special containment teams were trained to move into villages in order to stop outbreaks. Assessment teams then visited a sample of the villages to determine whether, in fact, the search had been properly per-

(Below left) Courtesy, Center for Disease Control, Atlanta; (right) John Moss—Black Star

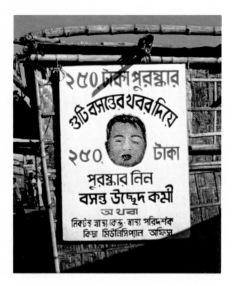

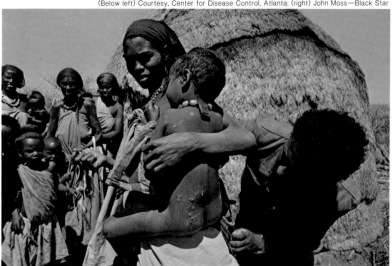

formed. To facilitate the discovery of cases, a reward was offered to anyone who reported a case. The reward initially was small, but as the number of cases declined, the reward was steadily increased. The result of these measures was a veritable explosion in recorded cases.

The experience in one Indian state, Uttar Pradesh, is a good illustration. Considerable work directed toward the improvement of reporting had been in progress for almost two years, but the state was large and had a population of about 100 million persons. During September 1973 between 100 and 300 cases were being reported weekly. During the first search week some 7,000 cases were discovered. Only later was it learned that during that first search only 50% of the villages had, in fact, been searched, and thus the true number of cases at that time was even higher. Once cases were discovered, however, they could be contained. The system of search and containment steadily improved and, eventually, assessments showed that in every state of India more than 90% knew that there was a reward for reporting a

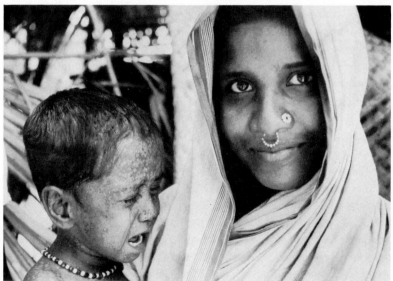

Courtesy, World Health Organization; photograph, D. Tarantola

case of smallpox and where to report a case. Knowledge of the reward resulted in literally hundreds of thousands of illnesses with rash of all types being reported to health authorities. Each of these had to be individually screened and assessed. However, as the smallpox incidence fell and small-pox cases disappeared, the fact that so many possible cases were being investigated provided increasing confidence that if a case were present, it would be discovered. The experiences in Bangladesh, Nepal, and Pakistan paralleled that in India.

In October 1974 the last known case of smallpox in Pakistan occurred; in April 1975, in Nepal; in May 1975, in India. The last known case of smallpox in Asia—the last known case of the severe form of smallpox, variola major, in the world—occurred in a three-year old girl, Rahima Banu, on Bhola Island, Bangladesh, in October 1975.

The final phases: Ethiopia and Somalia. The last battleground of the smallpox eradication campaign was Ethiopia, where the least severe form of smallpox, variola minor, was prevalent. Death rates owing to this form of smallpox were less than 1%. Several factors account for the persistence of smallpox in Ethiopia after it had disappeared from all other countries. For one thing the program there did not begin until 1971, three years later than in any other country. Until then the government's health resources had been almost totally committed to an unrealistically ambitious malaria eradication program, which ultimately foundered. Health staff were limited in number, and even with the addition of a cadre of U.S. Peace Corps volunteers, there were only a few more than 100 on the program staff during the first three years. These were few indeed to cope with a problem extending over an area three times the size of California. Moreover, political unrest was a serious problem; local rebel groups sometimes shot at the teams, and on several occasions national staff and WHO advisers were kidnapped and held hos-tage for days to weeks at a time. A large proportion of the population resided in houses and small villages widely scattered over the mountainous plateau of northern and western Ethiopia, and these villagers frequently resisted the unknown practice of vaccination. Too, roads were few in number and in disrepair; and heavy rains throughout the summer precluded work except in the few major towns and villages accessible by all-weather roads.

Beginning in 1975 nonprofessional staff were recruited and trained to augment the meager available resources. Helicopters were used to help supervise. Steadily the smallpox foci were eliminated, and finally, in August 1976, more than 2,000 Ethiopian local staff and WHO advisers searched the country for seven weeks; no cases could be found anywhere. It was then thought that the last case had been discovered and contained.

However, in late September 1977, cases were discovered in Mogadishu, the capital of Somalia, which lies adjacent to Ethiopia. Subsequent investiga-tion revealed that cases had been imported into Somalia as early as April or May of 1976 and, although discovered by lower level government health officials, reports of the cases had been suppressed.

The 1976 importations were not rapidly contained; not until late in the year were satisfactory measures finally applied. In mid-January 1977 transmis-sion appeared to have been stopped in Mogadishu. A limited search among

As eradication progressed, money was offered to anyone who reported a case of suspected smallpox. A poster in Bangladesh (opposite far left) announces rewards. Cash incentives inevitably generated vast reporting of all kinds of illnesses with rash. A worker in Ethiopia (right) checks a case and finds that it is chickenpox. Finally, in October 1975 three-year-old Rahima Banu (bottom) on Bhola Island, Bangladesh, had the world's last known case of the severe form of smallpox.

nomads in the vast Ogaden desert area surrounding the capital revealed no cases: again it was thought that the last case had been detected; again it was discovered later that smallpox had spread in at least three to four nomadic camps in the desert; and again some of these cases were known to lower level government health authorities but were not reported.

In March, as the rainy season began, the nomadic groups moved actively across the desert, often concentrating in agricultural development areas. The disease spread rapidly, causing the government to declare a state of national emergency. More staff from Somalia were deputed to the program, and additional WHO advisers were brought into the country. By June a major effort was under way: in all, more than 3,000 cases occurred. Finally the last known case developed smallpox rash on Oct. 26, 1977. An intensive search continued and, as in other countries, rewards for the discovery of a case were offered. Thousands of cases were screened and hundreds of specimens examined in laboratories, but none was smallpox. Meanwhile, in adjacent areas of Ethiopia, Kenya, and Djibouti intensive search operations were continued. An importation into Kenya had occurred early in 1977, but it was rapidly contained. No cases were found thereafter. The ten-year target date for eradication of smallpox was thus missed by only ten months.

Confirmation of eradication. To confirm that eradication has been achieved, two full years of intensive search will have to be conducted to be certain that transmission of smallpox is not still occurring. Only then can a

In 1967 smallpox was endemic in many parts of the world. By 1972 and 1975 dramatic progress in conquering the disease was evident. The final map (1977) indicates total eradication as the ten-year WHO program achieved its goal.

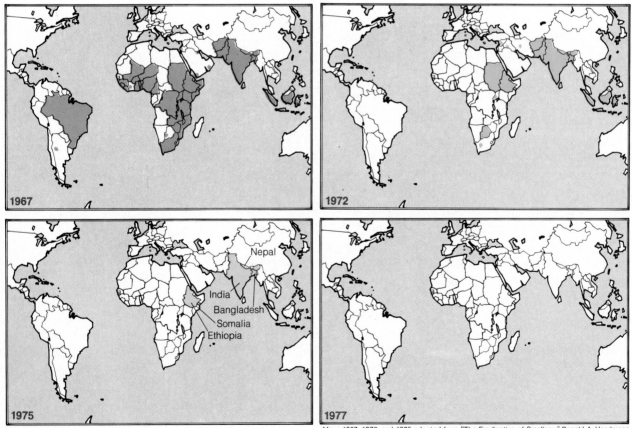

Maps 1967, 1972, and 1975 adapted from "The Eradication of Smallpox," Donald A. Henderson

WHO international commission be convened to determine through inspection of records and field visits that smallpox is no longer present. So far, WHO commissions have certified smallpox eradication in South America, Asia, and all but the eastern horn of Africa. The last areas will probably be certified late in 1979 or early in 1980.

Meanwhile, throughout the course of the program, many research studies have been conducted in an effort to discover a naturally occurring smallpox virus reservoir in nature. None has been found. The fact that during the past ten years every focus of smallpox in nonendemic areas has been able to be traced to known endemic regions is the most persuasive evidence that indeed no natural reservoir of smallpox does exist.

With the cessation of smallpox transmission, variola virus will be confined to research laboratories. Since 1975 WHO has been engaged in a special program to identify and register all laboratories retaining stocks of variola virus. Most laboratories have destroyed their stock of virus; it is expected that by 1980 not more than four laboratories will retain variola virus—and this under high security precautions.

Cost. Records have been maintained documenting all costs of the eradication program since 1967. By the time eradication is finally certified, approximately $110 million in international assistance will have been made available—approximately $8 million per year. The less developed countries themselves will have spent approximately twice that amount, but few will have expended much more than they were spending on relatively unsuccessful smallpox-control programs. With final confirmation of eradication, vaccination everywhere can be stopped; the savings worldwide on vaccination will be in excess of $1 billion annually.

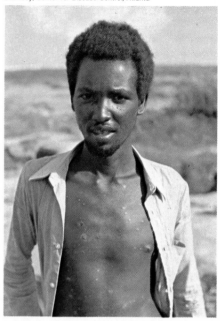

Ali Maow Maalin, the world's last known smallpox victim, in Merka, Somalia, October 1977.

Jenner's dream realized

The achievement of the eradication of smallpox itself represents a notable milestone in medical history. But the lessons implicit in the achievement are perhaps more important. The international mobilization of resources, the cooperation achieved among countries, and the subjugation of national interest to a common goal executed under the guidance of a United Nations agency offer hope for the future that equally ambitious enterprises are possible. The fact that it *was* possible to organize and execute a health program that extended into the most remote villages in some of the most under-developed parts of the world suggests that a longer-term program of health care capable of similar outreach is within reason. The savings achieved at such minimal cost dramatizes the potential of preventive medicine. Already in progress is a program whose goal is immunization of the world's children against six common diseases preventable by immunization—diphtheria, pertussis, tetanus, poliomyelitis, measles, and tuberculosis. And a worldwide cooperative program of research to find effective means for preventing the world's major tropical diseases is also under way.

Finally, a principal delegate to the World Health Assembly summed up the significance of the WHO smallpox eradication effort: "If the World Health Organization were to have achieved nothing other than the eradication of smallpox, it would have more than justified its existence."

FOR ADDITIONAL READING:

Dixon, Cyril W. *Smallpox.* London: J. & A. Churchill, 1962.

Henderson, Donald A. "Smallpox." In *Preventive Medicine and Public Health* [by] Maxcy [and] Rosenau. Edited by Philip E. Sartwell. 10th ed. New York: Appleton-Century-Crofts, 1973.

McNeill, William H. *Plagues and Peoples.* Garden City, N.Y.: Anchor Press, 1976.

World Health Organization, Geneva, Switz. "Smallpox Target Zero." *World Health* (October 1972).

The Acute Leukemias
by James F. Holland, M.D.

The acute leukemias are a group of cancers arising in the bone marrow that in their untreated state lead to death. They are to be distinguished from the chronic leukemias, which are characterized by white blood cells that mature more effectively to normal adult cells and which, in an untreated state, run a more protracted and irregular course to death. Although most authorities would agree on at least six types of chronic leukemia, the most common by far are chronic lymphocytic leukemia and chronic myelocytic leukemia.

Similarly, the acute leukemias represent several different cancers of the white cells that ordinarily populate the bone marrow. Many different subvarieties and subclassifications of the three principal types—acute myelocytic, acute lymphocytic, and acute monocytic—are recognized.

Leukemic cells are often individually indistinguishable from corresponding normal cells of the same age. Young white blood cells are, however, disproportionately represented in acute leukemia, and the failure to proceed through normal differentiation gives the appearance of a bone marrow populated by proliferating immature cells. There are several characteristics that distinguish them as a malignant population of young cells, not just an adaptive response to some overwhelming infection. These include the frequent appearance of chromosomes separating into two prospective daughter cells during mitosis; a large nucleolus or multiple nucleoli, recognizable structures in the nucleus of the cell where vigorous RNA synthesis is in progress; disproportion in the normal relationship between nuclear and cell diameters; and often larger amounts of cytoplasm (the protoplasmic substance of the cell outside the nuclear membrane) than would ordinarily occur. Cytoplasmic structures may also appear immature for the age of the cell as judged from its nuclear configuration.

James F. Holland, M.D., is Professor and Chairman of the Department of Neoplastic Diseases and Director of the Cancer Center at Mount Sinai School of Medicine, New York City.

(Facing page) Photomicrograph of the bone marrow of a person with acute myelocytic leukemia.

142

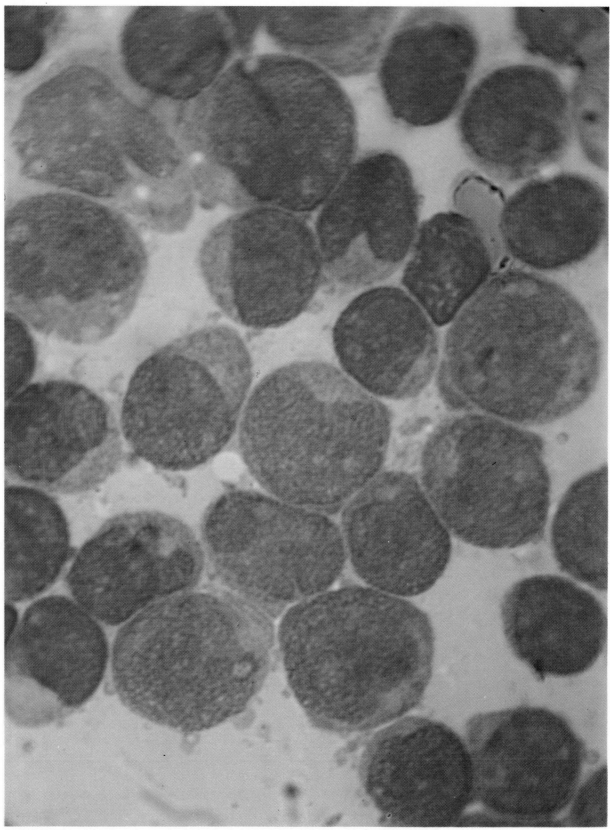

Hau C. Kwaan, M.D.

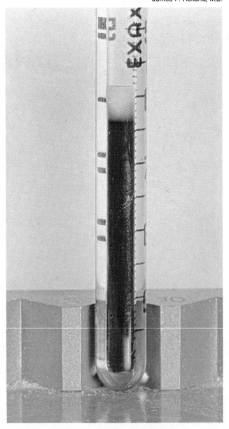

James F. Holland, M.D.

Leukemia *means "white blood." This centrifuged anticoagulated leukemic blood shows a much increased layer of leukocytes, or white blood cells, at the interface between the layer of red blood cells at the bottom and the plasma at the top.*

A composite interpretation of the pattern of cellular maturation, infiltration, and the individual cellular characteristics has met with disagreement among experts. There is no absolute minimum threshold above which acute leukemia can always be diagnosed with certainty. This phenomenon has given rise to such terms as preleukemia and dysmyelopoiesis (abnormal marrow function).

Acute leukemic cells originate in the marrow and may be so prominent there that they replace all other normal marrow elements, presumably by suppression of their formation and by occupying the space in which normal cells would ordinarily proliferate. Although under normal conditions immature cells rarely enter the circulating blood, by mechanisms not wholly clear such immature leukemic cells do traverse the walls of the vascular channels in the marrow and enter the blood. There they may be present in approximately the same numbers as normal leukocytes, or they may reach much higher numbers—as many as several hundred thousand cells per microliter (cubic millimeter) of blood. A normal number of leukocytes is from 4,500 to 10,000.

Despite the excess of leukemic cells in the marrow, blood, and tissues, leukemia is often principally manifest as a disease of deficiencies of normal blood function. Knowledge of the normal constitution and role of the blood provides a backdrop against which these deficiencies can be appreciated.

The normal blood

The marrow is an organ diffusely spread throughout the central cavity of bones, populated by the marrow stem cell and its progeny. The marrow stem cell functions as a self-reproducing seed crop that assures the integrity of its line. A stem cell, after reproducing itself, can reserve one daughter cell for perpetuation of the stem line. The other daughter cell multiplies repeatedly, differentiating into various kinds of blood cells: an erythroid precursor, which gives rise to red cells; a myeloid precursor, which gives rise to granulocytes; a monocytic precursor, which gives rise to monocytes; and a megakaryocytic precursor, which gives rise to megakaryocytes, large multinucleate cells whose cytoplasm becomes blood platelets.

Lymphocytes are cells that probably arise in the marrow from the hematopoietic (blood-forming) stem cell and circulate to the lymph nodes, spleen, tonsils, and lymphoid patches of the intestine, where further growth occurs. Lymphocytes that are present in the bone marrow and other distinctive sites are known as B cells. Some lymphocytes of the marrow circulate to the thymus, where they are processed, taking on special properties, and are known as T cells. A few lymphocytes lack markers for either T or B and are known as null cells. In addition to these cells that are formed in the marrow and that accomplish most of the normal blood functions, there are several other less common cell types of less certain function. The function of a normal quantity of erythrocytes is to carry oxygen to tissues and thus allow normal cerebral function, muscular work, exercise tolerance, and a feeling of well-being. Normally granulocytes kill random bacterial invaders of the bloodstream that may appear during dental extraction, tooth brushing, and even chewing; they also attack bacteria in the gut and bacteria from

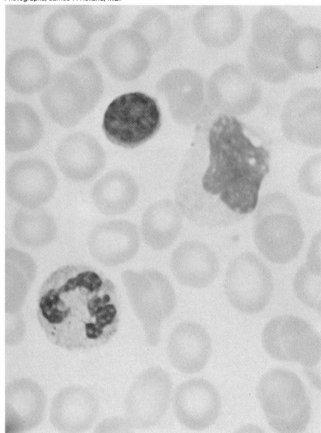

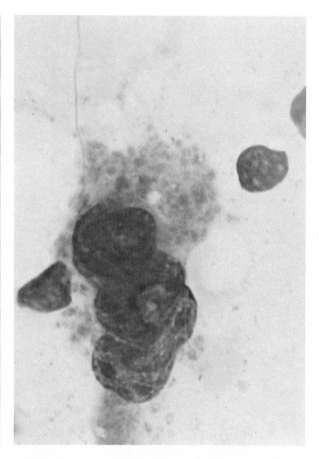

minor skin infections. Though monocytes are mobilized slower than and follow behind the granulocytes, they too are important in the defense against microorganisms in the tissues. Platelets adhere to the inner layer of cells that line the larger blood vessels and constitute the fragile wall of the capillaries. Platelets have the capacity to activate the clotting mechanism by aggregating locally, thus preventing or stopping bleeding through a ruptured capillary or vessel wall.

Lymphocytes are the mediators of immunity. The B cells produce antibody in small quantity and mature into plasma cells, which produce abundant antibody. T cells (and under special conditions B cells) interact directly with foreign cells and kill them. Lymphocytes can also be mobilized by foreign cells and by some fungal and viral infections.

Symptoms and signs of acute leukemia

The acute leukemias are explained almost entirely by the dysfunction of normal marrow and blood cells. Several blood cell deficiencies are common: anemia, granulocytopenia, thrombocytopenia, monocytopenia, and lymphocytopenia. Anemia, a deficiency of the red blood cells, may be manifest by pallor, weakness, easy fatigability, headache, ringing in the ears, dizziness, rapid heart action, and in the elderly or those with preexisting cardiovascular disease, inadequate oxygen-carrying capacity of the blood to supply the oxygen demand of the heart and thus angina pectoris or cardiac

(Left) Photomicrograph of normal circulating blood. Many red cells are seen in the background. The prominent cell at left is a granulocyte; the one in the center is a small lymphocyte; and the one to the right, a monocyte. The photomicrograph at right shows a normal megakaryocyte: the cytoplasm is intensely granular and at the periphery is pinching off to make platelets. The multilobed nucleus is characteristic of this type of cell.

145

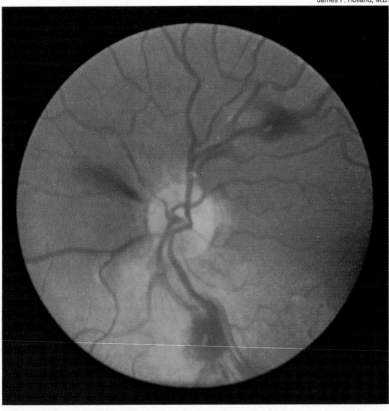

A deficiency of blood platelets may be a symptom of acute leukemia, sometimes manifest as bleeding into the eye. Here flame-shaped hemorrhages in the retina are visible; blood vessels of the eye are shown converging on the optic nerve where it enters the retina.

failure. Any and all of these symptoms of anemia may be present in acute leukemia. It is not uncommon that weakness, general fatigue, and an insidious loss of mental and physical capacities bring the patient to the physician in the first place. Granulocytopenia, a deficiency of granulocytes, leads to skin infections (boils), dental infection, bacterial pharyngitis, perirectal abscess, sinusitis, urinary tract infection, infections around the nails, and pneumonia. In the patient the first sign may be a common infection that may resolve with appropriate standard care. Repeated infections, however, are a hallmark of granulocytopenia. Thrombocytopenia, a deficiency of platelets, may be recognized by petechiae, small hemorrhagic spots, particularly in the lower extremities, where the gravitational pressure of the blood is greater. It may also be manifest as easy or spontaneous bruising, nosebleeding, gum bleeding, and, less commonly, as internal bleeding into the intestinal or urinary tracts or bleeding into the eye, into the brain, or into the meninges surrounding the brain.

Monocytopenia and lymphocytopenia, deficiencies of monocytes and lymphocytes, are not as readily recognizable and frequently do not have specific symptoms, although viral infection from herpes simplex in the form of fever blisters, sometimes exceptionally prominent at the onset of acute leukemia, may be a manifestation of impaired immunity.

In addition to these symptoms of deficiency, the accumulation of leukemic cells may cause a number of symptoms from their very bulk and from invasion of normal tissues. Leukemic cell invasion of the marrow may, in addition to the suppression of normal marrow function, lead to increased

146

intraosseous pressure (pressure within the bones) and pain. Acute leukemia in children has often been mistaken for rheumatic fever because of the bone and joint manifestations.

Leukemic cells that accumulate and proliferate in lymph nodes, the liver, and the spleen cause enlargement of these organs. An elevated leukocyte count in the peripheral blood is evidence of cells in transit out of the marrow. They may appear as infiltrations in other tissues; in the skin and mucous membranes infiltrates occur often at the site of trauma or infection. In cases of acute myelocytic leukemia with exceptionally high leukocyte counts, invasion of blood vessel walls in the brain may lead to fatal hemorrhage when the walls weaken.

A typical history of acute leukemia might include a few weeks of exceptional fatigue after ordinary activities, weakness, and avoidance of strenuous challenge. Queries by others about pallor and lack of energy may be punctuated by an unusual infection, often slow to heal. A failure to regain normal health and activity and a resolution to do something about it seem frequently to be triggered by a second infection or unexplained fever. Such infections often precipitate a shower of pinpoint hemorrhages in the lower extremities, usually unnoticed by the patient; in some cases excessive bruising from forgotten or nonexistent trauma has been observed. Dull aching that is hard to define is not unusual. When the patient recognizes that the total symptom train is not one of a lingering cold, medical examination is usually sought. Such examination may disclose a few enlarged nodes, possibly splenomegaly (enlargement of the spleen), evidence of minor infection, bruising, and petechiae. A blood count generally is done, which rarely is diagnostic but indicates the need for bone marrow examination.

Prognosis. In their untreated state, or when therapy is ineffective for a specific patient, the sequence of abnormalities in the acute leukemias continues at an ever more rapid rate, complications multiply, and death from overwhelming infection or bleeding into a vital organ often supervenes. Rarely, death is due to a tumor of leukemic cells invading a vital area.

Fortunately this once inevitable ending is no longer inescapable. Children with acute lymphocytic leukemia, particularly those whose leukemic cells demonstrate neither the B nor the T surface antigens but which fall into the more benign null cell group, have an overall prognosis for cure by modern treatment in approximately half of the patients. Those with the T and B cell subtypes of acute lymphocytic leukemia do not fare nearly so well. In children who die, however, the terminal event is sharply altered by treatment. Death may be characterized by all the phenomena described above or by markedly hypofunctional marrow—a result of the intensity of drug treatment required—with inadequate regeneration of normal marrow cells to sustain life. In patients with acute myelocytic leukemia survival patterns have improved over the past decade. Death may occur from uncontrolled disease or from marrow aplasia. The latter represents the failure of stem cells to repopulate the marrow in time to sustain life after a chemotherapeutic effort. Due to increasing resources and skills available to physicians, particularly platelet transfusions, bleeding is infrequently a cause of death; infection is the principal cause.

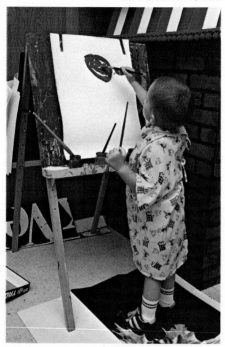

Approximately half the children with acute lymphocytic leukemia have an overall prognosis for cure with modern treatment. The leukemic child may be converted from profoundly ill to robust in a matter of weeks, and he or she is generally hospitalized only long enough to bring the disease under control; some may not be hospitalized at all. This young leukemia patient is in the Sidney Farber Cancer Institute in Boston.

Frequency. The frequency of leukemia at different ages varies markedly between the acute lymphocytic and acute myelocytic varieties. Acute lymphocytic leukemia reaches a peak incidence between ages 2 and 4, when 50 per million per year are affected. This falls to 20 per million by age 10, then below 10 per million per year at age 20 until after age 65, when it again climbs to 15. On the other hand, acute myelocytic leukemia is quite constant from birth through the first 10 years at about 10 cases per million per year. Then it rises to about 15 per million until age 55, after which the incidence progressively increases to 50 at age 75. This suggests cumulative injury from a ubiquitous toxic agent, presumably from elements in the environment. Clinically, 80 to 90% of children with leukemia have acute lymphocytic leukemia, and 80 to 90% of leukemic adults have acute myelocytic leukemia. This distribution may in part be related to cells that are actively growing when a leukemogenic stimulus is encountered. In mice it is possible to direct the type of leukemia that appears after viral inoculation. It has been demonstrated that removal of the thymus and spleen, organs with large lymphoid cell populations, decreases the ordinary frequency of acute lymphocytic leukemia and augments the incidence of acute myelocytic leukemia.

Causes of leukemia

The etiology of human leukemia has not been established. Several causes are known, but whether they work through a final common pathway or are totally independent in their mechanism of causing the cancer has not been clarified. The vast majority of patients with acute leukemia have not been exposed to a known cause, however.

Exposure to gamma rays or X-rays in the course of medical or industrial activities has led to substantially increased leukemia incidence. Survivors of the atomic bombings of Japan—Hiroshima and Nagasaki (1945)—also have a higher incidence of the acute leukemias. Survivors of cancer treated with radiotherapy, particularly if combined with chemotherapy that uses an alkylating agent, have a higher risk of acute myelocytic leukemia. Chronic administration of alkylating agents alone, as in patients with myeloma, ovarian cancer, and Hodgkin's disease, has led to increased incidence of leukemia. These latter cases may arise from direct genetic (chromosomal) injury or from the effect of the drugs causing major depression of marrow function. Certain other drugs that rarely cause major marrow depression such as phenylbutazone and chloramphenicol, after producing marrow injury, have been followed by reported instances of acute myelocytic leukemia. Benzene, a chemical that was once used widely for dry cleaning and is still used in the chemical industry as a reagent and solvent, can cause acute myelocytic leukemia; in Denmark the prohibition of the use of benzene in dry cleaning led to a decrease in the incidence of acute leukemia in workers.

RNA viruses are known to cause leukemia in fish, birds, mice, cats, dogs, monkeys, and gibbon apes. Some of these viruses may be transmitted horizontally (*i.e.,* via some route of contagion). This is a common phenomenon among felines. When cats showing overt or immunologic evidence of leukemia are removed from residential colonies, the appearance of new cases of leukemia is sharply reduced. Such horizontal transmission has also been demonstrated in feral mice. In other laboratory experiments conducted with artificially inbred strains, the RNA virus may be transmitted vertically (genetically) from mother to offspring.

Viral particles have been seen in human leukemic cells, and biochemical evidence of enzymes characteristic of viruses has repeatedly been observed in leukemic cells. There is no convincing proof that either of these observations indicates viral etiology of the human disease, however. Leukemic cells may provide a rich environment in which passenger viruses can thrive. Endogenous viruses that develop within the cell, apparently characteristic of mammalian cells, may be stimulated or released in leukemic cells. Such viruses are composed of RNA; the specific enzyme that allows RNA to serve as a template for the transcription of DNA—a sequence reversed from the normal process—is present. Thus, although some indication of viral infection is present in leukemic cells, it is not certain that such infection is the result of a virus that caused the leukemia. Additionally, it has been conjectured that the effect of radiation and chemicals on inducing leukemia might be explained by activation of a hypothetical virus.

The appearance of multiple cases of acute leukemia in clusters has been described in several outbreaks in the world. These are particularly provocative when children under six living within one mile of one another have contracted acute leukemia in a period of less than 90 days. When sought prospectively, however, in large and critically conducted epidemiologic studies, predicted clusters have not appeared. Environmental factors, coincidence, the presence of intermediate asymptomatic carriers, and the manifestation of leukemia as a clinical endpoint of a more benign viral infection in only a few of those affected are all possibilities that could affect the incidence. In addition to these potential causes that could affect previously normal individuals, some constitutional disorders characterized by chromosomal abnormality or instability, such as Down's syndrome (trisomy 21 or mongolism), have been associated with increased incidence of acute leukemia.

Treating leukemia

No successful method is known to bring about maturation of leukemic cells. Techniques to convert leukemic cells to normal do not exist. Although the administration of a derivative of a cellular hormone, dibutyryl cyclic adenosine monophosphate (cyclic AMP), has been shown to convert other types of cancer cells to normal appearing cells, these cells still have the neoplastic potential of cancer when inoculated into susceptible animals.

The goal of leukemia treatment then is to kill leukemic cells by selective poisoning. In order to attain therapeutic success, the treatment must have a more noxious effect on the leukemic cells than on the most sensitive vital normal cell line. This situation is optimized when the regenerative capacities of normal cells are more rapid than those of leukemic cells, thus allowing restitution of vital function by progressively decreasing the leukemic population and allowing normal cells to grow back. The most sensitive host cells to any leukemic medication are ordinarily the bone marrow stem cells. For

Photographs, James F. Holland, M.D.

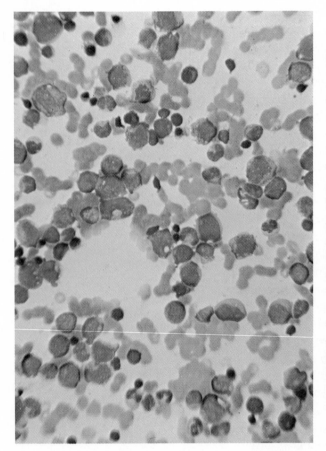 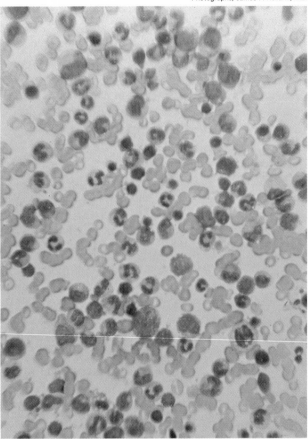

The photomicrograph (left) of a person with acute lymphocytic leukemia indicates a predominant cell type infiltrating the bone marrow before treatment. After the patient received five weeks of chemotherapy (right), normal marrow cell types returned and leukemic cells disappeared.

some drugs the mucous membranes of the entire alimentary canal (the digestive passage that extends from the mouth to the anus) are exquisitely sensitive. Profound toxicity to the mucous membranes of the alimentary canal or to the normal marrow stem cell, which does not allow recovery before the advent of fatal infection or bleeding, is one of the potential hazards of therapy.

Chemotherapy and remission. The usual procedure, after the diagnosis is determined, is to proceed with vigorous treatment designed to induce remission—a condition in which evidence of the disease disappears. In acute lymphocytic leukemia this can be accomplished in approximately 90% of patients using a combination of vincristine, prednisone, and asparaginase. These drugs are independently active, and by virtue of affecting the multiple subvariants of cells, which have less sensitivity to any single agent, the combination diminishes the likelihood of encountering resistance.

The induction of remission is a dramatic phenomenon. Fall in leukocyte count, shrinkage of enlarged lymph nodes, spleen, and liver, and regression of bone marrow infiltration may occur in 7 to 28 days. Emergence of an abundant, maturing, normal marrow from the normal stem cells that had been suppressed occurs next. The first sign of a remission is usually an increasing platelet count, increasing granulocyte count, and the patient's feeling of well-being. The child with acute lymphocytic leukemia may be converted from profoundly ill to robust and active in three to six weeks.

150

Complete remission of the disease is characterized by absence of detectable organ infiltration, normal values of the peripheral blood, and normal appearance and distribution of the marrow cells. It has proved impossible to cure children simply by continuing this induction treatment. However, shifting treatment to powerful antimetabolite drugs that interfere critically with the normal nutrition of the cell may kill the residual growing leukemic cells once they are below the threshold of detection. The presence of residual leukemic cells is known because premature cessation of treatment leads to relapse with cells identical to those present at the outset of the disease. Methotrexate and 6-mercaptopurine are the most important of these antimetabolites, although several other drugs have also been used in this maintenance phase. Too low a dose or too short a duration of treatment compromises therapeutic success. Periodic reinforcement with vincristine and prednisone, as used in the induction, has been shown to be of significant value.

Drugs used during the induction and maintenance phases reach high concentrations in the blood plasma and in the fluid between cells. This latter concentration alters the milieu to which most leukemic cells are exposed. The passage of drugs into the cerebrospinal fluid, however, is sharply restricted by the characteristics of the membrane that separates the blood from the brain and spinal fluid. Leukemic cells that may have entered the brain or meninges (membranes that envelop the brain and spinal cord) are thus protected as if in a sanctuary by escaping the lethal concentrations of drugs to which cells in the systemic circulation are exposed. Central nervous system leukemia is a characteristic complication in 50% of children. Control of this phenomenon has been approached by administration of methotrexate directly into the cerebrospinal fluid by a lumbar puncture needle and by the application of X-ray treatment to the entire cranial contents, or by a very high concentration of methotrexate given intravenously to promote its passage across the blood-brain barrier. The central nervous system leukemia attack rates can be reduced to less than 15% with these techniques. Recent evidence suggests that cranial radiotherapy in the doses used has adverse effects on the growing brain, and its use is currently being critically reexamined.

Results in children. Leukemia therapy in the U.S. has primarily emphasized combinations of drugs and their scheduling to gain maximum leukemic cell kill. Using these techniques survival has dramatically increased in children with acute lymphocytic leukemia. If one excludes T cell leukemias, the results are substantially better. The treatment of T cell leukemia is only transiently successful, and although rapid remission induction is achieved, relapse is early and frequent. In children between two and eight years of age with leukocyte counts below 30,000 per cubic millimeter, the prognosis is considerably better, but at older ages or in the presence of a higher leukocyte count, the prognosis for acute lymphocytic leukemia is worse. The recognition of an abundant amount of cytoplasm and either one prominent nucleolus or two or more nucleoli in the cells of a leukemic patient generally foreshadows an unfavorable outcome.

In Europe immunization of children with radiated leukemic cells from adult myeloblastic leukemic donors and the administration of attenuated tuber-

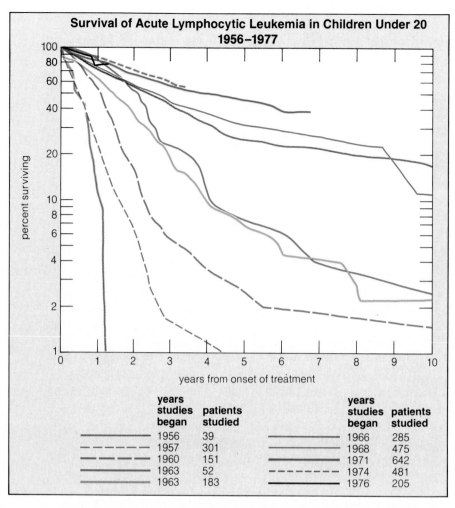

**Survival of Acute Lymphocytic Leukemia in Children Under 20
1956–1977**

percent surviving

years from onset of treatment

	years studies began	patients studied		years studies began	patients studied
	1956	39		1966	285
	1957	301		1968	475
	1960	151		1971	642
	1963	52		1974	481
	1963	183		1976	205

Great progress in the survival rates of leukemic children has been demonstrated over a 21-year period in studies by an organization known as Cancer and Leukemia Group B. Of children whose treatment began in 1956, none survived more than 15 months, while of those whose treatment began in the 1970s, more than 50% survived more than five years, and many are still alive.

culosis vaccine, BCG (bacillus Calmette-Guérin), has been repeatedly reported to prolong remission duration and survival. Confirmatory studies in the U.S. have not been done, perhaps because BCG alone has not worked and perhaps because increasing success in chemotherapeutic management with improving survival has curtailed interest in immunotherapeutic approaches.

Over 20 years ago a U.S. study conducted by an organization known as Cancer and Leukemia Group B demonstrated no survival beyond 15 months in children. That study, however, has been succeeded by progressively evolving investigations—now showing more than 50% of children apparently cured. Of children who were treated for eight months of intensive maintenance in 1966, 27% are alive and well ten years after cessation of chemotherapy. For them the term *cure* is warranted.

Results in adults. It is more difficult to induce remission in patients with acute myelocytic leukemia than in those with acute lymphocytic leukemia insofar as the myelocytic leukemic stem cell is more similar to the normal marrow cell than is the lymphocytic leukemic stem cell. Thus with the intensive drug treatments used, inevitable injury is inflicted on the normal marrow stem cells. Sharp reduction or absence of normal marrow cells may persist

152

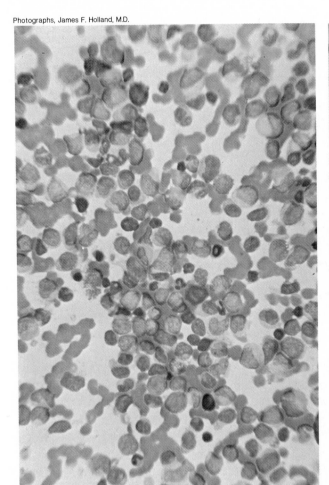

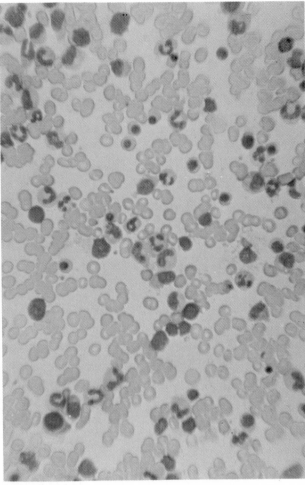

for weeks following destruction of the leukemic cells by combined chemotherapy. The most widely used combinations include cytosine arabinoside and often an anthracycline antibiotic, daunorubicin or doxorubicin (adriamycin). Bleeding and infection are common during the induction period. When treating acute myelocytic leukemia with these drugs, access to cellular replacement therapy is imperative. Platelet transfusions, granulocyte transfusions in the presence of sepsis or presumptive sepsis, and red cell transfusion may all be necessary. Regression of leukemic infiltration, progression of already profound depressions in leukocyte and platelet counts, the appearance of fever, and a plethora of lesser complications can and usually do appear. They make the weeks of remission induction in patients with acute myelocytic leukemia among the most complicated and challenging in all of medicine. Failure to attain total eradication of leukemic myeloblasts from the marrow after the first course of drug administration is not uncommon, and a second course must be initiated with a repetition of the entire sequence of events. It has been found that administration of cytosine arabinoside continuously for seven days with three daily injections of daunorubicin is more often effective than lower dose repetitive courses.

The appearance of platelets and granulocytes in the peripheral blood may

A monotony of cell type and an excessive number of cells characteristic of acute myelocytic leukemia are apparent in the photomicrograph of bone marrow before treatment (left). After three months of chemotherapy (right) there is a normal appearing marrow with a variety of cell types and evidence of normal maturation of cells.

153

herald a remission. Avoidance of infection during the induction period has been accomplished by isolating patients in laminar flow rooms—specially enclosed areas where the air is filtered to exclude bacterial contamination. Some observers have reported additional protection from the prophylactic use of oral nonabsorbable antibiotics, although this has not been a universal finding. Transfusions of platelets and of granulocytes are most effective in patients with acute myelocytic leukemia during remission induction; in some cases life-saving effectiveness has been demonstrated by such transfusions.

The remission duration and survival of patients with acute myelocytic leukemia are shorter than the comparable phenomena in patients with acute lymphocytic leukemia, in part because the differences between normal marrow stem cells and leukemic stem cells are so small that treatment applied during the maintenance phase must be restricted. Nonetheless, survival has increased appreciably from more effective application of the drugs at hand.

Pioneering treatment approaches

New approaches at the frontier of leukemia research are currently providing promising leads. One approach—repetitive intensive treatment, despite already having reached remission—has, according to some reports, caused greater remission duration than more gentle therapy with the same chemotherapeutic approaches applied on an ambulatory basis. The costs and risks of such aggressive treatment have not as yet been assessed, however, against the reported benefits.

Other workers have devoted sustained effort to marrow transplantation. This requires eradication of the leukemic population, which is ordinarily accomplished by supralethal doses of drugs and total body irradiation, and

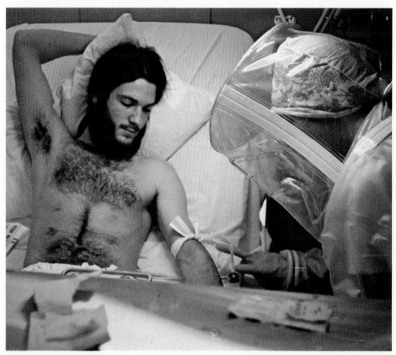

Patients have been isolated in specially designed laminar flow rooms to avoid infection during remission induction. Air is filtered at the head end of the room and blows bacteria-free over the patient's bed. Nurses and other personnel are technically outside the room at all times.

James F. Holland, M.D.

replacement of the marrow from a genetically compatible donor. Eradication and replacement are both extremely difficult to carry out. Early success has been attained by a few research groups, and indeed the procedure appears to be of use for that minority of patients who have a sibling with proper immunological characteristics. Since most do not, however, fundamental advances in transplantation across genetic barriers will be required before the procedure will be widely applicable.

Another approach is the application of chemoimmunotherapy, the combined use of drug treatment with attempts to stimulate immunity against one's own neoplasm by specific or nonspecific stimuli. Nonspecific immunization with BCG, a live attenuated tubercle bacillus vaccine, or with its nonliving derivative, MER—the methanol extraction residue or phenol-killed BCG—has been investigated. The benefits of these medications are hard to ascribe to a specific antileukemic effect but rather may be due to an increase in immunity against infection. Survival prolongation from BCG or MER alone is not yet firmly enough established to warrant widespread adoption.

It is known that the membranes of acute myelocytic leukemia cells elicit an immune response when injected into the skin of patients with acute myelocytic leukemia, a phenomenon that is not characteristic of all patients with respect to their own tumors or those of others. Furthermore, once patients with acute myelocytic leukemia have attained remission, the reac-

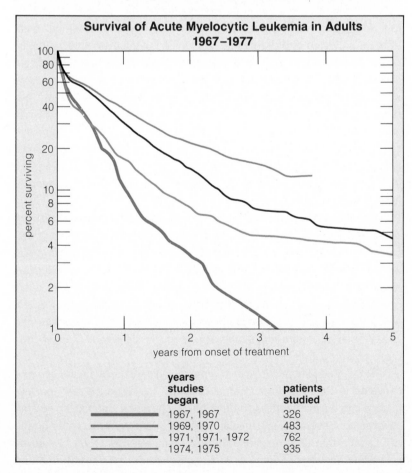

Studies in patients with acute myelocytic leukemia show a progressive improvement in survival rates reminiscent of the improved outcome in recent years for children with acute lymphocytic leukemia.

tion of their lymphocytes with their own myeloblasts shows evidence of immune stimulation. Several investigators have reported modest prolongation of survival by immunization with irradiated myeloblasts from another donor together with the administration of BCG. In these situations remission duration is not significantly prolonged, and the beneficial effect cannot be distinguished from a nonspecific immune stimulus that would protect the host against life-threatening infection. However, an approach that utilizes specific immunotherapy has evoked considerably greater interest and evidence of effectiveness.

Together with J. George Bekesi, his principal colleague in this research, the author has studied patients with acute myelocytic leukemia, randomly allocated to receive chemotherapy alone or chemoimmunotherapy in the remission phase. The chemotherapy is identical in the two arms of the research program. In the chemoimmunotherapy arm monthly immunizations are interspersed midway between the chemotherapy courses. The particular form of immunotherapy was adapted directly from model systems that proved effective in mice with transplanted and spontaneous leukemias. Leukemic cells harvested from an untreated volunteer patient are purified (separated from red blood cells and nonleukemic cells) and frozen in the vapor of liquid nitrogen. When a patient is in remission and ready for immunization, a reserved block of approximately ten billion donor cells is thawed. N-acetyl-neuraminic acid, a carbohydrate compound on the surface of cells, is removed from these myeloblasts by an enzyme, neuraminidase, that is obtained from *Vibrio cholerae* bacteria. In mice the removal of this carbohydrate compound was shown to propitiate markedly the ability of treated leukemic cells to elicit an immune response against subsequent challenge with viable leukemic cells. Presumably this is because the enzyme had removed a critical molecular linkage, thus exposing antigens on the cell surface against which the host could respond. Immunized mice could withstand 100,000 times the ordinary lethal dose of leukemic cells after a single immunization and after multiple immunizations 100 million lethal doses. The effect was far greater than found following immunization with radiated or formaldehyde-treated cells.

In man the administration of neuraminidase-treated myeloblasts has been optimized by giving them in multiple sites in the skin. Patients injected with neuraminidase-treated cells respond with a local immune response that may last for weeks. In laboratory tests stimulation of their reactive lymphocytes against the immunizing leukemic cells and against their own frozen leukemic myeloblasts has been observed. The most convincing evidence of effectiveness, however, is the prolongation of remission and survival among the group receiving chemoimmunotherapy, which is significantly longer than those of the controls.

Attempts to augment this specific immunologic response by the use of a derivative of BCG have not been successful. The evidence that immunotherapy can augment remission duration has, however, opened a new area of research. Several key questions arise: What are the substances on the cell surface that elicit response? Can the same response be elicited by cellular derivatives or synthetic compounds? And how can the effect be

156

broadened so that more immunized patients will respond to it? Since several patients have demonstrated freedom from disease for several years, our knowledge of how to determine when and if such a patient is cured is challenged. In mice a cure is obtained by chemoimmunotherapy under circumstances where chemotherapy alone or immunotherapy alone is not successful. Since it is impossible to continue chemotherapy indefinitely in patients, we are at the juncture where treatment can be stopped with legitimate hope (and expectation) that a cure has been obtained in some patients with acute myelocytic leukemia.

The future of leukemia research

Acute leukemia is a paradigm of advanced metastatic life-threatening cancer. It is disseminated from the outset and never a suitable disease for surgical eradication. Radiotherapy has been tested and does not work. The challenge to chemotherapy is clear, particularly since half of the children and the majority of adults still die. The evolution of research methods for clinical investigation of new drugs, new knowledge of how to use these drugs, and the new science of immunotherapy augur well for the future, however.

For many years leukemia has been a keystone of the efforts in cancer research, since quantification of the tumor can be accomplished reasonably accurately with great ease. The feedback loop from experimental approach to assessment of outcome is thus significantly shorter in leukemia than in other cancers. The progress in acute lymphocytic leukemia of children reflects the longest sustained research effort in clinical cancer chemotherapy. Acute leukemia has served as the model tumor that allowed scientists to forge our current chemotherapeutic weapons against cancer; the first remissions in acute lymphocytic leukemia of childhood were described in 1948.

Several principles that have dominated leukemia therapy are directly translatable to investigations of other metastatic cancers. These include combination chemotherapy; induction as a phase separate from maintenance; reinforcement and intensification of the maintenance treatment; unrelenting effort to achieve a complete disappearance of all clinical manifestations; regional therapy where the effects of systemic chemotherapy have not been well achieved, such as in the central nervous system; randomized prospective controlled clinical trials; and recently immunotherapy. The progress in acute lymphocytic leukemia already has spilled over into research into Hodgkin's disease, breast cancer, lymphosarcoma, and several sarcomas of children.

If our present dynamic acceleration in striving for curative chemotherapy and chemoimmunotherapy has already scaled a part of the mountain, what will the next 30 years bring? Given public support, given dedication of bright young scholars, given the cooperation of patients and practicing physicians who believe in living cancer research, given the financial resources to maintain staff and equip laboratories and clinical cancer research centers, the future looks dazzling for even greater accomplishments.

Living with Leukemia
by Morris B. Abram

Photographs by George W. Gardner

It may be a miracle that I have survived leukemia for five years. My disease is a particularly ferocious cancer that cannot be reached by surgery, as it lives in the marrow of every bone from skull to big toe. When my several hematologists, oncologists, and immunotherapists first became acquainted with me in June 1973, they no doubt looked upon my prospects as bleak, and statistics supported them.

Of course, I have contemplated at the oddest hours and in the most unusual places the reasons for my good fortune. And since the distinguished and caring physicians who have treated me are not at all sure why I have lived, I do not feel presumptuous in putting my own ideas forward. Moreover, none of the team of doctors that finally assembled to treat me could know, despite all their years of experience, the emotional conditions through which I passed during my drastic, unremitting, and often novel treatment.

Even in the face of morbid statistics, I resolved the night of diagnosis that I would not yield; I would not die; I would seek the most aggressive help available and take any risks for the chance, however small, to live.

An ominous diagnosis

I was, as accustomed, enjoying near perfect health when I arranged with my friend and family physician, Dr. Hyman Ashman, for a complete physical examination. The date picked was my 54th birthday, June 19, 1973. My complaints were a slight dizziness when I rose from a long sit in a rocking chair I have in my law office and repeated colds, which had lingered throughout the previous winter.

Dr. Ashman seemed not a bit disturbed after a thorough examination and dismissed me as he had many times before, but with an exception: he would call me when his lab had given him the results of my blood samples.

When he called in two days, I was astounded by his cautious phrasing: my hemoglobin, which had stood at a relatively normal 16.9 grams in 1972, was down to 11.6. Something was wrong, he said. Either the lab had made a mistake, or I was ill. I agreed to get a new complete blood count.

This time the hemoglobin was up to 12. Dr. Ashman called within minutes of receiving the second report: would I keep an appointment with a hematologist the following morning at 9 o'clock? I arrived at the hematologist's office feeling put out by the interruption in my schedule only to find the

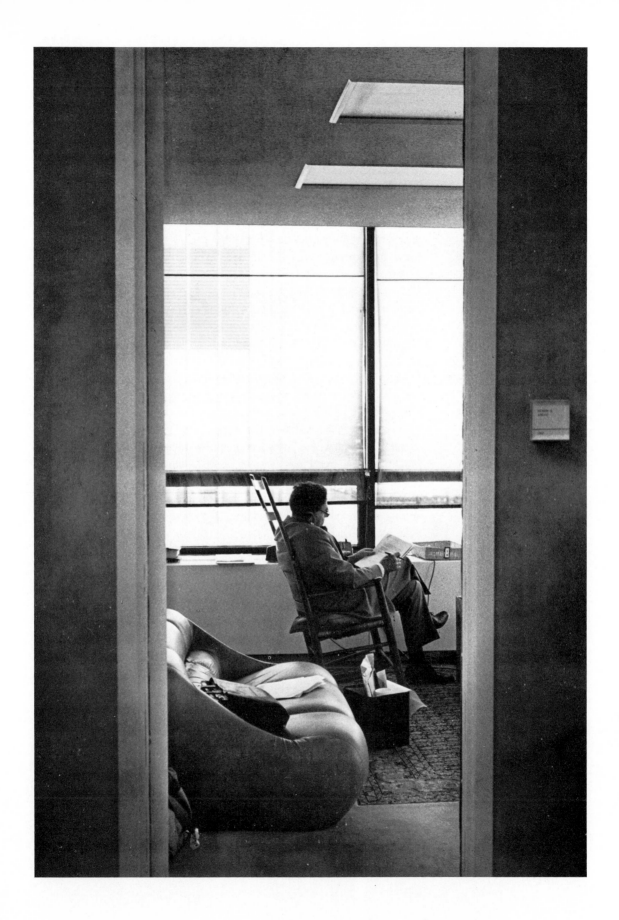

doctor late and his office full. I told his nurse after he had not appeared in a half hour that I was leaving. She pleaded with me to remain and promised I would be first. As soon as the harried man arrived and washed, he had me on his examining table approaching my breastbone with a collection of several small needles and one large one. He explained he was going to do a "bone marrow." I had had no idea that this was the purpose of my visit and remonstrated that I didn't have time for such a procedure. Upon his assurance that Dr. Ashman very much wanted it and that no more than ten minutes were required, I calmed down, and he proceeded.

After narcotizing pricks with small needles, the bone marrow was extracted after a crush through the bone itself by a large aspiration needle. The doctor approached my vital aorta with a deadly dagger. When the needle was in the marrow, he pulled back and I experienced a great sucking feeling as the deed was done.

I arose from the table and went to my office, relatively unalarmed by this peculiar course of events. Then a day later Ashman called in detectable anguish: could he see me at the close of the day? Instinctively I asked, "Do I have leukemia?" (My God, I wondered, where did that word come from? To my knowledge no person in my entire family had ever had cancer.) Ashman said, "We'll discuss the matter at 6 o'clock." The remaining hours dragged, and I could not shake off the ominous tone of Ashman's voice.

My reaction to the diagnosis, "acute lymphocytic leukemia," was terror, mixed with disbelief. (Later it was determined I had acute myelocytic leukemia.) My friend Ashman had seemed as rattled as I. The room was ill-lighted and as somber as the news he had to convey. For a short time we shared the anguish. Then I left his office to walk many blocks down Park and Lexington avenues into the gathering evening. I had a blind date that night, and thus a perfect stranger was the first to hear of the sentence that had been passed on me.

Ashman had wasted no words: the disease was fatal. One died of infection. The time left was unpredictable but minimal. "Was there any possibility of cure?" I had inquired. He replied that chemotherapy was the treatment being used. It was a crude, painful, horrendous therapy, which Ashman obviously regarded as a palliative and more likely to make the days remaining intolerable than do anything constructive. He had repeated several times: "These chemicals are dreadful poisons."

My recent contact with leukemia patients confirmed everything Ashman said. An Atlanta, Georgia, law partner had lost his wife after five weeks with the disease a few years ago, a New York partner his wife a year later; she had survived only three weeks after diagnosis. A college friend in Atlanta had recently died, and earlier my tutor from the University of Oxford, one year older than I, had died in his 40s after a month's bout with leukemia.

Chemotherapy

I was admitted to Mount Sinai Hospital, New York City, on Sept. 9, 1973. The treatment prescribed in my case was a new protocol for acute leukemia. I did not know at first but I soon understood that my doctors were not attempting to temporize and suppress this mortal enemy but to destroy it without at

Morris B. Abram *is a partner with the New York City law firm Paul, Weiss, Rifkind, Wharton & Garrison. He also serves as President of the Field Foundation, Inc., and as Chairman of the Board of the United Negro College Fund, Inc.*

George W. Gardner *is a free-lance photographer whose work appears in the permanent collections of the Museum of Modern Art, New York City, and the Art Institute of Chicago. He lives in Hillsdale, New York.*

the same time killing me. I gladly signed every kind of waiver explaining the dangers and possible risks of the drugs I was to receive. I was told of the threat to my heart and every other bodily organ. From the start I received a fairly new drug, daunomycin, a reddish horror of the antibiotic family, developed in Italy. I soon discovered its power when a few drops leaked into the tissues instead of being flushed into the bloodstream through the veins. My right arm to this day bears the scars of its dreadful potential to do harm as well as good. On three occasions quantities of this liquid, which resembled the color of the red clay of my native Georgia, were pushed into me. Meanwhile, 24 hours a day for seven days, cytarabine, another chemical, was driven through my veins. Intermittently, the receiving vein would collapse, or the needle or lines would become clogged, or irritation would require a new stick in a new vein or a new site.

After a few days I developed fever. I was now almost totally without resources (white cells) to fight infectious disease. So an intravenous setup was established in the free arm, and a continuous flow of powerful antibiotics was dripped into my bloodstream while the doctors took frequent samples of my blood in an attempt to culture and identify the presumed infection. (None ever was pegged.)

I cannot fully explain why I expected to survive the hospital stay. On one occasion my physician brother and one of my junior doctors, thinking I was asleep, discussed at my bedside what they agreed was a very controversial issue: whether it is better to let the patient go or inflict the horrors of chemotherapy in the face of lugubrious statistics of so many failures or very short successes. While I pretended sleep, I resolved to ignore their pessimism. The daily routine of chemotherapy so far seemed bearable, especially when measured against those dreaded days of the bone marrows.

By now bone marrows were being performed at least every ten days from the hip, where the bone was thicker and harder, but at least I did not see the needle poised over my heart. Marrow is extracted from the hip when one is in a face-down position. One feels first the shallow, followed by the deep, penetration of the needle carrying novocaine to the lining around the bone that will be assaulted. Then comes the plunge of the big needle through the narcotized flesh to the bone. One knows when the metal and bone have met because the doctor then begins a struggle to force the high-grade steel through the bone to its center, where the marrow flows. The fears are now four: will the needle break? will the doctor hit a "dry well," requiring the whole thing to be done again? will the pain be unbearable when he pulls back on the syringe plunger and sucks out the marrow? and finally, what will he find when he reads the "tea leaves"?

For two weeks I endured the hospital regimen as I watched fall materialize in Central Park, visible from my windows. I hoped so much to be released just to toss a baseball or football to my 11-year-old boon companion, my son Josh. Visiting me often, he averted his eyes from my bottles and bandages and looked at that park scene with, I thought, the same hopes.

Then on the eve of the third week I knew I was in crisis. I weakened with blood clots around my gums, my hair was coming out in globs, and the fever was unabating. My family had materialized from all corners of the country.

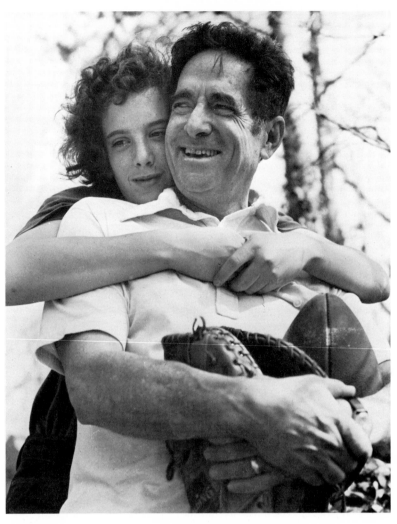

"*. . . that very afternoon we went to the park and tossed a baseball. On the weekend we went with friends to Pawling, New York, and played touch football. . . . I was weak but stupendously happy.*"

Morris Abram and his son Josh photographed by Lucinda Bunnen, a friend, in Atlanta in 1975, when Abram had been in remission for about 18 months.

Red cells were transfused into my body, which had grown pale and steadily more weary. Then came the bags of platelets, the cells that cause clotting, to replace the billions destroyed by the chemotherapy. These resembled liquefied raw pork. So at the end of September—98 days after diagnosis—I was being kept alive by other people's red cells and platelets, by antibiotics, and the blind luck that no infection had appeared.

The worse things appeared, however, the more optimistic I became, for I now was beginning to comprehend the theoretical magic of the treatment and could hope that in 1973 chemotherapy might succeed in my case despite the parlous record in the case of almost every other person afflicted with my disease. I lived on awaiting the day when my regenerated bone marrow could produce cells of its own—hoping, even attempting sometimes to pray, that the fresh white cells would be normal—in short, for a remission from leukemia. I wanted that new lease on life even if only for that game in the park with my son.

No matter how weak or ill I became, I was determined to keep up my spirits and my muscle tone. A dedicated tennis player and swimmer, I refused to give up my daily exercise: I attempted to sprint down the hospital hallways whenever possible, though that meant wheeling with me my complex of stands, bottles, and tubes, which were attached to my forearms with needles. I was a subversive cancer patient and a peculiar sight zipping through the corridors of Mount Sinai Hospital, first with one stand, later with two.

The joy of remission

In the middle of the second week of October another bone marrow was ordered. No one treated it as anything but routine. Indeed, one of my junior physicians had warned me that it was not likely that one course of chemotherapy would induce a remission. The day of this bone marrow was like all other days in the hospital, except that it was worse because of this procedure, and I was plain weary of the whole business.

That bone marrow was taken early in the morning. At 1 o'clock PM, Dr. Janet Cuttner, associate hematologist at Mount Sinai Hospital, came almost twinkling into the room. She exclaimed, "The megakaryocytes are back." I had no idea what the megakaryocytes were, but the way she sounded and the cheer in her face made me think, "The swallows have returned to Capistrano." She continued, "The bone marrow looks excellent. You are in remission."

I was past elation.

The next day my doctors began to discuss with me the course of treatment post-release. It seems that I was to return to the hospital in ten days for the first of continuous courses of "maintenance therapy," consisting of lesser doses of chemotherapeutic drugs administered in rotation.

So on October 5 I left the hospital. Josh soon joined me, and that very afternoon we went to the park and tossed a baseball. On the weekend we went with friends to Pawling, New York, and played touch football on the grounds of the local YMCA. I was weak but stupendously happy.

Looking back, I cannot in truth say that I expected to survive very long. I was determined to fight. I was resolved to agree to every known procedure to prevent the recurrence of the disease, but I was a realist. While I was not going to give up, it was still quite probable that leukemia would not give up, either. Though I was quick to order a $600 custom-made wig when my hair began to fall out, every time it was suggested that I buy a new suit, I resisted, speculating I would not need it long. Too, every time I contemplated any improvement in my living quarters, I elected to leave things as they were, feeling that the investment would be for too short a term. I was not able to surrender, but I was aware that I could be conquered. I awaited also the dreaded prospect of a return to the hospital for maintenance therapy.

The first course was performed in the hospital. That is, I slept there and received the morning and evening intravenous injections there. I worked at my office after checking out of the hospital each morning at about 11 o'clock, and I returned to the hospital at around 8 o'clock in the evening. But I was very apprehensive about the treatment. Would it prove physically disabling? Would it make my planned second marriage an unfair partnership? To my delight, the first maintenance went well. Best of all, I was not nauseated and did not feel particularly debilitated. I became confident that so long as the remission held, I could function at a satisfactory level.

163

Then in December there was another course of maintenance—this time performed outside the hospital. Each morning I went to the hematologist's office for a blood count and the intravenous administration of the scheduled drug. Each evening the physician or nurse visited my apartment to insert the evening dose.

When this planned course was finished, I felt washed out. On Monday, after the last dosage on the previous Friday, I went to the hematologist's office because I felt extraordinarily weak. The technician punctured my finger, and I could see, as she mixed several drops of blood in a vial containing a solution from which she read the hemaglobin count, that the red cells were down—very far down. In a few minutes a complete blood count was recorded, and I could tell by the look in the caring, tender face of the technician that she was concerned. Impulsively she blurted out, "You'll be going to the hospital." My white count was about 600; the normal is 5,000 to 7,000.

Soon Dr. Louis Wasserman, senior hematologist at Mount Sinai Hospital, appeared, and I asked if I was going to enter the hospital. I was surprised when he said, "Oh, no, that's the worst place for you; there are too many germs there. Go wherever you like." So I took the subway back to my office and, indeed, the next day, too, without any ill effects.

A few weeks later, when the blood count was up, Dr. Wasserman said, "We really clobbered you in the last maintenance; it was not intentional. You are extremely sensitive to these drugs, and we must learn to regulate the dosage." He went on to indicate that I had what in effect was somewhat akin to an inadvertent second remission induction. So there had occurred, and I had survived, without even an infection, another potent cancer-killing therapy. This is only one of the several cases in which the course of my treatment seems to have been influenced as much by serendipity as by plan.

Battling hepatitis

Several weeks later in Atlanta I knew something was wrong. I was simply worn to a frazzle, and no matter how much I slept I could not be refreshed. I was ill, and I knew it. Moreover, my urine was by now an orange color, and my stools were no longer brown but varying in color from a pale tan to near white. Immediately when I returned to New York I went to Dr. Wasserman's office and asked one of the junior physicians whether I might not have hepatitis. I don't know why I thought up this diagnosis, but I did know that I had received a lot of other people's blood components, and there seemed to me to be a yellow cast in my eyes. I was right.

Now I faced a terrible battle, one that frightened me to the core. I knew that I needed maintenance therapy, or at least the doctors thought I did, and I knew, too, that there was no possibility that while I was infected with hepatitis I could be treated for leukemia. I was also aware that hepatitis was no minor illness. There was nothing for me to do except wait and, as the doctors prescribed, rest and eat well.

Felled by hepatitis, unavailable for chemotherapy, I faced the new year of 1974 with trepidation. Moreover, I was very concerned about the scheduled trial of an important tax case in the United States District Court for the District

164

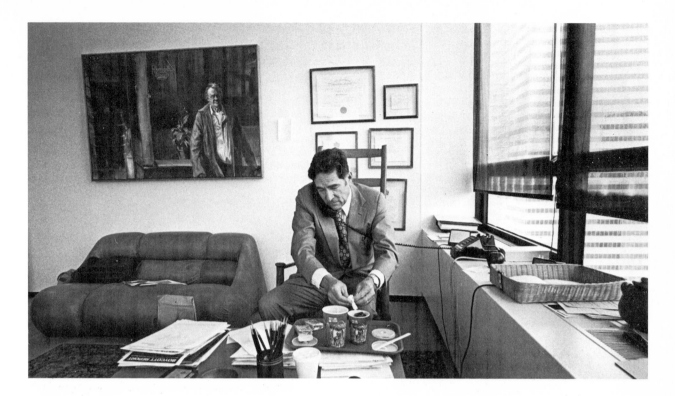

of Rhode Island, to commence on January 8. I had worked on the matter for two years, and I had been prepared to try it since I was first diagnosed as leukemic. After remission I felt that I was able to proceed, and my firm had planned no substitute on my assurance that I would be able to go ahead. That is, until I was hit with hepatitis. From the first evidence of this new invasion, I fretted over that case. The judge was old; we had waited a long time for the case to reach his trial calendar; the client of the firm wanted to try it now; and I alone of all the litigation partners was prepared. I asked my doctors, "Could I go to Providence to try the Textron case, which is estimated to last a week?" They were horrified. "Go to Providence in the snow, with hepatitis, and try a difficult case? Absolutely not." But as the day approached when we would either ask for a postponement or substitute a partner with limited acquaintance with the issues and the record, Dr. Cuttner saw my dilemma and weighed the medical equities. She finally said, "Go." I was grateful she was able to see that the anxiety of not being there would probably do me more harm than the physical stresses of the trial itself. The issues were complicated, but I rigorously litigated and won the case, and somehow for the four days required I found sufficient resources within my body despite its severely weakened state.

Some time in the early spring of 1974 the constantly monitored blood chemistries showed that hepatitis was receding. Blood counts, too, were returning to a level where it would be possible to resume chemotherapy. I suspect there never was a patient more eager to accept the unpleasant rigors of chemotherapy. And finally Dr. Cuttner said we would begin once more with cytarabine, as ever, and CCNU—for me a new drug, said to have a long-acting effect on the bone marrow.

"Looking back, I cannot in truth say that I expected to survive very long. . . . While I was not going to give up, it was still quite probable that leukemia would not give up, either. . . . I was not able to surrender, but I was aware that I could be conquered."

165

Immunotherapy: experimental frontiers

While I was still in the hospital during the early stages of my treatment, a friend and colleague from my days as president of Brandeis University brought me two pieces of intelligence from the frontiers of leukemia therapy. One was of a new general immunological agent, Methanol Extract Residue, "MER," developed by Dr. David Weiss of Hebrew University-Hadassah Medical School in Jerusalem. It had never been used in the United States but, I was informed, the results were promising. Israeli hematologists were reporting extended remissions in leukemia patients with the use of MER. I had also heard of the use of a specific immunological agent—radiation-treated leukemic cells—being administered to leukemia patients in remission at St. Bartholomew's Hospital in London.

Before I left the hospital in October 1973, I had raised the question of both auxiliary treatments with my doctors. I was told that at the time they were not prepared to recommend either. However, Dr. James Holland, a consulting oncologist, did tell me that at Roswell Park Memorial Institute in Buffalo, New York, where he had recently been on the staff, he and Dr. George Bekesi, an immunotherapist, had used leukemic cells treated with an enzyme, neuraminidase, in the same manner as British physicians had employed radiation-treated cells. However, Dr. Holland did not then have either the apparatus or the team necessary to use this therapy on me. He expected that it would become available but could not tell me when.

I began another course of chemotherapy on a Monday in March 1974. Nothing unusual occurred. On Tuesday morning I received the second intravenous dose of cytarabine. By 2 o'clock PM I was nauseated for the first time since chemotherapy had been administered in September 1973. I began to shake with chills as my temperature rose to 101°. I called Dr. Cuttner, who suggested that I go to a radiologist in the morning for chest X-rays. She wished to rule out a respiratory infection—a common curse of the leukemic.

Tests were negative, and after a day the cytarabine was resumed with no further ill effects. But for more than two years I had the "Tuesday sickness," which usually began between 1 and 2 o'clock in the afternoon on the second day of chemotherapy. But the nausea and accompanying chills and aches usually vanished by Wednesday morning.

At this time Dr. Weiss in Jerusalem, who was receiving reports of my case through a friend, recommended that I might benefit from his treatment. "A perfect case for MER," he'd said.

But there were two obstacles to my receiving MER in the United States. The Food and Drug Administration had not released it even for clinical trials, and my physicians were not convinced it was indicated.

In the spring of 1974 Dr. Weiss agreed to administer MER in Israel, and I was on the point of flying over. Then Washington authorities released the drug to Mount Sinai in New York, and Dr. Cuttner agreed to give it to me. However, when I reported to her for the initial dosage, she gave me a jolt: Dr. Holland was soon to begin a protocol at Sinai using treated leukemic cells. I could not be included if I began receiving MER before he was ready to proceed. Dr. Holland believed it would be best to do the two treatments in tandem.

166

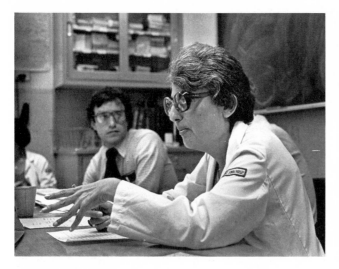

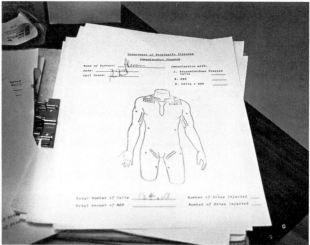

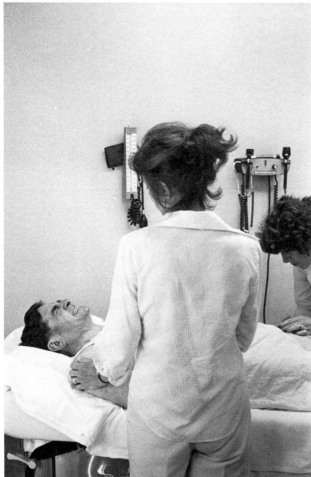

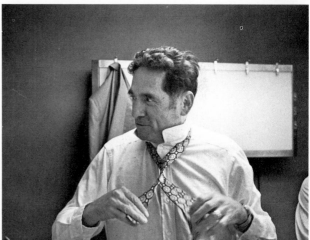

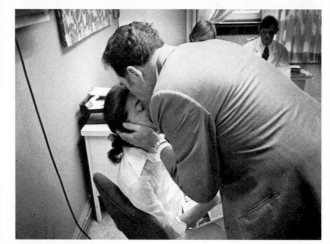

"I was, if I waited, to be the beneficiary of a new protocol whose utility was as yet unknown. I theoretically had a choice, but actually there was none. . . . I had decided to go for broke, to take any risk, to expose myself to any danger in the search of a 'cure' or a long remission."
(Top left) Dr. Janet Cuttner; (top right) diagram showing sites at which Abram receives immunotherapy; (bottom three pictures) undergoing immunotherapy with support from his wife.

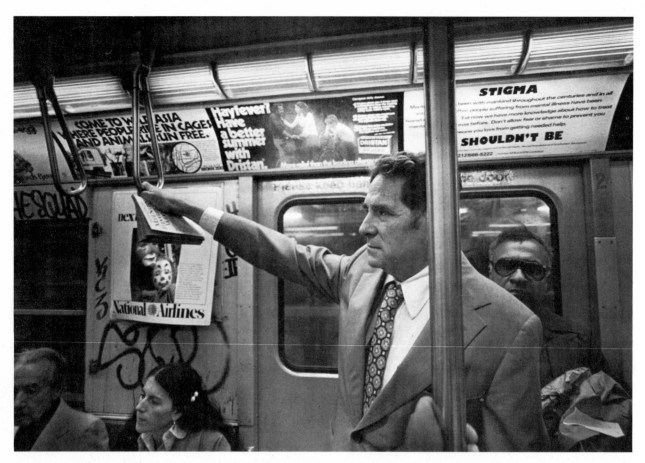

"Sometimes riding a subway through the Bowery in New York City, I see a drunk with glazed eyes, uncertain gait, and a flask. Momentarily I may catch myself saying, 'Why can't I have his normal bone marrow, which he puts to such poor use?' But I do not dwell on this."

Upon hearing that disturbing news I was shaken. Nevertheless, I instantly told Dr. Cuttner to put the MER vial back in the refrigerator. I was, if I waited, to be the beneficiary of a new protocol whose utility was as yet unknown. I theoretically had a choice, but actually there was none. As early as December 1973 I had decided to go for broke, to take any risk, to expose myself to any danger in the search of a "cure" or a long remission.

Each week I inquired as unobtrusively and as diplomatically as possible about the progress of Dr. Holland's efforts to set up his elaborate equipment and to recruit his colleagues, including physicians, nurses, and technicians necessary for the separation of leukemic cells from the diseased patients and the treatment and injection of these cells. During this period I never doubted that I had Dr. Holland's goodwill and sympathy. In fact, I had the sneaking suspicion that he wanted me as a patient as much as I wanted his novel therapy. I sensed that he saw in me the will to fight, a basically healthy constitution, and a willingness to take risks. He is and was an aggressive scientist, operating at the frontier of the current knowledge of a ravaging disease, and I an adaptable guinea pig; yet I felt the terrible dependency of the patient on the doctor, like a child on a parent, which too frequently characterizes the helpless in the presence of an authority figure. Thus, he became that figure, one to be propitiated lest, because of irritation or worse, he reject me as a beneficiary and exclude me from the group to be treated with this new "compleat" therapy.

168

Finally, Dr. Holland called and said, "Let's go; meet me in my office tomorrow at 3 o'clock." I went enthusiastically without the slightest idea of what awaited me. First, he said, he wanted to do a bone marrow. The thought of his doing a bone marrow froze me with horror, though I had to realize that he was not going to start treatment without having baseline proof that I was still in remission. But here was a very senior physician going to undertake a technical procedure usually performed by younger persons who do it routinely. So I could not resist asking, "Do you know how to do a bone marrow?" He took no offense and, laughing, replied that he never asked anyone to do that which he could not do himself.

The bone marrow examination showed that I was still in complete remission in June 1974 when Dr. Holland commenced the administration of treated leukemic cells and MER simultaneously. The cells were injected in about 50 separate lymph glands almost as a necklace around the collar area, in the groin, and the arms, producing an intense burning pain for a few seconds. At one time they were administered along the sternum, but that became too painful. The MER was injected in first five, and later ten, sites on the chest and legs; it did not hurt so much when injected, but the drug turns the sites into unsightly ulcers—some as big as quarters—and later scars.

In 1976 the blood studies indicated that I was saturated with MER and actually becoming sensitized to its powerful stimulation. Hence, I was taken off MER, but chemotherapy every other month and cells every month were routinely administered. I both believed in and was suspicious of my good fortune as monthly times for the bone marrow approached; I never ceased to be apprehensive, hovering in the doctor's office for the specimen to be stained, dried, and the results reported before leaving to go to work. I have never been able to endure the anxiety of standing by a midtown phone to wait out the doctor's schedule and interruptions, which might delay the news. And when the process takes longer than usual in the doctor's office, I grow nervous there. Is he disturbed by what he sees and reluctant to tell me? Does he wish confirmation of the bad news from someone else? Does the junior doctor who does the bone marrow wish the equivocal bad news to be delivered by the physician-in-chief? After more than four years of good reports, I still am anxious until the doctor says, preferably with a smile, "Your bone marrow is good." I even listen for the overtones. Once when a junior hematologist said, "I think everything's okay," I nailed him to the wall. "Is it different from the way it has been? What percentage of blasts [bad cells]?" I want to know everything, and I am skeptical when the bone marrow diagnosis is delivered in less than the enthusiastic tone of Dr. Cuttner when she first told me, "The megakaryocytes are back."

I call the examination of the bone marrow "reading the tea leaves" because in the marrow as viewed in the electron microscope is the clear story of my condition so far as a specimen of a previously diseased, flowing, and presumably uniform organ can reveal the state of the whole. By convention and practice the result is taken as definitive for the time.

When the tea leaves read favorably, as they always have in my case since 1973, I then focus on the upcoming five-day period of chemotherapy with

"While my doctors have performed miracles, and though I believe that death is a condition that always has to be held at bay by the will to live—which I have in abundance—I know that I am struggling against a powerful enemy, which sleeps but may awake.

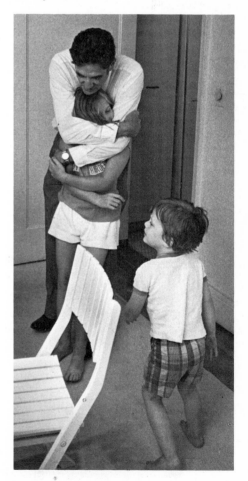

its aches, nausea, fever, chills, and general lassitude. But the good news that my bone marrow is clean outweighs the anxieties of the approaching chemotherapy.

A powerful will to live

Without a doubt I have been treated with great skill, and chemotherapy has been administered with fine tuning. As time goes by, and the disease does not reappear, I grow tired of this unpleasant bimonthly episode, which makes me nauseated, debilitates, and seems (to my uninformed opinion) less relevant than a nuisance. Still, who wishes to quarrel with success, particularly when no one knows what has produced it?

For five years I have never been free of the fear of dying from leukemia, but at no time have I actually accepted the prospect that my end was approaching. My psyche has certainly been deeply etched by the prospect of a shortened life. I have little doubt that the cause of death is likely to be leukemia or an associated illness. While my doctors have performed miracles, and though I believe that death is a condition that always has to be held at bay by the will to live—which I have in abundance—I know that I am struggling against a powerful enemy, which sleeps but may awake.

Ashman's diagnosis of leukemia found me unready to yield to its inexorable sentence of doom. In 1973 I felt a special responsibility to support, as much as a father can, an 11-year-old boy through the uncertainties of puberty and the turbulence of adolescence and a 17-year-old son just entering college. Also, while I was proud of my record as a public servant and an aggressive attorney, I felt unfinished.

Sometimes riding a subway through the Bowery in New York City, I see a drunk with glazed eyes, uncertain gait, and a flask. Momentarily I may catch myself saying, "Why can't I have his normal bone marrow, which he puts to such poor use?" But I do not dwell on this. It is not a thought that lingers long or consumes me.

While I believe I must accept fate—if by that one means forces absolutely beyond one's control—I hold and act daily on the proposition that some of these so-called forces can be affected by will and determination. To the extent that an earlier death was a possibility, I believe that my resistance has held that at bay.

From time to time I reflect that death is the frame around the painting of life. A painting on a canvas of infinite size, worked on eternally, would be without focus, meaning, and probably without beauty. A painting, as life, needs limits. While I have an almost insatiable craving for knowledge, I believe death to be the final and perhaps greatest teacher—the one that provides the key to the ultimate questions life has never answered. In my darkest hours I have been consoled by the thought that death at least is a payment for the answer to life's haunting secrets.

Finally, there is one thing of which I am sure: cancer is a battle between a disease and its host. This host wants to live. The cancer has not yet disclosed its final intentions. I am content to endure the contest in status quo.

170

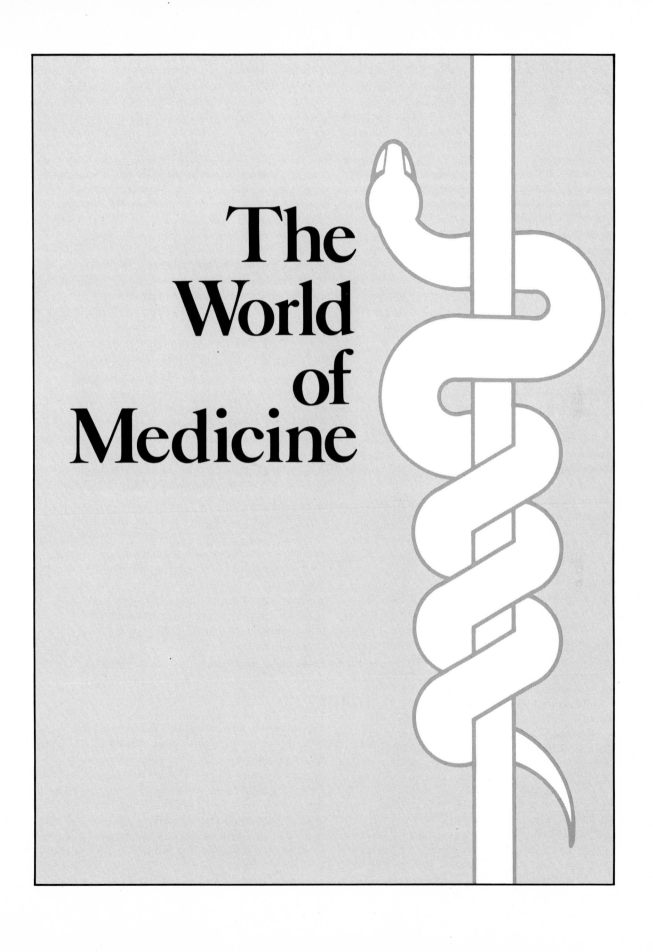

The World of Medicine

Contributors to The World of Medicine

François E. Alouf, M.D. *Mental Health* (in part). Associate Professor of Psychiatry, and Director of Education, Department of Psychiatry, Northwestern University Medical School, Chicago.

Edward L. Applebaum, M.D. *Ear Diseases and Hearing Disorders.* Associate Professor, Department of Otolaryngology and Maxillofacial Surgery, Northwestern University Medical School, Chicago.

L. Fred Ayvazian, M.D. *Lung Diseases; Lung Diseases Special Report: Update on Legionnaires' Disease.* Chief, Pulmonary Section, Veterans Administration Hospital, East Orange, N.J., and Professor of Medicine, College of Medicine and Dentistry, Newark, N.J.

Ellen Bernstein. *Trends in Medicine and Health Care Special Report: Medicine and Health on TV.* Editor, *Medical and Health Annual,* Encyclopaedia Britannica, Inc., Chicago.

Samuel S. Cardone, Ph.D. *Alcoholism and Drug Abuse* (in part). Region 2 Alcoholism Coordinator, Illinois Department of Mental Health and Developmental Disabilities, Chicago.

Charles M. Cegielski. *World Medical News.* Associate Editor, Britannica yearbooks, Encyclopaedia Britannica, Inc., Chicago.

Mary Ann Cleary. *Death and Dying Special Report: The Nurse and the Dying Patient.* Coordinator, Hospice at St. Luke's, St. Luke's Hospital Center, New York City.

Edward P. Cohen, M.D. *Allergy and Immunity; Blood and the Lymphatic System; Infectious Diseases.* Professor, La Rabida-University of Chicago Institute, Chicago.

Toba J. Cohen. *Health Care Costs* (in part). Former Executive Secretary, National Commission on the Cost of Medical Care; Director, Special Projects, Office of Public Relations, American Medical Association, Chicago.

Marc I. Davis. *Birth Control Special Report: Drug Information for Patients; Heart and Blood Vessels Special Report: Saving Heart Attack Victims.* Former Editor, *Physician's Management* magazine; free-lance writer, Chicago.

Lawrence R. Drury, M.D. *Emergency Medicine Special Report: Disaster Medicine* (in part). Staff physician, Denver General Hospital, Denver, Colo.

Ann Englander, Ph.D. *Alcoholism and Drug Abuse* (in part). Administrative Coordinator, Alcoholism Treatment Program, Institute of Psychiatry, Northwestern Memorial Hospital, Chicago.

Casimir F. Firlit, M.D., Ph.D. *Urinary and Genital Disorders.* Associate Professor, Urology and Physiology, Northwestern University Medical School; Head, Pediatric Renal Transplantation, and Attending Pediatric Urologist, Children's Memorial Hospital, Chicago.

Lee Gladstone, M.D. *Alcoholism and Drug Abuse* (in part). Assistant Professor, Northwestern University Medical School; Chief, Alcoholism Treatment Program, Institute of Psychiatry, Northwestern Memorial Hospital, Chicago.

Gerald Glick, M.D. *Heart and Blood Vessels.* Director, Cardiovascular Institute, Michael Reese Hospital and Medical Center, Chicago; Professor of Medicine, The University of Chicago, Pritzker School of Medicine.

Robert A. Goepp, D.D.S., Ph.D. *Teeth and Gums.* Professor of Oral Pathology, The University of Chicago.

Jeanne P. Goldberg, R.D. *Diet and Nutrition.* Instructor in Nutrition, Tufts University, Medford, Mass.

Norma Golumbic. *Cancer* (in part). Senior Science Writer, Office of Cancer Communication, National Cancer Institute, National Institutes of Health, Bethesda, Md.

John F. Horty, L.L.B. *Health Care Law* (in part). Partner, Horty, Springer, and Mattern; Editor, *Action-Kit for Hospital Law,* Pittsburgh, Pa.

Vilma R. Hunt, B.D.S. *Occupational and Environmental Health.* Associate Professor of Environmental Health, College of Human Development, Pennsylvania State University, University Park, Pa.

David Ingall, M.D. *Genetic Disorders; Pediatrics.* Professor of Pediatrics and Obstetrics-Gynecology; Chairman, Department of Pediatrics, Evanston Hospital, Evanston, Ill.

Ted Isaacman. *Health Care Law* (in part). Managing Editor, *Action-Kit for Hospital Law,* Pittsburgh, Pa.

Albert W. Isenman. *Pregnancy and Birth Special Report: Midwifery, Prepared Childbirth, and Home Birth.* Administrator of Special Projects, American College of Obstetricians and Gynecologists, Chicago.

Lynn E. Jensen. *Health Care Costs* (in part). Director, Center for Health Services Research and Development, American Medical Association, Chicago.

Robert J. Kastenbaum, Ph.D. *Death and Dying.* Superintendent, Cushing Hospital, Framingham, Mass.; Professor of Psychology, University of Massachusetts, Boston and Dorchester, Mass.

Warren A. Katz, M.D. *Joints and Muscles.* Clinical Professor of Medicine, and Chief, Section of Rheumatology, Division of Medicine, Medical College of Pennsylvania, Philadelphia.

Bernard Levin, M.D. *Gastrointestinal Disorders.* Assistant Professor of Medicine, The University of Chicago, Pritzker School of Medicine; Director, Gastrointestinal Oncology Clinic, The University of Chicago Hospitals and Clinics.

Nathan W. Levin, M.D. *Kidney Diseases.* Chief, Division of Nephrology, Henry Ford Hospital, Detroit; Clinical Associate Professor of Medicine, University of Michigan Medical School, Ann Arbor.

Mortimer B. Lipsett, M.D. *Glandular and Metabolic Disorders.* Director, Clinical Center, National Institutes of Health, Bethesda, Md.

Derek H. Miller, M.D. *Mental Health Special Report: Health Care for Teenagers.* Professor of Psychiatry, Northwestern University Medical School; Chief, Adolescent Program, Northwestern Memorial Hospital, Chicago.

John C. Norman, M.D. *Surgery.* Professor of Surgery, University of Texas Health Science Center; Director, Cardiovascular Surgical Research Laboratories, Texas Heart Institute of St. Luke's Episcopal and Texas Children's Hospitals, Houston.

Walter L. Peretz, M.D. *Eye Diseases and Visual Disorders.* Clinical Associate Professor of Ophthalmology, Cornell University Medical College; Attending Ophthalmologist, The New York Hospital, New York City.

A. Frederick Rasmussen, Jr., M.D., Ph.D. *Glandular and Metabolic Disorders Special Report: Hormone Discoveries of the 1977 Nobelists; Infectious Diseases Special Report: Antiviral Drugs.* Associate Dean and Professor of Virology, School of Medicine, University of California, Los Angeles.

Martin C. Robson, M.D. *Emergency Medicine.* Professor of Surgery, Director, Burn Center, Chief, Section of Plastic and Reconstructive Surgery, The University of Chicago, Pritzker School of Medicine.

Robert E. Rogers, M.D. *Pregnancy and Birth.* Professor of Obstetrics and Gynecology, Indiana University School of Medicine, Indianapolis.

Peter Rosen, M.D. *Emergency Medicine Special Report: Disaster Medicine* (in part). Director of Emergency Medical Services, and Program Director, Denver General Hospital/St. Anthony Hospital Systems Emergency Medicine Residency Program, Denver, Colo.

Allan J. Ryan, M.D. *Physical Fitness and Sports Medicine; Physical Fitness and Sports Medicine Special Report: Jogging Injuries.* Editor-in-Chief, *The Physician and Sportsmedicine,* Edina, Minn.

Marion B. Sulzberger, M.D. *Skin Conditions.* Professor Emeritus of Dermatology, New York University; Clinical Professor of Dermatology, University of California, San Francisco.

Edward A. Tyler, M.D. *Mental Health* (in part). Director of Professional Services, Tri City Comprehensive Community Mental Health Center, East Chicago, Ind.; Professorial Lecturer, The University of Chicago, Pritzker School of Medicine.

Louise B. Tyrer, M.D. *Birth Control.* Vice-President for Medical Affairs, Planned Parenthood Federation of America, New York City.

Arthur C. Upton, M.D. *Cancer* (in part). Director, National Cancer Institute, National Institutes of Health, Bethesda, Md.

Robert M. Veatch, Ph.D. *Medical Ethics.* Senior Associate, Institute of Society, Ethics and Life Sciences, Hastings-on-Hudson, N.Y.

McCay Vernon, Ph.D. *Health Care Law Special Report: The "Mainstreaming" Quandary.* Professor of Psychology, Western Maryland College, Westminster, Md.; Editor, *American Annals of Deaf.*

Harold M. Visotsky, M.D. *Occupational and Environmental Health Special Report: Stress on the Job.* Owen L. Coon Professor, and Chairman, Department of Psychiatry and Behavioral Science, Northwestern University Medical School; Director, Institute of Psychiatry, Northwestern Memorial Hospital, Chicago.

Philip L. White, Sc.D. *Diet and Nutrition Special Report: Recent Developments in Treating Obesity.* Director, Department of Foods and Nutrition, American Medical Association, Chicago.

Anita K. Wolff. *Trends in Medicine and Health Care.* Associate Editor, *Medical and Health Annual,* Encyclopaedia Britannica, Inc., Chicago.

John B. Zabriskie, M.D. *Neurologic Disorders.* Associate Professor, The Rockefeller University, New York City.

Alcoholism and Drug Abuse

Alcohol abuse is currently considered by most drug experts to be a more significant problem than all other forms of drug abuse. However, the popular perception of alcohol is not that of a drug but rather of a "social lubricant," an adjunct to social living, a medicine, or a psychedelic agent. It has been reported that many parents are "relieved" that their children are drinking alcoholic beverages rather than being "on drugs." Alcohol, however, is itself a drug, one that acts upon the central nervous system. It can function as a stimulant at low doses and as a central nervous system depressant at higher doses. Chronic use of alcohol results in a tolerance for it, whereby progressively higher levels of blood alcohol concentration are required to produce intoxication. An additional effect of steady, long-term drinking is physical dependence.

The question most frequently posed is: What constitutes responsible consumption of alcohol? A typical response usually relates to the rate at which alcohol is metabolized by one's system. A safe rule for the average-size person would be one drink (¾ oz of alcohol) per hour. This consideration should be influenced by: (1) the speed of the drinking, since rapid swallowing of alcohol results in a higher peak blood alcohol level; (2) presence of food in the stomach, since eating while drinking retards the absorption of alcohol; (3) the individual's drinking history, which affects the personal tolerance for alcohol; and finally (4) the body weight.

The misuse or abuse of alcohol is obviously the behavior that causes difficulty. There has been some attempt to differentiate between problem drinking and alcoholism. Problem drinking is thought to include such variables as frequent intoxication and binge drinking, psychological dependence, symptomatic drinking, and an interference with usual social interactions.

Knowledge regarding alcohol abuse and alcoholism is continually growing. For example, it is estimated that approximately ten million people in the United States are suffering from alcoholism. This group includes both men and women, of all ages. They represent a cross section of every socioeconomic, ethnic, educational, and occupational group. The stereotypic skid row bum associated more specifically with drunkenness accounts for a very small percentage—some 3–5%, in fact—of those individuals with an alcoholism problem. The majority are working class, probably employed or employable, and enjoy some type of family constellation or significant relationships in their lives. The ratio of men and women who are experiencing alcoholism problems is becoming more equalized. The number of women seeking treatment has increased significantly, and it is now speculated that the frequency and amount of drinking among women have also increased.

According to a ten-year study that involved 8,000 high school students in Kansas, Michigan, New York, Utah, and Wisconsin, the average American first tastes alcohol by age 10. The average age at which students reported having their first drink was 13–14, although they may have tasted alcohol prior to this age. One in four users claimed to have been "high" on alcohol at least once during the month prior to the survey in the Kansas, New York, and Wisconsin studies. One in ten users in these studies reported having been "drunk" in this same period. In recent times the media have consistently reported incidents of excessive drinking among younger people and the frequency and intensity of drinking among teenagers rising.

Alcohol abuse and alcoholism have had a dramatic impact on specific life situations. For the past several years it has been reported that alcohol plays a role in approximately 50% of all highway fatalities. Individuals with chronic drinking problems were responsible for about two-thirds of the alcohol-related traffic deaths. Half of all homicides and one-fourth of all suicides are alcohol related. Alcohol is a factor in approximately 50% of all arrests in the United States.

According to some surveys, more than 50% of the individuals experiencing an alcoholism problem are employed. The 1,000 occupational programs in the U.S. cover only 7% of the 90 million workers. An annual loss of $10 billion worth of work time has been attributed to alcohol problems of employees in business, industry, government, and the military.

The effect that the problem drinker or alcoholic has on others can be dramatic. There is evidence that drinking by an expectant mother can endanger the health of the fetus. Fetal alcohol syndrome is a specific pattern of physical, mental, and behavioral abnormalities that can occur in the offspring of women who drink heavily during pregnancy. Physicians suggest that a pregnant women limit her daily intake to no more than 1 oz of absolute alcohol (the approximate equivalent of two mixed drinks, each containing 1 oz of distilled spirits), two 5-oz glasses of wine, or two 12-oz cans of beer. One group of researchers recently reported that the frequency of birth defects or growth retardation among 42 offspring of mothers who were heavy drinkers was twice that of infants born to abstinent or moderate-drinking mothers. Within that group of 42 infants, there were 15 whose mothers were able to abstain from drinking or reduce alcohol intake during the third trimester; these 15 demonstrated fewer abnormalities than the 27 infants whose mothers had continued heavy drinking throughout pregnancy. (*See also* Pregnancy and Birth.)

The emphasis on treatment reflects an attitude change in the U.S. toward alcohol abuse and alcoholism. Historically, society's feelings toward this problem have been, at best, ambivalent, with a tendency toward viewing alcoholics as morally weak and criminal. In fact, public intoxication was treated as a crime in all states until 1967, when Congress removed it as a crime

174

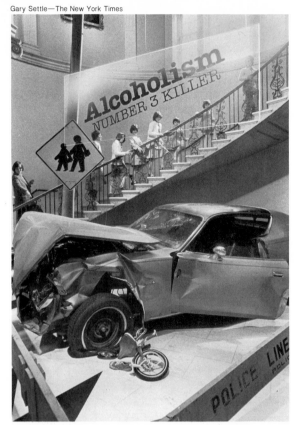

The Museum of the City of New York, New York City, mounted a series of dramatic exhibits to call attention to the consequences of untreated alcoholism.

in the District of Columbia. Similar action in most states followed the 1971 promulgation of the Uniform Alcoholism and Intoxication Treatment Act by the National Conference of Commissioners on Uniform State Laws. This act essentially stated that alcoholics and intoxicated persons may not be subjected to criminal prosecution because of their consumption of alcoholic beverages but rather should be offered a continuance of treatment in order that they may lead normal lives as productive members of society. By mid-1978, 27 states had adopted the Uniform Act, while 9 more adopted some form of comprehensive treatment legislation but do not have all the requisites of the Uniform Act.

In 1976 the Rand Corp. issued a report stating that some recovering alcoholics could engage in moderate, "social" drinking. The conventional wisdom had been to promote total abstinence because of the alcoholic's inability to control his alcohol intake. Two studies published in 1978 addressed themselves to aspects of the Rand Report. A *Journal of Studies on Alcohol* report of interviews of 244 alcohol rehabilitation patients found that the Rand Report did not have much influence on the patients. An analysis of alcohol abusers at 26 Oklahoma treatment centers found that those who tried to resume social drinking were three times as

likely to revert to uncontrolled drinking as those who abstained.

Research and evaluation continue to provide data upon which to examine the current status of alcohol abuse and alcoholism and, of course, to formulate a plan for the future. The National Institute on Alcohol Abuse and Alcoholism (NIAAA) has demonstrated support of this need by recommending funding for the establishment of Alcohol Research Centers.

Drugs and drug abuse

Drugs, licit and illicit, are misused by a large percentage of the population in all economic and social strata. Interested only in the mood change and sensations produced by the drugs, the misuser appears indifferent to and often ignorant of the physical effects on the body. An endless variety of drug compounds, in endless combinations, are experimented with, ranging from opiate derivatives (*e.g.,* heroin) and tranquilizers to exotic plants such as Jimson weed and hallucinogenic mushrooms. The drugs most commonly used are heroin, cannabis (marijuana), tranquilizers, cocaine, methadone, and the hallucinogen phencyclidine (PCP). Drug-related street crime continues to be perpetrated mainly by heroin addicts. Cases involving overdosage, many leading to death, are treated by the thousands in hospital emergency rooms.

The magnitude of addiction has increased the illicit drug traffic, resulting in turn in stepped-up government actions to prevent drug trade and smuggling—from the spraying of marijuana fields with paraquat in Mexico to attempted control of opium poppy agriculture in Turkey. The widespread misuse of drugs has also stimulated research to find substitutes for addictive drugs. Those that have recently been examined are LAAM (levo-alpha-acetyl-methadol) and groups of chemicals known as endorphins that are produced by the body.

Methadone-LAAM. Methadone is a synthetic narcotic originally produced during World War II by German chemists as a substitute for opium, which was not readily available in Germany during the war. Administered orally or by injection, it became widely used in the 1960s for detoxification of heroin addicts. The value of methadone is that it allows painless withdrawal from morphine or heroin, and its own withdrawal symptoms develop more slowly and are less severe than those of morphine or heroin. For those who felt they could not tolerate a drug-free existence, methadone-maintenance programs were developed. In these programs the addict either visits a clinic daily to receive his or her dose of methadone or, in some cases, is permitted to take home a certain amount of methadone to reduce the number of visits to the clinic. Although chemically unlike morphine or heroin, methadone produces many of the same effects when taken in higher than maintenance dosages. Thus the practice of allowing addicts to take methadone out of the clinics resulted in the development of a black market, which in turn led to many deaths from overdosage. Partly to eliminate the misuse of methadone and partly to eliminate the need for daily clinic visits, an injectable substance, levo-al-pha-acetyl-methadol, or LAAM, was developed. The value of LAAM is that its duration of action can be as long as 42–72 hours, in contrast to methadone's, which is only 24 hours. Thus the need for take-home medication is eliminated; the addict need visit a clinic only three times a week. Moreover, the reduction in the number of visits per week also reduces the individual's preoccupation with the drug.

Endorphins. A narcotic, or opiate (*e.g.,* opium, heroin, or morphine), is a drug that in moderate doses depresses the central nervous system, relieving pain and producing sedation and sleep. Endorphins, which are composed of chains of amino acids called polypeptides, are chemicals with opiate-like activity that are produced naturally by the body. The term *endorphin* is the combination of two words, *endogenous* (internal) and *morphine.*

Endorphins produced internally by the body and narcotics introduced externally function in the same area of the brain and perform in the same way. The area of the brain that accepts the chemical is known as a receiving, or receptor, site. The interesting aspects of endorphins are their analgesic (pain-relieving) quality and the fact that their receptor site appears to be the same as that of externally introduced narcotics. Thus nonnarcotic compounds such as endorphins and a narcotic compound such as morphine, although chemically dissimilar, fit into the same receptor site as keys fit into a lock. The structure and action of endorphins therefore suggest the possibility that a nonaddictive substitute for externally introduced narcotics (opiates) might be developed and used in the treatment of pain and addiction.

Marijuana. It is estimated that there are 13 million to 20 million marijuana users in the United States. Something of a panic, therefore, was created in early March 1978 when the Department of Health, Education, and Welfare announced that users were in peril of toxic effects from smoking marijuana that had been sprayed with the herbicide paraquat. The herbicide was used in a Mexican-U.S. cooperative effort to control the illicit drug—60% of the marijuana used in the U.S. is smuggled in from Mexico. However, marijuana growers found that they could salvage their crops by harvesting them immediately after the spraying had taken place. Paraquat-contaminated marijuana, in moderately heavy use (three cigarettes a day), can cause irreversible lung damage from pulmonary fibrosis and can also damage kidneys. Lesser use can also prove harmful. As the paraquat announcements were made, laboratories equipped to test for the presence of the herbicide were swamped with requests for analysis of marijuana samples, and home testing kits were soon appearing. And because the private use of marijuana had been virtually decriminalized in many states, the U.S. government was requested to stop funding paraquat spraying and to put pressure on the Mexican government to abandon paraquat altogether.

Phencyclidine (PCP, angel dust). In 1977 and 1978 phencyclidine emerged as a leading street drug: it was cheap, widely available, and easy to synthesize. It was estimated in 1978 that seven million people, mostly 12 to 25 years of age, had tried the drug; for many it was the drug of choice, the "heroin of the suburbs." Phencyclidine was developed by Parke, Davis & Co. in 1956 as an anesthetic. Because of the drug's severe and unpredictable side effects, it was discontinued for human patients but remained in use in veterinary medicine. In the mid-1970s its use as a hallucinogen began to grow. PCP, in liquid or crystal form, can be injected, inhaled, or ingested; most commonly it is sprayed or sprinkled on marijuana, tobacco, or

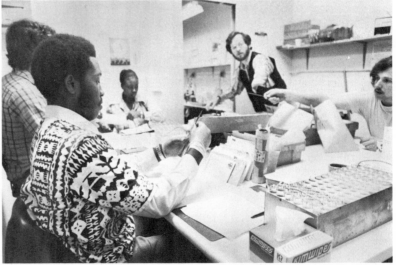

Technicians at Pharm Chem Research Foundation, Palo Alto, California, prepare to test some of the hundreds of marijuana samples they received following a March government announcement that much of the marijuana in use in the U.S. had been dangerously contaminated by the herbicide paraquat. Prolonged smoking of the contaminated marijuana threatens permanent, irreversible lung damage.

herbs and smoked. It is frequently used to enhance low-grade marijuana and is often sold as LSD or THC. Drug enforcement agencies began to become aware of the problems associated with the use of PCP when its users began to seek aid in hospital emergency rooms and in street drug clinics. The drug's severe psychological and physical side effects resulted in 100 deaths in 1977 and in a number of bizarre murders, suicides, and self-mutilations induced by self-destructive and paranoid-schizophrenic reactions. The psychological effects of a single dose of PCP sometimes persisted for a month. In February 1978 the Federal Drug Enforcement Administration reclassified PCP as a Schedule II drug, placing it in the same category as barbiturates. The National Institute on Drug Abuse launched a campaign of education on the drug's effects early in 1978.

Hypnotics and sedatives. In April Betty Ford, wife of former president Gerald Ford, announced that she was voluntarily entering a drug rehabilitation program, having become dependent on a combination of drugs, including alcohol and prescription drugs that she had been taking for several medical conditions. The revelation sparked a great deal of discussion of the abuse or overuse of prescription drugs, especially the most widely prescribed drugs—tranquilizers, sedatives, and stimulants, as well as analgesics. Figures released revealed that in 1976, 128 million prescriptions had been filled for sedative-hypnotic drugs—one billion doses. Tranquilizers and sleeping pills were implicated in 35% of all confirmed drug-related deaths. While these powerful psychoactive drugs have all been approved as safe in proper doses and under proper circumstances, many users increase dosage or take the drugs in combination or while using alcohol, an often dangerous complicating factor. It was also revealed that since women visit doctors more frequently than men and are more likely to express anxiety, they are more likely to receive mood-altering medications. In addition, there is a greater possibility that a woman's dependence on drugs can be hidden if she is able to remain in the home, where her altered behavior is tolerated or excused. In this way a woman may be protected from facing the reality of the depth of her problem. It was disclosed that the median age of white women who die of drug abuse is 43, as opposed to the median age of 28 for most segments of the population. The ultimate effect of the discussion of prescription medications was to encourage both doctors and patients to be aware of the drug interaction problem and the possibility of dependency. Physicians were urged to fully consider each prescription they wrote, and patients were advised to inform physicians of any ongoing drug therapy when new therapies were instituted.

—*Samuel S. Cardone, Ph.D.,*
Ann Englander, Ph.D., and
Lee Gladstone, M.D.

Allergy and Immunity

Asthma is a disease of allergic origin that affects the breathing. It can be a chronic, frustrating problem, but new treatments are giving asthmatics a more hopeful outlook.

The effects of asthma

Air passes into the inner regions of the lungs through the bronchi, or breathing tubes, to the alveoli, microscopic air sacs. In the alveoli oxygen enters and carbon dioxide leaves the blood across a fine capillary membrane. Air flows to and from the alveoli through the bronchi in a smooth, unimpaired stream, the diaphragm and chest wall moving rhythmically as a bellows. In an attack of asthma much of this changes: the bronchi are constricted to narrow passages and are partially obstructed with thick, sticky mucus. Passage of air through the asthmatic's partially obstructed narrowed bronchi results in a characteristic "wheezing" sound. The bronchial constriction in allergic individuals results from breathing what are for most people harmless protein-containing substances such as tree pollens, mold spores, and dust. In asthma the body reacts to these materials as if the lungs were being invaded by virulent viruses or pathogenic bacteria.

To fight infection the immune system forms antibodies, large protein molecules that combine with and help neutralize foreign organisms. Most antibodies circulate in the blood; one class of antibodies, termed Immunoglobulin E (IgE), attaches to specialized cells containing histamine and other pharmacologic mediators of the allergic response. These cells, called mast cells, are found throughout the body. They are present in fine muscles that encircle the breathing tubes. One part of the IgE molecule, the part that associates with foreign substances, is "exposed," projecting from the surface of the mast cell, enabling it to combine with bacteria, viruses, and other material. In allergic individuals IgE reacts to pollen and other harmless airborne substances. Each IgE reacts with only one substance— IgE for ragweed pollen does not react with grass pollen. A part of the IgE molecule without antigen specificity is anchored in the outer membranes of histamine-containing cells. Interaction of IgE antibodies with foreign material triggers histamine release from mast cells. In the asthmatic, substances such as ragweed pollen trigger histamine release in mast cells lining the bronchial passages. It is the histamine and other pharmacologic agents released from these cells that cause bronchial constriction and mucus secretion. Wheezing, shortness of breath, and, on occasion, death from suffocation result.

Treating asthma today

To counteract these effects doctors administer drugs that lead to bronchial relaxation and diminished mucus production. Foremost among such drugs is epinephrine (adrenaline), a hormone normally formed in and released from the adrenal gland in times of stress.

Muscle cells respond in two general ways to epinephrine: smooth muscles surrounding the bronchi relax, dilating the air passages, and mucus secretion in the bronchial mucosa diminishes. All this occurs through epinephrine's stimulatory effect on the level of cyclic AMP, a chemical substance in bronchial muscle (and elsewhere) that has profound effects upon the activity of the cells. Higher cellular levels of cyclic AMP lead to relaxation of bronchial muscle, lower levels to contraction. Newer drugs, such as terbutaline, have longer lasting, more profound effects than epinephrine.

Drugs that reduce the natural rate of cyclic AMP degradation have an effect on muscle contractility that is similar to those drugs that stimulate cyclic AMP formation. Also used are agents such as theophylline, which inhibit the action of cellular enzymes known as phosphodiesterases that degrade cyclic AMP. Physicians often prescribe terbutaline and theophylline together. Taken as prescribed, asthma patients feel relief for hours. Unfortunately, the disease is not cured by these treatments—the symptoms often return, requiring further medication.

Another new agent has been widely useful in the prevention of acute asthma; it is not effective in treating acute attacks once they have occurred. This agent, cromolyn sodium, appears to work through a mechanism quite different from that of agents affecting cyclic AMP levels. While its mode of action is not established with certainty, it is likely that cromolyn sodium prevents the release of histamine and other mediators of the allergic response from antigen-stimulated mast cells. The interaction of pollens and other foreign substances with IgE-coated mast cells is without effect if this substance is used. Thus, asthmatics use cromolyn sodium before an attack, preventing mediator release, not after the attack is under way. Once the mediators have been discharged, it is of no use.

Cromolyn sodium was discovered by an English scientist, Roger Altounyan, himself an asthmatic. Altounyan was surveying a variety of compounds for their effects on the treatment of asthma when he discovered that cromolyn sodium, extracted from the seeds of a plant from the eastern Mediterranean known as *Ammi visnaga,* prevented the release of mediators from pollen-stimulated mast cells.

The compound is administered as a fine white crystalline powder inhaled as a mist from a specially prepared dispenser. The mist of powder reaches the innermost regions of the bronchial tubes, where IgE-coated mast cells are found. Mast cells exposed to cromolyn sodium do not react if exposed subsequently to foreign antigens. Histamine and other mediators of the allergic response are not released; the asthmatic remains asymptomatic.

Cromolyn sodium dissolves completely in water. After coating the bronchial mucosa, it is gradually taken up by the blood, where it is carried throughout the body and is rapidly excreted in the urine by the kidneys and in the bile by the liver. The body is unable to metabolize cromolyn sodium—it is excreted in an unchanged form. This is an important positive aspect, since its inert character reduces the likelihood that it will cause serious side effects. Many thousands of asthmatics use it daily without ill effect.

Cromolyn sodium is most effective in treating asthmatics whose symptoms result from allergic reactions occurring in the lungs. Patients whose bronchospasm results from nonallergic causes, who have chronic bronchitis resulting from smoking or air pollution, rarely are benefited. Cromolyn sodium is useful as well in treating patients with allergic rhinitis—hay fever. The cellular mechanism is quite similar: IgE-coated mast cells in the nose fail to release their contents when stimulated with foreign antigens. In treating this disorder cromolyn sodium is sniffed rather than inhaled and patients can proceed through the hay fever season with minimal symptoms. While cromolyn sodium is used in the United States for treating asthma, its use for hay fever is not yet approved, although it is widely used for this purpose in Europe.

—*Edward P. Cohen, M.D.*

Birth Control

Voluntary sterilization has emerged as the world's leading contraceptive method practiced by married couples when the wife is older than 30. Today about 80 million couples currently use sterilization to put a permanent end to reproduction. This is an increase of 60 million since 1970. There are many reasons that account for this trend: it is the most effective contraceptive method available; it is available for either the male or female; it requires one procedure only, thereby eliminating the need for continuing motivation, checkups, and expenditures for contraceptives; it has a very low risk of complications, including mortality; it is the answer to many concerns about possible undesirable side effects associated with oral contraceptives and IUD usage; it is cost effective when amortized over the couple's remaining productive years; it is now a method acceptable to most physicians and policymakers.

It is most important, however, that couples be carefully counseled regarding the intended permanence of the procedure, that there be no coercion, and that informed consent be given, as the sterilization should always be considered to be permanent.

Vasectomy for the male continues to be the simplest and safest procedure and is performed on an outpatient basis with local anesthesia. As simplified female sterilization techniques have become available, however, the demand for them has risen. With the advent

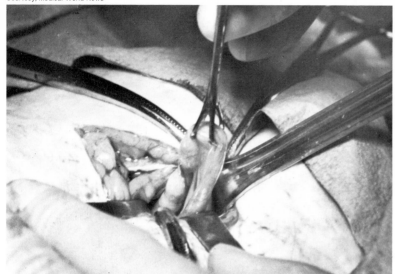

With sterilization gaining popularity as the birth control method of choice for married couples, the "mini-lap" technique for tying a woman's fallopian tubes has gained many adherents. It involves tying the fallopian tubes under direct vision through a small incision. The surgery can be performed on an outpatient basis and has a low rate of complications.

of laparoscopic tubal sterilization (commonly known as the "Band-Aid" operation), female sterilization can be performed in an outpatient surgical facility as well as a hospital and requires only a brief recovery period. The newest modification of this technique is open laparoscopy, whereby the laparoscope (a surgical instrument used to inspect and treat organs in the abdominal cavity) is inserted through a tiny incision next to the navel under direct vision. This further increases the safety of the operation, as it eliminates the risk of perforation of vital abdominal structures, which is possible with the traditional laparoscope. The fallopian tubes may also be approached through the vagina, avoiding a scar in the abdomen. With this approach, however, there is a slightly increased risk of complicating pelvic infection.

A newer technique, mini-laparotomy, is also widely utilized for tubal sterilization. It is usually performed under local anesthesia through a 2.5-cm (1-in) incision just above the pubic bone. By manipulation of a uterine elevator inserted through the vagina the fallopian tubes are visualized and closed, usually with a suture. Utilizing this simplified approach eliminates most of the rare but inherent risks associated with the traditional technique of laparoscopy.

Oral contraceptives

The Pill, the most popular prescription method of birth control, has come under increasing scrutiny as new data emerge about increased, albeit rare, risks associated with its use. For women under the age of 35 who have no complicating health risks it is considerably safer than pregnancy. However, data published in

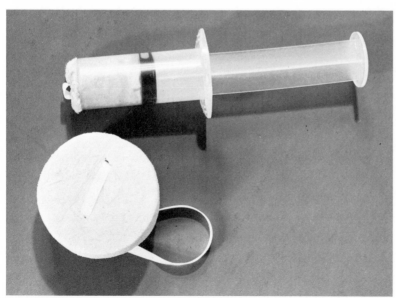

New mechanical means of birth control continue to be developed; many users consider them more desirable than chemical means such as the Pill and safer than IUD's. The collagen sponge (bottom) is inserted manually or with a simple applicator (top) and forms an effective mechanical barrier to the passage of sperm. In addition, the collagen has a natural spermicidal property that is enhanced by the addition of zinc. The sponge also inhibits the replication of herpes simplex virus, which can be venerally transmitted. Developers expect the sponge to be marketed by mid-1979.

Birth control

the British medical publication *The Lancet*, Oct. 8, 1977, increase the concern in regard to oral contraceptive use by women over 35, especially if certain other risk factors are present. The article revealed the results of a nine-year study of 63,000 British women. Among oral contraceptive users in England such risk factors as heavy cigarette smoking (over 15 cigarettes a day), diabetes, hypertension, hyperlipidemia, or obesity, when combined with oral contraceptive use, increased the risk of the occurrence of circulatory diseases in a multiplier effect (synergism)—the presence of more

In tests with hamsters, an egg (top) treated with an antipregnancy vaccine cannot be penetrated and fertilized by a sperm, as the egg at bottom has been. Developers estimate that a comparable vaccine for human use is about five years away.

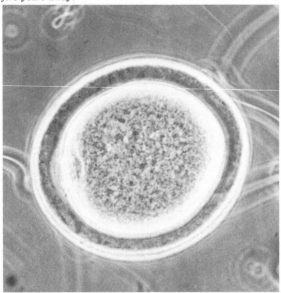

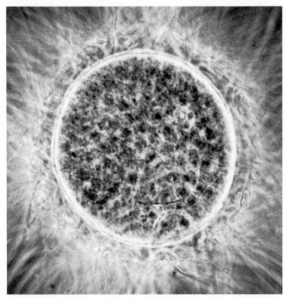

than one risk factor produced a higher risk than the expected total of the two risks added together. In the British study the increased risk of death from cardiovascular disease for Pill users as compared with nonusers was about one per 5,000, mostly in the age group over 35. Of the various risk factors, combining cigarette smoking with Pill use appears to contribute the highest percent of risk.

Additionally the study reports that oral contraceptive use of five years or more appears to increase the risk of developing circulatory disease, and that this risk may continue for an undetermined period after discontinuing the Pill's use. These latter two preliminary findings require further studies before confirmation.

The recommendations emerging from these authorities regarding Pill use by British women are as follows. For women under 30 years of age, emphasize the importance of stopping smoking, but make no recommendation of any change of oral contraceptive practice. For women aged 30–35, reconsider oral contraceptive use. Heavy smokers, particulary with five years or more of continuous Pill use, are at greatest risk and should choose between cigarettes and the Pill. Women over 35 should consult their doctors about the appropriateness of using another method of contraception, particularly if they have any of the additional risk factors previously mentioned.

Since women in England may be more prone to circulatory diseases than women of other cultures, the findings and recommendations for that population do not necessarily apply to other women of the world.

Search for new methods

An urgent need exists for a wider variety of safer and highly effective methods of birth control. Such methods are being tested; one is a long-acting injectable contraceptive, norethindrone enanthate. Since research has shown that it does not produce breast tumors in dogs, as does medroxyprogesterone acetate (Depoprovera), it may become available for human contraception. Another promising method is the vaginal ring, worn like a diaphragm, which has the advantage of minimal systemic side effects. The ring releases small but sufficient amounts of contraceptive hormones to induce local cervical and uterine changes with resultant contraceptive effects. Such a ring may also be developed to release an active spermicide. The collagen sponge vaginal barrier is now undergoing clinical testing, and the preliminary results are encouraging.

Preliminary work is also under way to develop a vaccine for immunization against pregnancy for use by women. Research in male methods includes various methods to arrest sperm production and valves implanted in the vas deferens so that male sterility can be reversible.

— Louise B. Tyrer, M.D.

Special Report:

Drug Information for Patients

by Marc I. Davis

Regulations promulgated by the U.S. Food and Drug Administration (FDA) now require pharmaceutical companies to issue detailed information and consumer warnings in the form of a patient package insert (PPI) to accompany certain prescription drugs. The drugs covered by the new federal regulations include products containing estrogen, oral contraceptives, certain inhalation preparations, and intrauterine contraceptive devices (IUD's). Approximately ten million women in the United States use oral contraceptives—the Pill—while more than three million use IUD's. In addition, five million women take estrogen preparations, most often for postmenopausal symptoms. Since for each of these women use is likely to continue over months and even years, it is essential that women know the risks involved and have enough information to choose intelligently between the available alternatives. Legislation is now being planned to cover a variety of other drugs in the PPI program. The patient package inserts are made available to pharmacies by individual manufacturers of the regulated drugs.

The PPI tells the patient about the medical risks in using each drug, lists possible side effects, and gives appropriate warnings on use and misuse of the product, storing information, and a general explanation of the specific medical use for each drug. The need for PPI's is based on the contention that physicians often do not adequately warn patients about potential adverse drug effects and that patients do not understand or remember these warnings if they are given. The information in the PPI is presented in a straightforward way and is written in language that is nontechnical and easily understood. For example, the PPI distributed with estrogen medications states: "Oral contraceptives increase the risk of blood clotting in various parts of the body. This can result in a stroke (if the clot is in the brain), a heart attack (clot in a blood vessel of the heart), or a pulmonary embolus (a clot which forms in the legs or pelvis, then breaks off and travels to the lungs). Any of these can be fatal."

Formulating the legislation

In 1975 a petition was filed by the Center for Law and Social Policy on behalf of various consumer groups requesting that certain prescription drugs be accompanied by consumer warnings. In response to the petition, the federal Food and Drug Administration (FDA) solicited comments from interested parties, collected appropriate information, and held joint discussions with consumer, medical, and pharmacy groups. The FDA also conducted a survey among users of oral contraceptives to determine if additional drug information was necessary and how it might affect consumer attitudes. The current form and content of PPI legislation and its future direction are based largely upon the recommendations and material acquired by these methods.

More than 1,000 comments were received by the FDA, detailing a variety of adverse side effects suffered by users of prescription drugs, most of whom claimed they were not adequately warned by their physician or pharmacist about the possibility of such effects. The responses listed complaints of temporary or chronic drug reactions, some serious, others mild, some of short duration and others long-term. Typical physical symptoms included headaches, nausea, vomiting, skin rashes, swellings, hypersensitivity to sunlight, impaired mental ability, and, in some cases, hallucinations. Some respondents reported narrowly avoiding serious accidents while operating automobiles or machinery in a state of drug-induced drowsiness. Adequate warnings might have reduced the potential hazards caused by these adverse drug reactions and alleviated the patients' anxiety after their occurrence. Numerous respondents, however, claimed that no such cautionary information was given them or their families.

Among physicians, pharmaceutical companies, pharmacists, and health professionals responding to the FDA, a portion opposed the patient package insert. Too much drug information, in their view, might confuse, bewilder, and alarm certain patients, many of whom are suffering disease-related stress. Neurotic patients might imagine they had the symptoms that are cited as possible side effects. Other frequently heard arguments against the PPI program included worries that the doctor-patient relationship might be compromised, fears that doctors might spend less time with their patients, and the belief that the cost of drugs would increase.

To supplement the comments on consumer-group petitions, a symposium was conducted by the FDA, the American Medical Association (AMA), the Pharmaceutical Manufacturers Association, and the Drug Information Association. While generally favoring the PPI, panelists advocated a cautious development of

Adapted from *The Journal of the American Medical Association,*
Dec. 5, 1977, p. 2505, table 2

Recall of Information in Insert and Booklet		
	Recall of Information	
Information Recalled	**Current Users**	**Former Users**
% of insert readers who remember item		
directions for use	69.2	68.9
side effects	49.5	46.6
dosage	19.3	24.2
precautions on use	23.0	20.1
composition	12.6	10.0
is you forget a Pill	23.2	...
other	14.7	12.9
don't know	9.7	17.3
% of booklet readers who remember item		
Pill effectiveness	29.7	28.8
Pill composition	13.6	11.4
how the Pill works	29.9	33.3
common reactions	59.9	40.4
blood clots	32.2	28.2
special health problems	7.9	8.5
directions for use	62.0	43.3
what to do if you forget a Pill	36.8	24.3
what to do if you miss a period	12.8	13.8
who should not take the Pill	8.0	9.0
about seeing physician	16.9	9.4
don't know	12.7	21.5

the plan. A recurring theme of symposium participants was the need for continued research and evaluation of the effects of the PPI program. A representative from the AMA recommended that only a limited number of drugs, closely monitored, be initially chosen for the program, so that results could be carefully evaluated.

It was proposed that the extent and nature of PPI information be limited—warnings were made against including data that encouraged the patient to exercise medical judgment. In addition to information on adverse reactions and steps to take if they occurred, it was proposed that the PPI contain explanations of the importance of taking the drug, reasons why discontinuing usage without the physician's consent would be detrimental, food, drugs, or activities to avoid while taking the drug, instructions on how to handle a missed dose or overdose, and instructions on drug storage and refilling the prescription.

Some panelists recommended that physicians and pharmacists retain the option of withholding information if they believed it would be injurious to the patient. A representative of the American Society of Hospital Pharmacists suggested that it was not necessary to provide a PPI for hospitalized patients taking the affected drugs since they are so closely monitored by physicians, nurses, and pharmacists. All the panelists agreed that the PPI should be simply and clearly written and easy to understand.

Implications of the PPI

Crucial scientific and legal problems implicit in the PPI program have yet to be resolved to the complete satisfaction of opponents of the plan. Still debated are the extent of legal liability of pharmaceutical companies for drug reactions that are not included in the PPI warnings and the standards of the clinical evidence that are applied in composing a list of indicated uses and in deciding which side effects are important enough to be mentioned.

Commercial considerations are also important. Before changing a label pharmaceutical manufacturers must conduct extensive research, file documents with the FDA, withhold the drug pending FDA approval, and print and distribute new labeling. The investment of time and money must be justified by potential profits.

Most importantly, the practice of medicine is concerned with unique, individual patients who often cannot be treated according to standardized routines. In many cases the physician chooses one of a variety of appropriate treatments after considering specific physiological, psychological, economic, social, and cultural factors. Some physicians fear that under the current PPI program such decisions will be made by government employees using general considerations not necessarily supported completely by clinical or scientific evidence.

Some critics of the PPI contend that the need for the program has yet to be fully established. Before a wider application of PPI's is undertaken, they suggest controlled scientific studies and comprehensive research to ascertain the influence of the PPI on prescribing patterns and volume and patient compliance and to determine potentially adverse consequences.

The FDA is now considering PPI labeling for progestin, metronidazole (Flagyl; used to treat vaginal infections), and the widely prescribed tranquilizers Valium, Librium, Miltown, and Equanil. A variety of antibiotic drugs have also been proposed for inclusion in the PPI program. An FDA proposal for expanding and developing the PPI plan was published in the *Federal Register* late in 1977, and again interested parties were asked for their comments. Meanwhile, both houses of Congress have been studying recently introduced legislation involving the PPI.

Joseph Onek of the Center for Law and Social Policy, the group that initially filed the petition requesting the PPI, has proposed that all drugs eventually be accompanied by descriptive labeling. At present, however, he urged that drugs with the most severe side effects have top priority, in addition to drugs used by patients not under the continuous care of a physician. The patient package insert, according to Onek, is not a panacea solving all problems connected with prescription drugs. It is only the beginning of a doctor-patient dialogue, serving the patient's right to know and to participate in the decision-making process.

182

Blood and the Lymphatic System

Researchers believe that certain types of cancer in humans are caused by viruses. The evidence for this is strongest in malignant diseases of lymphocytes (one type of white blood cell) such as leukemia and diseases of lymphoid tissues such as lymphoma.

Epstein-Barr virus (EBV) has been investigated most extensively as a possible cause of human lymphatic cancer. It is closely implicated as the inciting cause of Burkitt's lymphoma, a malignant disease of lymph glands that is found primarily, although not exclusively, among peoples of central Africa. EBV may also be the causative agent of nasopharyngeal carcinoma, a malignant disease of tissues of the back of the nose and upper regions of the throat. The virus also causes infectious mononucleosis, a nonmalignant, self-limiting disease of lymph nodes found primarily among young adults of higher socioeconomic classes.

The effects of EBV on cells

Like other viral agents, EBV is transmitted from an infected person to a susceptible noninfected individual. The belief that EBV causes human lymphoid tissue cancer is based upon a number of important observations. Lymphoid cells removed from the body (they are found in large numbers in the blood) and placed in test tubes and flasks live at most for a few weeks. After proliferating slightly, or perhaps not at all, they die and gradually disintegrate. In contrast, cells from the same donor that are deliberately infected in culture with EBV divide repeatedly, increasing their numbers and persisting indefinitely. The cells continue replicating as long as they are provided with sufficient amounts of fresh medium. They are converted by EBV infection from cells with limited life spans to cells with unlimited potentials for growth. They have been "immortalized." In cancer, malignant cells in the body, like transformed cells in culture, have an unlimited proliferative capacity.

Cells transformed *in vitro* (outside the living body under laboratory conditions) by EBV exhibit other growth characteristics of malignant cells. Before EBV infection densely populated nonmalignant cells exhibit contact inhibition; *i.e.,* they fail to divide in culture if they "touch" other cells. When infected with EBV, the cells behave as if they were malignant. They are no longer contact inhibited and proliferate without apparent regard for the presence of other cells.

Only lymphoid cells possessing specific surface receptors for virus attachment are susceptible to infection with EBV. Other cell types, such as those originating in liver, kidney, or muscle, are not susceptible. The DNA of EBV itself may be detected by special techniques inside transformed lymphoid cell types. It is detectable whether the infection occurs deliberately in cells in culture or naturally in human populations. Attempts to detect by similar means the presence of the

Courtesy, World Health Organization; photograph, H. Page

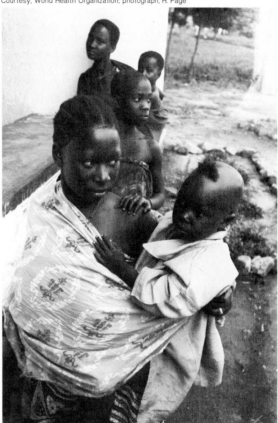

The Epstein-Barr virus has been implicated as the cause of Burkitt's lymphoma, a malignant lymph disease that mainly affects populations of central Africa. EBV research may unlock the mystery of viral causation of cancer.

viral nucleic acid among the tissues of normal noninfected individuals or among nonlymphoid cells of infected patients have been unsuccessful.

In most cells, viral DNA is a "passenger"—carried and replicated by the cell and doing no obvious harm to the body. In productively infected cells, *i.e.,* cells in which viral DNA has been activated and replication is occurring, the complete virus is readily seen with the electron microscope or by immunofluorescence identification methods. Cells "carrying" viral DNA are detected using DNA:DNA hybridization techniques involving the specific association of known viral DNA and "hidden" viral DNA in cells.

It might be argued that conversion by EBV of normal lymphocytes in culture to lymphocytes capable of replicating for indefinite periods really has little to do with malignancy of lymphoid tissues in humans. In humans the ultimate test of malignancy is to conduct research in which virally transformed cells are returned to their human source. Observations are then made to determine whether cancer develops. Obviously this is both dangerous and unethical, so research scientists use other means of investigation. A strain of laboratory mice, nu/nu, has a congenital deficiency of the immune system. These animals are quite susceptible to infection; associated with their lack of immunity is an inability to reject foreign tissues, including a wide variety of tumors from diverse sources, even human tissues. Normal, nontransformed human lymphoid cells, like cells in culture, grow for limited periods in such animals, gradually dying and disintegrating. Tumor cells, including lymphocytes from humans transformed *in vitro* by EBV, grow progressively as cancer cells in nu/nu mice. Their growth characteristics support the conclusion that EBV infected cells are converted to malignant types.

EBV is a virus infective for humans. While humans are primarily susceptible, some animal species may be infected as well. Here the evidence that EBV is a causative agent of cancer in lymphoid cells is the strongest. Owl monkeys and marmosets may be infected with EBV. Experiments that cannot be performed in humans have been performed in such susceptible animals, and the results are remarkable, supporting this cancer's viral etiology. Lymphoid cells are removed from normal, non-tumor-bearing animals and placed in culture. The cells are then infected with EBV and returned to the animal from which they originated. Lymphoid tumors develop. The animals eventually die from widespread malignancy induced by EBV. In these experiments cells treated in the same way but without exposure to the virus were returned without harmful effects—a procedure no different from removing and returning blood to the same individual.

Variable effects of EBV infection

One of the most intriguing aspects of this history is the observation that not all infections with EBV lead to malignancy. It points up the important role the host plays in preventing the emergence of cancer cells. Young adults from Caucasian middle-class homes who are infected with EBV develop infectious mononucleosis rather than neoplastic disease. Young adults from poor inner-city areas are most often immune as a result of an earlier infection that occurred with no clinical symptoms. Infectious mononucleosis is a self-limited, rarely fatal illness characterized by persistent low-grade fever, aching, fatigue, sore throat, and the enlargement of lymph nodes and spleen. Death, when it occurs, results most commonly from spontaneous rupture of the spleen, although serious secondary bacterial infections—pneumonia and the like—sometimes occur. Patients recovering from the disease have lifelong immunity. This rather common disease of young people has many features of lymphoid tissue malignancy. The fever, painful lymph node enlargement, and increased white blood count are also features of leukemia. In early stages leukemia and infectious mononucleosis, with so many similarities, often are mistaken for each other. In the case of mononucleosis,

however, the disease gradually subsides. Subtle differences between the morphology of lymphoid cells of leukemia and mononucleosis patients aid the physician in distinguishing between the two diseases.

It is significant that lymphoid cells from patients with infectious mononucleosis behave *in vitro* like malignant transformed cells. Lymphoid cells from the blood of infectious mononucleosis patients, obtained in the early stages of the disease, are immature—early forms found normally only in the bone marrow, the site of blood cell formation. Placed in tissue culture, these immature cells exhibit the capacity for unlimited proliferation. Unlike nonneoplastic cells they show no evidence of contact inhibition and grow in spite of high cellular density. Subsiding of the disease is accompanied by the appearance of a serum antibody that reacts, for unknown reasons, with the red blood cells of sheep!

Why is it that what appears to be the same viral agent causes a fatal disease among Africans and a benign self-limited disease among Americans? The answer is unknown. Africans live in an area in which malaria is endemic; most suffer from this and other parasitic diseases; in addition, many are poorly nourished. Whether the modifying effects of infection and poor nutrition are involved is not certain. Peoples in other regions of the world with similar health problems do not share the high incidence of Burkitt's lymphoma. A genetic predisposition may be involved, possibly involving the host's inability to recognize and destroy, by immunologic means, the transformed cells.

The cellular mechanics of EBV

The virus enters lymphocytes after associating with attachment sites or receptors on the surface membranes of the cells. The function of such receptors clearly is not to provide a site of virus attachment—the virus takes advantage of preexisting structures on the surfaces of the cells. Once inside the cell the virus is replicated, using in part cellular structures, cell nutrients, and so forth. Cells productively infected, actively producing virus, will die, usually within 72 hours after viral replication begins. The virus takes over all the "machinery" of the cell to provide for its own replicative needs. Not every cell infected with the virus immediately replicates the virus; only about one in 100 is involved at any moment. For most infected cells the virus is "silent," carried along by the cell. The cells producing the virus die in the process after thousands of new infectious particles are completed.

The relationship between the viruses of Burkitt's lymphoma and virally infected but nonmalignant cells of Western peoples is indicated by several means. In experiments involving the formation of hybrid nucleic acid molecules of DNA, the EBV DNA isolated from lymphoma is indistinguishable from that of infectious mononucleosis-infected cells. The virally specified proteins of productively infected cells are quite similar and may be identical. Several such proteins, detected with antibodies from mononucleosis patients, have been found—namely, an EBV-nuclear antigen, associated with the nucleus of infected cells; an EBV-derived capsid antigen, associated with the virus itself; EBV-induced early antigens, viral components present early in the course of productive infections; EBV-specified soluble antigens; and the EBV-determined membrane-associated antigen complex. Antibodies, appearing during the course of initial infection with the virus, react with these components. They are detected by "tagging" the antibodies with a fluorescent dye and viewing the stained cells in a microscope equipped with a source of ultraviolet light. Cells forming these virally specified components stain a brilliant green color, readily seen; noninfected cells, or cells that are not engaged in viral replication, do not react with the antibody and fail to stain.

To maintain viral replication in the presence of specific antibodies, productively infected cells appear to have evolved means of "escaping" immune defenses, surviving in the presence of active host immunity. One means some cells use to escape host immunity is to cease producing the membrane-associated proteins that are targets of immune attack. In this instance the membrane-associated targets actually disappear from the surfaces of the cells. Antibody-induced "stripping" of membrane-associated antigens is one means used by Burkitt's lymphoma cells to escape host immunity. After the cells are removed from the antibody-containing medium, the membrane-associated target of immune attack returns. The reaction is reversible.

Latent infection of cells with EBV leads to malignant transformation. This does not mean with certainty, however, that all individuals with infectious mononucleosis or childhood EBV infections will develop lymphoid cancer. Other host factors almost certainly are involved, preventing the emergence of malignant lymphoid cells. EBV capable of converting normal EBV human lymphocytes to malignant forms has been recovered from patients with infectious mononucleosis. Conceivably, the patient's immune system "cures" the potentially malignant disease.

Success of malignant-cell growth is dependent upon the capacity of the cancer cell to escape the ability of the host's immune system to seek out and destroy malignant cells. In Burkitt's lymphoma the malignant cells most often are derived from a single transformed cell; *i.e.,* the disease is monoclonal. In tissue culture there is no "immune system," and so exposure of normal lymphoid cells to EBV leads to the appearance of multiple clones of malignant cells. Patients with Burkitt's lymphoma as well as those with infectious mononucleosis possess high quantities of antibodies for EBV transformed cells.

— Edward P. Cohen, M.D.

Cancer

The National Cancer Act, which became law in 1971, has fostered programs in all aspects of cancer research. Basic research exploring the nature and behavior of cancer cells is producing a surge of knowledge in such cancer-related sciences as immunology and virology. Research into the causes and prevention of cancer embodies a growing recognition that environmental factors often play a crucial role in cancer development. Cancer therapy in recent years has witnessed marked advances, especially in the treatment of cancers that primarily afflict children and young adults; the information gleaned from this work with children is in turn being integrated into the treatment procedures for adults with common types of tumors. Many new programs have been created to ensure that knowledge newly emerging from the research sector is transferred into the everyday practice of medicine and becomes accessible to health professionals, patients, and the general public alike.

The National Cancer Institute's (NCI) *Cancer Patient Survival, Report No. 5* is the latest in a series of comprehensive reports on the survival experience of cancer patients. The report, which covers the period from 1950 through 1973, indicates that the overall survival rate of cancer patients has improved gradually since the early 1960s. The downward trend in cancer mortality continued until 1976, when the rates rose about 1%, chiefly because of a large increase (about 7%) in the number of deaths from respiratory, and primarily lung, cancer among women. The rate of cancer deaths among children and young adults has dropped 31% since 1960.

Treatment strategies

Chemotherapy. Of the family of approximately 100 diseases known as cancer, 11 can now be considered curable with anticancer drugs. These include acute childhood leukemia, cancers of the bone and kidney in children, a muscle tumor in children (rhabdomyosarcoma), Hodgkin's disease, which is a type of lymphoma, testicular cancer, a hereditary eye cancer, and a tumor of the placenta (choriocarcinoma). For another 11 types of cancer—including carcinomas of the ovary, breast, and lining of the uterus (endometrium), acute myelocytic leukemia in adults, lymphocytic lymphomas, and cancers of the prostate—drugs can produce complete remission in more than half of the patients, causing the illness to disappear temporarily, thus lengthening survival.

The current therapeutic concept of adjuvant chemotherapy involves systemic treatment—the use of drugs to track down and destroy cancer cells wherever they are in the body—combined with localized treatment by surgery or radiotherapy. This method of treatment evolved from the recognition that as many as two-thirds of the cancers that appeared to have been cured by surgery or radiotherapy in fact recurred because cancer cells had already been disseminated at the time of diagnosis.

The advantage of chemotherapy is that it is able to combat the cancer after it has spread, or metastasized. In metastasis a few cancer cells break off from the original tumor and may travel through the bloodstream or the lymph system to a new location, where they start a new growth. Localized treatment is used to remove or destroy the bulk of the tumor, and drugs are subsequently used to eliminate any cancer cells that escape.

Researchers believe that the current progress in the chemotherapeutic treatment of solid tumors is comparable to the important advances in the use of chemotherapy for hematologic malignancies ten years ago. The results from two four-year studies on breast cancer indicate that the use of drugs in combination with surgery effectively delays and may prevent recurrence of the disease, particularly in premenopausal women who are found during surgery to have metastases in the lymph nodes of the armpit. Ordinarily nearly half of these women would experience a recurrence of the disease within five years.

Small-cell carcinoma of the lung, which accounts for about 20% of all lung cancers and which is typically fatal within three to five months after diagnosis, has responded dramatically to chemotherapy, used either alone or in combination with radiotherapy. In about ten studies treatment has produced a complete remission in more than half of the patients, and in each of the studies a small fraction of patients have remained apparently free of any symptoms of the disease for an extended period.

Therapy for stomach cancer has also made advances. Although the incidence of this type of cancer has been reduced by more than half in the past 25 years, albeit for reasons that are still unknown, it was expected to strike about 23,000 persons in the U.S. in 1978. While surgery can often remove the tumor effectively, recurrence is common. Now studies indicate that combinations of drugs can lessen the incidence of recurrence, and researchers are optimistic about increasing the length of survival for persons with this type of cancer.

Chemotherapy has also produced favorable responses in some patients with brain cancer and with osteogenic sarcoma (a tumor of the bone). In the case of still other cancers, among them cancers of the colon, bladder, rectum, and cervix, drugs have produced a good initial response but are not yet known to have increased the patients' life-spans.

About 40 anticancer drugs are commercially available, and others have demonstrated anticancer activity in clinical trials. A cis-platinum compound has proved effective against cancer of the testes and ovary and shows promise in cancers of the bladder, cervix, head,

and neck. A drug called hexamethylmelamine is also effective against ovarian cancer.

Clinical trials have begun for three other new drugs. One is a plant derivative called maytansine, which has been effective against leukemia and a variety of cancers in laboratory animals. Another is chlorozotocin, which does much less damage to the bone marrow than related anticancer drugs. A third, called PALA, appears to be uniquely effective against solid tumors.

Because anticancer drugs kill normal cells as well as cancer cells, researchers are working to develop ways to offset their toxicity. One potent anticancer antibiotic, doxorubicin, is effective against many types of solid tumors but, because it produces damage to the heart muscle, it can be given only in limited quantities. Now animal studies have suggested that companion doses of vitamin E (alpha-tocopherol) may protect the heart muscle, allowing doxorubicin to be given in larger, more potent quantities.

Similarly, a clinical study has shown that when diuretics are given along with a cis-platinum compound, they speed the passage of the anticancer drug through the kidneys, thus reducing renal damage. This procedure allows patients to tolerate twice the usual dose of the anticancer drug.

Radiotherapy. Radiotherapy has been a mainstay of cancer treatment for decades. In recent years radiotherapeutic capabilities have been greatly expanded by the development of supervoltage machines like the linear accelerator, which produces high-energy X-rays, and the cobalt machine, which emits powerful beams of gamma rays.

The newest advance in radiotherapy utilizes high-energy subatomic particles such as neutrons, heavy ions, and pions. Because these particles deposit most of their energy at a specific point rather than all along their path, they make it possible to deliver a dose of radiation to a tumor in a relatively selective and precise manner. Neutron therapy is being administered in several cooperative clinical trials for patients with cancers of the head, neck, brain, and uterine cervix. The results of this experimental therapy will take from five to ten years to become conclusive.

Surgery. Studies on surgery, long another principal treatment for cancer, have recently focused on reducing the extent of surgery insofar as possible. Such restricted surgery would aim to remove all of the diseased tissue while limiting the amount of stress for the patient.

Nowadays more women with suspected breast cancer are electing a two-step procedure for their surgical biopsy, with the first operation limited to diagnosis. If the biopsy reveals the presence of cancer, the patient is able to discuss her options for various types of surgery with her physician and to prepare herself psychologically before undergoing a procedure to remove the remaining breast cancer.

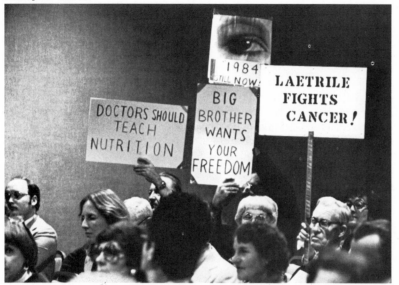

Laetrile advocates continue to support the substance's use in the treatment of cancer despite its rejection by the medical community and despite the absence of clinical data supporting its effectiveness and safety. Cases of cyanide poisoning and deaths from laetrile have been documented.

Sharing advances. As therapeutic advances have been pioneered, the benefits of proven techniques have been extended to cancer patients throughout the country. For example, a study that examined the records of 101 children with acute leukemia—representing all the cases diagnosed in 1972 in five different geographic regions—revealed that it took only one month on the average for these children to see a doctor after their first symptoms appeared, an additional week for diagnosis, and one more day for the first treatment. Moreover, the survival rates for these children were comparable to those of children receiving the best treatment available.

A number of steps have been instituted by the NCI to disseminate the latest techniques by enlisting community hospitals and primary care physicians in various programs. One group of networks, each of which involves approximately 100 community hospitals, has been set up to demonstrate the most effective therapies for specific types of cancer, such as Hodgkin's disease and breast cancer. To emphasize cooperative treatment efforts, a clinical oncology program has organized teaching hospitals into collaborative relationships with nearby community hospitals; the staffs of these community hospitals receive training, consultation, and assistance in administering the latest techniques in combination therapy from the teaching hospitals' cancer clinicians. Community physicians are also being encouraged to participate in clinical experiments. In addition, most of the nation's 19 Comprehensive Cancer Centers are conducting outreach programs, supplying specially trained health professionals to lecture and consult with hospital staffs as well as public audiences. All in all the NCI is bringing its influence to bear, directly or indirectly, on more than 1,700 of the country's 4,000 larger community hospitals and on the 60 million people they serve.

The continuing controversy over laetrile

Laetrile, also known as amygdalin and vitamin B_{17}, continues to create controversy. Despite the absence of scientifically sound data, its proponents contend that it will cure cancer. Animal studies of laetrile have demonstrated no anticancer activity, nor is there any documented evidence of this in human patients. NCI tests of the drug, a cyanide-containing extract of apricot pits, have shown it to be variable in composition, microbially contaminated, and hence unfit as a pharmaceutical product for human use.

Additionally, laetrile is known to be a potentially dangerous substance. When it comes into contact with enzymes in the digestive tract, the deadly gas hydrogen cyanide is produced. At least 37 cases of poisoning and 17 deaths from laetrile and cyanide-containing fruit kernels have been documented. Nevertheless, 14 states have voted to legalize laetrile. Moreover, a federal district court judge has ruled that terminally ill cancer patients have the right to import laetrile and that the Food and Drug Administration (FDA) may not interfere with interstate commerce of the substance.

To determine whether there is enough evidence of possible antitumor activity to justify a prospective clinical trial, the NCI is conducting a retrospective case review. The institute is soliciting evidence of favorable responses to laetrile, asking physicians or patients who know of such responses to submit their records for review. The goal of the study is to amass well-documented data on at least 200 to 300 of approximately 75,000 patients in the U.S. who have taken laetrile.

Detection and diagnosis

The screening for early cancers has long been encouraged by physicians since the sooner a cancer is discovered, the better the chances of effective treatment. Currently several programs are evaluating the

187

feasibility and effectiveness of screening large numbers of symptom-free individuals who are in a high-risk category for several of the most common cancers.

Lung cancer was expected to develop in approximately 102,000 persons in 1978, four-fifths of the cancers resulting from cigarette smoking; 92,000 were expected to die of the disease during the year. The recorded reduction in the number of adult smokers has not yet had time to affect the incidence of lung cancer, which continues to rise. In a five-year project, some 30,000 male cigarette smokers who are 45 years of age and older are being screened annually. These volunteers receive a special type of chest X-ray, and half of them additionally have periodic tests to see if their sputum contains any cancer cells. If cancer cells are found in the sputum despite negative X-rays, the physician uses a flexible fiberoptic bronchoscope, which allows him to look within the patient's lungs. Early data indicate that these techniques can reveal small lung cancers before they have spread. Individuals whose cancers are diagnosed in this way have greater survival rates than those diagnosed by conventional methods.

Cancer of the colon and rectum was predicted to strike some 102,000 Americans in 1978 and claim about 52,000 lives. Because it is believed that many patients could be saved by early diagnosis and prompt treatment, the efficacy of a screening technique that identifies traces of blood in the stool, an indication of colorectal cancer, is being field-tested. When the occult blood test, which detects blood that is present in very small quantities, is positive, the patient receives a complete battery of diagnostic tests to determine the cause of the bleeding. This test is being used in 30,000 people between the ages of 50 and 80; another 15,000 persons are participating as untested controls. By the time the first two-thirds of the participants had been recruited, 24 cancers had been detected and represented 13% of all those who had positive tests.

Breast cancer is the most common cancer among American women. In 1978, 91,000 new cases and 34,000 deaths were expected. To evaluate wide-scale screening, the NCI and the American Cancer Society jointly sponsored the Breast Cancer Detection Demonstration Projects (BCDDP). Beginning in 1973 the BCDDP offered five annual screenings at centers around the country to 280,000 women between the ages of 35 and 74. The techniques included recording of the clinical history; physical examination; mammography, or X-ray of the breast; and thermography, or the study of heat patterns emitted by the breasts.

The projects succeeded in discovering numerous breast cancers, many of which were small. Over one-third were smaller than one centimeter in diameter; at least 75% had not spread to adjacent lymph nodes. In such cases 85% of the patients can expect to survive at least five years.

However, several studies have suggested that radiation from annual mammograms might itself trigger breast cancer later in the women's lives. In September 1977 the National Institutes of Health and the NCI co-sponsored a Consensus Development Meeting on Breast Cancer Screening. A 16-member panel composed of scientists, clinicians, and lay persons met in an open forum to review the reports of several study groups and to hear testimony from a wide range of witnesses. Because the only scientifically sound data on mammographic screening available to date show decreased mortality only for women over the age of 50, the panel recommended that the BCDDP offer routine mammographic screening only to women 50 years of age and older or to those younger women with increased risk of cancer. The women in this latter category are, first, those aged 40 through 49 whose mother or sisters, or they themselves, had already had breast cancer and, secondly, those women aged 35 through 39 with a personal history of breast cancer.

The panel went to great lengths to point out that

The microwave thermograph detects the presence of breast tumors by sensing the heat generated by the increased blood supply associated with the tumor. Growths up to ten centimeters (four inches) below the skin can be detected.

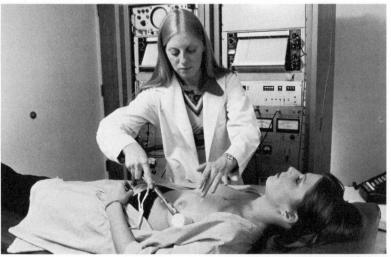

mammography used for screening is distinct from mammography used to diagnose or localize suspected breast cancer. They emphasized that the value of diagnostic mammography is indisputable and that a woman with symptoms should not hesitate to follow her physician's advice to have a mammogram.

Cancer of the uterine cervix is almost surely curable if it is discovered early while it is still *in situ*. It is easily detected before any symptoms occur with the Pap smear, a technique named after its developer, George N. Papanicolaou. Some 40,000 cases of *in situ* cervical cancer were expected to be discovered in 1978. These are so easily treatable that they are not even included in overall cancer statistics. However, another 20,000 women might be expected to have a diagnosis of advanced cancer, and 7,400 of these women would be expected to die.

Some 35 state and regional health departments are collaborating in an effort to motivate high-risk, hard-to-reach women to avail themselves of cervical screening services and to seek follow-up diagnostic care when needed. Thus far they have enlisted more than 1,300 hospitals and screened more than half a million women. In a screening population of just over a quarter of a million, the program has discovered almost 900 cases of uterine cancer, *in situ* in more than 600 women and invasive in the remaining 300.

Since its introduction several years ago, the process of computerized axial tomography (CAT), which combines computer capabilities and X-ray techniques to produce images of thin cross-sections of the body, has revolutionized the diagnosis of brain lesions. Now there is a similar device that can be used to study any part of the body. CAT scanning of the entire body is showing great promise in the diagnosis of deep-seated cancers, such as cancer of the pancreas, which are difficult to visualize by conventional means.

Diagnosis of pancreatic cancer is also being facilitated with the fiberoptic endoscope. This flexible instrument is passed through the throat and esophagus to obtain samples of pancreatic secretions, which can be analyzed for the presence of certain telltale enzymes and proteins. Fiberoptic scopes also are being used to diagnose cancers of the colon and the lung.

A similar instrument called a peritoneoscope can be inserted through a small incision in the abdomen to allow doctors to view the abdominal cavity and biopsy the liver. A recent study has shown that the technique is valuable in determining the extent of disease in patients with Hodgkin's disease. It is necessary to know the extent of disease in order to select the appropriate therapy, and the alternative for these patients until now has been major abdominal surgery.

The causes of cancer

While treatment is continually becoming more sophisticated and early detection is accelerating, the ultimate answers to the problem of cancer lie in its prevention. Efforts to discover the causes of cancer and to create ways to thwart its development are advancing on several fronts.

A major focus of preventive efforts is environmental, since many scientists believe that the majority of cancers stem from the environment in which we live, from our air, water, food, drink, smoking, drugs, workplace, home, chemicals, radiation, and viruses. To the extent that these factors may be found to be carcinogenic and their actions can be identified and controlled, many types of cancer may eventually prove to be preventable.

The number of chemicals in the world is estimated to exceed seven million, more than 30,000 of which have commercial importance. An additional 700 or more new clinical agents are introduced each year. Relatively few chemicals, some 16,000, have been tested to some extent for carcinogenicity in animals, and some evidence of carcinogenicity has been established for about 400 of these chemicals. Between 30 and 35 chemicals have been observed to be carcinogenic in humans, prime examples being components of tobacco smoke, asbestos, and vinyl chloride.

The bioassay program of the NCI tests about 100 chemicals in animals each year. Each animal test takes about four years and costs about $300,000. Animal tests can detect only the potential of chemicals to cause cancer in humans; their results cannot predict whether a particular chemical will actually cause human cancer. However, the carcinogenicity of chemicals in man correlates well with their carcinogenicity in animals. Most chemicals known to be carcinogenic in man are also carcinogenic in animals. Consequently, animal tests offer a logical approach for identifying chemicals that are potentially carcinogenic for humans.

When animal tests are completed and the results analyzed, the NCI publishes the findings in the Federal Register, informs the public through the media, and provides the information to appropriate federal regulatory agencies. Additional information is sent to physicians concerned with occupational medicine, industrial and labor organizations, and environmental and consumer groups. (*See also* Diet and Nutrition; Occupational and Environmental Health.)

One substance tested by the NCI, chloroform, was found to produce liver cancers in mice and kidney tumors in rats. Scientists suggested that the test findings signaled possible cancer-causing activity in humans, and the FDA subsequently banned chloroform from drugs and cosmetics, including toothpaste.

Smoking

Cigarette smoke is one of the most pervasive of environmental carcinogens. Several recent surveys, however, confirm that cigarette smoking is declining and

Cancer

that smokers in all segments of the population are now in the minority. Moreover, even among smokers nine out of ten say they would stop if they could.

Adults, especially men, are smoking less. Between 1964 and 1975 the proportion of male smokers in the population dropped from 52 to 29%. The proportion of women smokers also fell, although less dramatically, from 32 to 29%. Unfortunately, during recent years the percentage of teenage girls who smoke has risen from 22 to 27%, representing an increase of half a million girls. Four out of ten of these teenagers smoke at least a pack a day.

The NCI is now working on an anticancer campaign in collaboration with research, service, and public health agencies as well as with the tobacco industry. The joint effort of these groups is to develop programs to identify and modify the behavior of individuals most likely to develop smoking-related cancers, to modify smoking products, and to develop drugs to help high-risk individuals stop smoking or reduce the hazardous effects of the habit. A less hazardous, low-tar cigarette, developed under NCI auspices, is now in wide use. It is hoped such cigarettes will reduce the risk of developing lung and other cancers for those unable to forgo smoking. (*See also* Lung Diseases.)

Estrogens and cancer

It has been suggested that estrogens, the female sex hormones, may cause cancer when taken over a period of time. Estrogens are used by millions of women in oral contraceptives or for treatment of the symptoms of menopause.

Although the evidence is not conclusive, one study has suggested that oral contraceptives of the type that are on the market today increase the risk of breast cancer in women with benign breast disease. Other studies have found an increased rate of early uterine cervical cancer in women taking these contraceptives.

A very small percentage of the millions of women who have taken the Pill have developed liver tumors. Only a few of these tumors have been found to be cancerous; however, benign tumors are dangerous because they can rupture and cause fatal hemorrhage.

A type of oral contraceptive that is no longer marketed in the United States, the sequential oral contraceptive, has been implicated as a cause of endometrial cancer, or cancer of the lining of the womb. Women who take estrogens for menopausal symptoms have roughly five to ten times as great a chance of developing endometrial cancer as women who take no estrogen; the risk increases with length of use and possibly with increasing doses. In addition, one study has suggested that using menopausal estrogen may increase the risk of breast cancer 10 to 15 years later, especially in women with benign breast disease. The FDA requires that a special brochure accompany each prescription of menopausal estrogen, recommending that users be monitored closely by their doctors, that they use estrogen only as long as is necessary, and that they take the lowest effective dose to control symptoms. (*See* Birth Control Special Report: Drug Information for Patients.)

Taken during early pregnancy, estrogen may seriously harm the offspring. Nearly 30 years ago an estrogen-type hormone, diethylstilbestrol (DES), was prescribed for as many as two million pregnant women with the intent of preventing miscarriages. In recent years many of the daughters of these women have developed noncancerous vaginal irregularities and minor cervical changes; a small number of the DES-exposed daughters have also developed vaginal or cervical cancer. Abnormalities of the urinary and sex organs have been reported in DES-exposed sons.

The NCI has undertaken an extensive program to publicize this problem and is supporting a study at four institutions to determine the incidence and natural his-

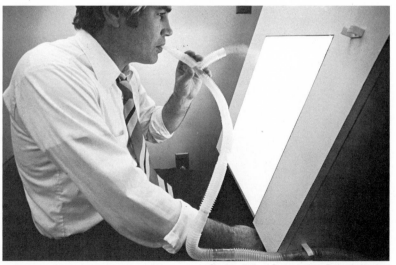

A device collects sputum from the air passages of the lungs. The secretions can then be analyzed for the presence of cancerous cells; lung cancers too small to be shown on an X-ray can thus be detected.

tory of the vaginal abnormalities in 2,000 of these young women. A question has been raised as to whether mothers who took DES do themselves incur an increased risk of cancer of the breast or sex organs. A task force within the Department of Health, Education, and Welfare has been formed to evaluate this and related issues.

Cancer prevention

Research has suggested the possible use of drugs to counteract the carcinogenic process. Synthetic compounds related to vitamin A, called retinoids, have been effective in preventing lung cancer in hamsters and also in preventing or delaying bladder and breast cancers in rats. The NCI plans to begin a clinical trial to investigate the effectiveness of a synthetic retinoid in preventing the development of new lesions in the bladders of persons who have had early bladder cancers removed surgically.

Research has provided information about another category of compounds that blocks cancer development in animals. These are antioxidants, chemicals that prevent substances from interacting with oxygen, and are used widely to prevent the deterioration of foods, rubber, and other materials. The mechanism by which they interfere with cancer development is not known, but when rats are fed an antioxidant at the same time they are given chemicals known to cause liver cancer, the cancer is diminished.

In a given situation an individual concerned about reducing the risk of cancer must weigh the potential benefits of a hazardous practice or substance against its potential risks. Even though exposure to a single potentially carcinogenic agent may be small, it must be remembered that human populations are rarely exposed to large doses of single carcinogens. It is more common for man to be exposed intermittently to many carcinogens in various combinations and at low doses. There are also substances called promoters that enhance the cancer-inducing effects of carcinogens. Because there are different kinds of carcinogenic agents, two or more of them acting in combination may be mutually inhibitory, additive, or multiplicative in their effects. Much research in progress is aimed at increasing the understanding of the multifactorial, multistage process involved in the development of cancer.

Cancer research

The study of the nature of the uncontrolled growth of cancer and the spread of cancer cells is fundamental to all other aspects of cancer research. Two important areas of cancer biology investigation are immunology, the study of the body's immune system, and virology, the study of viruses.

The immune system, which protects the human body from "foreign" attackers such as viruses and bacteria, also plays a role in susceptibility and resistance to can-

cer. Scientists are conducting research to understand the relationship of immunology with cancer and to develop immunologic techniques to assist in the prevention, diagnosis, and therapy of cancer.

Several antigens, foreign substances, have been identified in the blood or urine of persons with cancer and with certain other diseases. Because these antigens occur normally in the fetus, they are called oncofetal antigens. They include AFP, or alpha-fetoprotein, which occurs in cancers of the liver and testes, among others; CEA, or carcinoembryonic antigen, and a subfraction, CEA-S, which is elevated in patients with cancer of the colon and gastrointestinal tract; an ovarian tumor antigen; and another that is present in patients with cancer of the pancreas.

Because such antigens tend to recede as a cancer patient responds to treatment, researchers use them as "biological markers" to monitor the course of the disease and the effectiveness of therapy. It is hoped that eventually such markers will provide a useful and easy device for screening high-risk people.

Immunologic techniques are also being developed for treatment in combination with surgery, radiotherapy, or chemotherapy to enhance the immune defense system of cancer patients. Cancer patients with weak immune defense systems have a worse prognosis than patients with strong immune defense systems. Furthermore, a patient's immunocompetence declines as the disease progresses.

One approach under study is to develop a specific antitumor vaccine, using cells from the patient's own tumor or a similar tumor from another patient. In other studies researchers are attempting to boost natural immunity by treating patients with BCG (bacillus Calmette-Guérin), which was developed originally as a vaccine against tuberculosis and which appears to stimulate the body's overall immune response. Studies have been conducted in which living BCG organisms were implanted into the chest cavity following surgery to remove lung cancers. Early observations suggest that these patients have fewer recurrences and live longer than patients treated by surgery alone. A large-scale study of this approach is now getting under way.

A major recent advance in basic immunological research was the discovery that the immune system, like other complex biological systems, is controlled by a series of negative as well as positive regulatory mechanisms. One type of small white blood cells called lymphocytes is the T cell. It has been found that there are both "helper" T cells and "suppressor" T cells. The former assist in the production of antibodies, the protein substances that bind and inactivate antigens, whereas the latter block such production.

Disorders in this regulatory system have been found in association with a variety of diseases. For example, patients with some immunodeficiency diseases incur a high risk of developing cancer. It has been found that some of these patients have either an abnormal number of, or abnormally acting, suppressor T cells that block an adequate immune response. A similar situation has been found in experimental animals with tumors. Studies have shown that after suppressor T cells were removed, the animals effectively fought off the tumors. Research with AFP from human fetuses has shown that this protein stimulates the production of suppressor T cells. These suppressor T cells in the fetus function to prevent the mother's body from recognizing the fetus as "foreign" and rejecting it.

Research is continually revealing new aspects of the immune process. For example, it has been found that T cells as well as other cells are capable of killing tumor cells directly. Moreover, a whole new class of lymphocytes has been identified. These lymphocytes seem to play a critical role in the destruction of tumor cells and are being called NK cells, or "natural killer" cells.

Another recent development has made it possible to distinguish between the two major classes of human lymphocytes, T cells and B cells. Preliminary studies in patients indicate that this advance is likely to have early clinical applicability. Antisera have been developed to distinguish between T cell and B cell leukemia, a distinction that eventually may be important in choosing the appropriate chemotherapy.

The possible role of viruses in the development of cancer has been the subject of extensive research. Since the 1950s scientists have found that a variety of viruses are capable of producing tumors in almost every species of animal, including subhuman primates. This phenomenon is so widespread that although no human cancer-causing viruses have been conclusively identified, it seems likely that viruses will be found to play a role in some forms of cancer in man. (See also Skin Conditions.)

Cancer induction is a complex process, however, and a number of factors are known to interact with viruses to influence their activity within the cell. These include host factors such as genetics, hormones, and immune responses as well as environmental factors such as chemicals, X-rays, and ultraviolet light.

The emphasis in cancer virology has recently moved from the search for cancer-causing viruses to the study of ways in which the virus affects the growth and regulation of cells. Viruses have thus become one of the major tools for studying the carcinogenic process.

It is now known that a tumor virus contains genetic materials that integrate with the hereditary materials of a cell to cause changes that transform a normal cell to a malignancy. It has been found that a whole virus need not be present to induce the change to cancer. Rather, all that is necessary is a single gene, the basic unit of heredity, or a small number of genes from a tumor virus. It appears that one gene in the absence of any other signs of viral activity is capable of specifically transforming a normal target cell to a cancerous one.

Furthermore, for some tumor viruses scientists have been able to isolate the gene sequences that are involved in cell transformation. It has subsequently been shown that these sequences are activated not only in naturally occurring rat tumors but even in chemically induced rat tumors that show no other evidence of viral activity. These sequences thus indicate that carcinogenic agents as different as viruses and chemicals share a common step in the process of cancer development.

Spreading the word

The cancer act of 1971 gave new impetus to the education of the health professions and the general public about the disease. In fulfilling its responsibility to interpret, disseminate, and promote up-to-date information on the causes, prevention, diagnosis, and treatment of cancer, the NCI has developed a variety of programs and has established working arrangements with many community and health-related groups. Among the organizations with which the NCI now works are the American Academy of Family Physicians, the American Society of Clinical Pathologists, the Association of Community Cancer Centers, and the American Cancer Society.

To heighten the awareness of cancer risks, the NCI has supported educational programs alerting health professionals and the public to the dangers of radiation, tobacco, asbestos, vinyl chloride, and the drug estrogen. NCI has an interagency agreement with the Occupational Safety and Health Administration for an occupational cancer information and alert program. The purpose of the program is to make available information and training aimed at reducing the occupational risk of cancer among workers.

In another activity the NCI has launched a campaign to alert both persons who received radiation treatment years earlier and their physicians about thyroid abnormalities. Beginning in the 1920s radiotherapy was used to treat patients with such conditions as enlargement of the thymus gland in the neck, oversized tonsils and adenoids, and acne. The long-term result of this head and neck radiation has been an increase in thyroid cancers.

A new avenue for conveying information to health practitioners and the public is the Cancer Information Service (CIS). Located in most of the country's Comprehensive Cancer Centers, CIS offices offer a toll-free telephone service for answering cancer-related inquiries. To back up the regional system there is a national toll-free line to the NCI, which operates 24 hours a day, seven days a week. In its first year of activity CIS handled nearly 100,000 calls, most of them from patients, individuals with symptoms, or their families.

Another new activity is the Cancer Information Clearinghouse. The clearinghouse was established to collect and disseminate information on services and materials relating to patient, public, and professional information and education. Organizations involved in cancer communications, such as the cancer centers, professional associations, service, educational, labor, and industrial organizations, and government agencies with cancer-related programs can both contribute to and draw upon information in the clearinghouse.

The NCI also distributes publications on various aspects of cancer and on the National Cancer Program in response to thousands of requests and through supermarket and consumer distribution services. Approximately six million publications are distributed each year. So without question the word about cancer will continue to spread.

– Arthur C. Upton, M.D., and
Norma Golumbic

Death and Dying

It is sometimes said that "nothing is certain but death and taxes." The association may be even closer if we believe that every life owes nature its death. But on closer examination we realize that much is *uncertain* about both death and taxes: neither enters the same way into the life of every individual, nor do their circumstances remain the same from one time and place to another.

Death in the past

Through most of human history the lives of the very young have been in particular jeopardy. Early death was common from preliterate times until the present century. The visitor to an old graveyard in the United States or Europe will find numerous markers attesting to the brevity of life. On Burial Hill in Plymouth, Mass., for example, we read of F. W. Jackson, who died in 1799 at one year of age:

> Heav'n knows What man
> He might have been. But
> He died a most rare boy.

Women brought many babies into the world, knowing that a relative few would survive to maturity. The prospects for a life of moderate length improved considerably once a person was fortunate enough to survive the hazards of infancy and childhood. When vigor began to fail, however, the individual was once again exceptionally vulnerable to the ravages of infectious disease and other threats to life. The biblical specification of three score and ten years has become a realistic expectation only after the public health advances of the 20th century—and a long life-span is still limited to citizens of nations that have been able to provide a relatively high level of nurturance and protection.

Many of our ancestors on this planet knew a short, hard life in which people dear to them perished all too soon. Physicians often were helpless in the presence

of afflictions that today have been brought under substantial control. Furthermore, the sufferings of terminally ill persons were sometimes increased by methods of treatment founded on misconceptions. Today some elderly people hold deep memories of brothers, sisters, and parents dying at home, where all could share the grief but few if any could take effective action.

Death was experienced in those days as an immediate reality, not as an abstract concept. The average person, then, grew up with many exposures to death: the physical reality of seeing a loved one dying; the emotional reality of living with the sorrow and loss. Sermons insistently reminded the congregation of their mortality. Religious faith and the belief in a joyous hereafter often seemed a better source of support than anything the physician could offer. One could not depend upon a long life here on earth, nor an easeful death. It made sense, then, to discipline thoughts, feelings, and actions so that death might be a blessed release into a superior realm of being.

Death today

The conditions of both life and death are rather different for many of us today. Public health and medical advances have tended to move death to the fringes of both the community and our own minds. We look to the health care establishment with ever increasing expectations for prevention and cure of life-threatening afflictions. The increased life-span has made it possible to reduce family size but has also emphasized the association between aging and death. We have come to expect the young to survive, and most people expect to enjoy a period of retirement—itself a fairly recent and remarkable concept in the light of human history.

A century ago the word *death* might have brought to a person's mind the image of a young person caught in the crisis of an acute illness. Today one is more likely to think of an aged person beset by a combination of chronic impairments and degenerative processes, moving almost imperceptibly from life to death. Furthermore, this process is likely to be taking place "somewhere else" (*e.g.,* in a hospital or nursing home), rather than in one's own home.

There is some objective reality in the growing association between aging and death, but there is significant distortion of fact as well. The mental link between aging and death overlooks the fact that there are more vigorous, healthy old people in the population today than ever before. *Old* by no means equals *dying* or *ready-for-death*. Yet we sometimes succumb to the temptation to believe that death is "natural" for the aged and for nobody else. Have you ever heard a death described as "tragic and untimely?" What was the age of the person involved? Almost without exception, phrases such as this are applied to the young, betraying an assumption that death is "timely" for the old person and not nearly the loss that is represented

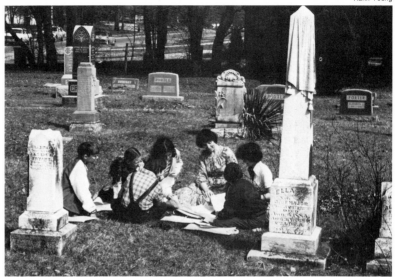

Hank Young

A sixth-grade class in Prairie Village, Kansas, holds a discussion in a cemetery. Schools are increasingly offering courses to help students discover their own feelings about death, confront society's treatment of the dying, and deal with the awareness of their own mortality.

by the death of a young person. Such an assumption can lead us to miss opportunities to work for survival of the old person, and in addition leads us to block out of conscious awareness the fact that death is a possibility at any age.

In the 1960s Americans were being told that they had an evasive, denying attitude toward death. Mortality was a taboo subject, avoided by health care professionals as well as by the general public. There was some validity to these observations, and one still encounters otherwise mature and forthright people who seen unable to relate themselves to the realities of dying and death. However, winds of change have already been felt. Death education courses are now offered in many schools, especially in high schools and colleges; both scientific and popular writings on the subject have increased remarkably; and the medical community has addressed itself more systematically to providing psychological and physical comfort to the terminally ill. It is no longer rare to find professionals and nonprofessionals working together to create hospice systems through which terminally ill people and their families can find skilled and sensitive support to maintain a high quality of life despite the inroads of illness and the nearness of death.

Many serious problems remain, some of them peculiar to our own generation. How can we create a balance between the personal integrity of the terminally ill person and the improved technical resources at the disposal of the medical establishment? Attacks are often made against impersonal and insensitive applications of modern medicine—where the dying person is surrounded and invaded by equipment instead of resting undisturbed in a pleasant environment where family and friends can feel at ease and offer support. Yet those with long memories would not want a return to situations in which comfort-bringing medi-

cation and nursing techniques were not available. The cure versus comfort issue is not always easy to resolve. Should one more course of medical action be taken in an attempt to halt the terminal process, even though the probability of success is low—or is it time to concentrate on relief of distress in order to enable the individual to use his or her remaining days in ways of greatest personal value?

Social scientists point out that an improved climate of communication between the terminally ill person, the family, and the health care providers is necessary if decisions such as these are to represent the best interests of everyone involved. Too often a mutual pretense situation exists: each individual knows what is really happening but conceals this knowledge from the others. Physicians and family members may think they are protecting the terminally ill person by evading or denying the facts. This has been often found to have an isolating and depressing effect on the dying individual, and can deprive him of the opportunity to communicate his own wishes, needs, and preferences. It may be said, then, that we are entering a distinctive phase in relation to death, one in which our assumptions and our patterns of interaction are critical determinants of how wisely the advanced medical technologies can be applied to alleviate distress.

Thinking about death

How a person thinks about death not only influences his behavior and experience at the time of his death but also affects the total organization of his personality throughout life. Some people organize much of their lives around death themes (Edgar Allan Poe is but one of the many examples), while others appear to organize their lives to avoid all reminders of mortality. Whether or not a particular individual develops an extreme death-embracing or death-avoiding pattern of

194

life, his own orientation starts to develop in early childhood.

Even the youngest child is sensitive to the possibility of separation. Many small separations and returns are experienced every day—Mother goes away, Mother comes back. Infants and young children are dependent upon adults for their survival and well-being, and they do not yet have an understanding of time that might allow them to distinguish between a short, a long, and a permanent separation. This means that any separation could potentially arouse an anxious state. It is many years before the child develops an adult concept of death. But one primary component of the adult view —death as separation—can already be appreciated by the young child. Loss and separation are experiences that are quite within the young child's range even though he may not be able to distinguish firmly between temporary and permanent separation.

Children often notice death and withering in the world about them: the leaves and blossoms that flutter down, the bird that will no longer fly. These small experiences can make a lasting impression. They are recognized as something important and special and help to arouse a more general curiosity about life. Parents who try to protect children from knowledge of death have set themselves a difficult, if not impossible, task, and one that is perhaps ill-advised as well. The normal child is interested in "where things go" as well as "where things come from." Adults who are comfortable enough with their own death-related feelings to share their children's discoveries can contribute much to their open and vigorous mental development. The child who learns that he is not supposed to notice death in any of its forms or talk about it carries an extra burden in his progression toward developing his understanding of the world.

Although even very young children can notice death and show sensitivity to separation and loss, it takes many years before complete comprehension of death is reached. Psychologist Maria Nagy found that the preschool child usually does not comprehend the finality of death. Being dead is like being less alive. The dead do not get hungry—but maybe just a little. Dead people may be thought of as bored, lonely, and sad. It is not unusual for the young child to believe that the dead person will return, as people usually do after being away.

Somewhere between the ages of five and nine most children grasp the idea that death is final (although this understanding may seem to come and go in the same child for a while). It is often easier for the child to recognize the finality of death than to appreciate the fact that all living creatures eventually die. If somebody is hit by a truck, for example, then this person might die, completely deprived of life. But a person might be lucky enough not to have an accident or to catch a dangerous illness. Death is still seen as somehow "outside"

the individual. If lucky or clever enough, one might evade death.

By about age nine or ten, however, most children recognize that death is inevitable as well as final. It is seen as both a general phenomenon, applying to all of life, and in personal terms: the child himself will die some day. The discovery of personal mortality is one of the most important psychological events in human development. Many children take this discovery in stride along with the other aspects of the world and themselves that they are beginning to understand. However, the meaning of personal mortality often generates questions and concerns throughout the individual's entire lifetime.

In adolescence, for example, the individual often begins to think seriously about the future. Who-I-am seems very closely related to who-I-will-be. Those who have particular problems in coming to terms with thoughts of personal mortality in adolescence also are more likely to have problems in thinking of the future in general. Both life and death are "out there" in the years ahead, and it is difficult to think of one without the other. It cannot be said that there is one typical or normal adolescent view of death—people at any age level have wide variety of attitudes and feelings on this subject. But research does suggest that adolescents have a greater tendency to fluctuate between extreme attitudes. A teenager might express a cool, distant attitude as though death could not really touch his life but in another situation show a sense of great vulnerability and apprehension as though his life might quickly come to a catastrophic ending. It is not unusual for healthy adolescents to contemplate the possibility of dying young. Experiments with drugs and with other forms of risk taking, such as reckless driving, are seen by some psychologists as ways of trying to master death anxiety by courting disaster and hoping to survive it. Other adolescents are able to explore the meanings of their own deaths by reading and writing poetry, having long talks with best friends, and turning over in their own minds the philosophical and personal challenges raised by knowledge of mortality. The thoughtful teenager or young adult recognizes that mortality of self and loved ones somehow must be integrated into his general view of life.

The fact that more and more people are surviving well beyond middle age influences the meanings of death in adulthood. A person of 30, 40, or even 50 years of age may not have experienced the death of people very significant to him. This circumstance was highly unusual in the past but is becoming more common. It is also becoming more common for people to report that death had not struck home to them emotionally until their mothers or fathers died, often at an advanced age. The individual may have grasped the finality and inevitability of death at age 10 and thought about it from time to time since. But it was not until loss of a parent in midlife that personal mortality fully engaged his thoughts and feelings. The sense of being more closely involved with death often develops in the 40s and 50s as one's own friends and acquaintances prove mortal. Even the deaths of people one did not know well begin to take on more personal relevance. While the adolescent may think of 40 as an advanced age, the parent may shake his head when reading in the newspaper that a well-known person has died—"and he was only 40!"

This heightening awareness of death probably has always been present for people who were moving into the middle and later years of life. But new elements have come to the fore today that give this awareness a somewhat different character. The expectation that medical science can win battle after battle with death (and, some believe, the "war" itself) can make acceptance of personal mortality more difficult than in the past. Hope for miracle cures has been expressed over the centuries but never has been as firmly interwoven into society's expectations as it has become in our own times.

Furthermore, the causes of death have shifted. Environmental and life-style factors are being recognized as critical influences. According to many physicians, psychiatrists, and social scientists, premature death is related to the stress of contemporary life. Competition, pressure, insecurity, and lack of deep satisfaction have been linked to life-threatening conditions such as heart disease, hypertension, and ulcers. Stressful life patterns are also seen to lead to excessive eating, drinking, and smoking, as well as to suicide attempts. The possibility that environmental pollution, including hazards associated with a number of occupations, may also be shortening our lives has been suspected for several decades. The information is not always easy to obtain or evaluate, but it is likely that environmental hazards of human origin will be increasingly recognized as factors leading to death. The adult confronted either with his own death or that of a loved one may now have to come to terms with the likelihood that individual and social patterns are among the most critical factors. It is not as simple as having "caught" an illness or suffered an "accident." In other words, as some of the traditional hazards to human life have been brought under control, death increasingly appears to be related to how we live as individuals and as a society. This poses a challenge to our understanding and feelings, as well as to our inclination to reshape our life patterns.

Bereavement and feelings about those who have died

Changing conditions of life have also created new challenges in our relationship to the dead. Thoughts and feelings about another person do not end with that person's death. In the past most societies recognized this psychological fact through elaborate rituals that made it legitimate for the survivor to retain a sense of contact with the deceased. Some of the world's most impressive edifices, such as the Taj Mahal, were conceived as monuments to the dead, and some of the most powerful music ever composed has been in the form of the requiem or mass for the dead. Religious and ethnic traditions have provided guidelines for the appropriate behavior of the bereaved person and have encouraged support of the bereaved during the mourning process.

There are many indications today, however, that the entire process of memorialization is being weakened. A pattern of legalistic and economic objections to acknowledgment of death is emerging. There is pressure to ban funeral processions because they are slow moving and hold up traffic, refusal to grant permission for new cemeteries and pressure to convert existing burial grounds to more "efficient" use, and criticism of funerals as both too expensive and "too emotional." The spirit of the times perhaps can be seen also in the new emphasis on organ donation, in which attention is directed to the possibility of saving somebody else's life rather than upon the sorrow associated with the death itself. Specific points such as these can be argued in practical terms, but the pattern is wider and cuts deeper. It includes a reduced social tolerance for the person who is in mourning. In the past a person who had lost a significant loved one held a special status. The widow, for example, might wear austere clothing and withdraw from much of her customary social life. People expected different things of each other during the mourning period. By contrast, today there often are very few acceptable ways by which a bereaved person can indicate his or her status. The pressure is for people to be "strong" and return to normal life patterns as soon as possible.

Specialists in dying and death see these phenomena as related to society's discomfort with the idea of death. The dead must be quickly forgotten, or our lifestyle, which depends so much upon death evasion, will come into question. Furthermore, the fast tempo of society and its time-is-money emphasis work against the traditional patterns of support for the bereaved person. The concern is growing that depression, anxiety, psychophysiological disturbances, accident-proneness, and suicide tend to increase when the bereaved person is too quickly forced to "snap back" and when society does not share somehow in the sense of loss. Widow-to-widow programs have sometimes proved effective as means of support, and professional counselors are beginning to realize the scope of bereavement-related problems and to offer appropriate services. In general, society appears to be in a transitional state. New patterns of behavior are developing that can meet the need for sensitive understanding when we are confronted by the death of a loved one.

—*Robert Kastenbaum, Ph.D.*

Special Report:

The Nurse and the Dying Patient

by Mary Ann Cleary, M.S.

The attempt to conquer and eradicate disease has called forth the stalwart virtues of courage, insight, and ingenuity. Medicine and science have devoted vast sums of public and private money toward this goal. So when disease prevention or curative measures fail, people afflicted by disease become reminders of failure. Doctors can react to "hopeless" patients in a personal way, through mechanisms of rejection and denial. Rejection is evidenced by the lack of follow-through in the care of the chronically or terminally ill; physicians feel it is useless to spend energy and time on their care. More often the ultimate rejection is the denial that such people need the skills and expertise of modern medicine. These patients are rather relegated to the care of their families, without appropriate professional support. When patients and families are thus abandoned, stress is a likely outcome. The patient becomes depressed because no one cares, and the family finds it increasingly difficult to cope with the ill person and reacts by seeking institutionalization for custodial care. The patient becomes an outcast from society at large and from loved ones in particular, unloved, unwanted, and burdensome. The family is troubled by a tremendous sense of guilt.

In this atmosphere dying becomes a process to be ignored by society and by science. Only in the past ten years has the subject of dying and death become of significance in American culture. The health professions have begun to evaluate their roles dealing with death. The nurse has traditionally been the health professional most central to patients and families confronted with imminent death. In hospitals and nursing homes the nurse is involved in the personal care of the terminally ill; community-based public health nurses and visiting nurse services attempt to assist the dying at home. The focus of nursing care is comfort and reassurance for families and the use of therapeutic skills to maintain body integrity and functioning for the patient. The most problematic dimension of care, the need of both patients and families to talk of the experience of dying, has been less a part of nursing care.

The most unfortunate outcome of avoiding discussion of dying is that society, families, patients, and health care providers avoid learning about death as a natural and inevitable biologic process. The work of Elisabeth Kübler-Ross attests to the fact that the dying can teach the living while personally benefiting and receiving appropriate support. It is hoped that acceptance of Kübler-Ross's work, coupled with the importation of the British "hospice" program of care for the terminally ill, will both aid dying people and provide physicians and nurses with reassurance that the experience can be a positive and satisfying interaction.

Hospice care for the terminally ill

The hospice is a concept derived from ancient times, connoting a place where travelers, pilgrims, the sick, wounded, or dying could find rest and comfort. Its contemporary meaning implies a program of care offered to people completing their journey through life—a way station for the terminally ill. The philosophy of the hospice is provision of palliative and supportive care to dying patients and to their families, with emphasis on symptom control and preparation for and support during and after death. The aim of hospice programs is to improve the quality of the remaining life. In many instances supportive care is provided in the home, allowing patients to die in familiar surroundings. When this is not possible or feasible, the dying person is cared for on an inpatient basis with the family encouraged to participate in the care.

Although England is perhaps the best-known country providing hospice care, the United States has begun to accept and apply the concept of the hospice, primarily to those dying from cancer. The British have provided this care in facilities that are noted for bright, cheerful environments, where comfort and compassionate understanding are the guiding precepts. In this manner the hospice is viewed simultaneously as structure and process. St. Christopher's Hospice in Sydenham, England, is perhaps the best-known example of an institution devoted exclusively to this end. At the Royal Victoria Hospital in Montreal, hospice patients are admitted to a specific unit within the general hospital where palliative measures and nursing care consistent with the hospice concept are provided. This Palliative Care Unit is able to utilize the resources of the hospital when appropriate to the needs of patient and family. A consultative team to other in-hospital patients is also provided.

Perhaps the most controversial approach to inpatient hospice care exists at St. Luke's Hospital Center in New York City. Hospice patients requiring symptom control and nursing care are admitted to this acute care facility on any unit, similar to the admission of any other type of patient in need of hospitalization. Hospice care is provided by a Symptom Control Team, primarily on a consultative basis, an approach that recognizes the knowledge and skills of nurses and physicians currently caring for the terminally ill while providing additional expertise in situations where symptom control has been difficult to achieve. Regardless of structural differences, all hospice programs are committed to the belief that dying need not be a painful, agonizing process and that the universal experience of death requires support and assistance. The quality of care provided by hospice programs attests to that belief.

Symptom control

The aims of hospice care are founded upon anticipated events that occur to patients and families affected with the life crisis of terminal illness.

1. Provision of emotional support by recognizing that chronic illness affects all aspects of family life.

2. Reinforcement of the belief that patients and families experiencing the progression of a disease beyond cure need, and are entitled to, expert medical and nursing care.

3. Provision of professional expertise for specific problem areas in the event's physical, psychological, interpersonal, spiritual, and financial aspects.

In cancer, the major symptom to be controlled is pain. Over 60% of all terminally ill cancer patients experience some degree of pain. This pain may be directly related to the disease process or may be a manifestation of the anxiety, depression, or anger underlying the realization that death is imminent. In this sense pain is anguish. Often pain is a combination of both dimensions, each exacerbating the other, both drastically reducing the individual's ability to participate in the activities of living. Hospice doctors and nurses view pain as an undesirable and, in most instances, unnecessary experience. To control pain and the ever present fear of its return is not an impossible task. The use of around-the-clock, regular administration of oral analgesics or narcotics can obviate pain. When the strength of the dosage is calculated on an individual basis, the medication allows the patient to be free of pain and mentally alert, able to participate in meaningful activities and relationships.

Concern that the patient will become addicted to the drug fades into meaningless rhetoric when pain control is the issue with terminally ill hospice patients. Fears of psychological dependence are unwarranted; in a retrospective study of over 500 hospice patients at St. Christopher's, the data show that in many instances the dosage of narcotics does not significantly increase over time; once pain is controlled, patients can be stabilized on reasonable doses, and in some cases dosages can be decreased.

The role of the nurse in hospice care

Hospice programs provide care through many disciplines—medicine, nursing, social work, religion, psychiatry, and related fields; in addition, all programs make use of the talents and interests of volunteers. But at the core of all hospice programs is the nurse and the provision of nursing care. Historically and scientifically, nursing is the single profession that has as its essence holistic, compassionate concern for the individual. Nursing's social welfare commitment affords its practitioners the knowledge base to provide effective care in all situations, from health maintenance to supportive care for the dying. Nurses involved in hospice programs have the opportunity to provide comprehensive care in the physical, psychosocial, and spiritual dimensions of life. Whether the patient is cared for at home or in a hospice, the nurse functions as the major provider and coordinator of direct and indirect patient care services.

While the patient is being cared for in the home, the nurse is a teacher, instructing family members how to minister the physical care necessary to promote comfort. The nurse guides the family as they learn how to position, feed, ambulate, and attend to the functions of elimination. The nurse encourages family participation, knowing that this involvement draws the patient and loved ones together in mutually sharing and caring activities while reducing the feeling of helplessness that the family often feel during this phase of the illness.

Whether the patient is at home or in a hospice facility, the nurse has a major role in strengthening communications between patient and family. The nurse listens to each person's concerns and supports his or her efforts at talking about the eventuality of death and what it means to the patient and the relatives who survive. The nurse must also be attentive and responsive to the spiritual needs of the hospice patient and family, apart from any help offered by the clergy. The framework of these needs is the individual's perceptions of factors necessary to reconcile his religious beliefs to his illness or impending death and to derive reassurance and comfort from these beliefs and to conduct his last days in congruence with them.

The primary goal of hospice nursing care is to provide the patient and family with a secure feeling and to minimize fear of abandonment as death approaches so that all involved become more hopeful for a comfortable and peaceful death. By providing nursing and medical care, hospice staff afford patients the physical and psychological comfort to enjoy their remaining days by encouraging personal growth. Hospice care planned and administered in this way reaffirms the value of life.

Diet and Nutrition

At first glance nutrition would hardly appear to be a controversial subject. No one really questions the general objective that everyone should know what constitutes an adequate diet, one that promotes health and, insofar as possible, prevents disease. Nor would anyone question the idea that it is desirable for both government and industry to keep the food supply safe. In practice, however, neither of these objectives is easy to achieve, and disagreements arise as experts try to define an optimal diet or to set standards that ensure safety of food without gratuitously disrupting the food-processing industry.

The saccharin debate—continued

Perhaps no substance in our food supply has evoked more controversy than saccharin, which was discovered just 100 years ago, in 1879, by Ira Remsen and Constantin Fahlberg, chemists at Johns Hopkins University. A chemical that Fahlberg had synthesized from a coal-tar derivative accidentally got on a piece of bread, making it taste very sweet. That chemical, of course, was saccharin. By 1900 saccharin had been patented, and it has been available commercially ever since.

From the very beginning, however, there were questions about its safety. In fact, until 1938 saccharin was available to diabetics as a drug but was banned from foods. And until 1959 it was considered either a drug or a dietary supplement and was carefully monitored by the Food and Drug Administration (FDA). At about that time a dietary change came about—Americans began to consume diet soft drinks in increasing quantities. In the U.S. the per capita intake of noncaloric sweeteners —three-fourths of which are consumed in soft drinks— rose from one pound in 1960 to eight pounds in 1976. Since 1970, when the cyclamate ban went into effect, all of the artificial sweetener consumed in such beverages has been saccharin.

Then in March 1977 Canadian scientists reported a study linking saccharin to malignant bladder tumors in 200 laboratory rats. The incidence of tumors was even higher in second generation rats whose mothers were given saccharin during pregnancy and who were themselves fed saccharin from the time they were weaned. On the basis of these findings, the Canadian government immediately banned the use of the substance as a food additive. When the FDA attempted to do the same thing in the U.S., however, there was an enormous public protest.

As a result, in November 1977 Congress passed the Saccharin Study and Labeling Act. Under its provisions the FDA's ban on saccharin in food was postponed for an 18-month period. However, all saccharin-containing foods shipped in interstate commerce were required to carry the following label warning: "Use of this product

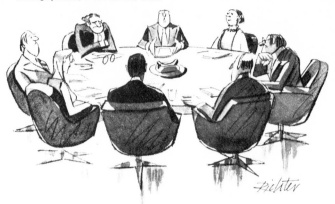

"Granted the public has a right to know what's in a hot dog, but does the public really want to know what's in a hot dog?"

may be hazardous to your health. This product contains saccharin which has been determined to cause cancer in laboratory animals." Warning statements must also be displayed in retail stores selling saccharin-sweetened products. Other provisions of the law mandate a broad range of studies not just of saccharin but of other issues involved in food safety. These studies are being carried out by the National Academy of Sciences, with reports to Congress and the FDA to be available by February 1979. Finally, the FDA itself, in cooperation with the National Cancer Institute, is conducting a nationwide epidemiologic study of the relationship between saccharin and other substances and the development of bladder cancer. Evidence currently available simply does not allow us to predict the potential risk of saccharin-induced bladder tumors in humans, nor do we yet know whether there is a safe maximum dosage. These are questions that must be answered.

Nitrates and nitrites

Nitrates and nitrites, which occur naturally in both water and food, have been used for centuries as additives in the process of curing meat and poultry. They inhibit the growth of microorganisms that have not been killed in processing and are a particularly important weapon against *Clostridium botulinum,* the organism that causes botulism poisoning. Nitrates and nitrites also impart some of the characteristic taste, texture, and color that consumers have come to expect in cured foods. The problem is that nitrates can be converted to nitrites, and nitrites combine with substances called secondary amines—which are found in many foods, beverages, and drugs—to form nitrosamines. Some nitrosamines have been shown to cause cancer in laboratory animals.

Unfortunately there are no acceptable alternatives to nitrates and nitrites. Without them such foods as hot dogs and bacon are highly perishable and could be

199

quite dangerous. Recognizing the potential hazard, the United States Department of Agriculture (USDA) has in recent years reduced the amount of nitrate and nitrite allowed in cured products and has continued to study the problem. In 1973 the secretary of agriculture established an Expert Panel on Nitrates, Nitrites and Nitrosamines, which was to advise him whether the use of nitrates and nitrites in the curing of meats and poultry constituted a public health hazard and, if so, whether such use should be restricted or prohibited. The panel has recently submitted its report, together with minority dissenting opinions. It did not call for a ban on nitrates and nitrites but set recommendations for what it regarded as acceptable levels of nitrates, nitrites, and ascorbates used to inhibit nitrosamine formation in various cured meats. It also recommended that the USDA closely monitor carcinogenic nitrosamines formed during food processing or preparation and that efforts be taken to reduce such formation to undetectable levels within three years. The USDA must now decide how it will act on the recommendations.

Together with the FDA, the USDA has also requested that manufacturers provide more data. And they are jointly reviewing both the need for and the safety of nitrates and nitrites in certain types of poultry products. The debate over the use of nitrites is far from resolved and, because of the wide variety of foods that are affected, is of major importance to the food industry.

Finally, one technological advance in increasing the safety of nitrites appears imminent. Bacon has long posed a particular problem because nitrosamines are formed during the frying process. According to both the USDA and the American Meat Institute, it appears that it will soon be possible to produce a nitrosamine-free bacon that is still safe from spoilage.

Sugar in breakfast cereals

The growing concern over the high amount of sugar in the average American diet has focused attention on processed foods containing large amounts of sugar. At the present time the average annual per capita consumption of sugar and other sweeteners in the U.S. is 126.4 lb per year. Three-fourths of this comes from prepared foods, including presweetened cereals. Sugar has, of course, been definitely linked to tooth decay. Some evidence also suggests that a high sugar intake may contribute to the development of diabetes in genetically predisposed individuals. And high sugar consumption can contribute to excessive caloric intake, often resulting in obesity and an increased risk of certain serious diseases. The cereal industry has put forth many arguments in defense of their presweetened products, including the fact that several studies have failed to link presweetened cereals with tooth decay. It should be noted, however, that these are relatively short-term studies, which may not reveal long-term effects on cariogenic activity.

Some manufacturers have voluntarily begun to label the sucrose (table sugar) content of their products, so that consumers can make their own informed decisions. An independent analysis done a few years ago found only eight cereals containing less than 5% sucrose and glucose, 23 with combined sugar levels between 10 and 25%, and 24 with 25 to 50% sugar. Eleven contained more than 50% added sugar, including one with a level of 70.8%. The FDA recently determined that it has the authority under the Federal Food, Drug and Cosmetic Act to require the labeling of the sweetener content on the labels of ready-to-eat breakfast cereals. And the commissioner of the FDA has directed the Bureau of Foods to prepare a procedure for implementing that authority.

Dietary goals for the United States

From its creation in 1968 until its termination at the end of 1977, the Senate Select Committee on Nutrition and Human Needs concerned itself with a broad spectrum of problems related to diet and nutrition in the U.S. Led by Sen. George S. McGovern (Dem., S.D.), the committee investigated the most urgent problems of poverty and inadequate diet, guided the development and expansion of food programs, and examined the relationship between nutrition and preventive health care. Several months before it disbanded (its work has been transferred to the Senate Committee on Agriculture, Nutrition and Forestry), the committee released a report entitled *Dietary Goals for the United States.* This marked the first time that any branch of government outlined goals for national nutrition planning as well as for individual nutritional practice.

Publication of these goals generated widespread debate. Many nutritionists, as well as a number of professional organizations, supported the goals, pointing out that they were to a great extent an expansion of the prudent diet they had been recommending for some time. Some criticized the report for its failure to include recommendations for reduction of alcohol consumption, reduction in total caloric intake for overweight Americans, and an increase in physical exercise. Still others disagreed with some of the actual dietary allowances recommended; for example, it was felt that a limit of three grams of sodium per day might be unrealistically low.

Among the opponents of the concept, however, perhaps the most vigorous argument offered was that there simply is not enough evidence to set such goals. Michael C. Latham and Lani Stephenson of Cornell University provide a rebuttal to this view, pointing out, in the *Journal of Nutrition Education,* that people cannot stop eating while nutritionists decide what they should or should not eat; goals are needed, and nutritionists should play a role in establishing them, in changing them on the basis of new knowledge, and especially in helping to achieve their adoption.

Courtesy, Dr. Ira L. Shannon, Oral Disease Research Laboratory, Veterans Administration Hospital, Houston; from the *Journal of Dentistry for Children*

Sugars in Breakfast Cereals

Cereal	% sucrose	% glucose	Cereal	% sucrose	% glucose	Cereal	% sucrose	% glucose
Shredded Wheat (large biscuit)	1.0	0.2	Rice Crispies (Kellogg)	10.0	2.9	Super Sugar Crisp	40.7	4.5
			Raisin Bran (Kellogg)	10.6	14.1	Cocoa Puffs	43.0	3.5
Shredded Wheat (spoon size biscuit)	1.3	0.3	Heartland (with raisins)	13.5	5.6	Cap'n Crunch	43.3	0.8
			Buck Wheat	13.6	1.5	Crunch Berries	43.4	1.0
Cheerios	2.2	0.5	Life	14.5	2.5	Kaboom	43.8	3.0
Puffed Rice	2.4	0.4	Granola (with dates)	14.5	3.2	Frankenberry	44.0	2.6
Uncle Sam Cereal	2.4	1.2	Granola (with raisins)	14.5	3.8	Frosted Flakes	44.0	2.9
Wheat Chex	2.6	0.9	Sugar Frosted Corn Flakes	15.6	1.8	Count Chocula	44.2	3.7
Grape Nut Flakes	3.3	0.6	40% Bran Flakes (Post)	15.8	3.0	Orange Quangaroos	44.7	0.6
Puffed Wheat	3.5	0.7	Team	15.9	1.1	Quisp	44.9	0.6
Alpen	3.8	4.7	Brown Sugar-Cinnamon Frosted Mini Wheats	16.0	0.3	Boo Berry	45.7	2.8
Post Toasties	4.1	1.7	40% Bran Flakes (Kellogg)	16.2	2.1	Vanilly Crunch	45.8	0.7
Product 19	4.1	1.7	Granola	16.6	0.6	Baron Von Redberry	45.8	1.5
Corn Total	4.4	1.4	100% Bran	18.4	0.8	Cocoa Krispies	45.9	0.8
Special K	4.4	6.4	All Bran	20.0	1.6	Trix	46.6	4.1
Wheaties	4.7	4.2	Granola (with almonds and filberts)	21.4	1.2	Froot Loops	47.4	0.5
Corn Flakes (Kroger)	5.1	1.5	Fortified Oat Flakes	22.2	1.2	Honeycomb	48.8	2.8
Peanut Butter	5.2	1.1	Heartland	23.1	3.2	Pink Panther	49.2	1.3
Grape Nuts	6.6	1.1	Super Sugar Chex	24.5	0.8	Cinnamon Crunch	50.3	3.2
Corn Flakes (Food Club)	7.0	2.1	Sugar Frosted Flakes	29.0	1.8	Lucky Charms	50.4	7.6
Crispy Rice	7.3	1.5	Bran Buds	30.2	2.1	Cocoa Pebbles	53.5	0.6
Corn Chex	7.5	0.9	Sugar Sparkled Corn Flakes	32.2	1.8	Apple Jacks	55.0	0.5
Corn Flakes (Kellogg)	7.8	6.4	Frosted Mini Wheats	33.6	0.4	Fruity Pebbles	55.1	1.1
Total	8.1	1.3	Sugar Pops	37.8	2.9	King Vitaman	58.5	3.1
Rice Chex	8.5	1.8	Alpha Bits	40.3	0.6	Sugar Smacks	61.3	2.4
Crisp Rice	8.8	2.1	Sir Grapefellow	40.7	3.1	Super Orange Crisp	68.0	2.8
Raisin Bran (Skinner)	9.6	9.3						
Concentrate	9.9	2.4				**Mean—25.1% sucrose, 2.3% glucose**		

The table above shows the sugar content of 78 widely sold breakfast cereals. The sucrose content is considered the more significant, as sucrose must be broken down in the mouth into glucose and fructose. This action makes sucrose the best known fuel for the bacteria that cause tooth decay.

After the release of the first report the committee continued to solicit opinions of leading experts in nutrition and held additional hearings. In December 1977 the second edition of the *Dietary Goals* was published. The second edition included a revised list of goals along with suggestions for food selection and preparation.

The revised goals are:

1. In order to avoid overweight, consume only as much energy (calories) as is expended; if overweight, decrease energy intake and increase energy expenditure.

2. Increase the consumption of complex carbohydrates and "naturally occurring" sugars from about 28% of energy intake to about 48%.

3. Reduce the consumption of refined and processed sugars by about 45% to account for about 10% of total energy intake.

4. Reduce overall fat consumption from approximately 40% to about 30% of energy intake.

5. Reduce saturated fat consumption to account for about 10% of total energy intake, and balance with polyunsaturated and monounsaturated fats, which should account for about 10% of energy intake each.

6. Reduce cholesterol consumption to about 300 mg a day.

7. Limit the intake of sodium by reducing salt intake to about 5 g a day.

The report also recommended a decrease in the consumption of animal fat and an increase in fruits, vegetables, and whole-grain cereals.

The liquid protein diet

The latest—and possibly most dangerous—in a long succession of fad diets, the liquid protein diet, received increasing attention from both physicians and the news media during the past year. About 50 different brands of the liquid—a predigested protein mixture, artificially sweetened and flavored—were available without prescription, and many persons were following the diet without medical supervision. Initial reports linking some 40 deaths to the diet were deemed inconclusive and inaccurate by government researchers, but studies at the Center for Disease Control confirmed some 10–15 cases in which the diet was a contributing factor. Most of the deaths associated with the use of liquid protein were caused by cardiac problems, particularly irregular heartbeat. The FDA announced in November 1977 that it would request manufacturers to include a warning on the labels of all such substances and would seek to ban their over-the-counter sale.

—*Jeanne P. Goldberg, R.D.*

Recent Developments in Treating Obesity

by Philip L. White, Sc.D.

According to a recent study by the National Center for Health Statistics, Americans today are not winning "the battle of the bulge." Men and women in most age and height groups weigh *more* than they did 15 years ago; at least 70 million people in the United States are overweight. Obesity is a complex problem, but some notable progress in treating it *has* been made by medical science.

The object of obesity treatment is to force the body to draw on its fat reserves. This can be accomplished in two ways: by reducing energy intake below total requirements and by increasing energy expenditure beyond energy intake. Nearly all methods of treatment are concerned with reducing food intake, abstinence from food, or interference with nutrient absorption. While regular strenuous physical exercise as a means of expending energy is increasing in popularity, it is infrequently incorporated into medical regimens.

Obesity is generally defined as "the accumulation of fat in undesirable excess." While many attempts have been made to find more precise terms, there is as yet no universally acceptable definition that appropriately describes standards for both sexes, all age groups, all somatotypes (body types), and both physically active and inactive people. Physical measurements such as height and weight, fatfold thickness, and limb and trunk circumferences are essential parts of the definition but do not take into account age and health risk and therefore do not have public health significance. Weight (in kilograms) over height squared (in meters)—the weight-height index—is gaining in popularity as a measurement for obesity, even though it also has drawbacks. Accepted indicators of obesity for this system are 27 or over for medium framed men and women and 30 or over for large framed men and women. The most common practice, however, is to derive weight in pounds (in indoor clothing) according to height and small, medium, and large frames from Desirable Weight tables prepared by the Metropolitan Life Insurance Co. and to define obesity as 20% above that weight. Some have suggested that better values are obtained by using the upper limit of the large frame size as the reference point. From the latter it is possible to define obesity in men when body fat equals or exceeds 28% of body weight and in women when body fat exceeds 36.4%.

Obesity has many causes and is often accompanied by physical and medical problems that can jeopardize health and emotional and physical comfort. To date there is no consensus that obesity is an inherited trait; there is, however, little doubt that strong familial factors influence trends in weight gain. In all likelihood, individual response to one's social and physical environment exerts great influence on ultimate body weight. Obesity is often described as the malnutrition of excessive caloric intake, but this says nothing definitive about the cause or causes of excess.

A thorough understanding of the precipitating events is essential to the proper treatment of obesity. Without this understanding and appropriate reorientation of the patient's concepts about self, food, drink, and eating, the probability of the successful reduction and maintenance of weight is minimal. One possible exception may be found with procedures involving surgical intervention, which will be described later. Such interventions serve, for the most part, to take matters out of the control of the patient.

It is well to bear in mind several accepted generalizations about the management of obesity.

1. The probability of successful weight reduction decreases in proportion to the degree of obesity.

2. The longer the time that obesity has been established, the lower the probability that weight reduction will be achieved, particularly if the obesity is of childhood onset.

3. The probability of success decreases in any given patient as the number of his previous failures increases.

4. Significant weight loss carries with it the potential for physiological and psychological harm that may place the patient in greater jeopardy than would perpetuation of the obese state.

5. There is no public health measure to cure obesity; therefore, more emphasis must be given to its prevention.

6. The only successful program of weight control is the achievement of a "desirable weight" and long-time retention of that weight.

Methods currently in use for weight reduction can be categorized as *moderate* or *aggressive*. The more moderate methods that involve modest caloric restriction (*i.e.*, caloric deficits up to 1,200 cal per day) are applicable to all patients; the aggressive methods should be reserved for those patients who are mas-

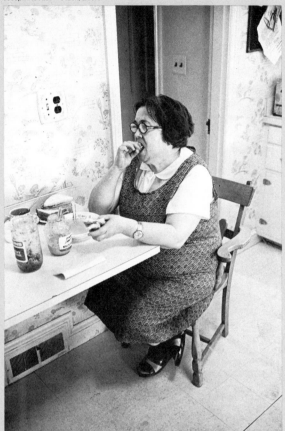

Overweight is the most important nutritional disorder in the U.S.; treatment is difficult and often requires alteration of lifelong habits.

sively obese (*i.e.,* more than 100% above desirable weight or 100 lb overweight). Aggressive methods should be used only when there is medical justification for rapid weight loss because such methods are not without risk. There is little, if any, justification for employing the aggressive methods on individuals who are 10 or 15 lb overweight and probably no justification for their use on children.

Moderate methods

Energy deficits of 500–1,000 cal per day produce rather rapid initial weight loss due to the early loss of body water, particularly if carbohydrates are restricted. Dietary regimens that contain less than 50 g of carbohydrate are good examples of the phenomenon, since sodium and water excretion are the rule on low-carbohydrate diets. However, the unprepared dieter may become discouraged when after a few weeks the average loss will be only one or two pounds per week. This is a satisfactory but often disillusioning rate of loss. The ever popular high-protein, high-fat diets cause ketosis —an abnormal amount of ketone bodies in the blood and urine, commonly associated with the diabetic state

—if carbohydrate is severely restricted. There is some evidence that ketosis may inhibit appetite, which with the high satiety effect of fat and protein, greatly assists the dieter to achieve caloric deficit. However, the cost, discomfort, and lethargy that often accompany such diets discourage many from long adherence.

There are many variations of diets, based on the reduction of all three of the macronutrients (fats, carbohydrates, and proteins) that make up the major portions of food we eat (other than water) and are necessary sources of energy. Thus, one finds diets that restrict carbohydrate, or carbohydrate and fat, and even one variation that restricts protein and fat! After the initial effects of dehydration, all of the diets produce a rate of weight loss that is proportional to the caloric deficit; *i.e.,* the particular combinations of foods permitted or forbidden have little to do with the rate of loss, although dieters may find one regimen easier to follow than another.

Weight control clubs, such as Weight Watchers International Inc., are evolving programs that include an educational component; carefully constructed diets comprised of a wide variety of foods, which provide adequate amounts of nutrients; weight maintenance regimens that are designed for long-term use; and group reinforcement. Members are schooled, usually at weekly meetings, to adhere to the program. While large numbers of dieters join, there is little available information for judging success rates. However, for those who choose this method of weight control, some measure of comfort may be derived from the knowledge that the dietary regimens are well designed and can be counted on to provide proper nourishment even if weight loss is minimal.

A variation of conventional weight reduction diets may be found in the diabetic exchange diet. This diet features six groups of foods with size and number of servings allowed carefully designated. The diet is easily adapted to weight reduction since weight loss is frequently an important aspect of diabetic control.

Another variation may be found in the so-called prudent diet, which is designed to control blood lipids and cholesterol for those at risk of coronary artery diseases. The diet has been well tested by the New York City Bureau of Nutrition through its Anti-Coronary Club. Calorie balance for weight control is a very important part of a program to reduce the risk of coronary heart disease. The prudent diet and its more recent counterparts—1,200- and 1,800-cal modified diets devised by the American Heart Association, and regimens developed by the National Heart, Lung and Blood Institute— stress a low-saturated and high-unsaturated fat content and limited amounts of sugar; they restrict red meat and stress poultry and non-oily fish.

Meal replacements and calorie-controlled foods for weight control have enjoyed mixed acceptance in recent years. The formula diets, such as Metrecal, pro-

A Losing Battle Against Fat
Average Weights for Men and Women by Age and Height, 1960–62 and 1971–74

	18–24		25–34		35–44		45–54		55–64		65–74	
Men	'62	'74	'62	'74	'62	'74	'62	'74	'62	'74	'62	'74
5' 2"	135	130	139	141	147	143	146	147	146	143	142	143
5' 3"	138	135	143	145	150	148	150	152	149	147	146	147
5' 4"	142	140	148	150	154	153	154	156	153	153	149	151
5' 5"	145	145	152	156	158	158	158	160	156	158	152	156
5' 6"	149	150	157	160	162	163	162	164	160	163	156	160
5' 7"	152	154	161	165	166	169	166	169	164	168	159	164
5' 8"	156	159	166	170	169	174	171	173	167	173	163	169
5' 9"	159	164	170	174	173	179	175	177	171	178	166	173
5' 10"	163	168	175	179	177	184	179	182	174	183	169	177
5' 11"	166	173	179	184	180	190	183	187	178	189	173	182
6' 0"	170	178	184	189	184	194	187	191	182	193	176	186
6' 1"	173	183	188	194	188	200	191	196	185	197	180	190
6' 2"	177	188	192	199	192	205	195	200	189	203	183	194
Women												
4' 9"	114	114	110	118	129	125	127	129	136	132	130	130
4' 10"	116	117	114	121	132	129	130	133	139	136	133	134
4' 11"	118	120	118	125	134	133	134	136	142	140	136	137
5' 0"	120	123	122	128	136	137	138	140	145	143	140	140
5' 1"	123	126	126	132	138	141	141	143	148	147	143	144
5' 2"	125	129	130	136	141	144	145	147	150	150	147	147
5' 3"	127	132	134	139	143	148	148	150	153	153	150	151
5' 4"	129	135	138	142	145	152	152	154	156	157	154	154
5' 5"	132	138	142	146	147	156	156	158	159	160	157	158
5' 6"	134	141	146	150	150	159	159	161	162	164	161	161
5' 7"	136	144	150	153	152	163	163	165	165	167	164	165
5' 8"	138	147	154	157	154	167	166	168	168	171	168	169

vide 225 cal (and corresponding quantities of nutrients) in one serving. These liquid or solid foods are consumed four times a day; thus they are 900-cal diets. More recently a variation on this theme appeared in the form of protein-rich powdered supplements, such as PVM and Slender Now, which, when mixed with a juice, yield a few hundred calories and represent one meal. Most plans suggest two such meals followed by a planned meal of conventional food providing approximately 1,200 cal a day. There is little evidence that these plans have any advantage over reducing diets composed of conventional foods. However, for some, the elements of monotony, ritual, and reduced decision making are helpful.

An extremely popular moderate method for treatment of obesity is the low-carbohydrate, high-fat, and high-protein diet popularized by Alfred Pennington, Herman Taller, Irving Stillman, and Robert Atkins. These regimens restrict sugars and starches to a minimum by stressing meats, poultry, fish, and cheeses. The effect on the body is to produce ketosis and dehydration; thus initial weight loss may be marked, building up great expectations in the dieter. However, the richness of the diet may produce adverse effects related to the excretion of large amounts of uric acid and other nitrogenous end products and to the high saturated fat content of the diet. Studies suggest that even though calories are not counted, the usual caloric intake is reduced on such diets because most are unable to adapt rapidly to the marked change in dietary composition, which accounts for the weight loss obtained after ketosis is established and fluid balance stabilizes.

Behavior modification is a procedure of reorientation of eating behavior. Essentially, every cue associated with eating, particularly the environmental signals that invite the thought of food and consequent eating, are isolated and dealt with by removing or subordinating them. For example, one who consumes large quantities of food while reading establishes separate times for meals and reading and never combines the two. Or one who has a habit of eating cookies before bed finds a new, pleasurable activity to replace the bedtime snack, such as taking a walk, keeping a diary, doing yoga, etc. The procedures for meal planning, preparation, and consumption are studied, and behavior is changed to ensure that overeating is not encouraged. The place in which meals are eaten, the manipulative aspects of eating, and distractions while eating are carefully controlled. The ultimate objective is the relearning of eating behavior by the development of a new consciousness about food and elimination of the unconscious or uncontrolled consumption of food and beverage. This procedure, carried out under the guidance of a psychotherapist, may be used as the sole approach to weight control or may be incorporated into other programs for weight control in order to retrain the subject to maintain good nutritional practices after weight loss has been achieved.

Dietary fiber is a general term for indigestible carbohydrates that make up the cell walls of plants. Many foods contain fiber, but it is found most abundantly in raw vegetables, fruits, seeds, nuts, and grains. Plant fibers, either as bulking agents or for their suspected action in interfering with lipid absorption or bile salt recycling, have received attention recently. The evidence that fibers per se exert much influence on calorie deficit is weak. When there is an effect, it is probably because foods that are high in fiber are generally lower in calories than many processed foods. Moreover, high-fiber foods take longer to chew and are often more filling than other foods. But the value of high-fiber breads and other foods that are promoted as being useful in weight control remains to be demonstrated.

Fasting may consist of skipping a few meals or going a few days or weeks without food. This method has not been found to be effective for obese individuals but may serve the needs of those with just a few pounds to lose. Fasting for any extensive period is not without hazard and when practiced requires medical supervision. Fasting and starvation are not synonymous regimens. Obviously both involve abstinence from food; starvation means that the body's metabolic functions have shifted to the catabolic (destructive) state, which depends primarily on the body's fat as fuel. This conversion may require up to 12 days, a period longer than the usual fast. Fasting has not been found to be a very effective way to control weight over a long period of time.

Aggressive methods

Perhaps the only advantage of obesity is the ability to withstand starvation. Man's ability to store fat must be a teleological holdover from his feast-and-fast days as a forager. Recently, total starvation in an institutional setting (usually a hospital) has been used to produce massive weight loss. This is an expensive procedure— the patient normally is hospitalized for 47–121 days— and certain risks, not the least of which is unforeseeable death, are involved. Most physicians would prefer to manage patients with 800-cal diets that are safer although slower.

Awareness that the body "adapts" to starvation with mechanisms that "conserve" body protein has led to development of the concept of protein-sparing modified fasting. In principle just enough protein is fed to meet or slightly exceed protein (nitrogen) excretion, without otherwise upsetting the metabolic pathways of starvation; i.e., utilization of fat as fuel with little or no dependence on exogenous sources of carbohydrate. This modified fast presently takes three forms: (1) an amount of lean meat, poultry, or fish that provides 1.5 g protein per kg of ideal body weight (300–700 cal); (2) 25 g egg albumin and 40 g carbohydrate (260 cal); (3) 45 g egg albumin or other high-quality protein and 30 g carbohydrate (300 cal). Supplements of potassium, other minerals, and vitamins may be employed in conjunction with the protein-sparing modified fast.

Although four deaths have been recorded by one investigator in four years of experience with 1,200 patients (three probably due to coronary occlusion not directly related to the regimen and one due to blockage of the esophagus), the protein-sparing modified fast is accepted as a very promising method for the treatment of obesity. Incorporation of behavior modification, nutrition education, and exercise helps prepare the patient to return to normal foods and life-styles when sufficient weight has been lost. The method is suited for the truly obese individual but is *not* recommended for those with only a few pounds to lose.

A popularized version of this regimen employing liquid hydrolyzed collagen enjoyed great support in the U.S. until some 40 deaths were reported to have been associated in some fashion with the so-called liquid protein diet. As a result, interest waned rather quickly. The deaths, a majority of which occurred in young women, have not been adequately explained.

Two surgical intervention procedures have been developed that control the amount of food ingested and presented for digestion and absorption (gastric pouch or gastric bypass) or that reduce the amount of absorptive tissue in the intestinal tract (jejuno-ileal bypass). These are drastic surgical procedures that take matters out of the control of the patient. The bypass operations effectively limit the absorption of food energy and induce significant weight loss. However, intestinal bypass can interfere with some normal liver and renal functions and create electrolyte abnormalities, among other metabolic difficulties. It is the most drastic method of weight control, yet it has enjoyed more than modest attention, probably because it is a procedure of last resort. Because of the hazards associated with it, rigid criteria have been established that candidates must meet in order to be considered: (1) weight in excess of 100 lb over standard weight; (2) abject failure of other methods of weight control; (3) the presence of a life-threatening obese condition or the possibility of severe debilitation due to obesity; (4) the absence of severe heart, liver, kidney, or bowel diseases. In some instances massively obese patients have been subjected to weight-reduction procedures in preparation for bypass surgery because they exceeded the upper limits for acceptance. There have also been stories of patients who intentionally *gained* weight to meet the minimum weight criterion.

Several variations of bypass surgery are employed that involve connecting a short segment of jejunum (a section of the small intestine) directly to the end of the ileum (a part of the small intestine that connects the jejunum and the large intestine) or to a shorter segment with the "unused" or bypassed portion of the jejunum draining into the cecum (a cavity of the large intestine) or colon (the part of the large intestine that extends from the cecum to the rectum).

The shorter the segment of intact intestine, the more rapid the weight loss but also the greater the risk of complications such as nutritional inadequacies, liver dysfunction, diarrhea, and other metabolic problems. Careful follow-up care is required, including liver biopsies every six months. Weight loss on the order of 30–50 lb is common during the first year, followed by a gradual fall in the rate of loss thereafter. In some instances weight gain has occurred after a few years perhaps because of the gradual accommodation of the intestine by enlarging in diameter and increasing its effective absorptive capacity. The high initial weight loss followed by a tapering off also suggests that food intake may be greatly curtailed until the patient has become acclimated to his or her changed intestinal situation. A complication of the jejuno-ileal bypass is the loss of undesirable amounts of *lean* body mass along with the sought-after fat loss.

A more recent procedure, gastric exclusion, leaves the intestinal tract intact but greatly reduces the available size of the stomach, thereby limiting food intake. Approximately 10% of the upper portion of the stomach is sutured to form a pouch and connected appropriately to the jejunum, leaving 90% of the stomach in suspended animation. Great care must be taken to train the patient to eat very small amounts of food at one time. Although the rate of weight loss is slower than that following ileal bypass, the complications are much less severe. It has been reported that lean body mass loss is much less, while the amount of fat loss may be identical to the experience with the jejuno-ileal bypass. More time is needed to evaluate the long-term effect of both forms of obesity intervention; since both are quite recent developments, continued follow-up is necessary.

Jaw wiring to prevent the passage of food has been tried in some obese persons. The subject is fed a liquid formula diet or homogenized food by tube. There appears to be only moderate interest in this method since the patient can easily ingest any amount of formula or other high-calorie liquids, defeating the system. Unless the patient responds to the reeducation of eating behavior, the weight may be quickly regained once the jaws are freed.

Acupuncture has been advocated for weight control, based on a theory of "hunger points" in the ear, but clinical trials have failed to find any effect. Ear staples to reduce appetite or needles manipulated in the ear, once popular forms of acupuncture, appear to have passed their zenith.

There is an increasing awareness of the adverse effects of amphetamines and amphetamine-like adrenergic drugs used as anorexiants (causing loss of appetite). The use of such products has been curtailed greatly, and physicians are encouraged to reserve their use for the most difficult treatment situations or to use other pharmacologic agents. Other anorexiant agents such as fenfluramine and mazindol appear to produce more central nervous system depression than stimulation. Appetite suppressants may be used for short-term adjunctive treatment as part of a total program of weight control. They should not, however, be used as the sole form of therapy.

Over-the-counter preparations such as phenylpropanolamine are ineffective in the dose provided (25 mg), although promotion for the product continues. Diuretic agents are used only when the degree of edema (water retention) is significant or when other indications for use are indicated. Diuretics have no role in the conventional management of obesity.

Human chorionic gonadotropin (HCG), a hormone produced by the placenta and excreted in the urine of pregnant women, coupled with a 500-cal diet, enjoyed considerable notoriety several years ago. The hormone has been used clinically in boys for treating underdeveloped secondary sex characteristics, and many boys have been observed to lose weight during such therapy. However, obese patients who received HCG injections did not appear to lose weight because of the action of the hormone alone. Failure to confirm clinical usefulness and problems that arose from careless patient management brought a timely end to popularity.

The search continues for safe and effective appetite suppressants and for hormonal agents that may safely increase metabolic rate without inducing concomitant loss of lean body mass, including protein and bone. Thyroid preparations are used cautiously, if at all, in weight reduction for the above reasons and because of the ability of the thyroid gland to compensate and decrease endogenous hormone secretion, defeating the purpose of therapy.

Of all the aggressive forms of obesity treatment, the protein-sparing modified fast with appropriate behavior modification and nutritional and exercise retraining has produced the best results and, so far, the best record for weight maintenance.

Meaningful strides are being made toward the definition of obesity and of its risks. Understanding of the causes and treatment of obesity is evolving slowly. There is still a long way to go. The rather discouraging results in treating obesity to date make more imperative coordinated efforts to prevent the onset of obesity and to arrest modest amounts of unnatural weight gain before the pattern becomes established.

Ear Diseases and Hearing Disorders

Approximately 14.5 million persons in the United States suffer from impaired hearing. Over 3 million of these are school-age children. Hearing acuity tends to deteriorate as a person grows older; 5% of the population has experienced some hearing loss by age 65. After that age most people are affected to some extent.

Treating hearing loss requires an accurate and precise diagnosis of the extent of the impairment. A basic diagnostic tool is the audiogram, a graph that is made of the perception of sound in a wide range of frequencies and decibel levels. Dysfunctions of particular components of organs of hearing show characteristic results on the audiogram, which, combined with other information in the medical history, makes accurate diagnosis possible.

Until the 20th century the extent of hearing loss in a patient could be estimated only by evaluating responses to spoken and whispered voices, bells, whistles, tuning forks, and other noises. Electronics technology made possible the development in the 1930s of contemporary clinical audiometry, whereby hearing is measured in response to speech or pure-tone signals carefully calibrated in frequency and intensity. Although the test signal became refined by the application of sophisticated electronics technology, the actual evaluation of hearing still depended on the full cooperation of the patient, who would signal the reception of a test sound by raising a hand or pushing a button. This "behavioral response" of the patient precluded the accurate assessment of hearing in infants and young children as well as in those whose cooperation could not be had because of mental retardation, emotional instability, or desire to feign a hearing loss. The limitations imposed on audiometry by the behavioral response have encouraged the development of objective audiometric methods in which the role of the patient is a passive one.

An early-20th-century attempt at objective audiometry employed the electrical measurement of skin resistance changes in response to sound signals. The responses in skin resistance were due to the changes in the amount of perspiration present and could be "conditioned" by the use of mild electric shocks. Because of the discomfort produced and a lack of accuracy, this method has been abandoned.

Electric waves (potentials) evoked from the auditory system were noted in electroencephalographic (brain-wave) recordings in 1939. During the next two decades attempts were made to improve the extraction and isolation of the minute auditory potentials from the background electrical activity generated by the brain, heart, and muscles. This testing method became known as evoked cortical response audiometry. Unfortunately, it proved difficult to recognize the auditory electrical response on a consistent basis, and the problem was complicated further by the effect that varying degrees of alertness had on the recording. These disadvantages limited clinical application of the technique.

The development and improvement of the response-averaging computer during the past 25 years have made electric response audiometry a practical tool. This type of computer has the ability to isolate the small electrical signals generated by the inner ear and brain stem from the background "noise" of other electrical activity and to amplify these signals. The computer is synchronized with the auditory stimulus. Auditory evoked electrical responses occur at regular intervals following the stimulus and are recognized and enhanced by the computer, while the randomly occurring background electrical activity is averaged out and diminished.

Patients are usually tested in quiet, electrically isolated rooms. The test signal is delivered by an earphone or speaker, and one of two types of electrode placement—needle or surface—is used to detect the electrical response evoked by the auditory signal. Electrocochleography measures the electrical responses generated by the inner ear and auditory nerve via a needle electrode that is usually inserted through the tympanic membrane. Brain stem electric response audiometry uses surface electrodes on the scalp to detect responses presumably generated by the auditory nerve and brain stem. Both recording techniques have the advantage of not requiring active participation by the patient. The patient need only remain motionless to ensure good recordings. If that degree of cooperation is not possible, sedation or anesthesia may be administered that will not interfere with the evoked electrical activity. Electrocochleography is an "invasive" technique requiring the passage of a needle through the eardrum. Sedation or anesthesia (local or general) is usually required. Brain stem electric response techniques have the great advantage of being noninvasive and therefore produce no discomfort and require no sedation or anesthetic. In electrocochleography the recording electrodes are closer to the electrical generating sites of the inner ear than in brain stem electric response audiometry, and a more accurate assessment of inner ear function is produced. However, as experience is gained and recording technology improved in the noninvasive technique, there will be a diminishing need for the invasive electrocochleographic method of electrode placement.

It is now possible to assess the hearing of patients previously considered impossible to test. In the case of infants, early detection and accurate quantification of hearing loss are extremely important to minimize the effects of the handicap and enable the child to make maximum use of the remaining hearing. Furthermore, the analysis of electric response waveforms is providing new diagnostic information to help localize defects in the auditory system. For instance, tumors pressing on the auditory nerve have shown distinctive changes in waveform.

The ideal method of objective audiometry has not yet been developed. However, contemporary techniques utilizing the recording of auditory evoked electrical responses are an important development in the progress toward that goal.

—Edward L. Applebaum, M.D.

Emergency Medicine

The burn injury can be one of the most serious and devastating forms of trauma a human being can sustain. Approximately two million people seek medical attention for burns in the United States each year. Of these, 80,000 to 120,000 require hospitalization and about 12,000 die. Injuries to children are frequent: one child is burned every four minutes. The patient with a major burn may spend $500 to $1,000 a day for hospitalization; approximately $6,000,000 a year is spent on care for burn patients in the United States. The economic loss to the nation exceeds $41,000,000 annually, in addition to the permanent loss of millions of productive work years.

Thermal destruction of the skin produces severe and diverse local and systemic physiologic alterations. A successful treatment requires a recovery period extending over a period of months or even years. The major advance in understanding the burn injury and treating the burn patient since the 1950s has been the recognition of the need to develop highly specialized burn teams and burn care facilities.

The physiology of burns

Within the limits of biological variability, human skin will tolerate reaching temperatures up to 40° C (104° F)—a few degrees above the normal temperature for blood—for brief periods of time. Temperatures above this level result in a rapidly multiplying increase in tissue damage irrespective of the time of exposure. The depth of burning—the number of tissue layers affected—is determined by the combination of the burning agent, temperature, and time of exposure. There is a concentric decrease in the severity of burning extending outward from the site of injury. In the center of the injury, at the point of contact with the heat, cells are immediately destroyed by coagulation. Next, there is a zone of injured cells, which may under ideal circumstances survive, but which usually progresses to tissue death in 24 to 48 hours. Finally, there is a zone of tissue that is minimally injured but will recover over a period of seven days.

In addition to damage to the skin at the site of burning, local and systemic changes also occur. Among the most immediate and severe of these are changes in the heart and blood vessels. The cardiac output drastically declines, and blood vessels develop permeability. This leads to a massive fluid shift, with the vascular volume that is normally inside the blood vessels exuding into the surrounding tissue. These changes lead to the state of shock, which in turn causes imbalances in each of the body's physiologic systems.

The function of all organ systems will eventually be altered by a major burn. Some of the changes are in response to the stress of injury; some are related to burning itself; but most are due to alterations in the functional capacity of the skin. The depth of burning is therefore important. Although in an actual burn the depth will vary tremendously, it is conceptually easier to view a burn as a uniform injury. The superficial or first-degree burn is characterized by redness and discomfort only. Within a few days, the outer injured skin cells peel off from a totally healed burn with no scarring. The second-degree burn is best divided into two subsections: superficial partial thickness and deep partial thickness. The superficial partial-thickness injury is characterized by blisters. Removal or breaking of the blisters results in weeping of fluids from the burn surface. Since the basal layers of the skin are not destroyed, regeneration is prompt, and superficial partial-thickness burns usually heal in 14 to 17 days if no infection develops. The deep partial-thickness burn is more severe and has many areas of severely injured tissue. This skin will survive and heal only under the most optimal conditions. Finally, the third-degree or full-thickness burn contains totally destroyed skin. This is the most severe type of burn and cannot heal itself. Total-thickness skin loss can be restored only by application of skin grafts from nonburned portions of the body. In the most severe burns damage may go below the skin to muscles and other deep tissues.

Diagnosis of burn severity and determination of care

The first thing to be done in treating the burn patient is to determine the severity of the injury so that the level of expertise necessary to care for him can be decided. The ultimate determinant in burn injury is the volume of tissue destroyed. Although it is difficult to accurately determine depth, the extent of the burn area can be assessed by careful observation. It is customary to record extent in terms of percent of body surface area. Any burn, regardless of degree, that affects in excess of 20% of body surface area (5–10% in children) requires special care in a hospital.

The depth of burn is almost impossible to estimate correctly. However, some guidelines exist: scald burns other than those due to immersion tend to be more superficial than flame burns; burns in small children or the aged tend to be deeper; chemical and electrical burns may be deep even though they sometimes initially appear to be superficial. Any burn thought to constitute a full-thickness injury over more than 2% of the body surface may require hospitalization.

The age of the patient determines the natural thickness of the skin and also dictates the amount of stress the patient can withstand. Burns in people under the age of 3 or over the age of 60 can be quite severe. Special areas of the body exist in which the burn is considered major by location alone. These areas are the head and neck, hands, feet, and genitals.

The inhalation of smoke increases the severity of all burn injuries. Similarly, the existence of nonassociated serious medical illnesses make the burn more grave. Social factors may also affect the decision to admit a burn patient to a hospital. Among these are the inability of a patient or family to care for the burn properly at home. Injuries occurring as results of suicide or homicide attempts or as a result of child abuse also cannot be cared for outside the hospital.

Treatment of the burn patient

Regardless of whether hospitalization is required or whether the patient is to be treated on an ambulatory basis, several emergency measures should be taken.

Early measures. The burned part should be cooled. This is best done by soaking the burned part in ice water or wrapping the area with towels soaked in ice water. To be effective, this measure must be performed within the first 30 minutes after injury. Although ice water is beneficial, ice itself is detrimental.

It must also be quickly determined if the patient is able to breathe properly. At times, burns around the chest area produce an unyielding leathery condition of the skin that limits chest expansion during breathing. This condition may be severe enough to cause acute respiratory distress and necessitate emergency re-lease of the constricting tissue. The releasing procedure, termed an escharotomy, is often necessary in major burn injuries associated with breathing difficulties. Even without chest burns, respiratory distress can occur from inhalation of smoke. The problems associated with smoke inhalation are insidious and result from the incomplete products of combustion, which are toxic to lung tissue. Because the effects of smoke inhalation may not be acute when the patient is first seen, the suspicion of impending inhalation injury requires admission to the hospital and care of the patient's airway, with supplemental oxygen and, in some circumstances, mechanical ventilatory assistance.

Once the injured part has been cooled, if the criteria for admission are not present, the patient will be treated on an ambulatory basis as an outpatient. The treatment will consist of safeguards against tetanus, prevention of infection, and local care of the burn wound itself. In the United States tetanus prophylaxis is usually quite simple and consists of a booster shot for a patient previously immunized against tetanus and who has not had a booster in the previous five years. In patients not previously immunized, human immune antitoxin is given in addition to the tetanus toxoid.

The most common infection of burn wounds is due to β-hemolytic streptococcus bacteria. The nature of the burn wound, with edema from the fluid seeping into the tissues, eliminates the skin's natural defense against streptococci. Therefore, infection prevention is aimed against this organism, and penicillin or erythromycin is given during the three-day phase of the injury when edema is present. Antibiotics with a broad spectrum against all bacteria can cause dangerous imbalances in the burn patient and, therefore, are contraindicated.

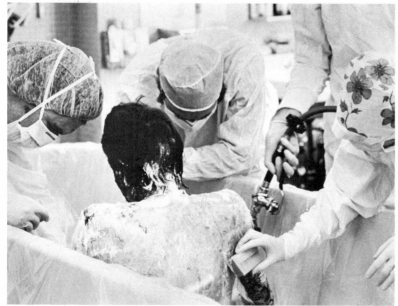

Once a burn patient's vital signs have been stabilized, treatment of his wounds can begin. The patient here has been placed in a tub of water, and dead tissue is being washed away. The procedure helps doctors assess the nature of the damage and removes a breeding ground for the bacteria that can cause massive infection, the most serious problem facing the patient.

Dan McCoy—Rainbow

In caring for the wound, care must be taken to: (1) do no harm to the wound, (2) prevent infection and allow survival of all remaining viable tissue, and (3) obtain the best functional and aesthetically attractive coverage as quickly as possible. The burned area is first washed with a bland soap, and blisters are cleaned of foreign particles and nonviable skin. A dressing is then applied to the injured area. The functions of the dressing are: (1) to protect the wound from further mechanical trauma or bacterial contamination, (2) to absorb any external drainage from the wound, and (3) to immobilize the injured part.

The burn victim who is treated as an outpatient is usually seen 24 hours after the initial treatment and then seen periodically for dressing changes until all wounds have healed. If the diagnostic criteria applied to the burn patient dictate admission to the hospital, the treatment becomes more complicated. The fluid shifts that occur in a burn that covers 20% or more of the body surface area in an adult may be associated with circulatory collapse and shock. Impending shock must be treated immediately by the intravenous administration of buffered isotonic salt solutions. The weight of the patient, the type of the burn wound (*e.g.,* scald *vs.* flame), and the percentage of the body burned help to determine the amount of resuscitation fluid that is required. Evaluation of successful resuscitation is made by determining the rate of urine output. This must be maintained at 30–50 ml per hour in the adult or 1.2 ml per kilogram of body weight in the child. To maintain such an exact measure of urinary output, it may be necessary to place a catheter in the bladder. The loss of plasma and fluid occurs to the greatest extent during the first 12 hours after burning and then continues much more slowly for another 36 hours. Replacement, therefore, must be at the greatest volume immediately and then can be slowed to correspond to the rate of loss. After 48 hours intravenous replacement can usually be discontinued. However, the increased metabolic rate in a burn victim will continue until all the burn wounds are healed or have been covered by skin grafts. Great amounts of fluid and calories must therefore be given to the patient throughout the course of treatment.

The indispensable element in the management of the burn patient is wound closure. Ideally, the burn wound should be excised immediately after injury and replaced by a skin graft from an unburned part of the body. Unfortunately, this is impossible in all but the very small and isolated full-thickness injury. In a major burn it is an arithmetical impossibility, since it has been estimated that 6,000 sq cm (930 sq in) of skin are required to resurface a 50% full-thickness burn in an adult. The management of the burn patient may be largely equated to the management of the burn wound itself. Certainly, the main concern in the care of the patient after resuscitation is the care of the wound and the need to prevent infection while simultaneously preparing the wound for closure.

Preventing infection. Since the realization that the prevention of infection involves the maintenance of an equilibrium between the ever present bacteria and the patient's powers of resistance, the early care of the burn wound has been aimed toward preventing the numerical proliferation of bacteria. As bacteria proliferate within the burned skin, they surround and occlude blood vessels, causing clotting of the vessels and death of the skin. This discovery explained the unresponsiveness of infected wounds to systemic antibiotics and showed that the topical application of antibacterial agents was required. The most common topical antibacterials in use today are silver sulfadiazine, silver nitrate, mafenide acetate, gentamicin sulfate, and povidone-iodine, applied either in solution or as water soluble creams.

All of the commonly used topical antibacterial agents have advantages and disadvantages. None is the panacea for burn wound sepsis, but none has disadvantages that rule it out as an effective agent under particular circumstances. New agents are continually being developed and evaluated, among them cerium nitrate, silver zinc allantoin, silver lactate, and zinc sulfadiazine. However, even as these new agents are being discovered, the bacteria that infect burn wounds continue to change so that at no time will the mythical "topical antibacterial agent of choice" be available for treatment of the burn patient.

The threat of infection in the burn wound is always present despite the continued use and development of antibacterial agents. Thus, the goal must be to rid the patient of nonviable tissue as quickly as possible. This can be done in several ways. Obviously, full-thickness skin loss can be excised. Skin damaged in partial thickness can be tangentially removed or removed by enzyme preparations capable of differentiating between living and nonliving portions of the skin. Tedious bathing and selective removal of necrotic (dying) tissue can also be done. All of these techniques may be used simultaneously in the same patient to remove tissue incapable of survival.

Skin grafts. Once the nonviable tissue is removed from the injured portions, replacement can take place by skin grafting. Certain areas of the body have priority for grafting. These are the face (especially the eyelids) and neck, the hands, and other areas containing flexion creases; *e.g.,* the elbows and knees. Permanent replacement of burned skin can occur only by transplantation of the patient's own skin from nonburned areas of his body. In the case of massive burns, temporary wound coverage can be obtained by using skin from the patient's relatives, cadaver skin, animal skin, or fetal membranes. None of these skin substitutes is permanent, but they are often a life-saving temporary measure.

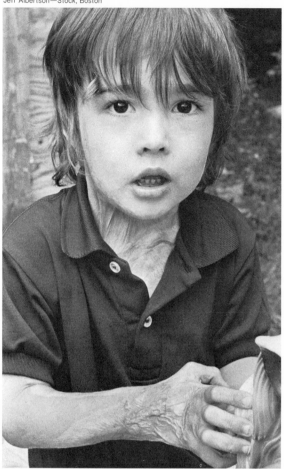

A child who has been badly burned may face a years-long series of skin grafts and plastic surgery to restore maximum use and improved appearance to the burned areas.

Skin grafting does not complete the treatment of the burn patient. Successful grafting achieves wound closure only. The grafts must be protected and controlled during their maturation phase. Continued pressure during this phase by specially constructed elastic garments prevents the hypertrophic (enlarged) scarring so often associated with burns in the past. Correct positioning, splinting, and exercises will maintain the range of motion of all joints and prevent the contractures of muscles and deformities all too often associated with injuries from thermal trauma. To be effective in this rehabilitation period, once resuscitation is complete, the physical therapist, occupational therapist, and other members of the burn team must assist the patient in both an active and passive exercise program to maintain function.

Controlling pain. Throughout the course of burn treatment, from the scene of the injury through the emergent and convalescent phases of care, anxiety and pain control are very important. The fear and, at times, the pain that are present in a patient who has been burned can be extreme. There is fear of dying, fear of pain, and fear of living with deformity. To a degree this fear is realistic and healthy. If present to an excess it hinders treatment. Therefore, mood-modifying drugs and tranquilizers are often useful.

Pain, although usually not manifested at the time of injury, may become severe during the acute phase of treatment and may remain so through rehabilitation. Dealing with pain is the responsibility of every member of the burn team. Narcotics administered intravenously control pain during the resuscitation. Following this time many methods are used to maintain comfort for the burn patient. Among these are psychological counseling, diversionary measures, hypnotism, anesthesia, and analgesic drugs. Since pain and anxiety are closely related, a compassionate staff that is honest and realistic with the patient often provides the best control of these emotions.

Some burn centers have allowed the patient and his family to assist in determining to what extent measures will be used to salvage the patient. In a very small, select group of adult patients who have been burned so severely that there is no previous record of any comparably burned person surviving, the patient and the family may elect to use drugs to minimize pain and anxiety but to withhold further treatment of the burn. (*See* Medical Ethics.)

Complications

Success in the treatment regime outlined above is not necessarily reflected in survival statistics. Functional rehabilitation and social acceptance must constitute the measure of success in treatment of the burn patient. Despite the efforts of the burn team to achieve success as measured in these terms, complications can occur throughout the treatment course and even into the postrecovery phase. Among these, some have previously been alluded to: cardiac failure, pulmonary insufficiency, pneumonia, renal failure, and wound or systemic sepsis (spreading the infection). Others are not as clearly related to the burn but are indeed due to the altered physiology of thermal trauma. These include changes in the stomach, intestines, liver, adrenal glands, bones, joints, and blood cells. Finally, psychiatric complications can develop in patients undergoing the prolonged physical trauma of a major burn.

Treating burn victims with a concept of total patient care requires a knowledge of the physiology of thermal injury, the judgment and ability to carry out the needed treatment, and the recognition of the many complications that can occur. A comprehensive and quality management program requires the knowledge and skills of the entire medical team. A further, most important aspect of burn medicine is prevention of burns before they occur, through education and protective legislation.

—Martin C. Robson, M.D.

Special Report:

Disaster Medicine

by Lawrence R. Drury, M.D.,
and Peter Rosen, M.D.

At 8 AM on Oct. 30, 1972, the emergency department of the University of Chicago's Billings Hospital received a phone call asking for help for a train crash that had just occurred. As is often the case, the caller was excited and failed to give any useful information other than a general location near Michael Reese Hospital and a sense of urgency, while conveying some sense of the magnitude of the disaster. A team of doctors, nurses, paramedics, and administrators quickly assembled and drove to the Illinois Central (IC) Railroad tracks, where they found the wreck in an open field directly east of Michael Reese. A rush-hour commuter train crammed with passengers had overshot its stop and was backing to the station when it was hit by the following train.

The medical team found the scene truly Dantesque. Many of the mildly injured had walked away from the wreck and were pouring into the emergency departments of Michael Reese and nearby Mercy Hospital. Other rescue workers were arriving on the scene. The city fire department was present and securing the wreck, although flame risk had been minimized by cutting off electric power to the tracks. The police were controlling traffic access to the area as well as attempting to set up a route for emergency vehicles.

The Billings team quickly set up a medical command post and in conjunction with the fire department physician began to take control over patient evacuation. Before control was achieved, there had been a chaotic removal of casualties with no accurate assessment of casualty priorities or notion of destination. As a result approximately 80% of the casualties ultimately ended up at either Michael Reese or Mercy Hospital. This situation, of course, caused a tremendous overload of these facilities and proved the need for a well-designed system of patient dispersal.

As in many civilian disasters, many of the most seriously injured victims were trapped in the wreckage, and it required a number of hours of extrication efforts to remove them. By then the scene was well under control, and the open disaster site enabled helicopter evacuation of these critical casualties. Although some treatment had been given in the field, many victims were trapped in inaccessible locations where steel bulkheads had to be removed before victims could even be seen. Others were in positions that prevented or hindered effective treatment. For example, one young woman who was pinned in a car could be reached by crawling under the train, but it was impossible to treat her effectively until firemen could break through into her section of the wreckage and free her. Oxygen administration presented a particularly difficult problem, both in terms of its delivery to individual patients and its safe use around the acetylene torches being used in the extrications.

Even the most experienced medical personnel cannot help but be shaken by the horror of such scenes, which resemble nothing short of the carnage of war. This response, of course, adds to the difficulties of effective disaster management, not to mention to the psychological trauma of the victims.

Ultimately all victims of the train wreck were removed and cared for, but the final toll of 45 dead and several hundred injured does not begin to include the shattered lives and many years of rehabilitation still being experienced. Nor has the final monetary toll, both from direct cost as well as subsequent litigation and damage costs, been assessed.

Minidisasters

For all of its horrors, economic effects, and stunning frequency, the kind of crisis described above still represents what can be classified as a "minidisaster." Such calamities involve a relatively small number of victims, usually less than 1,000 people. The most frequent causes of minidisasters are transportation accidents and fires; however, disasters at rock concerts, sports events, political conventions, professional meetings, and other large gatherings of people are occurring more often. Biological causes can also precipitate such disasters; for example, a large jet aircraft received contaminated food that incapacitated most of the passengers in one of the sections. Another serious cause of so-called minidisasters on the increase is the terrorist's bomb or machine gun.

What is constant to most minidisasters is the rapid onset of the inciting cause of injury, followed by a period of delay, which allows approach to the victims for extrication, initial assessment and treatment, and evacuation for definitive care.

A minidisaster can be described both in terms of the number of casualties and by the terms *close-ended* or *open-ended*. In a close-ended minidisaster, such as the IC train crash, the casualties are generated over a short period of time. The number of casualties usually can be accurately assessed and planned for. In contrast, open-ended disasters, such as fires or weather-related disasters, will generate an unknown number of casualties over an unknown period of time.

Maxidisasters

On the other end of the disaster scale are the so-called maxidisasters. While, fortunately, these are rare, when they do occur they frequently destroy the resources generally used to respond to minidisasters. Maxidisasters, too, can be open- or close-ended. Unfortunately a great potential for maxidisasters exists in our industrial society, and it will probably be only a matter of time before the world experiences a maxidisaster other than earthquakes or upheavals in weather. For example, in 1974 a cloud of chlorine gas formed from an industrial leak on the South Side of Chicago. Fortunately the prevailing winds blew the gas over Lake Michigan, but it is estimated that had the gas settled over the city, it would have caused at least one million deaths as well as millions of serious injuries. Clearly, neither Chicago nor any other city has the resources to deal with a problem of this magnitude, especially when many of the city's hospitals would have fallen under the poison cloud.

Maxidisasters in our times have usually been ecological: earthquakes, volcanoes, tornadoes, or floods. While uncommon in Western society, infectious disease epidemics are still experienced in other parts of the world, and these ravages of disease can be considered disasters.

The clearest potential for maxidisaster—experienced over and over in past and recent history—is the military conflagration. Conventional weaponry has induced unfathomable horrors in the past; today's advanced weaponry provides the capacity to create an almost universal maxidisaster.

Disaster preparedness

It is probably impossible to truly prepare for a maxidisaster. Certainly such planning cannot be carried out with the resources of any single community and, in fact, in some cases entire nations may have to come to each other's aid. It is difficult to comprehend why the People's Republic of China refused assistance during the aftermath of its massive earthquakes of 1976, which took a reported 655,000 lives and caused an estimated 779,000 injuries.

Today, however, the resources and know-how are available to prepare for minidisasters. Emergency medical systems as well as effective internal disaster plans for medical facilities, now common in many U.S. cities, can handle disasters in a relatively orderly manner, and patient dispersal can be carried out in such a way as to not overload any individual facility, as happened during the Chicago IC wreck.

Cooperative efforts. The first priority in preparing for disasters is mutual cooperation and understanding among agencies that are charged with controlling patient assessment, managing the disaster site, and informing the public. (These may include fire departments, police, medical teams, Red Cross, Salvation Army, and local media.) One agency must assume primary control for overall disaster responsibility. This will probably vary with the source of the individual disaster. In most civilian disasters the fire department has over-

The 1972 crash of two crowded Illinois Central commuter trains in Chicago created a chaotic situation for nearby hospitals and revealed to city officials the need for a well-organized disaster plan.

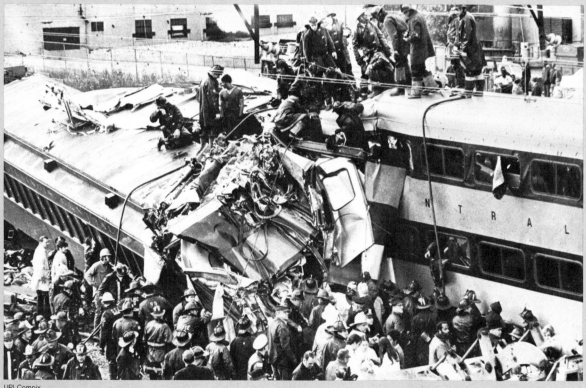

UPI Compix

all site responsibility, but obviously if the source were to be insurrection or terrorism, the police department or even federal or military authorities would have to take charge. Prior planning to contemplate what variety of disasters is most likely to occur in a particular area is essential. Establishing contingency responsibilities, so that time delays can be averted at the critical point of dealing with the real crisis, is also a must. Next there must be a definition of the limits and specific responsibilities of each agency involved.

The medical agencies responsible for management should be clearly identified and a system of mutual cooperation developed. In any community there are a finite number of resources and usually a very small number of facilities possessing the resources capable of instantaneous response 24 hours a day. These institutions will have the role of primary responders. The remaining facilities can be drawn into utilization as needed. The emergency departments in hospitals designated as primary responders should be the coordinating centers in those institutions.

Communications. Communication is the hub of effective response. Many cities have installed 911 emergency telephone systems, which can provide rapid and effective response to a disaster as well as confirm the location of the call for help. However, any plan must also include the realistic possibility that normal communications systems will be destroyed by the disaster event, and alternative emergency links must be ready

Thousands of citizens slept in the streets during the series of earthquakes in China in 1976; urban dwellers in crowded areas face special problems from natural disasters.

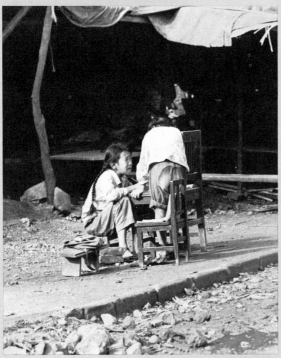

Sygmachine

and functional. Therefore, a backup system that is portable and can generate its own power will be needed. Central to effective communication is the ability to identify individual teams as well as to coordinate the agencies involved. A central communications vehicle that can monitor as well as link each involved agency is indispensable. In addition, however, it is imperative to have two-way radios or some similar communication device that the teams can use to keep in touch. With effective communication from site to hospital, accurate information about the number of predicted victims can be transmitted, allowing a hospital to continue normal functions as it prepares to gear up for the disaster. Many hospital emergency teams have had experiences in which the initial number of victims was predicted to be much greater than the number that actually materialized. A plane crash at Chicago's Midway Airport, where most of the victims were trapped in the plane and died there, is an example of this.

Managing the scene. The first workers on the scene are usually firemen or police. Their responsibility is to secure the safety of the area as well as to set up routes of access to the disaster site. The first medical team to arrive will usually be an ambulance squad, and only later (30–60 minutes) will physicians and nurses arrive. The first medical responsibility is to establish a command area and to assess the kind and approximate number of injuries that will be transmitted to the primary responding medical facilities. The second medical responsibility will be to begin initial assessment of the victims. In most disasters there will be a discrete time lag between the onset of the disaster and access to the most critical patients. In certain kinds of disasters where there is risk of continuing fire or explosion (*e.g.,* a plane crash), victims will have to be evacuated from the site before assessment is safe.

Triage is a term developed from military experience meaning to separate victims into three categories. In most civilian disaster situations four or five classes are used. (Class I: life or limb threatened; class II: serious but life not threatened, stretcher required; class III: walking wounded; class IV: alive but chance of survival minimal; class V: dead.) In most minidisasters a response to each class can be made on the basis of the most serious coming first. However, as the number of casualties becomes great, a different approach must be adopted, or salvageable lives will be lost owing to wasted efforts to treat the unsalvageable. Fortunately, in most minidisasters the walking wounded generally create a self triage, and there is time to establish control over the other classes of patients.

In addition to the functions of sorting victims into categories and beginning initial therapy, there is the equally important triage function of identifying each victim, placing an identification tag on that person, and keeping a log of the victims and the medical facility to which they are transported. It is imperative to have a log of where victims are being transported in order to not overload any one facility. In the hours and days immediately following the disaster a log will be invaluable in uniting family with the victims or informing family members of a victim's death. There is also a curious phenomenon observed in large cities after many disasters: more victims show up to claim injury and compensation than the disaster actually generated. However, the opposite will also happen: emergency workers may be unable to locate the victims that are reported to be involved. The identification tag should include as much information about each victim as possible. If a name is unavailable, then the physical characteristics of race, sex, age, etc. are used. Special problems occur in the identification of victims of fires and floods, in which identifying physical features can be obscured. In these cases dental characteristics may be all that is left to provide identification.

Treating victims. The ability to render definitive care in the field is quite limited and, in fact, efforts are generally more profitably directed toward rapid evacuation. However, there is a finite period of time required to effect dissemination of victims, and during that time some will require treatment as well as protection from the environment. It is estimated that had the IC crash occurred two months later, during the severe winter weather, the number of deaths would have doubled.

There should be supplies available for transport to disaster sites stored at various convenient locations and regularly inspected to ensure utility. No city has adequate numbers of ambulances if only public vehicles are utilized. Therefore, private ambulance companies will be involved. They must, however, be willing to subordinate to medical command; otherwise true chaos can ensue.

Unfortunately, no matter how effective the police force, there will always be onlookers and other interested bystanders to add to the disorganization. There also seems to be no way to escape the ubiquitous presence of the news media, whose efforts to provide responsible coverage frequently interfere with medical efforts to get the job done.

Individual hospitals' responsibilities are best defined in advance of any individual disaster, and if there are well-organized systems of patient distribution in an emergency medical services system, they will be effectively utilized in the disaster, especially if the disaster incapacitates or destroys one or more of the participating hospitals. No matter how extensive or well prepared any single facility is, it has a finite capacity to respond to numbers of critical patients. Thus the most effective utilization of all facilities will come in a timed dispersion of patients to multiple facilities.

Denver's disaster plan

The disaster plan for Denver, Colo., can serve as a model of how an effective emergency medical system works. Denver has a great potential for airplane disasters since it is the tenth busiest airport in the U.S., and indeed it has had a number of such emergencies.

The plan goes into effect when an airplane notifies the control tower that it is in trouble. A "yellow alert" is called, which notifies the fire department, the police, and medical services to stand by. If a disaster develops, a "red alert" is called, and the fire department is at the site to control the fire and to move victims away from the potentially explosive aircraft. The police will immediately secure the area and establish entrance and exit lanes for fire and ambulance vehicles. The nearest ambulances to the disaster will go immediately to the disaster site. They will coordinate with the fire department and police to set up a command post, which will control all operations at the disaster. After this, they will assess the magnitude of the disaster, inform the ambulance dispatcher of the number of victims expected, and then begin triage of victims.

At the time of the red alert Denver General Hospital, which is the agency charged with coordinating medical care, will initiate its three-part disaster plan. First, the emergency department, then the rest of the hospital, is notified that the disaster plan has begun. Second, a triage team of physicians, nurses, and clerks for transport to the disaster site via ambulance is assembled. Third, a disaster telephone network that links all the area hospitals is activated. Each hospital is informed that the disaster has occurred, and each is asked what its capabilities are for caring for the five categories of patients.

The initial ambulance on the scene will begin triage of victims to the hospitals. This will be coordinated through the ambulance dispatcher, who keeps a running log of hospital capability and patients received. When the triage team arrives on the scene, the ambulance is relieved of its triage function. The triage team immediately coordinates with the command post so that groups are not working at cross purposes. The team will have available a limited number of medical supplies so that a minimal amount of care and stabilization can be given to victims while they wait for transportation to the hospital.

After all victims are assessed and transported, the disaster situation is technically over, but the work is far from finished. The log of victims transported must be cross-referenced with each receiving hospital to ensure that each victim is accounted for. The Red Cross or Salvation Army generally handles notification of families. When all are receiving care in hospitals or are released after treatment, the final step is a thorough critique of the management of the disaster by the individuals and agencies involved so that subsequent emergencies can be better provided for. By virtue of proper planning, cooperative organization, and a generous dollop of luck, it *is* possible to minimize, accept, and manage the unknown.

Eye Diseases
and Visual Disorders

There have been encouraging advances in the treatment of diabetic retinopathy in the past few years. These advances arrived at a time when the incidence of this disease had been increasing rapidly. Ironically, good medical practice is responsible for this increase. With better knowledge and treatment of diabetes mellitus, the life span of diabetics has been prolonged. And with these additional years, the late complications, which are a function of the duration of the disease, have become more prevalent. One of the most devastating complications of diabetes is the vascular change in the eye known as diabetic retinopathy. In recent years it has become the second leading cause of adult blindness in the United States. There is a 50% incidence of diabetic retinopathy in individuals who have had diabetes for 10 years, 75% incidence after 15 years of diabetes, and over 95% incidence after 20 years.

How diabetic retinopathy develops

Diabetic retinopathy is a disease of the blood vessels of the retina. It starts with alterations in the basement membrane of the vessels—the delicate inner layer of the blood vessels—that lead to progressive narrowing and obliteration of retinal capillaries and terminal arterioles (tiny arterial branches). The volume of blood perfusing the retina is decreased, thus decreasing the supply of oxygen. In an attempt to supply additional oxygenated blood, there is a dilation of adjacent vessels and shunting of blood. However, the new but weaker blood vessels do not deliver enough additional oxygen to satisfy the needs of the retina. At this point, in an abortive attempt to form other new blood vessels, small outpouchings, called microaneurysms, occur along capillaries. These can be observed as small, dark red spots. Because microaneurysms and other newly formed vessels are thin walled and weak, they eventually leak whole blood and serum into the retina. If the leaked materials cover the central portion of the retina known as the macula, there can be marked reduction of vision at this early stage. When this leakage is absorbed, it can leave behind exudates—precipitates of fatty materials, lipids, and lipoproteins—which appear as hard yellow deposits in the retina.

With continued deterioration of the retinal vessels, a cycle of occlusion, new vessel formation, bleeding, swelling, and scarring occurs. Eventually fresh blood spills into the central cavity of the eye and mixes with the vitreous body, the clear gel-like substance that fills most of the eye. As more blood mixes with it, the vitreous humor loses its clarity, and a reduction in vision results. The vitreous may contract, pulling on the retina and the newly formed blood vessels. This can produce a massive hemorrhage if vessels are torn, or it may pull the retina toward the central cavity with resultant detachment. With new techniques, however, individuals with diabetic retinopathy can expect more than a 50% chance of improving the course of the disease process. Two of the more important of these advances are photocoagulation of the retina and vitrectomy.

Diagnosis and treatment

The characteristic defects of the retina in a diabetic person can be easily observed with an ophthalmoscope. Diabetic retinopathy is the most readily visible manifestation of the disease process. With the technique of fluorescein angiography, however, changes in the retina can be demonstrated even before they become visible by direct observation. This aid in the early diagnosis of diabetic retinopathy enables early treatment.

Photocoagulation of the retina has developed into a low-risk treatment of diabetic retinopathy. The procedure consists of applying a controlled burn to the retina by means of an adjustable light source. The two most widely used light sources are the xenon light and the argon laser. The xenon light is white and utilizes the entire visible spectrum, while argon is a monochromatic green-blue light. Although the light sources are somewhat different, both of these methods depend on thermal, or heat, effects to place burns in the retina.

The argon laser is more popular for several reasons. The coagulation it induces can be finely controlled in both intensity and area. The laser has a lesser effect on the retinal nerve fibers. Since only eye drops are necessary for anesthesia, the procedure can be performed on an outpatient basis. A wide range of magnification can be used, and almost all of the retina can be reached. Xenon photocoagulation delivers larger doses of energy and is used where more extensive destruction of retina is indicated. The light beam, preset for intensity and size, destroys leaking blood vessels, microaneurysms, neovascular tissue, and zones of poorly oxygenated retina. If photocoagulation is successful, the abnormal areas will atrophy and dry up. The destroyed areas require less oxygen, and stimuli for new blood vessel formation are thus reduced. The remaining retina functions more adequately, and vision remains stable. When renewed activity occurs at indeterminate intervals, additional photocoagulation may be performed.

Vitrectomy, a method of removing and replacing the vitreous, is the newest method in treating another aspect of diabetic retinopathy. At present this technique is being assessed by several study groups throughout the U.S. There have been preliminary reports of a success rate up to 65% in restoring some degree of vision. Episodes of bleeding into the vitreous humor can be small with only slight diminution of vision, and such episodes can occur sporadically, with clearing of vision in the interim between small hemorrhages. If the bleed-

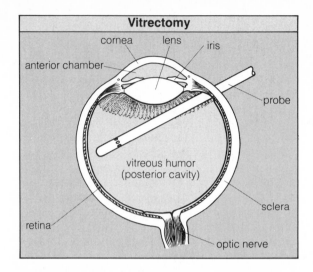

Vitrectomy

cornea
lens
iris
anterior chamber
probe
vitreous humor
(posterior cavity)
sclera
retina
optic nerve

ing occurs more frequently and faster than the blood can be absorbed, vision will deteriorate. A large hemorrhage can result in immediate loss of useful vision, which may take months or even years to clear. The consistency of the vitreous usually becomes fibrous and organized if the blood is allowed to remain. An attempt to remove the vitreous should be made before this change occurs. In vitrectomy a probe is introduced into the large posterior cavity of the eye that contains the vitreous. A built-in suction apparatus pulls the vitreous into the tip of the probe. Simultaneously, a blade chops the vitreous into small pieces and, as it enters the probe, it is removed and replaced with clear saline solution. Eventually almost all of the opaque vitreous is replaced with clear fluid. The procedure is performed with the aid of a microscope focused through the dilated pupil. If the fluid remains transparent, vision is restored, although the degree of acuity depends on the condition of the retina.

—*Walter L. Peretz, M.D.*

Gastrointestinal Disorders

Newly developed methods of diagnosis and treatment as well as increased understanding of basic physiological processes have contributed to recent advances in the treatment of gastrointestinal disorders. Among the areas of current interest are the effects of certain disease conditions on the body's metabolism of vitamin D, new understanding of hepatitis, and new approaches to the management of upper gastrointestinal hemorrhage.

Vitamin D in health and disease

It has long been recognized that severe lack of vitamin D causes rickets, a disease in which bone calcification is retarded. Only recently, with more sophisticated understanding of the metabolism and synthesis of vitamin D, correlated with bone mineral formation, has it been

possible to understand and correct the more subtle alterations that occur in a number of other disease states.

Vitamin D is derived from foods and is also produced in the skin from the action of ultraviolet light. The relative importance of these sources depends on dietary intake and exposure to sunlight, but quantitatively, synthesis in the skin is probably more important in most normal individuals. Ingested vitamin D is absorbed predominantly in that portion of the small intestine known as the proximal jejunum by a process of simple diffusion. Bile salts derived from the liver are required for absorption. Biochemical activation to more active substances begins in the liver, where vitamin D is converted to 25-hydroxyvitamin D. A feedback system regulates the activity of the enzyme system involved in the formation of 25-hydroxyvitamin D; enzyme activity is enhanced in vitamin D deficiency and suppressed during the vitamin-replete state. 25-hydroxyvitamin D is the major form of the vitamin in blood serum, in which it is transported by specific binding proteins.

In the kidney 25-hydroxyvitamin D is further metabolized into 1,25-dihydroxyvitamin D, which is the form of the vitamin that is most active in stimulating intestinal calcium absorption. This conversion is stimulated by parathyroid hormone and by low levels of inorganic phosphate in the bloodstream.

A number of gastrointestinal and liver diseases can interfere with vitamin D metabolism at various levels: inadequate dietary intake of vitamin D because of lack of appetite; malabsorption due to intestinal disease or lack of bile salts; impairment of the formation of 25-hydroxyvitamin D as a result of certain liver diseases; failure of a diseased small intestine to respond to 1,25-dihydroxyvitamin D. New techniques for the measurement of tiny amounts of these circulating vitamins have helped to determine the specific abnormalities in these disease states.

It has been recognized recently that osteomalacia, or severe bone demineralization due to lack of vitamin D, can be detected at an early stage by bone biopsy techniques that can be performed in an outpatient clinic. A special needle is used to obtain the bone sample. The tissue is then stained by methods that permit analysis of the amount of calcification, which in turn can be correlated approximately with levels of circulating 25-hydroxyvitamin D.

From the standpoint of therapy, these new techniques for evaluation enable the physician and nutritionist to tailor the correct doses of vitamin D in the diet to an individual's needs. The most logical approach is adjustment of vitamin D dosage to maintain normal vitamin D and serum calcium levels.

Hepatitis

Since the discoveries of the Australia antigen (hepatitis B virus) and of the hepatitis A virus, these microorganisms have become distinguishable by specific blood and immunological tests.

Hepatitis A virus is usually spread by the fecal-oral route, commonly by close contact, and infection occurs readily in conditions of poor sanitation and overcrowding. In developed countries, however, food and water-borne transmission are not major factors that enable the infection to persist in the populace. However, ingestion of shellfish cultivated in water contaminated by infected sewage is associated with a high risk of hepatitis A. The spread of infection is reduced by simple general hygienic measures and sanitary disposal of human waste.

Hepatitis B virus is associated especially with transmission by the transfusion of infected blood and blood products. In addition, a variety of body fluids such as saliva, menstrual and seminal fluid, and breast milk have been implicated in the spread of infection. The B virus is associated with chronic liver diseases such as chronic active hepatitis and cirrhosis, and in some parts of the world infection by this virus may predispose to the later development of primary liver cancer. This form of viral hepatitis is an occupational hazard among certain health care personnel, such as those in renal dialysis centers. High rates of infection have been reported in homosexuals, prostitutes, and drug abusers.

A further type of hepatitis, in which no agent has yet been identified, has been called "non-A, non-B hepatitis." Now that hepatitis B positive donor blood can be excluded by appropriate serological tests, non-A, non-B hepatitis represents a high proportion of the cases of post-transfusion hepatitis in the United States. Uncommonly, other viruses such as cytomegalovirus or Epstein-Barr virus can be incriminated in hepatitis following massive transfusions, but these viruses can also be detected by blood tests.

Until recently there have been only indirect indications that an infectious agent is responsible for non-A, non-B hepatitis. These indications are: (1) a variable but defined incubation period (about 6 to 12 weeks) intermediate between that of type A and type B hepatitis; (2) a positive correlation between the development of non-A, non-B hepatitis and the source of donor blood (as in the case of type B hepatitis, non-A, non-B hepatitis is more common after transfusion of paid donor blood than of volunteer donor blood); and (3) patterns of liver cell inflammation and destruction that can be virtually indistinguishable from those seen in types A or B. Recently two groups of investigators have demonstrated more directly that this type of hepatitis is caused by one or more infectious agents. By transfusing plasma from patients with acute or chronic non-A, non-B hepatitis into laboratory animals, they were able to show biochemical changes of liver cell inflammation in the blood and evidence of liver cell destruction. A detailed study of this animal model will undoubtedly further the understanding of the biology and control of non-A, non-B hepatitis. The development of a vaccine remains an important long-range goal to aid patients who may require multiple transfusions.

Upper gastrointestinal hemorrhage

Gastrointestinal bleeding is one of the more common serious clinical problems; determining the specific cause and administering appropriate therapy can be difficult. Significant mortality occurs in instances of massive hemorrhage, particularly in the debilitated or elderly, whose cardiovascular systems are not able to tolerate sudden decreases in perfusion pressure. Upper gastrointestinal bleeding may be profuse and is manifested by the vomiting of blood either bright red or brown, resembling coffee grounds and due to the action of stomach acid on the blood, and/or by the passage of tarry black, sticky stool with various amounts of red blood interspersed. Causes of significant upper gastrointestinal hemorrhage include peptic ulcers, stomach cancer, and erosive gastritis (severe inflammation of the inner lining of the stomach).

The diagnosis of gastrointestinal bleeding has been revolutionized by fiberoptic techniques—which enable the physician to see inside body cavities—with a specific diagnosis being made in over 80% of patients. In many instances, however, despite improved accuracy of diagnosis, the rate of survival after a major hemorrhage has not changed much for the past two decades. In part this may reflect limitations of current treatment approaches. Because fiberoptic endoscopy permits visualization of the bleeding site in most patients, direct application of agents to promote blood coagulation and healing or direct coagulation of the bleeding site seems feasible. A number of methods of coagulation have been proposed; some have been tested in animals and even in human subjects. These methods include electrocoagulation, heater probes, suture clips, chemical injections, and photocoagulation by means of lasers.

Ophthalmologists have successfully used visible light to photocoagulate abnormal vessels in the retina that occur, for example, in diabetic retinopathy. (See Eye Diseases and Visual Disorders.) In the past decade several sources of monochromatic, coherent light (laser) have been developed. These have been adapted for delivery through the fiberoptic endoscope. An argon laser beam is transmitted along a single, flexible quartz fiber that is encased in a polyethylene catheter. The catheter can be inserted through the biopsy channel of a standard gastroscope. The endoscopist can see the blue-green laser as it is emitted and can guide it to the bleeding point. In a number of laboratories in the U.S. and Europe, teams of physicians and electronic engineers are studying the effects of laser photocoagulation on normal tissues and on experimentally induced ulcers in animals. A recent report outlined the use of the argon laser in controlling hemorrhage in almost 100 small bleeding gastrointestinal lesions in humans.

The future of these new techniques remains to be determined. Standardization of the methods is required as well as demonstration that the results of treatment are superior to those of conventional medical and surgical management. Currently patients with prolonged bleeding or repeated episodes are subjected to surgery, the type of operation being determined by the source and site of bleeding. Patients who stand to benefit most from these types of endoscopic therapeutic techniques are those for whom surgical treatment would be either unsafe or ineffective.

— Bernard Levin, M.D.

Genetic Disorders

Exciting and provocative advances in the fields of cytogenetics, biochemical genetics, and cytology have expanded the potential for diagnosis and prevention of a variety of developmentally disabling conditions. Amniocentesis and prenatal diagnosis are important aspects of comprehensive obstetric care. In this context it is now possible to diagnose Duchenne muscular dystrophy and neural tube disorders early in pregnancy. Hypothyroidism is now detectable by neonatal metabolic screening programs. Some notable new associations of human diseases with HL-A antigens have been established. Through the powerful new tools of chromosome banding techniques and a successful replacement therapy of a missing enzyme the impact of genetics is felt in clinical practice.

Prenatal diagnosis

Duchenne muscular dystrophy (DMD), a progressive and fatal X-linked recessive disorder, is the most common of the muscular dystrophies affecting children. High concentrations of creatine phosphokinase (CPK), a muscle enzyme, are found in the blood of patients with this disease. Fetoscopy, a direct visualization of the fetus and the placenta, had previously been useful in obtaining samples of fetal blood cells necessary for diagnosing hemoglobinopathies—blood diseases such as sickle-cell anemia that are caused by genetically determined changes in the structure of hemoglobin. Through the use of the same technique, elevated levels of CPK were found in the plasma of a 20-week-old fetus later confirmed to have DMD. This technique is still experimental, but the potential for improved diagnosis is great.

The neural tube is the portion of the embryo from which the brain and spinal cord arise. Neural tube defects (anencephaly, myelomeningocele, and so on) were previously diagnosed using ultrasonography and X-rays. The presence of alpha-fetoprotein (AFP) in the amniotic fluid in increased concentrations has been more dependable. AFP is produced in the yolk sac,

liver, and gastrointestinal tract of the embryo. Present normally during fetal life, its function is not known. It is detectable in serum of the embryo at six weeks and rapidly disappears during the first month of life. The presence of AFP in increased concentrations in amniotic fluid not only has heralded the existence of neural tube defects but has served as a marker for a variety of other congenital anomalies, among them omphalocele, Turner's syndrome, congenital nephrosis, and intestinal obstruction. It may also signal that the fetus is in distress or has died.

Disorders permitting seepage of fetal fluid to amniotic fluid (*e.g.,* myelomeningocele) or involving altered amniotic fluid dynamics (*e.g.,* increased production) can be diagnosed prenatally using amniocentesis and AFP determination. Ultrasonography is recommended before performing amniocentesis for two reasons. The first is to locate the placenta in order to avoid contamination of the amniotic fluid by blood. The second is to confirm the gestational age of the fetus, since the measurement of AFP in the amniotic fluid correlates with the normal range for a stated gestational age.

Only one out of ten neural tube defects occurs in a family with a history of such defects. Consequently, the utility of measuring AFP in maternal serum has interested investigators, particularly those in the United Kingdom. Available evidence suggests that screening of maternal serum at 16–18 weeks of pregnancy is practical and reliable. Multiple pregnancy, disturbed fetal homeostasis, molar or ectopic pregnancy, and Rh disease may be associated with elevated levels of AFP in maternal serum. When these conditions are excluded, raised serum AFP warrants further investigation by amniocentesis and ultrasonography.

Newborn screening

Routine screening of newborns for a variety of metabolic disorders ranging from phenylketonuria (PKU) to maple syrup urine disease represents one of the major developments in medicine. The results of such screening have provided a better comprehension of the incidence of metabolic disorders as well as an appreciation of the variability of their biochemical aberrations. Early diagnosis of specific diseases allows the prompt institution of therapeutic measures, preventing serious central nervous system disturbance. In addition, appropriate genetic counseling can be provided, and enlightened family planning can proceed.

With a broadened understanding of the function of the thyroid in the fetus and the newborn, and with the development of sophisticated laboratory methods (radioimmunoassays), screening for congenital hypothyroidism is now feasible. Although fetal skeletal maturation may be somewhat impaired, the fetus does not seem to need thyroid hormone in order to grow and develop normally. Infants with congenital hypothyroidism rarely are recognized at birth or during the first few months of life. It is difficult to recognize the disorder, as the tentative signs that may occur are subtle and nonspecific (lethargy, poor feeding, weak sucking, constipation, skin mottling, prolonged jaundice, hypothermia, respiratory distress, edema, and a large posterior fontanelle). However, in the weeks after birth, thyroid hormone seems to become essential to ensure normal brain growth and development. Biochemical identification of sporadic congenital hypothyroidism as soon as possible after birth allows the institution of thyroid replacement therapy, minimizing the effects of low thyroid hormone levels on the infant. (*See also* Glandular and Metabolic Disorders.)

Both congenital hypothyroidism and PKU are associated with mental retardation. Congenital hypothyroidism occurs sporadically and is two to three times more common (one in 5,000 births) than PKU. It is the most common type of potentially preventable mental retardation. In a regional screening program laboratories can be centralized, supporting sophisticated technology and establishing expertise in the performance of thyroxine and thyrotropin radioimmunoassays. Once a range of normal values is established, screening information can be subject to computer analysis. A system of routine follow-up and retrieval will enhance the screening process, permitting confirmatory testing and thyroid replacement therapy.

The health of a developing fetus can be monitored by ultrasound: high-frequency sound waves beamed toward the fetus; the information is visualized on the screen of an oscilloscope (below). Details of development and position can be determined, enabling the physician to anticipate possible complications in delivery.

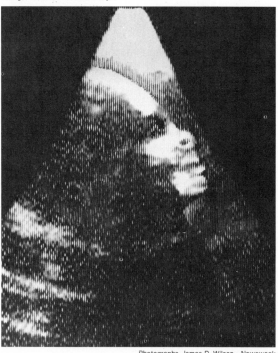

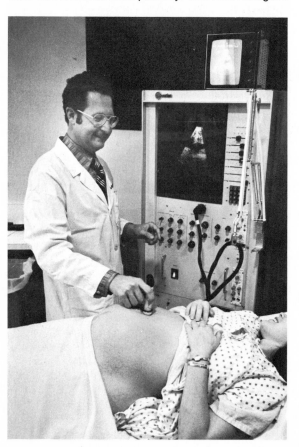

Photographs, James D. Wilson—Newsweek

HL-A antigens and susceptibility to disease

The primary importance of the histocompatibility (HL-A) antigen complex has been related to organ transplantation. The success or failure of a transplant is, to a considerable extent, dependent on the similarities or differences of the HL-A antigen system of the donor and the recipient. Attention has now been directed to the association of the individual HL-A makeup and the risk or susceptibility of developing certain diseases.

HL-A refers to the protein molecules that have been found on the surfaces of human nucleated cells. They form the basis for the recognition by the body's immune system of antigens of a group different from the host's. Determination of HL-A antigens is essential for tissue compatibility typing, not only for organ transplantation but also for leukocyte and platelet transfusion.

The genetics of this system involves four separate, closely linked loci (locus A, locus B, locus C, locus D—a locus being the position of a gene on a chromosome) on the small arm of chromosome 6. Since humans have two sixth chromosomes, the gene complex of histocompatibility consists of four paired alleles (forms of a gene at the same locus) that are inherited from generation to generation without one becoming dominant and the other recessive.

The association of specific HL-A antigens with disease has received wide publicity. The HL-A antigens are viewed as valuable genetic markers capable of providing researchers with profound epidemiologic and biologic insight into the occurrence of a variety of disorders of hitherto unknown origin.

For example, the HL-A B-27 locus is correlated with a rheumatic condition called ankylosing spondylitis. This is a striking correlation since B-27 occurs in less than 10% of the Caucasian population but in almost 90% of Caucasians with this disorder. Individuals with B-27 show a lesser but significant susceptibility to other rheumatic conditions, such as juvenile rheumatoid arthritis, Reiter's syndrome, acute anterior uveitis, psoriatic arthritis, and reactive arthritis (arthritis caused by bacterial infection by such agents as *Yersinia*, *Salmonella*, and *Neisseria gonorrhoeae*).

Gastrointestinal, neurologic, endocrine, and cutaneous problems have been associated with HL-A B-8. Gluten-sensitive enteropathy, chronic active hepatitis, myasthenia gravis, Graves' disease, Addison's disease, juvenile diabetes mellitus, and dermatitis herpetiformis are the most important conditions correlated with the B-8 locus.

About 50 diseases have now been associated with specific HL-A antigens, but the significance of this relationship remains unclear. Altered immune function has been postulated, yet most of the disorders have no documented cause. They do not represent genetically determined entities, although family clustering has been reported. Several hypotheses have been proposed as explanations of the genetic influence of these antigenic markers.

An initial concept of molecular mimickry suggested that the HL-A antigens had immunochemical similarities to antigens of infectious agents, resulting in impaired or depressed immunological response. A second view postulated that the HL-A complex was a potential receptor for specific viruses, thus facilitating infection in the host. A hypothesis that is currently popular is that additional genes, important for the immune response, are located in proximity to the HL-A antigen. Verification of this hypothesis awaits further study.

Chromosome banding techniques

The introduction of a variety of banding techniques has extended understanding of chromosome structure and function. Chromosome banding techniques enable researchers to identify each human chromosome. In addition, microscopic realignments and breaks can be detected. More than 30 disorders have been detected by use of a banding technique through which a specific abnormality seen in clinical practice is consistently associated with a specific chromosomal defect.

Replacement therapy

Severe combined immunodeficiency disease (SCID) represents a group of inherited disorders characterized by an increased susceptibility to infection, ultimately resulting in death. Within this group is one entity associated with deficiency of a specific enzyme, adenosine deaminase (ADA).

Clinically, SCID with ADA deficiency appears in infants before they are six months of age. There is failure to thrive, chronic diarrhea, and severe and recurrent infections (*e.g.,* pneumonia) due to bacteria, viruses, or fungi. Skeletal X-rays may show characteristic abnormalities including concavity and flaring of the anterior ribs, abnormal articulation of the posterior ribs with the transverse processes of the spine, abnormal pelvis, and flattening of the vertebrae. The relationship of the bony abnormalities to the rest of the syndrome is unclear but, at present, ADA deficiency is thought to cause the SCID.

In the past, therapy for SCID with ADA has consisted of histocompatible bone marrow transplantation and fetal liver transplants, both of which have restored normal lymphocyte function, thereby boosting the immune response; however, the technique does not correct the enzyme deficiency. More recently, monthly transfusions of irradiated red blood cells, which contain ADA, have replaced the missing enzyme. Dramatic and continued improvement in immune function and freedom from infection have followed repeated transfusion. Although the mechanism underlying the success of this approach is uncertain, it provides an opportunity to clarify the relationship of the enzymatic deficiency to the increased susceptibility to infection.

—David Ingall, M.D.

Glandular and Metabolic Disorders

Hormones are chemical substances whose primary function is to preserve the well-ordered status of the whole body. They regulate metabolism—the combined chemical processes of the body. Hormones are catalytic agents, produced and released by various endocrine glands, causing either the inhibition or the acceleration of the body's activities.

The understanding of the intricacies of the endocrine system as well as hormones and prostaglandins (fatty substances with hormonelike actions) has led to major advances in the treatment of many disorders. Research in hormones and prostaglandins continues to provide some of the most significant developments in the biomedical sciences.

The synthesis of somatostatin by recombinant DNA techniques

The discovery of somatostatin and the use of recombinant DNA techniques were joined this year in a scientific achievement of great potential importance. There has been a long-standing need for greater amounts of certain protein and polypeptide hormones for clinical testing and treatment purposes. For example, insulin, a polypeptide hormone required by diabetics, must be isolated from pig or cow pancreases, and supplies are barely keeping pace with demand. Chemical synthesis of this polypeptide, which has a molecular weight of 6,000, is expensive and time-consuming. Similarly, the growth hormone that is used to treat hormone-deficient dwarfs must be isolated from human pituitary glands—a very limited source of supply.

Two years ago Roger Guillemin and his collaborators at the Salk Institute, near San Diego, Calif., isolated and characterized a 12-amino-acid protein from the hypothalamus. Because this new protein hormone inhibited the secretion of growth hormone, they named it somatostatin, which comes from the Greek words for "body" and "stop." This achievement and others led to the award of the Nobel Prize to Guillemin in 1977. (*See* Special Report: Hormone Discoveries of the 1977 Nobelists.) It was found subsequently that somatostatin could turn off the secretion of pancreatic hormones and other hormones. Somatostatin has the potential of preventing some of the diseases that accompany long-standing diabetes and for treating some patients with acromegaly, a disease caused by a growth-hormone-secreting tumor of the pituitary gland. But presently somatostatin is difficult to synthesize chemically in large amounts; therefore extensive clinical trials have not been possible.

During the period of discovery and testing of somatostatin, biochemists were learning how to alter the genetic code of bacteria. *Escherichia coli,* the common bacterium of the human intestinal tract, carries a single circular chromosome with the genes that contain the information necessary to direct the synthesis of all essential bacterial proteins. In addition it often carries

Plasmid DNA, shown here in a laboratory flask, is a basic material that can now be used to synthesize hormones for use in treating human disorders.

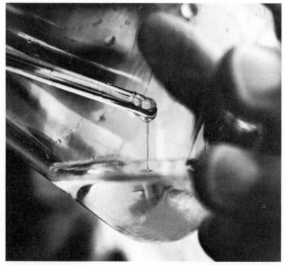

extra circular pieces of genetic material, called plasmids, that function like miniature chromosomes to provide the bacterium with other, sometimes very useful proteins. Using a variety of newly discovered enzymes (biologic catalysts), biochemists have learned how to equip a free plasmid with a piece of DNA (the genetic information) that has been either chemically synthesized or taken from another organism and then to insert the plasmid into a bacterial cell. This new information in the bacterium would permit synthesis of proteins corresponding to the inserted DNA.

Since somatostatin contains only 12 amino acids, it was possible to compose its corresponding gene chemically, attach it to a plasmid, and then insert the plasmid into the *E. coli* cell, producing a bacterium now capable of synthesizing a human hormone. In order to guard against the remote possibility that this new bacterium could escape the laboratory, infest humans, and synthesize somatostatin in excess (which could have dangerous consequences), the bacterially manufactured somatostatin emerges attached to another protein and is thus inactive. However, a simple chemical step can release somatostatin. This bacterial manufacture of somatostatin is important in its own right since it will permit large-scale clinical trials. But one reason this process is considered a breakthrough is that the same principle and techniques of recombinant DNA research can be used to synthesize large amounts of any protein hormone and other proteins such as antibodies and enzymes.

Detection of cretinism in the newborn

The central nervous system in the human does not complete its development until after six months of life. This process is dependent upon the presence of adequate thyroid hormone synthesized and secreted by the body's thyroid gland. Should the gland be congenitally deficient and the condition not be detected quickly, irreparable damage to the brain results, leading to idiocy in the extreme and mental retardation at best. Since congenital hypothyroidism is not rare, it was important to develop a screening test for it.

In the simplest terms the secretions of the thyroid and pituitary glands are related in a negative feedback loop. Thus, when the level of thyroid hormone in the blood falls, the pituitary gland secretes a protein hormone, thyroid-stimulating hormone (TSH), which signals the thyroid gland to secrete more thyroid hormone, thereby restoring the blood level. Conversely, when the level of thyroid hormone in the blood increases above normal, the pituitary gland stops secreting TSH, and the thyroid gland reduces its secretion of hormone. If an infant is born without a thyroid gland, the pituitary gland will secrete TSH at a high rate and the amount of TSH in the blood will be increased greatly.

It has been difficult to measure even this large

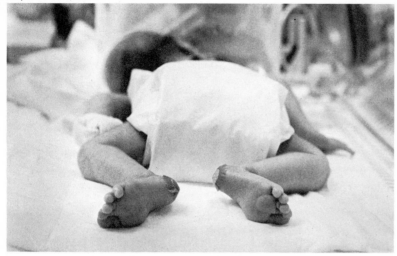

A tiny sample of blood taken from the heel of a newborn infant can now be used to screen for the presence of congenital hypothyroidism so that treatment can begin immediately, minimizing the effects on the child.

amount of TSH, and large volumes of blood were required. The discovery of the radioimmunoassay technique—the identification of a substance that has been radioactively labeled—permitted the measurement of billionths of a gram of hormone, a sensitivity never previously achieved. Further specific refinement of this technique for TSH enabled physicians to measure TSH in a small amount of blood obtained from a tiny puncture of the heel in a newborn infant. It has thus become possible to screen large numbers of infants, recognize congenital hypothyroidism quickly, begin treatment promptly, and improve mental development.

Estrogens—benefit and risk

It has recently become possible to assess the benefits and risks of the use of estrogens (female sex hormones), which have been the source of intense controversy. Estrogens have now been shown to have a major benefit—slowing the development of osteoporosis (thinning of bone) in older women. This disease develops after the menopause in most women and is characterized by loss of calcium with a consequent weakening of the bone. It is this decrease of bone strength that is responsible for the loss of height occurring in old age and for the greatly increased ease of fracture of ribs, vertebrae, and hips. Throughout life bone is in a dynamic condition, with calcium being deposited at some surfaces and reabsorbed at others. In middle-aged adults the rates of deposition and absorption are the same. In aging, and particularly after the menopause in women, both rates decrease, but the decrease in rate of deposition of calcium is proportionately greater, leading to a net loss of calcium and a thinning of bone. When estrogens are started within a year of the menopause and continued, the rate of thinning of bone is slowed so that severe osteoporosis takes longer to develop.

However, this positive effect of estrogens needs to be balanced against some serious side effects. The use of estrogens after the menopause has been associated with a four- to eightfold increase in the chances of developing cancer of the uterus, the risks increasing with the duration of estrogen treatment. There may also be an increase in the risk of developing cardiovascular disease. Optimal doses and methods of treatment with estrogens have not been established, and the decision to use estrogens must be based on individual judgments and consultations between women and their physicians.

Loss of menses and infertility due to pituitary tumors

Prolactin is the pituitary hormone necessary for lactation and is secreted in large amounts during and immediately after pregnancy. In nonpregnant women only small amounts of prolactin are released because pituitary secretion of prolactin is inhibited by dopamine, a factor of small molecular weight secreted by the hypothalamus. Occasionally, small benign tumors of the pituitary gland secrete excessive amounts of prolactin. This results in loss of menses and infertility. This loss of menses (amenorrhea) is the same as that seen in lactating women since it is due to prolactin secretion. The tumors are often so small that they have no effects other than the cessation of menses.

The development of a radioimmunoassay for prolactin made its measurement possible in small samples of blood. As a result, some women with amenorrhea and infertility have had pituitary tumors diagnosed. These small tumors may be removed by a neurosurgeon without damaging the rest of the pituitary gland. It is also possible to suppress prolactin secretion by these tumors and thereby induce menstruation and fertility by the use of a drug that has the same prolactin-inhibiting activity as dopamine. Dopamine itself cannot be used for this purpose because it does not penetrate into the central nervous system.

—Mortimer B. Lipsett, M.D.

223

Special Report:

Hormone Discoveries of the 1977 Nobelists

by A. Frederick Rasmussen, Jr., M.D., Ph.D.

The Nobel Prizes for Physiology or Medicine for 1977 were awarded to Rosalyn Yalow for her discovery of a biochemical technique—the radioimmunoassay—and, jointly, to Roger Guillemin and Andrew Schally for their discoveries that the hypothalamus at the base of the brain secretes hormones that control the secretion of other hormones by the anterior pituitary gland.

The three Americans were honored for their pioneering research and related discoveries in the role of hormones in the chemistry of the human body. Their achievements could mean a new era in endocrinology and a new outlook on the causes of human disease.

Yalow's research

Since 1950 Yalow—the sixth woman to win a Nobel Prize in science—has been a physicist in the radioisotope service of the U.S. Veterans Administration Hospital in the Bronx—a service that was established to provide the diagnostic and therapeutic services of a new subspecialty of medicine, nuclear medicine. This medical specialty evolved from the discovery by an earlier Nobelist, Ernest Lawrence, that radioactive chemical isotopes could be produced by electron bombardment of nonradioactive molecules in the cyclotron. The introduction of radioactive atoms into a variety of biologically reactive molecules, which could then be detected by radioactive emissions, was a development that was followed by extensive application of laboratory procedures based on this phenomenon to the study of normal and pathological functions and to diagnosis and treatment of diseases.

Laboratory diagnostic and research procedures based on immunologic reactions between molecular groupings or antigens and the antibodies produced in response to them have been widely used in experimental medicine and in the diagnosis of disease since the turn of the century. Widal's test was introduced to detect antibodies against the typhoid bacillus by observing the aggregation or clumping of suspensions of the bacilli when they were mixed with blood serum from patients who were recovering or who had recovered from typhoid. Similar tests for antigens in solutions were based on the visible precipitate that formed between antigens and their specific antibodies. Because such direct tests for antigens or antibodies were not always possible, indirect tests based on the same principle—the combination of an antigen and its specific antibody—were successfully introduced. These indirect tests greatly extended the sensitivity and range of practical applications but were still not sensitive enough for many diagnostic needs.

It was Yalow and her associate, medical scientist Solomon Berson, who combined the use of radioactive tracer techniques with antigen-antibody methodology to provide a procedure that could be used to detect and measure very small amounts of biologically reactive substances in health and disease and, indeed, to discover and measure active principles that had hitherto been either unknown or relegated to largely futile speculation. In this procedure, now commonly called the radioimmunoassay (RIA), a known radioactively labeled molecule competes with the unlabeled molecule that is to be identified or measured.

Berson and Yalow demonstrated the power of their new procedure in their classical studies on insulin resistance in diabetics. The troublesome fact that many patients with diabetes required larger and larger doses of insulin to control their diabetes and, indeed, became resistant to insulin therapy was a well-known therapeutic problem. That insulin resistance could be due to an immune response against insulin by the patient had been proposed but rejected because it had not been possible to demonstrate by conventional techniques that there were antibodies to insulin. Berson and Yalow successfully resolved this problem by first showing that insulin-resistant diabetics did have insulin-neutralizing antibodies in their blood and by then demonstrating that the addition of unlabeled insulin to a mixture of unlabeled antibody and radioactively labeled insulin resulted in displacement of the labeled insulin. The radioactivity of the displaced insulin could then be measured and thus the amounts of insulin in an unknown sample could be accurately determined. The solution to the problem of insulin resistance was a very significant achievement, but the wider application of the radioimmunoassay to measurement of amounts of enzymes, hormones, and other substances has had a far-reaching impact on our knowledge of biological processes. Berson and Yalow were jointly honored for their discoveries until Berson's death in 1972. Yalow has continued to extend the applications of the RIA through collaborative research with many investigators around the world.

Research in endocrinology has been spectacularly

facilitated because of the greater sensitivity and rapidity of RIA's for hormones, which can be completed in a matter of hours in contrast to traditional bioassays, which can require days, weeks, months, or even years. In no area of endocrinology has the impact of the RIA been more dramatic than in the elucidation of the system controlling the pituitary hormones.

The pituitary or master gland is about the size of a small walnut. It sits in a bony cup at the base of the brain, an inch or so above the uvula—the fleshy mass hanging from the soft palate above the root of the tongue. From this central position in the head the pituitary secretes its battery of hormones—hormones that control the operation of other major glands and tissues. The posterior lobe of the pituitary consists of nervous tissue and develops from and remains directly connected to the brain. The anterior and intermediate lobes arise from the roof of the mouth and are not directly connected to the brain.

Yet the anterior pituitary controls growth through the growth hormone it produces, regulates the secretion of thyroxin by the thyroid by secreting thyroid-stimulating hormone (TSH), regulates the female reproductive cycle by producing luteinizing and follicle-stimulating hormones, and controls the adrenal cortex through the secretion of adrenal corticotropin (ACTH).

Guillemin's and Schally's discoveries

It was this latter mechanism that Roger Guillemin and Andrew Schally undertook to elucidate in the mid-1950s. Guillemin, a native of Dijon, France, and Schally, of Wilno, Poland, met in Montreal, where Guillemin worked in the laboratory of Hans Selye, the noted researcher who has devoted much of his study to the problems of stress. Schally obtained a Ph.D. from McGill University. Between 1957 and 1960 Guillemin and Schally worked together at Baylor University in Houston, Texas. Guillemin has been a scientist at the Salk Institute for Biological Studies in San Diego, Calif., since 1970, and Schally has been at the New Orleans Veterans Administration Hospital and Tulane University since 1962.

The problem that Guillemin and Schally attacked separately in Montreal, together in Houston, and again separately when Schally left Baylor for New Orleans was the identification of the factor controlling the release of ACTH. This factor, called corticotropin releasing factor, or CRF, was one of several hormones postulated by a number of endocrinologists and particularly by Geoffrey Harris. Harris, an Englishman, and his associates had shown that cutting a system of blood vessels called the portal vessels, which flow from the hypothalamus to the anterior pituitary, depressed ACTH secretion. From this discovery Harris proposed that the hypothalamus, a small area at the base of the brain just above the pituitary, secreted neurohormones that were carried by the portal blood vessels to the

(Top) UPI Compix; (middle) Keystone; (bottom) Wide World

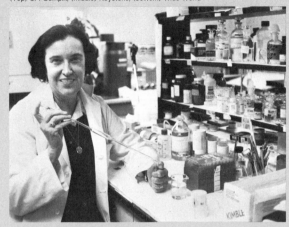

Rosalyn Sussman Yalow

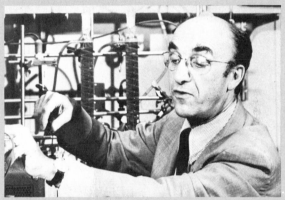

Roger Guillemin

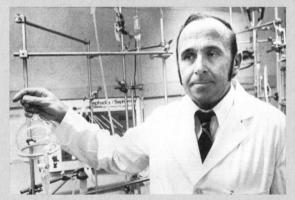

Andrew Schally

pituitary and, thus, controlled secretion of the anterior pituitary hormones. Harris attempted to isolate these hypothetical hormones without success, but he persuaded others to undertake this formidable challenge, among them Guillemin and Schally. Schally (with Murray Saffran) and Guillemin independently achieved initial success by demonstrating CRF in the hypothalamus. A key experiment achieved by both Guillemin and Schally was the demonstration that cell cultures of anterior pituitary will produce their usual

225

hormones only if fragments of hypothalamus are cultured with them. However, Guillemin's, Schally's, and others' heroic efforts to purify and chemically characterize CRF proved to be futile.

One of the problems of Harris and other workers was the time required to assay the potency of their preparations in animals. This problem was resolved by the RIA. An even more formidable problem, which the RIA could not resolve, was that the chemical characterization of CRF required milligram amounts of highly purified material, while the amounts in the hypothalamus are present in nanogram (one billionth of a gram) quantities. Guillemin and Schally tried to solve this problem by organizing networks of slaughterhouses where the brains of freshly slaughtered sheep and swine could be removed and the hypothalamuses dissected out before the hormone was destroyed by autolytic enzymes released by dying cells. This required the development of carefully trained, well-organized teams—an enormously costly effort. Even with the significant expenditures, by research laboratory standards, the chemical identity of CRF continued to be elusive.

In the meantime, other hypothalamic neurohormones had been detected by bioassays in animals and RIA's. Guillemin and Schally, working independently, then turned their attentions to these other factors at a time when the scientific community had become alarmed at the large amounts of money spent without dividends. Some influential scientists maintained that Guillemin and Schally were pursuing an impossible goal. But success was at last achieved, and in 1969, after seven years of fruitless effort on CRF and another seven to eight years of work on the thyrotropin releasing factor, TRF, Roger Burgus working with Guillemin reported the isolation of TRH. From thousands of kilograms of sheep hypothalamus they were able to recover a few milligrams of TRF, barely enough to allow structural determinations. The structure turned out to be surprisingly simple; the TRH molecule was a tripeptide containing the three amino acids—histamine, proline, and glutamic acid. Schally and his team, who had been very close to this structure three years earlier, followed within a few weeks with a report that TRH from swine hypothalamus had the same composition.

This achievement confirmed Harris' long-defended hypothesis that the hormones of the anterior pituitary were controlled by neurohormones produced in a part of the brain, the hypothalamus, and were carried to the pituitary by the portal blood vessels. It also allowed for the chemical synthesis of TRH, thus providing an economical source of this previously expensive hormone, which, in turn, allowed much more definitive studies on its function. Even more significantly, the characterization of TRH stimulated increased efforts, no longer in want of research funding, on the other hypothalamic neurohormones. Thus Schally in 1971 and shortly thereafter Guillemin determined the struc-

ture of luteinizing hormone releasing hormone (LHRH). (LHRH is the hypothalamic hormone that stimulates the anterior pituitary to secrete a second hormone, which stimulates the corpus luteum of the ovary.) The knowledge of the chemical structure of LHRH immediately facilitated an important advance in reproductive endocrinology by showing that luteinizing hormone (LH) and follicle stimulating hormone (FSH), previously thought to be under the control of different hypothalamic neurohormones were, in fact, both controlled by LHRH. Other important developments are rapidly following because of the availability of synthetic analogues of LHRH, which may have important uses in therapy of reproductive disorders or contraception.

The third hypothalamic hormone to be characterized, again by Guillemin and his associates, was the growth hormone release inhibiting factor (GIF), which was shown to be another polypeptide, considerably larger than FRH or LHRH, and which is now known as somatostatin. As was true of TRH and LHRH, the availability of somatostatin in pure form has allowed important advances in knowledge of its function. Somatostatin inhibits the action of TRH on the anterior pituitary to release thyrotropin. TRH also inhibits some secretory activities of the pancreas and the stomach. These discoveries suggest that somatostatin or its synthetic analogues may be useful in treatment of diabetes, growth disorders, and even peptic ulcers.

New roads opened for future medical research

The frontiers opened by the discoveries of Yalow and of Guillemin and Schally will no doubt continue to expand rapidly and in as yet unpredictable directions. One of the most important areas that have been opened up by the RIA is neurochemistry, and particularly the chemistry of opiate analgesia and of opiate addiction. Intensive current research on naturally occurring substances, the endorphins, which have morphine-like actions on the brain, promises to add a whole new dimension to our understanding of brain functions concerned with and influenced by sensations. Extension and amplification of the new knowledge of hypothalamic neurohormone function have already led to new discoveries with important applications in interactions of hormones not only in the brain and anterior pituitary but also at peripheral sites.

The 1977 awards have been greeted with enthusiasm in the scientific community not only because they recognize very significant advances in medical science but also because, in the case of Guillemin and Schally, they recognize the virtues of perseverence. It is unfortunate and sad that Solomon Berson, who might have shared a Nobel Prize with Rosalyn Yalow, died in 1972. Geoffrey Harris, who had contributed so much to the concept that the anterior pituitary gland was controlled by hormones coming through the blood from the hypothalamus, died in the previous year.

Health Care Costs

A quick solution to the increasing cost of health care—certainly one of the major public health issues of the last few years—continues to elude policymakers. For the most part opinion is polarized, with one group favoring increased federal regulation and the other favoring retention of the current system with modifications. A few signs of conciliation have emerged recently, however, and the beginnings of cooperative efforts can be seen. The success of these endeavors will play a major role in short-run decisions and long-range programs, both public and private.

Before considering various cost control strategies that are gaining support, it may be helpful to review some of the factors that have affected the delivery of health care in the U.S. in recent years. Evaluating experiences of the past is a necessary step that can provide needed perspective for understanding current situations and proposals for change in the health care system.

The health care marketplace

The health care marketplace in the United States does not fit the economist's prototype; it is not a market in which consumers determine how much of what kind of product or service they are willing to purchase while providers determine what to sell, with the prevailing price in the market serving as the principal economic regulator of behavior. Rather the consumer, or patient, usually relies on the provider, or physician, to determine the majority of the purchasing decisions. Furthermore, the services are most often paid not by the consumer but by a third party—a public or private insurer. The result of this interaction, in which neither consumer nor provider is given direct incentive to be particularly conscious of prices, is a tendency for overutilization of health care resources and an accompanying increase in health care prices.

The recent increase in malpractice suits has made insurance coverage for the physician one of his major yearly overhead expenses. The increased premiums are passed along to the patient in higher fees charged. And in order to protect himself from charges of laxity, the physician frequently orders costly confirmatory tests and X-rays to document the completeness of a regimen of treatment should his procedures be called into question.

An overview of the health care marketplace is not complete without a discussion of the effect of economy-wide inflation. Hospitals, which represent the single greatest category of health expenditures, purchase a market basket of goods such as food, plastics, and paper products—items that have experienced significant price increases in recent times. Because of the nature of the services provided, hospitals have little control over the prices of these commodities and only a small degree of control over the amounts used, particularly in view of an increased demand for hospital services.

Furthermore, hospitals are a labor-intensive industry and, until recently, paid lower wages on an average than many other industries. An extension of minimum wage legislation to hospital workers, combined with an expanded role for unions and collective bargaining, has resulted in a substantial increase in labor costs for hospitals.

Since physicians admit patients to hospitals, oversee their care, and decide when they are to be discharged, they play the key role in hospital utilization. In this role physicians are responding in part to an increased demand for more sophisticated health care. However, physicians are also in a position to have major influence on the level and composition of hospital utilization. In fact, the physician is the primary decision maker for more than 70% of health care services, and he or she is under unprecedented attack for the current cost scandal.

Trends in health care costs

A look at cost trends in the health care sector in the U.S. over the last decade and a half shows a dramatic increase in aggregate expenditures and begins to explain the so-called health-cost crisis. In fiscal 1960 expenditures totaled $25.9 billion, or $141 per person; in fiscal year 1976 the corresponding amount was $139.3 billion, or $638 per capita. This increase was the result of greater utilization of services as well as higher costs for services.

In 1960 just under one-third ($8.5 billion) of the total health care expenditure was spent on hospital care; in 1976, 40% ($55.4 billion) was spent. As hospital costs were increasing at an unprecedented rate, expenditures on physicians' services as a proportion of the total health costs showed a relative decline—dropping from 21.5% in 1960 to 19% in 1976.

Expenditures in other categories, though not as relevant to the current situation, are of interest. Dentists' services reflect a pattern similar to that of physicians; totals for dentists' services were $1.9 billion in 1960 and $8.6 billion in 1976. Drug and drug sundry expenses tripled over the past 16 years from $3.6 billion in 1960 to $11.2 billion by 1976. Nursing home expenditures showed the greatest growth of any single category; in 1960 they claimed only $500 million, but by 1976 they had grown to $10.6 billion.

Public funding, particularly from the federal government, increased over the period under consideration. In 1960, 21.7% of all personal health expenditures were publicly financed; slightly less than half of this amount was paid by the federal government. By 1976 the portion financed publicly had grown to 40.2%, with the federal government paying for 28% of that amount.

Conversely, direct, or out-of-pocket, payments have

227

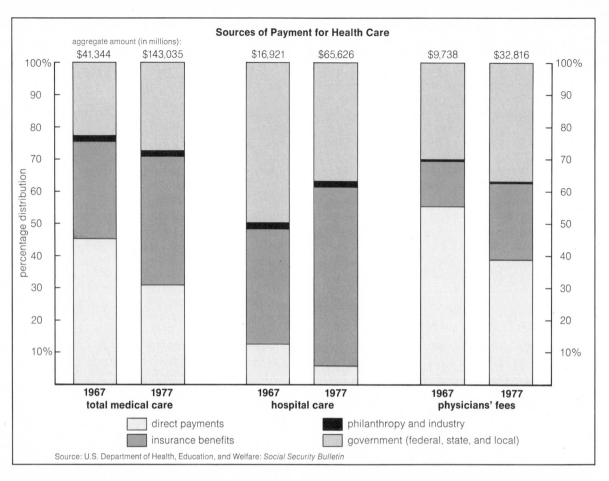

Sources of Payment for Health Care

aggregate amount (in millions):

| $41,344 | $143,035 | $16,921 | $65,626 | $9,738 | $32,816 |

| 1967 | 1977 | 1967 | 1977 | 1967 | 1977 |
| total medical care | | hospital care | | physicians' fees | |

direct payments

insurance benefits

philanthropy and industry

government (federal, state, and local)

Source: U.S. Department of Health, Education, and Welfare: *Social Security Bulletin*

dropped as a proportion of private expenditures. In 1960, 70.7% of all private expenditures were direct payments, compared with 32.5% in 1976. Third-party payers—private insurers and government—paid for less than 50% of all personal medical expenses in 1960; they now account for 68%.

The demand for health services

Since 1960 there have been substantial changes in the factors that determine the demand for and supply of health care services in the U.S. Demographics have played an important role in the demand for services. The population increased from 179 million in 1960 to 215.1 million in 1976. Meanwhile, the number of individuals with hospital insurance coverage grew from 122.5 million, or 68% of the population, in 1960 to 168.4 million, or 79.3% of the population, in 1976. Along with this increase in insurance coverage, there was a rise in the per capita disposable income rate—from $1,934 in 1960 to $5,493 in 1976.

In order to meet the ever growing demand for services, the health care sector has altered the type and method of delivery, including the number and kinds of physicians, dentists, hospitals, nursing homes, and allied health personnel. In 1963 there were a total of 276,475 physicians, or 146 per 100,000 population. Since that time there has been a 48% increase to 409,446 physicians, or 190 per 100,000 population. During this same time 29 additional medical schools—an increase from 87 in 1963 to 116 in 1976—were opened, while the capacity of existing schools was also increased. This expansion will first be fully felt in 1980, when there will be about 15,000 medical school graduates, compared with the approximately 7,000 who received degrees in 1960. A count of osteopathic practitioners, who are integral to the availability of medical care, has remained constant at approximately 14,500, or 8 per 100,000, over the period. The number of U.S. schools that train osteopaths has increased from 6 to 10.

Allied health care personnel—including registered nurses, occupational therapists, physical therapists, laboratory technicians, psychologists, licensed practical nurses, and others—were last counted in 1968. At that time the National Center for Health Statistics put the total at 3.5 million but did not include those professionals who work in physicians' offices, in industry, or in part-time employment.

The American Hospital Association currently lists 7,082 hospitals of all kinds, of which 5,956 are short-

228

term general hospitals ranging from 100-bed facilities to large medical center complexes. While the number of for-profit hospitals has declined since 1960 from 856 to 752 in 1976, the number of beds in these hospitals has increased from 37,000 to 76,000. This trend reflects the change in ownership from one or two physicians to investor-owned corporations.

The public utilized the increased availability of health professionals by increasing the rates of physician and hospital visits. The number of patient visits since 1963, the first year a nationwide attempt was made to count visits per person to physicians, has risen from 4.5 per year to 4.9. The average daily census of short-term general hospitals was 477,000 in 1960. By 1976 the census count was 715,000. The expense per patient-day over the same span went from an average of $32.23 to $151.28. Outpatient visits to general hospitals have shown a staggering increase of more than 1,000% between 1966 to 1976.

Price trends

The price of health care, reflected in expense per patient-day statistics, has skyrocketed over the past two decades. This span is often divided into four easily identified periods: pre-Medicare, 1960–65; Medicare, 1966–71; economic stabilization, middle 1971 to early 1974; and post-economic stabilization, 1974 to the present.

The Consumer Price Index (CPI) provides a useful means of measuring changes in the price of health care and of comparing health-related changes with those in the economy as a whole, particularly because it is the most widely used and quoted measure.

During the early 1960s, the pre-Medicare period, health care prices were lower than today but still above the "all items less medical care" index and the "all services less medical care" index. (Medical care includes all health care prices.) It can be assumed that there were already forces in the economy to cause a relatively rapid increase in health care prices.

From 1966 to 1971, the Medicare period, advances in health care prices averaged 7.3% per year, up from 2.2% over the preceding five years. While part of this climb was due to the increased access and utilization brought about by Medicare legislation, the economy in general showed large price increases as well.

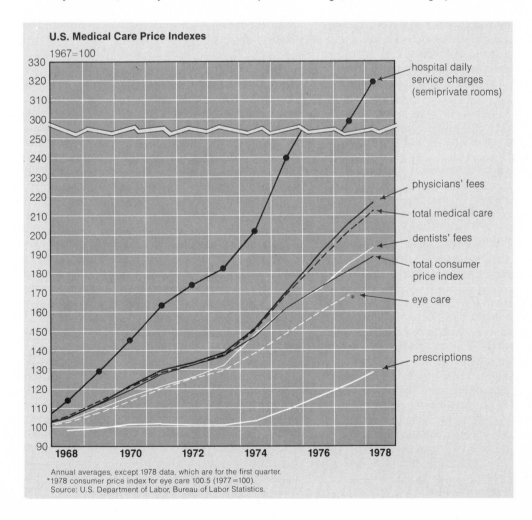

U.S. Medical Care Price Indexes

1967=100

hospital daily service charges (semiprivate rooms)

physicians' fees

total medical care

dentists' fees

total consumer price index

eye care

prescriptions

Annual averages, except 1978 data, which are for the first quarter.
*1978 consumer price index for eye care 100.5 (1977=100).
Source: U.S. Department of Labor, Bureau of Labor Statistics.

Health care costs

The economic stabilization period, when wages and prices were "frozen," brought an abrupt slowing of prices throughout the economy. (While most prices were held to a small range of change, other aspects of the nation's economic behavior experienced substantial disruption, and shortages developed in many key areas of the economy.) In the health care sector, prices were held to a 3.2% increase in the first year.

As economic controls ended for various segments of the economy, post-economic stabilization prices increased more rapidly than before controls. Prices for health care outstripped the rise in the economy, swelling 12% over the last year of economic stabilization. While the rate of increase has fallen since 1975, the CPI figures for the medical care segment are higher than the CPI overall.

Hospital cost containment plans

To counteract rapidly increasing health care costs, many of which are attributable to the rise in the cost of hospital services, in April 1977 the federal government proposed hospital cost containment legislation, or the so-called hospital cap bill. The government wants to set a ceiling on total inpatient hospital revenues by limiting payments from each third-party payer (insurer). The increase in revenue would be limited to about 9% in the first year of the program. The proposed bill would tie the rate of hospital inflation to a measure of overall inflation in the general economy, and allowance would be made for a moderate expansion of services and a steady improvement in their quality. The bill calls for a national limit of $2.5 billion for capital spending—a significantly smaller amount than is currently available. Each state's limit, allocated on the basis of population, would be a portion of this total amount. The authors of the tough government bill state that the intent of this limitation on capital spending is to restrict investment in expensive equipment and bed capacity (in areas already overbedded). A further intent of the bill is to provide incentives to hospitals to make better use of present resources, encourage greater use of ambulatory care, and foster the development of alternative forms of health care delivery, such as group practice.

Government figures claim that the program would result in a substantial reduction in the nation's hospital bills. In the first year alone, according to Department of Health, Education, and Welfare (HEW) figures, it could produce a reduction in excess of $2 billion. By fiscal 1982 the annual reduction could grow to $17 billion, and the total cumulative amount would exceed $43 billion. HEW is also seeking a long-range program to take over when the short-term goals are met.

The private sector—including hospitals, physicians, and others—sees some distinct problems with the hospital cap approach. The American Medical Association (AMA), testifying before the congressional Subcommittee on Health, Committee on Ways and Means, stated that at least a significant portion of the recent inflationary increases in hospital charges and the general increase in health care costs are a reaction to previous ceilings imposed on rates of increase in the health sector. Examples of such ceilings are reduced payments for services rendered under Medicare and Medicaid and the wage and price controls of the early 1970s. The extension of controls under the proposed hospital cost containment bill singles out only one segment of the economy for cost controls.

Furthermore, to implement the second part of the bill—the limit on hospital capital expenditures—the secretary of health, education, and welfare would be required to establish a national ceiling for the supply of hospital beds and a national standard for the rate of occupancy of hospital beds to be applicable to each geographic area. The bill defines the ratio of 4 hospital beds per 1,000 population and rate of occupancy for hospital beds of not less than 80% as the national standards. The effect of these two procedures could have a negative impact on the quality and availability of hospital care. With a cap on expenditures and the numbers of beds, care may simply become unavailable in some areas.

The alternative, offered by the private sector, is a voluntary effort for cost containment among hospitals, physicians, insurers, hospital supply manufacturers, and consumers to lower the rise in hospital costs by two percentage points per year over two years. This program was implemented in late 1977. Since the current rate of price increases is based on figures that show a gap of five percentage points between hospital expenditure increases and increases in the gross national product, the end product of a two-year effort would bring hospital expenditures into line with the rest of the economy.

Implementation of this program is being accomplished primarily through action at the state level. The leadership of the hospital associations, medical societies, and representatives of investor-owned hospitals in each state jointly created state-level voluntary cost containment committees. These local committees are developing cost containment programs based on the national goals and objectives, allowing for flexibility to meet varying local needs.

Part of the voluntary effort program is designed to establish a screen to identify for review any hospital with a rate of increase in its budgeted revenues or expenditures that is not at least two percentage points below the rate of increase in the previous fiscal year. Further, hospitals whose revenue increases are among the top 15% in a state will be screened and reviewed by the state committee. In keeping with the objectives of the government program, the voluntary effort would also observe the capital expenditure goal program. Two national objectives have been set: there should be no net increase in the nation's total stock of hospital beds, and new capital investment during the two-year period should be reduced to no more than 80% of the price-adjusted expenditure average of the preceding two years. Another goal is to expand programs to improve significantly the productivity of hospitals, preferrably by two percentage points per year over the two years. Also included are ongoing utilization review and the acceleration of current trends to improve the health delivery system through combining hospital systems and sharing services.

In mid-1978 the administration's hospital cap program was under revision and had not been passed by Congress. By contrast the voluntary effort has been implemented in a majority of states. If the voluntary approach shows progress, Congress may forestall the stiff regulatory cap measure.

National health insurance plans

Cost containment proposals do not stop with the hospital cap bill and the voluntary effort. In 1977 Congress saw more than 12 national health insurance (NHI) bills introduced. Of these, several were modified and reintroduced in 1978 to the Congress. Through various uses of private and public dollars, each is designed to make health care more widely available. Some bills would retain the present system of health delivery to a greater extent than would others. One would replace the present system and provide care through a program totally financed and administered by the federal government.

The principle underlying the plans that would retain some aspects of the present delivery system is that most persons in the U.S. today have health care cost insurance coverage through employers. The need for government financing, therefore, would be limited to those persons not covered through the private insurance system. Those who are unemployed, self-employed, or unable to meet the cost of health care insurance would receive special provisions. Comprehensive coverage would be available to the medical indigent through general revenues.

Of the major proposals, the AMA and the AHA plans would require that employers offer insurance to their employees and their families and that the employer pay a greater share of the premium than the employee. The proposal of the Health Insurance Association of America (HIAA), while advocating employment-based insurance, makes employer participation voluntary under a set of specific guidelines.

The bill proposed by Sen. Edward Kennedy (Dem., Mass.) and Rep. James Corman (Dem., Calif.), which would replace the current system with a federally financed and administered system, is currently under review and may be revised to contain some features that resemble those contained in the AMA, AHA, and HIAA plans. The Kennedy-Corman plan would add billions of federal dollars to the national budget. To avoid

this use of public dollars, which would result in an inflationary effect through the national budget, the administration has proposed that private insurers and therefore private dollars be used to a greater extent than in the original bill but that the administrative task would be carried out by the government.

Under the Kennedy-Corman plan, funds collected through taxation would be divided regionally and allocated to health service areas as defined by the National Health Planning Act of 1974. All participating physicians and providers would be under contract to the federal government. Consumers would be required to enroll for one year at a time in a prepaid group practice, such as a health maintenance organization, or with private practitioners. Services would be provided by a primary-care physician, and the services of a specialist would be accessible by referral only. However, since guidelines contained within the Kennedy-Corman bill are likely to change as it is further debated, the proposed plan may be altered before a final bill is submitted.

Other plans submitted to Congress would provide health benefits to limited segments of the population or would provide benefits only if health care expenses proved catastrophic to a family. For example, the maternal and child health care plan offers comprehensive benefits for children under 18 and maternity benefits for women during pregnancy and for 12 weeks immediately following the pregnancy. The program would be financed through Social Security taxes. A so-called catastrophic bill would provide major medical coverage; payments would begin when the person covered had spent $2,000 or had been in the hospital for 60 days. Employers and employees could choose to join a federal insurance program financed by HEW or could buy private insurance from federally approved carriers under HEW supervision.

A private sector initiative plan

Despite the plethora of NHI bills, there are a growing number of professionals who believe that the cost of health care can be reduced without federally legislated programs. The most comprehensive approach of this type has been released by the National Commission on the Cost of Medical Care—an independent 27-member commission sponsored by the American Medical Association—with representation from business, labor, the health care delivery sector, academia, the consumer area, and government. After nearly two years of study beginning in mid-1976, the commission has released 48 recommendations that outline a process for strengthening consumers' and providers' price consciousness. In addition, the report calls for complementary regulation that would result in the revitalization of a market for health services. The 48 recommendations are divided among seven broad categories, each of which helps to put in place a working system within which to deliver cost-effective, quality health care to the widest possible population.

The categories addressed by the commission report are: strengthening price consciousness; private sector cost containment initiatives; guidelines for regulation; cost containment measures within medical practice; supply and distribution of health care providers; research guidelines; and consumer and patient education. The commission report has received wide distribution. The various groups involved—the insurers, providers, and purchasers of health care—are currently acting on the report, while appropriate agencies of the government are also considering the report's recommendations. As with other proposals for containing health care costs, it will be some time before success in implementation can be measured. In the long run, however, many believe that this type of multifaction, voluntary approach, to slow the rate of health care costs will be more successful than a regulatory one. The reason given is that the delivery of health care has been, for the most part, responding to the needs and wants of society for many years. The guidelines under which health care is delivered should continue to be flexible enough to meet the shifting needs of the society it serves. The commission report concludes that a market system is more likely to fill that objective than a national regulatory scheme, which cannot readily adapt to changing requisites.

Finally, if efforts to contain health care costs in the long run are to be successful, they must adequately take into account society's needs and concerns with respect to the quality of and access to medical care and services. And whether health care policy is ultimately determined by the public or private sector, the problem of skyrocketing costs is likely to remain one of the most important issues facing medicine and society for some time.

—Toba J. Cohen and
Lynn E. Jensen

Health Care Law

Recent changes in the functions, capacities, and responsibilities of health care providers have had far-reaching legal implications. And, in turn, legislation and court decisions concerning hospitals and physicians have further altered the roles and liabilities of both institutions and individuals. A major factor in precipitating these changes has been the increase in governmental regulation of the U.S. health care system. A major result has been a vast proliferation of legal specialists versed in health care concerns.

Over the past five years, for example, the number of lawyers who were members of the American Society of Hospital Attorneys, an affiliate organization of the American Hospital Association, has grown from a few hundred to more than 2,000. Another group of health

care legal specialists, the National Health Lawyers Association, was formed only in 1971 and already numbers more than 1,300 members. Among the burgeoning number of law firms in Washington, D.C., is at least one that was formed about five years ago to deal exclusively with cases in the health care field. That firm, Epstein & Becker, which started with two partners, now includes four partners and three associates; one of the principals says he expects 15 to 20 lawyers to be employed in the firm within five years.

The regulatory tide

The birth and growth of the Washington firm demonstrates a major reason for the rise of health care law as a legal specialty. Among the firm's clients are many Health Maintenance Organizations (HMO's), Professional Standards Review Organizations (PSRO's), the American Association of Professional Standards Review Organizations, and the American Health Planning Association. Although the planning organization has been active for many years, none of the firm's other clients even existed five years ago. In other words, the increase in the number of legal practitioners in the field has paralleled the growth in the number of laws and regulations applying to it.

As with many trends affecting the health care industry, the regulatory tide began with Medicare and Medicaid. Although the federal government had been previously concerned with hospitals and other health care providers, notably in the disbursement of construction grants under the Hill-Burton program, it was the enactment of Titles XVIII and XIX of the Social Security Act that injected large amounts of federal money into the health care system and fostered the detailed directions and stipulations that inevitably accompany such large-scale funding.

The immediate effect of these programs was to put government (the federal government in the case of Medicare, and both state and federal governments in the case of the jointly funded Medicaid program) and hospitals at loggerheads over the determination of equitable payment for patient services. As the money expended on the programs grew beyond original congressional expectations and became a major factor in the federal budget—nearing the $50 billion mark in the latest Carter administration proposal—the original formula for determining proper reimbursements to providers of care was successively revised.

The initial formula, for example, allowed hospitals a 2% "override" to cover unforeseen cost factors. When the total cost of the programs began to rise precipitously, however, the Department of Health, Education, and Welfare (HEW) rescinded the 2%—which had been a sort of "cost plus" addition to the reimbursement formula—on the grounds that it was not legally justifiable. A few years later a similar differential for the nursing care of elderly patients also was withdrawn.

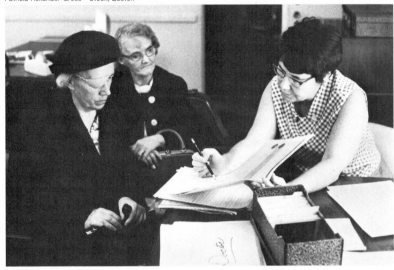

Federal involvement in health care, while upgrading the care available to many segments of the population, has created a huge volume of paperwork hedged around by numerous bewildering regulations.

The effect of these and other administrative actions has been to make the relationship between providers, physicians as well as hospitals, and the governments a contentious one. Appeals against the decisions of the paying agencies, the so-called fiscal intermediaries who carry on the day-to-day business of implementing Medicare and Medicaid, are now commonplace and follow a standard route running through various government agencies and, in some cases, into the courts.

In addition to the hospital's major concern of receiving fair payment for services rendered, there has also been an extensive effort by all hospitals, organized in associations and other groups, to alter and amend health care laws and regulations. Much of this initiative takes the form of lobbying in both federal and state legislatures and executive departments. But some of it takes the form of litigation.

As the costs of federally funded health care programs rose, the Congress attempted to stem the fiscal tide by the only method it knew: more legislation. Among the programs and promotions supported by this new wave of legislation are Professional Standards Review Organizations, an apparatus for checking the "appropriateness" of the care dispensed to Medicare patients by physicians; Health Maintenance Organizations, federally envisioned prepaid group practices whose cost of providing care is thought to be less than that of conventional medical practices; and Health Systems Agencies, creatures of the National Health Planning and Resources Development Act of 1974, whose goal is cost reduction through elimination of duplicate services and facilities and equalization of care throughout the country. Each of these legislative actions, as well as others, has spawned ever more regulation and, correspondingly, more litigation.

The American Medical Association (AMA), on behalf of its physician members, unsuccessfully challenged the constitutionality of the planning act by suing the government. Nonetheless, the AMA and its counterparts serving other professional groups have continued to contest provisions of these new laws, and such legal actions seem unlikely to cease. It is becoming clear that whenever new programs or policies appear to threaten a health care group, the decision on the program's legality and applicability will more likely be rendered by a judge than a bureaucrat.

An example of the seemingly never-ending cycle of legislation, regulation, and lawsuit is the recently promulgated health planning guidelines issued by HEW under the health planning act. The guidelines would establish standards for various types of hospital services such as the number of beds per thousand population in the area served, the number of births per obstetric unit within each hospital, the number of treatments per radiation therapy unit, and so on. Should a hospital fail to meet the set quotas for utilization of facilities, the local planning body (the Health Systems Agency) and its state parent would be expected to restrict or to eliminate from the hospital the service in question. Although the guidelines are couched in terms that suggest local flexibility of application, most observers believe the intention is universal and rigid adherence to the standards. The legal battle lines are just now being drawn over the standards, but if the past is a reliable indicator, it is virtually certain that these standards will ultimately be tested in a courtroom.

Even when hospitals attempt to regulate themselves, they fall prey to modern legal hazards. The Joint Commission on Accreditation of Hospitals (JCAH) is an organization, governed mutually by the major hospital and medical associations, whose purpose is the continual inspection of hospital facilities to assure their ability to provide high-quality care. Until a few years ago JCAH surveyors, following published standards, concentrated on such care-related factors as staffing, patient care procedures, equipment, and safety-related items such as electrical connectors and medical gas supply lines. In the past two years, however, the commission has been urged by federal authorities to emphasize building and fire code regulations, areas generally within the domain of other inspection agencies. These regulations are now pegged in some cases to JCAH accreditation, opening another avenue for appeals and other legal procedures.

The legal perils of technology

Advances in technology have also been the source of new or newly uncovered legal problems. While policies and programs of the past decade have radically altered the hospital outlook, machinery and personnel undreamed of only a few years ago have caused equally important changes. The intensive care unit, to cite one of the more familiar routine services of many hospitals, was born of recent developments in electronics that revolutionized monitoring techniques. Respiratory therapy did not emerge as a distinct department until only a few years ago.

Each new apparatus—and the personnel who operate it—exposes the hospital to a new series of legal perils. Foremost, of course, is the increased exposure to liability that accrues from more radical treatment. The possibilities of error in operation and patient misunderstanding raise the potential for allegations of negligence, lack of consent, and other grounds for litigation associated with significant medical measures. To some extent, the huge increases in malpractice insurance premiums over the last few years reflect this escalation in legal risk.

Accidents and miscalculations are not the only legal hazard posed by complex equipment. The decision to employ—or to withdraw—life-sustaining treatment has also emerged as a pivotal legal issue. The case of Karen Quinlan focused attention on the hospital's ability to provide continuing life support for the young New Jersey woman who was in irreversible coma. The legal situation concerning such patients has not been clarified by the various state court rulings. In New Jersey, for example, the courts eventually left the decision to discontinue life support to a medical committee, while a Massachusetts court demanded that only a judge should issue such an order in the case of a patient who is unable to make an informed decision. This latter ruling reportedly angered many physicians who feel that a court is ill-equipped to render such decisions. Nevertheless, in Massachusetts, at least, hospital attorneys may now spend a good deal of time petitioning courts for direction on patient treatment.

Medicine and labor law

The growing number of hospital technicians who operate complex equipment, and of other hospital employees, as well, poses another source of legal entan-

glement. Although some urban hospitals have a long history of labor relations, union organizing in hospitals is a fairly recent development. The floodgates for organization were lifted in 1974 when the hospital exemption from the National Labor Relations Act was rescinded, thus placing not-for-profit health care institutions under the jurisdiction of the National Labor Relations Board (NLRB). Since then, rulings regarding bargaining units, legality of organizing efforts, and limitations on picketing and information dissemination have flowed freely. Several unions consider hospitals, with their large numbers of nonsupervisory workers, to be fertile ground for union growth, and it can be expected that hospital cases will continue to represent a sizable portion of NLRB activity.

Legal status of the hospital

At the root of many changes that have forced hospitals and hospital care into a legal framework is the altered position of the hospital in the legal arena. Little more than a decade ago hospitals were viewed as charitable trustees of the public good. A series of major legal decisions has, however, reversed the untouchable status of the hospital and assigned to it direct legal responsibility. As the Nevada Supreme Court stated in one ruling, "Hospitals and their governing bodies may be held liable for injuries resulting from imprudent or careless supervision of members of their medical staffs." The notion of the hospital's responsibility for the doctors who practiced there was a new and far-reaching concept. It not only exposed the institution to the consequences of physician negligence; it also established an antagonistic position between hospital management and members of the medical staff. And, not surprisingly, this situation has produced a profusion of lawsuits. Furthermore, the trend in court decisions to assign responsibility directly to the hospital has, in turn, affected the process of litigation. It is likely that a patient who feels aggrieved or mistreated will name the hospital as well as his physician in any suit he will press. And where the action is filed against a hospital employee, such as a nurse or technician, it is a reflex action to include the institution as a defendant.

What of the future? Almost certainly the hospital will be enmeshed even deeper in legal processes. Current discussions of cost containment, whether by a national standard or state regulatory agencies, the imposition of a national health insurance program, more detailed planning activities, and so on, inevitably will make more work for health care lawyers. Other issues—the rights of mental patients, the availability of controversial drugs such as laetrile, the denial of abortion to Medicaid patients, to name but a few—promise certain expansion of the growing body of law that deals with health care.

—John F. Horty, LL.B., and
Ted Isaacman

Special Report:

The "Mainstreaming" Quandary

by McCay Vernon, Ph.D.

The most controversial legislation in the history of special education, Public Law (PL) 94-142—the Education for All Handicapped Children Act of 1975—is now being implemented. It will be the major educational factor in the lives of at least a generation of handicapped children. The intent of the law is above reproach as indicated by its statement of purposes:

> It is the purpose of this Act to assure that all handicapped children have available to them . . . a free appropriate public education which emphasizes special education and related services designed to meet their unique needs, to assure that the rights of handicapped children and their parents or guardians are protected, to assist States and localities to provide for the education of all handicapped children, and to assure and assess the effectiveness of efforts to educate handicapped children.

To bring about these idealistic goals, the law provides for some federal funding through the state to the local district for every handicapped child. The amount of that funding is based on a percentage of the average amount spent per pupil in public elementary and secondary schools in the U.S. and on the ratio of local handicapped children to the total number of handicapped children in that state. Under the law each state is required to provide full educational services for *all* its handicapped children regardless of their degree of disability. Individual educational plans must be worked out for each child in conjunction with the parents. All of this, including the education, is free to the child, and parents can appeal if they feel the provisions for their child are inadequate. The law also provides for the removal of architectural barriers and mandates the hiring of qualified handicapped persons in programs assisted by the act.

Problems posed by the law

When seen in terms of its sweeping purposes and broad features, PL 94-142 seems to create a utopian situation for the handicapped child and his or her family. However, the specifics of the law, especially the "mainstreaming" and funding features, make the seeming utopia more closely resemble Dante's Inferno.

Peggy Denton has 30 fourth graders. For years she had taught her classes with more than average success. However, since the passage of PL 94-142 Mrs. Denton's class has had four handicapped children placed in it. One child, Jeffrey, is severely mentally retarded, nonambulatory, and must be carried to and assisted in the bathroom. Thus, several times a day Peggy Denton leaves her 29 other students by themselves while she carries Jeffrey to the toilet and serves as a nurse.

Mrs. Denton is expected to provide an individual educational plan (IEP) for Jeffrey and each of her 29 other children, even though Jeffrey requires one-to-one personalized instruction. Among the three other handicapped children, for each of whom is required an IEP as well as personalized instruction, one is profoundly deaf, one cerebral palsied, and one mildly retarded. Mrs. Denton has a teacher's aide for one 45-minute period per day.

The reason these four handicapped children are in Mrs. Denton's class is the controversial mainstreaming provision of the law, which says that, to the maximum extent appropriate, handicapped children are to be educated with children who are not handicapped, and that special classes and separate schooling should occur only when the nature or severity of the handicap is such that education in regular classes with the use of supplementary aids and services cannot be achieved satisfactorily.

In practice the danger is that when handicapped children are educated in regular classes, schools will be forced, by virtue of unavailable staff and funds, to ignore the real nature and severity of a child's handicap. Furthermore, the financial provisions of the law allocate only a small proportion of the actual costs of adequately educating many types of handicapped children. Prior to the passage of the law, at least one million severely handicapped children were totally excluded from public schools. Most of these children had handicaps as profound as or more extreme than Jeffrey's. While the law's intent to serve these children is commendable, are regular public school classrooms such as Mrs. Denton's the place to do so?

Another problem posed by PL 94-142 results from the provision for removing architectural barriers to the handicapped. In essence, this section of the law mandates that every academic program be accessible to all students in public colleges and schools. For example, if the University of California at Berkeley has a nuclear physics class involving first-hand instruction on the construction of nuclear reactors, the nuclear reactor

235

Photograph, Nanda Ward Haynes of The Council For Exceptional Children, Reston, Virginia

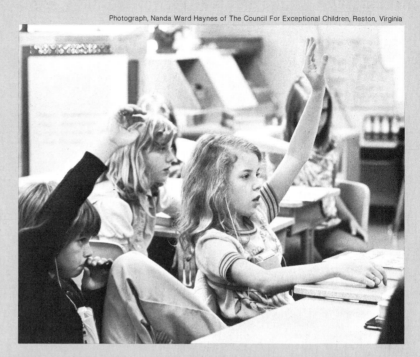

The child who is deaf or hearing-impaired faces special problems in school that are not shared by other handicapped children, who may be better able to communicate with the teacher and the other students. Some ordinary schools, with well-disposed teachers and special supplementary classes, may give the deaf child the type of total education he needs, but most cannot.

site must be made fully accessible to any quadriplegic student wishing to take the course. The cost for an adaptation of this sort for a single student could run into several million dollars. Furthermore, if another wheelchair-dependent student preferred to take the same course at San Francisco State College just a few miles away, the very same adaptations would have to be made there as well. In other words, it is not enough that a state provide the handicapped student a course in nuclear physics in a barrier-free college. Instead, such facilities must be provided in all colleges that such students wish to attend. The colleges must either make their course entirely accessible to the handicapped student or drop the course from their curriculum.

Such accommodations obviously entail billions of dollars in construction costs. Among the architectural requisites will be special ramps, elevators, the total redesign of scientific laboratories to make them usable from wheelchairs, special bathrooms, and so forth. And there will be mass duplication of expensive architectural adaptations in colleges within a few miles of each other to permit the handicapped student the same "access to program" as the nonhandicapped student. The cost for educating a single handicapped student in the small college, which may not have more than one such student in a decade, could be excessive.

"Mainstreaming" deaf children

A major feature of the new law is mainstreaming, an educational approach that should be carefully examined. As an example, consider the situation of the child handicapped by deafness.

Mainstreaming is not a new idea. In fact, deaf children have been mainstreamed for three decades. In the past this system was called "integration," but recently, to make the concept more palatable, it has been renamed "mainstreaming."

Historically, mainstreaming or integration has involved one of several basic approaches, the most common being to simply place deaf children in classes with hearing children. The deaf children are given hearing aids and told to sit in the front of the room. Usually they have a resource teacher who will see each child regularly, whether once a month or once or twice a day. That teacher may have from 5 to 40 deaf students in this arrangement.

What does this mean for a deaf child? He or she sits in classrooms with hearing children, unable to hear or understand what the teacher says. Even if the child is a good lipreader, only 5 to 20% of what the teacher says can be grasped, and that only if the teacher's lips can be seen. How then can a deaf student learn history, mathematics, or English if this small percentage of classroom lectures is all that can be grasped? When student discussion takes place, the situation becomes virtually impossible. By the time the deaf youngster locates the student who is speaking, someone else has started to talk, and the deaf child completely loses the train of discussion.

To compound the problem, the average deaf child is at least three to five years behind his hearing classmates in academic achievement, especially in reading and language arts. Thus, in addition to not understanding the teacher during class, the deaf student is often unable to read the textbooks.

Despite the gross inappropriateness of mainstreaming deaf children, it is undoubtedly the most prevalent approach in the United States today for educating deaf

Dennis Breo—*American Medical News*; published by the American Medical Association

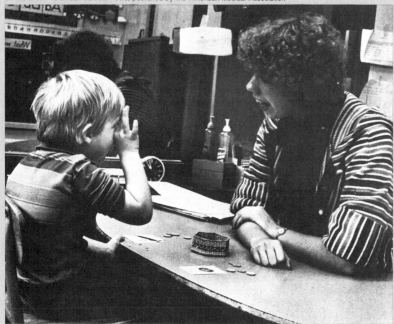

A deaf child needs individualized instruction to make maximum use of any existing hearing. Sign language and lipreading must also be taught and used continually to help the child develop his use of language to convey his thoughts and understand the thoughts of those around him. At the John Tracy Clinic in Los Angeles preschool deaf children get specialized training at a young age to develop manual and oral language skills.

children, especially teenagers. In every state in the nation there are large numbers of deaf students reading at the second or third grade level who spend all day in junior high and high school classes with hearing children and fail to progress. Often the only break for the deaf child in this frustrating, noneducational routine is an occasional speech therapy session. Many of these students quit such mainstreaming programs every year but are then left to face the world as functional illiterates.

Another form of mainstreaming practiced for many years separates deaf children attending regular public schools into special classes except for certain periods during the day when they are integrated or mainstreamed. Some students mainstream just for lunch, recess, and physical education, while others may be integrated for art, industrial arts, or an occasional academic subject. The rest of the day is spent in self-contained classes for the hearing impaired or in self-contained heterogeneous classes of children who may be mentally retarded, have certain learning disabilities, or have numerous other handicaps unrelated to deafness.

While this system of self-contained classes and part-time mainstreaming is preferable to literally dumping the deaf child into regular classes without adequate supportive services, it is still not mainstreaming in its original sense since the deaf children do not actually mix in a meaningful social or educational way with hearing children. For example, on a visit to programs of this type one usually finds all the deaf students eating together at lunch and playing together at recess. Generally they are engaged in noticeably different and more childish games than hearing children of the same

age. Little positive interaction occurs between the deaf and the hearing youngsters. The children are really integrated or mainstreamed only in terms of physical proximity.

The final system of traditional mainstreaming is one in which the deaf child initially spends the elementary school years in self-contained classes with other deaf children. Subsequently, when the child is of junior high or high school age—and usually academically behind by three to six years—he or she is mainstreamed under the first plan mentioned, which is to say, placed into classes with hearing students with periodic visits by a resource teacher. Placing a deaf youth in such a situation is obviously a terrible educational error; yet approximately 30% of deaf children currently spend part of their school years in programs of this type.

The systems of integration or mainstreaming described above have existed in the U.S. for 30 years or more and have roundly failed to educate the overwhelming majority of deaf children. Nowadays, however, because these programs are termed mainstreaming instead of integration, because the federal government legislates them, and because state legislators mandate local education, the practice of mainstreaming is sweeping the country.

The issue is not whether the principle of mainstreaming is good or bad. Rather, the issue is that the mainstreaming systems that have evolved in the overwhelming majority of schools are grossly inappropriate to the needs of hearing impaired students.

Alternative to mainstreaming

In contrast to traditional mainstreaming, a model program called the Holcomb Plan has been gradually developed in recent years. This plan grew out of Roy Holcomb's experience in education for the deaf in California, where he was director of a mainstreaming program that had at first been very traditional. This new plan makes use of total communication with each deaf student whenever possible. Total communication involves the simultaneous use of finger spelling, speech, amplification (the use of hearing aids), lipreading, some form of sign language, reading, and writing.

Extensive research has shown total communication, which combines oral and manual skills, to be a far more effective method of teaching deaf children than is the traditional, uniquely oral approach. Through total communication deaf children have the opportunity to fully understand what their teachers and fellow students are saying. They need no longer be thoroughly frustrated by the sheer difficulty and inevitable confusion of lipreading.

Under the Holcomb Plan the deaf child is put in a class with hearing children only when there is a tutor-interpreter available to translate into sign language what the regular classroom teacher is saying. The tutor-interpreter also helps in the classroom by tutoring the hearing students as well as the deaf children. Thus, instead of being deposited into a class of 30 hearing children with no means of understanding the teacher, the deaf child is given the necessary support of interpretation and tutoring needed to enable him or her to grasp what is going on in class.

This one innovation, the tutor-interpreter, is the core of the Holcomb Plan of mainstreaming. This model program provides the fundamental basis for a meaningful effort to mainstream deaf children and has already proved successful at the college level.

Another feature of the plan is that all hearing students are given the chance to learn finger spelling and sign language. Many are fascinated by manual communication and become very skilled in it, while other students do not bother to learn. In any case, enough hearing children do learn total communication to bring about meaningful social and educational integration on the playground, in class, and outside of school. Far more interpersonal interaction routinely occurs among deaf and hearing children under the Holcomb Plan than is ever seen with traditional mainstreaming.

This is not to say the Holcomb Plan results in full integration. There is not and will never be full social or educational mixing of deaf and hearing children or adults. However, the deaf child and the hearing child who want to integrate can do so. With traditional mainstreaming they are rarely able to integrate despite their wishes. What the Holcomb Plan has demonstrated in Delaware and California is that for the integration of deaf and hearing people to occur, the hearing person must also make an effort. While the deaf child tries to learn to speak and lipread to communicate with the hearing child, the hearing child must also go halfway by trying to learn to sign and finger spell. Under the Holcomb Plan total communication is also taught to parents of deaf children, regular teachers of hearing children, and other interested members of the community. Another important aspect of the Holcomb Plan is an effort to educate teachers of the regular schoolchildren, teachers of hearing-impaired students, interpreter-tutors, hearing and deaf students, and members of the community about the meaning of deafness and the nature and effects of mainstreaming.

The law's myopic approach

Although PL 94-142 has been interpreted by most educators, parents, courts, and legislators to mean that all or nearly all handicapped children should be mainstreamed, that is not what the law actually says. To quote the legislation:

Special classes, separate schooling, or other removal of handicapped children from the regular educational environment occurs only when the nature or severity of the handicap is such that education in regular classes with the use of supplementary aids and services cannot be achieved satisfactorily.

The benevolent intent of the law is to free the handicapped child from the severely restrictive environment that has tried to accommodate his or her special needs in the past and has as a consequence traditionally kept the child out of the mainstream. However, a close look at the educational and developmental problems of the child who is born deaf or becomes deaf in the first few years of life provides insight into how the new law unwittingly contributes to creating a different but equally restrictive environment for the deaf child.

The deaf child's plight with speech may be compared to that of a student learning a foreign language in school. It is difficult to learn to speak the language even though the student can hear and monitor his or her own voice and efforts to speak. Even the student who has done well by classroom standards soon finds out how unintelligible he actually is if he has to depend on his language skills in foreign travel. If this student was unable to hear his own voice or if he got only partial feedback while learning the foreign language, his situation would reflect the problems and limits that the deaf child encounters with speech.

Because of the difficulties involved in learning to speak when deaf, few persons who were prelingually deafened—95% of the school-age deaf population—develop speech that can be understood in most social situations. Traditional mainstreaming tends to ignore this rather unpleasant fact and deals with deaf children as though the fact did not exist.

The problems that lipreading presents for the deaf were explored in studies by the John Tracy Clinic at the University of Southern California in Los Angeles. It was found that hearing college sophomores who had never studied lipreading were better at it than deaf children and adults to whom it had been taught for most of their school lives. The reason for this unfortunate irony was that the sophomores had a solid language base, that is to say, a thorough familiarity with a syntax and vocabulary, which enabled them to readily guess the words that they could not lipread. Since at least half of the sounds in the English language are homophonous, or look similar in their lip formation to other sounds, a person lacking the language base needed to fill in the gaps understands very little. In fact, even the best lip-readers in a one-to-one situation are able to understand only 26% of what is said, and many bright, otherwise capable deaf children grasp less than 5% when lipreading. Thus it is senseless to mainstream the deaf child without a sign language interpreter.

Knowledge of sign language and finger spelling eliminate for the deaf the inherent problems of ambiguity in lipreading as well as the difficulties of self-expression that characterize their efforts to talk. These manual language skills enable them to communicate fluently with deaf and hearing persons who are also familiar with manual communication. Thus for the average deaf student, and especially for those few who can keep on an academic par with their hearing peers, mainstreaming must involve a signing interpreter.

Statistics on the educational achievement of deaf children indicate that, despite the fact that their IQ's follow the normal distribution, these children face an awesome educational handicap. The average gain in reading skills from ages 10 to 16 for deaf children is only eight months, compared with six years for children with average hearing. When leaving school at age 16 or older, deaf children have a rate of functional illiteracy estimated at 30%, and only 5% are able to read at ninth grade level. Thus reading remains a severely limited resource for most deaf students.

In view of the educational and communicative limitations imposed by deafness, the regular classroom with normally hearing children provides an extremely restrictive environment for the overwhelming majority of deaf students. It is the unfortunate irony of the new law that, although designed to provide less restrictive education, it actually increases the restrictive nature of education for the deaf. By contrast, it is the residential school, large day school, or well-graded, self-contained classes, and not the mainstream setting, that offer the least restrictive program for all but a tiny number of deaf children.

Unanswered questions

How the problems of mainstreaming are resolved will affect the lives of thousands of deaf young people and their families for years to come. Numerous questions on the fundamental issues of mainstreaming remain to be answered.

Is the mainstreaming program actually intended only for the child who is hard of hearing rather than for the deaf youngster, or is the degree of hearing loss in fact not a major issue? Must the hearing-impaired child be at the grade level of the hearing students in his or her class? At what grade level is mainstreaming most effectively executed? In what subject areas is mainstreaming most appropriate? Obviously many variables are involved in finding answers to these questions, and the ultimate decisions regarding mainstreaming should ideally be determined individually for each child. Nonetheless, meaningful guidelines for making appropriate decisions must be developed.

Another as yet unknown, though significant, factor in mainstream planning is that of cost. To properly mainstream a deaf child, many supportive services unavailable in regular public schools are needed and will undoubtedly prove very costly. However, until these costs can be estimated, meaningful planning and budgeting for education are virtually impossible.

The reason these costs are difficult to estimate is that no one has yet determined the exact nature and extent of supportive services needed. In the case of the unique kinds of specialists needed for this program, for example, the interpreter-tutors, no precedent exists for setting their salary levels and specifying the necessary formal qualifications. But until these are determined, it is impossible to know how much the special services will cost the school for each handicapped child and how many handicapped children will have to be served by each specialist for the plan to be economically feasible.

In summary, PL 94-142 has monumental implications for handicapped children. Although well intended, it fails to deal realistically with the scope and nature of the problems it addresses. For example, the law makes rigorous stipulations that all handicapped children be educated yet provides only a token portion of the funds required to do this. Its emphasis on mainstreaming, while an appropriate program for many mildly handicapped children, will do great harm to vast numbers of profoundly disabled youngsters. Many parents of children in this latter group find the law's insistence on mainstreaming appealing because it accommodates, albeit falsely, their desire to make their children "normal." In fact, mainstreaming further amplifies their children's abnormalities. In addition, the inordinate financial requirements of the law's architectural barriers provisions alone are already creating a massive backlash among educators and legislators, which may do more harm than good for the handicapped.

As court decisions are rendered giving fuller interpretation to the law, we will better understand its manifold ramifications. Additional clarification will be provided as state and local plans for implementation are submitted to the federal government for approval. Meanwhile, there is likely to be a period of lengthy and confusing transition before the impact of PL 94-142 is fully and finally known.

Heart and Blood Vessels

Problems posed by diseases of the cardiovascular system constitute a major threat to health in the United States. As pointed out in the 1977 annual report of the director of the National Heart, Lung, and Blood Institute, diseases of the cardiovascular system have been the major cause of death in the U.S. since the 1920s. In recent years more than 50% of the deaths in the United States have been attributed to diseases of the heart and blood vessels, including heart attacks and strokes. More than two-thirds of the deaths of people over the age of 65 result from cardiovascular causes; about 160,000 people below the age of 65 die annually from these causes. The major cardiovascular diseases include hypertension, which afflicts 27 million people; coronary artery disease, which strikes 4 million; and rheumatic heart disease, which affects 1.8 million. Congenital heart disease occurs in 8 in 1,000 births, with half of those affected dying before their first birthday. The economic impact resulting from the deaths and the incapacity produced by heart disease has been estimated to exceed $40 billion annually.

Declining cardiovascular death rates

Despite these grim statistics, figures from the last decade suggest that a marked improvement has occurred in the medical outlook relating to heart and blood vessel disease. From 1950 to 1975 a decline of 29.7% took place in the death rate attributable to cardiovascular disease, compared with a fall of 17.5% for deaths from noncardiovascular causes during the same time period. Even more striking are the figures for the years 1970–75. During this period deaths from all forms of cardiovascular disease fell 13.6%, approximately twice the decline observed in the death rate from noncardiac causes. The major single cause of death, coronary artery disease and consequent myocardial infarction (heart attack), fell during this same period by 13.2%. This improvement was seen to a similar extent in both men and women and in both blacks and whites. In 1974, for the first time since 1967, fewer than one million people died of major cardiovascular disease, despite the growth of the total population. Strokes, which result from abnormalities in the circulation to the brain, decreased as a cause of death by 17.5% during this time.

The reasons for the decline in the death rate attributable to cardiovascular disease have not been definitely established. It seems likely, however, that the decline stems from a number of causes, including improved control of hypertension, reduction in cigarette smoking, better dietary habits emphasizing reduced cholesterol and fat intake, the introduction of cardiac care units in hospitals, reducing the in-hospital mortality rate from heart attacks by more than 50%, and other as yet undefined causes.

Coronary bypass surgery

Atherosclerosis involving the coronary arteries is the major cause of death in the United States, with approximately 640,000 people dying annually from heart attacks. Atherosclerosis is the deposition of fatty material in the wall of an artery, which leads to narrowing of the channel (lumen) through which blood flows. The coronary arteries are the arteries that supply blood to the heart muscle itself. Therefore, if these arteries become unduly narrowed, the needs of the heart for blood may not be met, and a heart attack, a lethal abnormality in the heart beat, or chest pain (angina pectoris) may result.

Because the abnormalities in the coronary arteries are frequently localized at sites along the initial length of the artery, surgeons have developed a technique to bypass the obstruction. This technique, termed the coronary bypass operation, involves removing a large vein (saphenous vein) from the thigh and using it as a conduit connecting the aorta to the coronary artery beyond the area of atherosclerotic narrowing. Before such an operation can be carried out, the patient

Cardiac catheterization, a technique in which a fine tube is introduced into the heart through a major blood vessel, enables the condition of the heart to be assessed before surgery takes place.

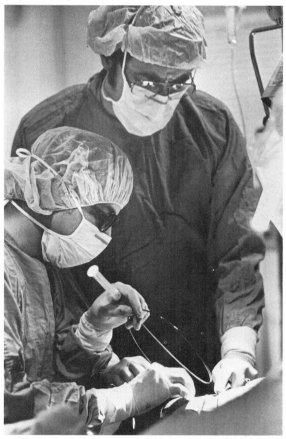

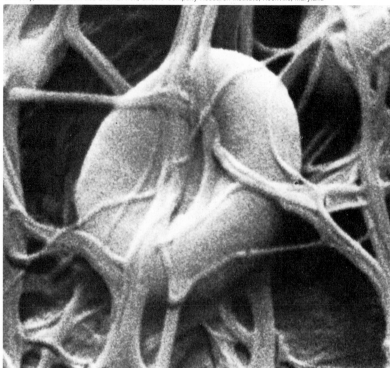

A red blood cell is enmeshed in strands of fibrin in a blood clot found in an intravenous catheter that had been implanted near the heart; the role of blood platelets in cardiac blood clots is currently under intense investigation.

first must have a cardiac catheterization so that the extent and location of the disease process in the coronary arteries can be determined. In cardiac catheterization a fine tube is introduced into the heart by moving the tube along a major vein or artery to be used as an aid in determining heart function.

For those patients suitable for surgery, a plan is then formulated to bypass as many of the involved blood vessels as possible. Experience with this operation over the last decade has shown that this operation can generally be done with a mortality rate between 1 and 3%. Function of 85–90% of the bypass grafts remains good for long periods of time; if a graft is open a few months after the operation, it usually stays functional thereafter. It is important to remember that the operation does not affect the underlying process of atherosclerosis itself. The patient who has had a coronary bypass should observe the same avoidance of risk factors (*e.g.,* smoking, high blood pressure, and high cholesterol intake) as the patient who has not had an operation. Such a program would probably minimize progression of atherosclerosis in the coronary arteries and in the graft.

At present, a major uncertainty exists as to which groups of patients benefit from the coronary bypass operation. Thus far, two groups have been identified for whom the operation appears beneficial. The first group includes patients with severe angina pectoris who do not respond adequately to medical treatment. The coronary bypass operation produces marked or complete improvement in symptoms in 85–90% of these

cases, but it has not been proven that the surgery will prolong life in these patients. The second group of patients includes those who experience symptoms and have a major obstruction in the left main coronary artery. This coronary artery branches into the left anterior descending coronary artery and the left circumflex coronary artery. Together with the right coronary artery, these blood vessels provide the heart's blood supply. Because the main volume of coronary blood flow passes through the left main coronary artery, the function and viability of the heart will be jeopardized if the lumen is reduced by more than 75% of its cross-sectional area. It appears that coronary bypass operations in this second group of patients will prolong life.

Whether the bypass operation will increase the lifespan, prevent sudden death, or forestall myocardial infarction in other groups of patients with coronary artery disease is a subject of great controversy at this time. Comparable groups of patients who have been treated by modern medical management and by bypass surgery have not been studied thoroughly to determine which treatment mode has been most successful. Enthusiasts for the operation point to the fact that patients with multiple-vessel coronary disease who have successful coronary bypass operations show a survival curve similar to the life expectancy curves derived by life insurance companies for the population at large. This comparison fails to take account of the fact that the life insurance statistics include patients who die from many other causes, including cancer, lung disease, kidney disease, etc. Patients

241

with these complicating diseases are not operated upon for coronary artery disease, and therefore, the group operated on does not display important risk elements that are present in the figures from the insurance companies. The importance of resolving this question becomes evident when it is realized that 80,-000 to 100,000 operations will be performed this year at a total cost approximating $1 billion. Indeed, the coronary bypass operation may become the most commonly performed elective operation in the United States. (See also Medical Ethics.)

Drugs reducing cardiac death rates

A major advance in the medical management of patients with a recent myocardial infarction was reported in 1978. It has been suspected that platelets, which along with red blood cells and white blood cells constitute the formed elements in blood, may have an important role in the formation of blood clots in the coronary arteries—platelets are known to be involved in the process of atherosclerosis. A number of drugs are known to alter platelet function, and three—aspirin, dipyridamole, and sulfinpyrazone—are currently undergoing widespread clinical trials. In the past, sulfinpyrazone (Anturane) has been used for the treatment of gout. In a well-controlled study involving 26 centers in the United States and Canada, it was shown that sulfinpyrazone, when administration was begun shortly after the patient's myocardial infarction, reduced the annual cardiac death rate from 9.5% in the control group to 4.9% in the treated group, which represents an observed reduction of 48.5%. The clinical trials of aspirin and dipyridamole have not been completed. If further studies prove that antiplatelet drugs are indeed effective, then a major breakthrough will have been achieved in the battle against coronary artery disease.

Impact of modern technology

Modern technology has altered drastically the manner in which cardiology is practiced. With the advent of this technology new diseases have been discovered, and a better appreciation of well-recognized problems has been obtained.

Echocardiography. This technique uses reflected ultrasound to view the motion of the heart wall as it contracts and relaxes and the movement of the heart valves as they open and close. A small probe is placed against the front of the chest. A sound beam generated by the probe is directed toward the back. As the beam of sound hits against substances that have different acoustic properties (*e.g.,* blood in the chambers of the heart versus heart valves or heart wall), echos are produced that are reflected back to the probe, where they are detected and analyzed. Echocardiography equipment allows instantaneous visualization of cardiac motion. The original echocardiogram machines generated a narrow beam of sound that produced a

view of a narrow cylindrical portion of the heart. More modern echocardiogram machines rotate this beam of sound at the rate of 30 to 60 times a second across an arc of about 60°, thereby visualizing a much larger plane of the heart. This is called a two-dimensional or cross-sectional echocardiogram. Because this test is done without the placement of catheters within the heart, it is a noninvasive test. Consequently, it can be used with greater safety to screen large numbers of people with suspected heart disease. Echocardiography has helped to define several cardiac problems, including idiopathic hypertrophic subaortic stenosis and the prolapsed mitral valve syndrome.

Idiopathic hypertrophic subaortic stenosis (IHSS), which is also known by such names as hypertrophic cardiomyopathy or asymmetric septal hypertrophy, began to be understood and diagnosed about 20 years ago. Because a cardiac catheterization was generally necessary to make the diagnosis a certainty, IHSS was considered to be a relatively uncommon disease. Echocardiography, however, has shown that the incidence of IHSS is much greater than had been thought previously. Indeed, approximately 50% of first degree relatives (*i.e.,* brothers, sisters, children) of patients with the disease have some evidence of a similar type of cardiac involvement. The disease itself is characterized by marked thickening or hypertrophy of the wall (septum) between the right and left ventricle. Obstruction to the outflow of blood from the left ventricle occurs when, during contraction (systole) of the heart, one of the leaflets of the mitral valve abuts against the enlarged septum, thereby blocking off the outflow of blood from the heart. In contrast to the obstruction to blood flow seen in patients with a fixed narrowing of the aortic valve (aortic stenosis), in IHSS the obstruction to outflow is varying and may change between examinations and even from beat to beat. The echocardiogram in IHSS patients shows the abnormal thickening of the septum and also shows the movement of the mitral valve as it hits up against the septum during systole. Although some patients with IHSS eventually must have surgery to relieve the obstruction to the outflow of blood from the heart, most patients with the symptoms of chest pain, shortness of breath, and fainting do well with medical management. In a small percentage of patients sudden death occurs despite currently available surgical or medical treatment.

The prolapsed mitral valve syndrome, or the systolic click-murmur syndrome, is another cardiac problem that has been delineated by the echocardiogram. For years cardiologists have heard certain cardiac murmurs and extra sounds (clicks) when they have listened to the hearts of apparently normal patients. These murmurs and clicks were a puzzle because they could not be related to known forms of heart diseases. Although the first clues to their origin came from studies during cardiac catheterization, the full magnitude of this potential problem was not realized until echocardiography became widely employed. It is now recognized that the extra sounds result from the mitral valve, which separates the left atrium from the left ventricle. During contraction of the heart, normally the two leaflets of the mitral valve come together to prevent the backflow of blood from the ventricle to the atrium. In this syndrome, however, the mitral valve prolapses or billows back into the left atrium, which causes the click sound, and if the valve no longer prevents the backflow of blood into the atrium, the murmur of mitral regurgitation is heard. In some serious symptoms occur. These include arrhythmias (abnormalities of the heartbeat), chest pain, the possibility of infection of the mitral valve, and even sudden death. Currently a number of different types of medication are used for the treatment of symptomatic persons, but none is entirely satisfactory.

Nuclear cardiology. Nuclear cardiology represents another incursion of technology into the field of cardiology. Depending on the radioisotope used, it provides a variety of noninvasive studies. Until 1975 these studies could not be done at the patient's bedside because the necessary equipment was bulky and immobile. Now mobile gamma cameras and miniaturized computers are available, allowing equipment to be brought to the bedside of critically ill patients. In patients with recent myocardial infarctions, radioisotopes (*e.g.,* technetium-99m) can be injected that localize preferentially in the area of damaged muscle, thereby producing hotspot images. Thus it is possible to confirm the diagnosis of myocardial infarction in doubtful cases and, in addition, to provide a measure of the size of the area of heart muscle involved. From such information it may become possible to determine the effectiveness of various medications.

Other radioisotopes (*e.g.,* thallium-201) are distributed to the heart muscle in proportion to the blood flow to various parts of the heart. If an area of the heart receives less blood than it needs to satisfy its requirements for oxygen (as occurs during attacks of angina pectoris), this underperfused area will show up as a cold-spot image. The sensitivity of this test is enhanced by the comparison of images obtained at rest with the images obtained during exercise. A cold spot present during both rest and exercise signifies a scar, probably the remnant of an old myocardial infarction. The development of a cold area only during exercise suggests sudden, relative underperfusion of a temporary type, which is characteristic of angina pectoris.

The marriage of computer technology with imaging of radioisotopes that remain in the bloodstream allows visualization of the cavity of the left ventricle. Computer processing of thousands of separate images results in a motion picture that displays the movements of the heart wall. Consequently, physicians can now evaluate regional abnormalities of heart wall motion, both at rest and during exercise. Because the coronary arteries are involved to varying degrees by the process of atherosclerosis, the ability of different parts of the left ventricle to contract forcefully will be affected in a nonuniform manner. This nonuniformity of contraction in patients with significant involvement of the coronary arteries is especially evident during the stress of muscular exercise. In addition, the percentage of blood ejected from the left ventricle with each cardiac contraction (*i.e.,* the ejection fraction) can now be determined, and is an important measure of the heart's reserve capacity.

Cardiac pacemakers. During the last decade electrical pacemakers have been developed that allow artificial pacing of the heart when the natural sequence of pacing is either temporarily or permanently impaired. An electrical pulse generator and battery pack, about half the size of a pack of cigarettes, is implanted under the skin of the chest wall or abdomen.

Originally the pacemakers were set at a fixed rate, without any attention to the heart's natural rhythm. As technology advanced it became possible for the pacemaker to sense the heart's rhythm, and when the rate of the natural rhythm is faster than the rate of the pacemaker, the artificial pacemaker is inhibited. When the rate of the natural heart rhythm becomes slower than the rate of the pacemaker, the artificial pacemaker takes over and paces the heart at a normal rate. More complex pacemakers are also available. These include programmable pacemakers, which allow external control of the demand pacing rate so that the heart rate can be varied with an external programmer according to the patient's needs. Pacemakers that produce sequential atrioventricular stimulation have been developed that permit the atria and ventricles to be stimulated in a normal sequence (the common pacemakers stimulate only the ventricles).

Until recently the power requirements have been furnished by mercury-zinc cells. These batteries had an expected life of two to three years, at which time the implanted generator-battery pack had to be replaced. Recent improvements in design have increased the life of these batteries to more than five years. Lithium iodide batteries are now used widely, with an expected life of six to eight years. Thus the need for repeated operations for battery failure is markedly reduced. An atomic power source has also been developed that allows about ten years of use.

The development of pacemaker follow-up units has made it possible to care for patients with artificial pacemakers in a safe and convenient manner. Patients can have the function of their pacemakers checked by transmitting their electrocardiograms over regular telephone lines. Such transtelephonic monitoring can detect when a battery pack begins to fail and allows ample time to schedule an operation for replacement of the generator.

—Gerald Glick, M.D.

Special Report:
Saving Heart Attack Victims

by Marc I. Davis

New and powerful weapons in the war against heart attacks are reducing the death toll from the number one killer in the United States. Modern technology and medical science have teamed up to save countless lives through the professional expertise, speed, and mobility that typify the new paramedics and the emergency medical services they provide. Of the 650,000 annual heart attack fatalities in the United States, about half die within the first hour after being stricken. With prompt paramedical treatment on the site and en route to the hospital, survival rates for heart attack victims have been increasing steadily. Throughout the U.S., cities with emergency medical services have been reporting impressive results.

In Chicago, for example, considered to have one of the best emergency medical systems in the country, the survival rate for heart attack victims treated by paramedics is now higher than 50%. Before the system was begun in the mid-1970s the rate was much lower—some 35% of heart attack victims admitted to hospitals in the 1960s died while hospitalized. Since then survival rates in Chicago have increased by 50%. Advances in medical science and emergency medical services (EMS) share the credit for saving these lives. Other cities with similar EMS programs also report substantial survival rate increases.

The elements of the system

The Chicago Emergency Medical Services system is regarded as a model of efficiency and organizational sophistication. Thirty-six mobile intensive care ambulance units currently serve the city, based in strategically located neighborhood fire stations. Three fire department helicopters stand by on alert at Meigs Field, a lakefront airstrip. By dialing 911 (the emergency police-fire telephone number) a citizen may report an apparent heart attack. An EMS team is instantly dispatched by radio, and trained paramedic personnel arrive on the scene in a mobile emergency room that in effect brings the hospital to the patient. The emergency van usually arrives in three to six minutes, and often much more quickly.

The ambulance is a converted Chevrolet van with a crew of three certified paramedics. Aside from the standard emergency medical equipment, each ambulance carries a portable electrocardiograph machine that can send a victim's electrocardiogram (EKG) to

the nearest hospital that has facilities to receive the transmission. An attending physician in the receiving hospital analyzes the EKG and transmits back appropriate instructions to the paramedics. Through this radiotelemetry device the patient's heartbeat can be constantly monitored and the patient continuously treated en route to the hospital. Since 25 to 33% of all fatalities occur instantly or within minutes after onset of the heart attack, prompt paramedical attention is essential if the victim is to survive the first critical moments.

Paramedics first determine if the victim is conscious and alert. If a patient responds to questions or if a pulse is evident, the heart is obviously still beating. The portable EKG machine is set up and a reading is taken. Moments later the EKG is transmitted to the hospital, where it is read by a physician. If the heartbeat is erratic (arrhythmic) or has stopped, defibrillator paddles may be used to administer electric shock to restore normal rhythm or restart the heart. Death or irreversible damage occurs to the brain if it is deprived of oxygen for about four minutes—the stopped heart must resume beating soon if a patient is to survive. Closed-chest massage—the rhythmic pressing on a patient's breastbone—may be used by paramedics to force an arrested heart to start pumping again. A dextrose solution may be administered intravenously along with lidocaine, a medication to combat arrhythmia. Suction devices and endotracheal airway tubes may be used to facilitate the patient's breathing.

Still in contact with the physician as they drive to the hospital, paramedics may be instructed to use additional defibrillation procedures and administer more medication. On arrival at the hospital emergency room—often within two minutes—a team of physicians, interns, and nurses takes over. The time saved by on-the-spot treatment by paramedics using the latest equipment assures the heart attack victim a better than even chance for survival.

Paramedic training

Emergency medical services personnel in the Chicago system are intensively trained for six months at participating hospitals and at the Chicago Fire Department Academy. Training complies with national guidelines and includes courses in cardiopulmonary resuscitation (CPR) techniques, anatomy, physiology, medical terminology, psychology, drug effects, cardiac arrest, and emergency childbirth. Paramedical instruction at Chicago's Northwestern Memorial Hospital is conducted by staff physicians who are also Northwestern University faculty members. Cardiac arrest is probably the most frequently encountered emergency, and paramedics are thoroughly trained to handle it until the victim is brought to the hospital.

Assignment to the Chicago paramedical corps is made by means of a combination of testing and a rigid merit system. In 1978 the Chicago Fire Department had a force of 275 in the paramedical division, a career service with the same benefits as those earned by regular uniformed firefighters.

In 1977 Chicago Fire Department paramedics responded to some 170,000 emergency calls, of which one-third were false alarms. The city's EMS system is currently handling some 12,000 emergency calls per month. In 1976 a single ambulance responded to 7,651 calls, an average of more than 20 calls per day all year long. Not all of the incidents were heart attacks, of course. Paramedics also respond to automobile accidents, fires, emergency childbirths, accidents in the home—a variety of situations that may or may not turn out to require emergency care.

The city of Chicago has also been training city workers and civilian employees who work in the downtown area in CPR techniques. CPR may keep a heart attack victim alive until paramedics arrive. By early 1978 over 13,500 people had completed the course given by the city. Some 50,000 other Chicagoans have taken CPR courses elsewhere. A 1977 city ordinance exempted persons trained in CPR from civil suits when they provide emergency medical care. Courts in other cities have upheld similar laws. The ordinance is intended to encourage people trained in CPR to use the techniques without fear of subsequent civil action. The use of CPR complements the work of paramedics and further contributes to the declining death rate.

A national emergency program

Emergency medical services were officially recognized as a national necessity in 1966 with passage of the Highway Safety Act, which required states to develop such systems. Failure to comply could have cost each state as much as 10% in lost federal highway construction funds. The subsequent emergency medical care system set up in Chicago became the blueprint for the 1973 Emergency Medical Services Systems Act.

The Chicago program was begun by David R. Boyd, director of Emergency Medical Services for the U.S. Department of Health, Education, and Welfare (HEW), who was at one time a resident physician at Chicago's Cook County Hospital. First-hand observation of the high fatality rate for heart attack victims, accident cases, and other emergency injuries motivated Boyd to create the system.

There are now 27,500 mobile intensive care ambulances in service nationwide, most in compliance with the American College of Surgeons' design standards. In previous years most private ambulances were operated by mortuary establishments and civilian companies that did not provide adequately trained personnel. Many of these ambulances were not properly equipped and did not contain two-way radio systems. Consequently the death toll was high. Since 1968, however, the dead-on-arrival rate for accident victims has fallen by 19%.

A completely outfitted paramedic van costs approximately $40,000 and contains a radiotelemetry system that can transmit a patient's electrocardiogram to a hospital, where a physician can analyze it, make a diagnosis, and transmit instructions for treatment back to the attending paramedics. A full spectrum of life-support equipment generally carried by each mobile intensive care unit includes stretchers, boards for supporting patients with possible injury to the spine, inflatable splints, a Lifepak (electrocardiogram machine to monitor heartbeat and to administer defibrillation shock), an ambu bag (for forcing air into a victim's lungs), a standard first aid kit, an aspirator, oxygen, clean linen and blankets, drugs, a crowbar, emergency lights, a fire fighter's costume, and miscellaneous diagnostic equipment.

There are now 287,000 certified emergency medical technicians in the U.S. Some 20,000 paramedics have been trained intensively at participating hospitals in courses of 81 to 480 hours of instruction on all facets of emergency care.

Major cities around the country with first-rate EMS systems include Seattle, Wash., Los Angeles, Calif., Charlottesville, Va., and Baltimore, Md. HEW, under its EMS division, is now creating regional EMS networks. Each unit in the network may comprise several counties, rural communities, or only a single large city. The U.S. Department of Transportation and HEW have already allocated $188 million to finance statewide EMS systems.

Early in 1978 about 100 local EMS systems were operating in scattered locations in the U.S. HEW officials hope 200 more such systems will be created. According to predictions, by 1982 EMS systems should blanket the country. The objective is to ensure that heart attack and accident victims will be treated by trained paramedics and swiftly transported to hospitals or trauma centers no matter where they are stricken or injured.

Research studies have not yet established with any accuracy the widespread effects of EMS programs. But fatalities are definitely declining in areas where EMS programs have been established. Many people who would otherwise be dead are now recovering from severe heart attacks and accidents because of professional paramedical care.

Infectious Diseases

In the days before antibiotics, pneumonia was a killer. About one of every three young, otherwise healthy patients with lobar pneumonia (so-called because characteristically segments of the lung are affected) would die from the disease. Mortality among the elderly, infants, and the chronically ill was considerably higher. The doctor was helpless—sitting by the bedside until the patient either recovered or died. With antibiotic agents such as penicillin the picture has now improved, but the problem has not been solved. Approximately 500,000 persons will get the disease each year in the United States. Of those who succumb despite antibiotics, surgery, intensive care, and the like, about one in 20, or 25,000 of the total, will die. Improved treatments have brightened the picture for the young and healthy, but those still most susceptible are elderly, debilitated, or suffering from some chronic illness such as kidney disease, heart disease, chronic bronchitis, or emphysema.

Pneumonia is the fifth leading cause of death in the United States. Those surviving pneumonia may require a period of hospitalization and a long convalescence. Surgery to drain lung abscesses may be necessary; permanent damage sometimes occurs. The costs to the patient and to society are considerable, amounting to many millions of dollars yearly.

Treating pneumonia

Until recently no attempts had been made to prevent the disease. Even though vaccines are used with great effectiveness for diseases such as smallpox, polio, measles, tetanus, and other contagious illnesses of both viral and bacterial origin, prevention of pneumonia by immunization had not been applied. In 1978, however, the United States Food and Drug Administration approved a new vaccine to combat pneumonia. This vaccine, recommended for use by high-risk patients, has been tested in more than 30,000 people. It protects against 14 of the most common types of pneumococcal organisms.

As many as 80 types of *Diplococcus pneumoniae,* the bacterial organism responsible for the disease, have been identified. They are distinguished from each other by the structure of their external capsule, the polysaccharide coat that surrounds them. Other types of *Diplococcus* have been identified that lack this protective coating; they are not pathogenic (disease-causing) in man. Pneumococcal organisms also cause middle-ear infections, meningitis, and bacterial arthritis.

Polysaccharides are large molecular structures consisting mainly of carbohydrate residues—glucose is an example. The capsule of the type 3 pneumococcus, one of the most common causes of pneumonia, consists of repeating units of D-glucose and D-glucuronic acid; they act as antigens, causing the formation of antibodies in horses, goats, and other animals, including man. Each type of pneumococcus forms a structurally different capsule. To induce the formation of specific antisera, bacteriologists isolate the antigenic polysaccharide capsule of various pneumococcal types and inject them into antibody-forming animals. Animals injected with one pneumococcal type form antibodies that react primarily with that pneumococcal type and not with those of the other types.

In 1881 Louis Pasteur discovered pneumococcal organisms; they were identified shortly afterward as the causative agents of lobar pneumonia. As an early form of treatment providing a passive type of immunity, antiserum, raised in horses, was injected into patients with pneumonia. So that the pneumococcal type causing the patient's illness could be identified the organisms were isolated from the typical "rusty" (blood-con-

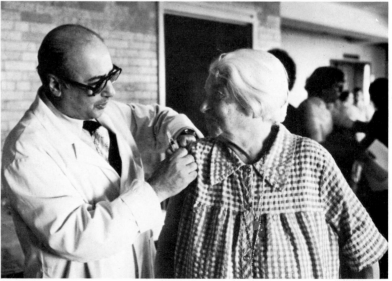

In 1978 the Massachusetts Department of Public Health directed the vaccination of 200 residents of a nursing home in East Boston, Mass., with the new Pneumovax pneumococcal pneumonia vaccine. The elderly are especially at risk from bacterial pneumonia.

taining) sputum of patients; its serological type was determined using antisera specific for each of the various pneumococcal polysaccharides. Horse serum containing high titers, or concentrations, of pneumococcal antibodies was administered to the patient, usually by a rather painful intramuscular injection. (Intravenous injections of foreign serum may cause blood clots.) Often the patients benefited. Horse antibodies combined with the pneumococci, aiding the patient's defense system in their destruction. Eventually, with time, the patient produced antibodies of his own; further serum therapy was no longer required. However, a serious complication of serum therapy sometimes occurs. The patient develops antibodies to the horse serum itself, often neutralizing its pneumococcal antibodies and thus reducing the effectiveness of subsequent injections. Many patients receiving "foreign" serum develop "serum sickness"—bloody urine and kidney damage, fever, and arthritis resulting from the presence of large quantities of antigen-antibody complexes consisting of horse protein and patient antibodies. The Arthus reaction, a painful reaction with tissue destruction at the injection site, often occurs after antiserum injection.

Antibiotic and antigenic therapy

In spite of these serious complications of treatment, pneumonia is such a life-endangering disease that serum therapy was practiced widely until the advent in the 1930s of bacteria-destroying antibiotics such as penicillin. Pneumococci are readily killed by penicillin and other antibiotics.

Antibodies to pneumococcal polysaccharides, produced by the patient himself or administered passively by serum therapy, attach to the capsules of the pneumococcal organisms. Antibody-coated pneumococci are readily engulfed by the body's phagocytic cells, which contain potent digestive enzymes that attack the capsule and the organism itself. The pneumococci are destroyed by the body's cellular defenses. Capsular organisms without antibody coatings, on the other hand, resist phagocytosis, remaining viable and proliferating rapidly in the lungs and elsewhere in the body.

The body's defenses against pneumococcal pneumonia are ordinarily quite strong. Epidemics of pneumonia rarely occur. Many people, entirely well, have disease-causing pneumococci living in their throats with no apparent ill effects. These organisms, kept in check by the presence of large numbers of different types of bacterial flora, sometimes gain access to the lungs, where they are effectively trapped by the mucous coating of the bronchi. Trapped organisms are carried by the action of ciliated cells to the back of the throat, where they are swallowed. Organisms reaching the stomach are destroyed by strong acid and digestive enzymes. Occasional organisms entering the inner regions of the lungs or the bloodstream itself are destroyed by large numbers of macrophages—large phagocytic cells found throughout the body.

Pneumococcal pneumonia becomes a threat to life in instances in which a second illness is ongoing. In these cases the bacteria often gain access in large numbers; in addition, host immunity may be depressed. In instances in which the mucous linings of the bronchi are injured, as during gas anesthesia or in chronic bronchitis, a heightened incidence of the disease is seen. Pneumonia is also a common aftermath of influenza. In cases of chronic heart failure the diseased heart, unable to pump blood as efficiently as the body requires, causes the accumulation of excessive quantities of fluid in the lungs—a suitable breeding ground for the growth of pneumococcal organisms. The work of phagocytic cells is impaired in fluid-filled body cavities; the pulmonary stasis occurring in the chronically ill, bedridden elderly may be a sufficient predisposing cause of pneumonia. An older patient forced to bed because of, say, a broken hip may die of pneumococcal pneumonia.

Organisms that do cross outer protective linings to the bloodstream are trapped and destroyed by phagocytic cells in the spleen, a major organ of immunity. Individuals who have had their spleens removed or damaged have a much higher incidence of pneumonia than healthy, normal people. Surgical removal of the spleen is a common treatment in certain illnesses such as Hodgkin's disease or hemolytic anemia. Patients whose splenic function is diminished as a consequence of their illness are also prone to pneumococcal pneumonia. The most common example of a disease process leading to a disruption of normal splenic function is sickle-cell anemia, in which normal splenic tissue is gradually replaced by scar tissue.

An effective vaccine

In an effort to protect patients with diminished splenic function from infection with pneumococci, Arthur J. Ammann and his colleagues from the Department of Pediatrics of the University of California, San Francisco Medical Center, administered as a vaccine the purified pneumococcal polysaccharides from eight common disease-causing types to 77 patients with sickle-cell anemia and 19 patients whose spleens had been removed. Another 106 age- and race-matched persons with sickle cell disease were followed without immunization as a control group. Within two years eight pneumococcal infections had occurred in the control group; none in the immunized group. Pneumococcal polysaccharides are a suitable vaccine for protecting patients with a heightened risk of disease. Pneumococcal vaccine became available for widespread use early in 1978. It is a polyvalent vaccine, effective against 14 major pneumonia-causing strains.

—Edward P. Cohen, M.D.

Special Report:

Antiviral Drugs

by A. Frederick Rasmussen, Jr., M.D., Ph.D.

Few advances, if any, in medical research have been of greater value in treating human diseases than the development of sulfanilamide, penicillin, and other chemotherapeutic agents. As a whole, chemotherapy has proved highly successful against such bacterial infections as pneumonia, tuberculosis, and syphilis, and against most of the important human diseases such as malaria that are caused by animal parasites. By contrast, the search for effective drugs for treating diseases caused by viruses until very recently has been very disappointing. This has not been due to a neglect of research in this field. Indeed, the dramatic success in discovering drugs effective against bacterial infections has stimulated intensive worldwide efforts receiving generous support from governmental agencies, private philanthropy, and industry. Failure to find effective antiviral agents has been due, rather, to the intimate relationship that viruses have with their susceptible host cells.

Although bacteria and other more highly organized infectious agents do parasitize their hosts and in some instances are completely dependent on host tissues for nourishment, they have essentially independent mechanisms for growth and reproduction. In contrast, viruses depend for all of their vital functions upon the host cell's own enzymatic, genetic, and nutritional systems. It has been very expensive and extremely difficult to find chemical agents that would effectively suppress the multiplication or transmission of viruses without at the same time causing intolerable damage to host cells and tissues.

The first antiviral drug to show a reasonable degree of selective efficiency in inhibiting the growth of a virus is isatin (thiosemicarbazone). This compound suppresses the growth of poxviruses, including smallpox, in cell cultures and in animals. During one of the last severe smallpox outbreaks in India, it also showed promise in preventing the disease in exposed persons. It was not an effective treatment, however, once symptoms had developed. Fortunately, vaccination appears to have eliminated this dread disease.

The second antiviral compound of proved efficacy and the first to be licensed for human use in the United States is amantadine, which has been shown effective against the influenza A viruses but not against influenza B. Although this narrow range might appear to indicate that the compound has very limited usefulness,

influenza A viruses are the major cause of epidemic influenza, and amantadine treatment of individuals exposed to these strains affords significant protection. Although effective vaccines against specific strains of influenza A viruses have been developed, influenza A viruses tend to undergo mutation to the extent that vaccines prepared from previously prevalent strains are not effective against new varieties. Hence, the availability of a chemical prophylactic agent could be invaluable if influenza A should ever recur in pandemics like that of 1918. Treatment of influenza with amantadine once symptoms have developed is also effective, but less so than when done for prevention.

It has long been known that tuberculosis, a bacterial infection, results in an enhanced responsiveness of the body's immune system to diverse antigens, including viral antigens. The possibility that immunologic responsiveness against human tumors could be enhanced by this mechanism is receiving great attention, and the approach has now been extended to experimental viral infections. Bacillus Calmette-Guérin (BCG), the live-bacteria vaccine used against tuberculosis, clearly enhances resistance to a number of experimental viral infections in animals. The chemical isoprinosine, a substance of very low toxicity, also has been shown effective in stimulating certain immune reactions in viral infections and, indeed, has been shown to have a protective influence on the course of the infection, presumably by strengthening the host's own immune response. This promising approach to treatment of viral disease needs cautious development, however, because of the possibility of side reactions.

Interferon research

Another approach to viral therapy became possible with the discovery that cells infected with some viruses produce a substance that itself has antiviral activity. This substance, called interferon, has been the subject of intensive study since its discovery in 1957. Interferon can be recovered from infected tissues or from cells in culture that have been experimentally infected with one of a number of viruses. Sendai virus, a respiratory virus related to mumps virus, is commonly used. To be effective, interferon must be prepared from cells of the same species in which it is to be used. Thus, for treatment of humans, interferon must be prepared from human cells, and the availability of sufficient supplies of human cells becomes a limiting factor in interferon production. For this reason experimental clinical trials have been greatly handicapped, and production of amounts of interferon sufficient for general use is not in sight.

Clinical studies have been conducted and are continuing with interferon prepared from leukocytes (white blood cells) harvested from human blood. White cells, which are lighter than red cells, can be separated by gentle centrifugation from blood that has been collected for blood transfusions. This type of interferon is described as exogenous interferon to distinguish it from the endogenous interferon produced in the cells of the animal or person infected with a virus. Exogenous interferon prepared from human white cells or other human cells has been effective in the experimental treatment of ulcers of the cornea of the eye caused by herpes simplex virus, the virus that causes the common cold sore. It is one of a group of related organisms called herpesviruses. Interferon has also shown promise in the treatment of one form of hepatitis and in treating influenza and herpes zoster (shingles). Exogenous interferon is essentially nontoxic, but it has caused reactions characterized by fever; however, these may be due to impurities. Hypersensitivity reactions have also been observed.

Because of the difficulties in producing exogenous interferon in practical amounts, thought has been given to methods that might stimulate the patient with a viral infection to produce more endogenous interferon. Viruses vary greatly in their capacities to stimulate interferon production as well as in their susceptibilities to the substance. In fact, a number of viruses that are poor interferon inducers are highly susceptible to its antiviral effects. The possibility of using a relatively harmless but effective interferon-inducing virus has been explored in animals but has been rejected for human use because of the danger that such a virus might become capable of causing serious disease.

A number of compounds, however, including synthetic polynucleotides, particularly double-stranded RNA's, have also been shown to be very effective inducers of interferon in experimental animals. Although this approach is being actively pursued, it has not yet been possible to develop effective interferon inducers that could be used successfully to treat human viral infections.

Chemical antiviral weapons

Among the first compounds to be studied in the search for antiviral drugs were purine and pyrimidine antagonists. Purines and pyrimidines are chemical constituents of nucleotides, which in turn are essential components of both RNA and DNA. All viruses have one or the other of these nucleic acids as their genetic material. As early as 1946 some purine and pyrimidine antagonists had been shown to inhibit growth of some viruses in culture, but none proved to be therapeutically useful until 1959, when idoxuridine (IDU), a pyrimidine compound, was synthesized and subsequently studied for possible use in the treatment of cancer. In experimental trials with tumor cells, IDU appeared primarily to inhibit the enzyme DNA polymerase, which is essential for the assembly of DNA from its constituent parts.

Further studies with IDU showed that this compound also inhibited virus-specific enzymes. In addition, the topical application of IDU on rabbit corneas infected with herpesvirus protected against the severe ulcers that this virus causes in both natural and experimental infections of the eye. Extension of these studies to treatment of human corneal ulcers caused by herpesvirus was also successful. Although subsequent studies indicated the tendency for the virus to develop resistance to the compound, drug resistance has not proved to be a problem in the topical treatment of herpetic ulcers of the eye. IDU was not effective, however, in treating systemic forms of herpes infection and has been disappointing in treating herpetic ulcers of the skin and of the genital mucous membranes.

In the meantime, another pyrimidine compound, cytosine arabinoside, was shown to inhibit the growth of herpesvirus in cell culture and to show some promise in the treatment of experimental infections in animals. Early experiments with this compound in the treatment of herpetic encephalitis, a viral invasion of the brain and one of the most severe forms of herpes infection, appeared to be successful. Subsequent studies, however, showed that the apparent success had been due to the variable course of this disease and that cytosine arabinoside was not an effective agent against herpetic encephalitis and other systemic herpes infections in man.

Within recent months, however, a closely related compound called adenine arabinoside (arabinosyladenine or ara-A) has been shown effective in the treatment of encephalitis caused by herpes simplex virus and in the treatment of a disseminated form of herpetic infection with characteristics of chickenpox and shingles (varicella-zoster) in patients whose immune mechanisms had been suppressed during treatment of leukemia and related malignant diseases. Infection of the brain with herpes simplex virus is the most common cause of nonepidemic, severe, and fatal encephalitis in the U.S. Its adverse effects are manifest by a high fatality rate and by a high incidence of severe brain damage in patients who live.

Because of the misleading and disappointing experience in earlier trials with IDU and cytosine arabinoside, which at first had appeared to be of benefit in poorly controlled trials, a very carefully controlled collaborative study of ara-A was undertaken under the sponsorship of the U.S. National Institutes of Health (NIH) to determine if experimental treatment of severe herpetic infections of man, including herpes simplex encephalitis, could be successful. This study received its major financial support as well as significant facilitating administrative help from project officers in the National Institute of Allergy and Infectious Diseases of the NIH. Scientific coordination was centered in the department of pediatrics of the University of Alabama School of Medicine in Birmingham. In order to have a sufficient number of patients for treatment and for controls within a reasonable period of time, it was necessary to enlist the collaborative support of departments of pediatrics or of infectious diseases at several other universities and hospitals. Rigorous standards for an unequivocal diagnosis of herpes encephalitis, including recovery and identification of herpes simplex virus from infected tissues, were established. Confirmation of the diagnosis of herpetic infection was of crucial importance because encephalitis caused by viruses that are not susceptible to ara-A are clinically indistinguishable from encephalitis caused by herpes simplex.

The design of the experiment, which included treatment of a control group of patients with placebos, was carefully explained to all patients who participated in the study and to their families so that informed consent could be obtained. Patients were examined daily for progression of disease. Clinical observations were recorded at five-day intervals for one month following onset or until death. Follow-up examinations of surviving patients were performed at 2-, 3-, 6-, 12-, and 24-month intervals with the help of local neurologists. These latter studies were designed to determine the degree of resolution of brain damage or of further deterioration of function.

Fifty-two patients completed the study. Two of the 52 were excluded from analysis for statistical reasons. Of the 50 remaining, 29 received ara-A and 21 received the inert placebo. Of 28 patients in whom the diagnosis was confirmed by recovery of herpes simplex virus from infected tissue, 18 were treated with ara-A. In this group of 18 the mortality rate was 28%, compared with 70% in the placebo-treated control group.

As soon as the reduction in mortality in the ara-A-treated group became statistically evident, placebo treatment of the control group was terminated for ethical reasons. Statistical evaluation of the effect of treatment on degree of recovery from brain damage in the placebo group was not possible because only three placebo-treated herpes-confirmed patients survived. However, 7 of the 18 herpes-confirmed patients treated with ara-A either recovered completely as determined by their ability to return to school or to work at their previous level of performance or were able to perform at a gainful level even though hampered by some brain damage. By contrast, only two of ten placebo-treated patients infected with herpes achieved this degree of recovery. There were six survivors in the ara-A-treated group, three adults and three children, who had very severe residual damage. The three

adults died between four and six months after treatment. The three children survived for the first year without substantial resolution of brain damage. Thus, it is apparent that even with promise of a substantial decrease in mortality following treatment with ara-A, a significant number of patients who survive may have very serious residual disability, which would include personality changes, partial paralysis, epileptiform seizures, and difficulty in speech and in controlling bowel and bladder functions.

This result is, of course, both encouraging and discouraging and raises concern as to the ultimate value of ara-A treatment. Follow-up data, however, must be regarded as generally encouraging because survivors of untreated herpes simplex encephalitis experience the same range of residual disability. In the reported study the quality of life in treated survivors was at least as good as that of survivors in the untreated controls. Termination of placebo treatment of the control group, although unquestionably necessary from an ethical standpoint, has left a number of very important unanswered questions.

Because of the very real danger of undesirable side effects, the daily dosage and duration of ara-A treatment chosen were conservative and clearly safe. The possibility remains that somewhat larger doses might have been used safely and that the duration of treatment, ten days, could have been longer. These considerations are particularly important in light of the possibility that more intensive or more prolonged treatment might reduce the residual brain damage among survivors. Another difficult problem revealed by the ara-A study was that treatment was uniformly discouraging in patients who had progressed to coma by the time treatment could be instituted. In contrast, those patients who had progressed only to a lethargic state when ara-A treatment was started responded much more favorably. Among seven lethargic, ara-A-treated patients all survived, and six had minor to moderate residual damage.

On the basis of this experience, ara-A will continue to be used. The collaborative group mentioned above and future ones will make careful observations on patients treated with ara-A, and intensive efforts will be made to establish a clear virologic diagnosis in as many patients as possible so that the unanswered questions may be answered through cumulative experience, even though the variable course of the untreated disease will make evaluation difficult. Intensive efforts to develop methods of early diagnosis must also continue.

For the immediate future, the prospect of recovery for patients with this dread disease is greatly improved, even though those who are severely maimed will constitute a continuing challenge. Progress can also be anticipated in the search for effective agents against other viral diseases.

Joints and Muscles

The musculoskeletal system is comprised of bones, joints, muscles, ligaments, tendons, and bursae (serum-filled sacs) surrounding the joints. Connective tissue, a collective term for tissue peculiar to each of these structures, is composed of varying degrees and types of protein fibers (collagen), complexes of amino-acid sugars bound to protein (proteoglycans), and the cells that elaborate these substances (fibroblasts).

Rheumatologists, specialists who care for victims of musculoskeletal disturbances, also treat patients with so-called connective tissue diseases. Sometimes referred to as collagen diseases or collagen-vascular diseases, diseases of connective tissue can be serious and may inflame the lungs, heart, skin, brain, kidneys, and other organs. Systemic lupus erythematosus is the prototype of these disorders.

Rheumatic diseases

Rheumatism is a vague term applied to any musculoskeletal ache or pain, particularly if persistent or recurrent. Arthritis, which can be either an inflammation of the lining membrane (synovium) of the joint or a destruction of the cartilage making up the joint surfaces, is but one type of rheumatism. Broadly speaking, rheumatism and arthritis have come to be used interchangeably when referring to musculoskeletal problems, particularly chronic ones. Osteoarthritis (osteoarthrosis) is familiar as the wear-and-tear disease of the middle-aged and older.

Nonarticular rheumatism. Characterized by rheumatic pain outside the joints, nonarticular rheumatism in any of its varieties affects men and women of all ages. Bursitis, tendinitis, and tennis elbow are examples of localized rheumatic pain syndromes sometimes precipitated by injury. These conditions may temporarily disable the patient but rarely cripple. Fibromyositis, fibromyalgia, and fibrositis are interchangeable terms for a more generalized condition in which pain arises from the soft tissues surrounding a joint. Fibromyositis is of unknown cause, but it tends to affect people under stress. It is sometimes confused with more serious forms of rheumatism and may be present with tendinitis or bursitis of multiple parts of the body. The disease is difficult to treat successfully, although it may disappear spontaneously. Little research has been performed on nonarticular rheumatism. However, one investigator noted that human subjects deprived of non-REM (rapid-eye-movement) sleep developed a fibromyositis-type syndrome.

Polymyalgia rheumatica is a common disease of the elderly yet truly appreciated only within the past few years. Most patients with this form of nonarticular rheumatism complain of pain all over the body, particularly in the neck, shoulders, upper arms, low back, buttocks, and thighs. Fatigue and depression may be pro-

found. As a measure of generalized inflammation, the erythrocyte sedimentation rate (the rate at which red blood cells settle in a tube of drawn blood) is almost always elevated. Inflamed cranial blood vessels sometimes accompany polymyalgia rheumatica, and blindness may ensue if this condition is not properly recognized. Polymyalgia rheumatica and its complications are treated effectively with certain corticosteroid drugs such as prednisone. Spontaneous remissions may take place after one to three years.

Rheumatoid arthritis. Rheumatoid arthritis is a generalized, often progressive disease that has potential for joint destruction, crippling, and disability. Inflamed joints are painful, swollen, and often limited in motion. Morning stiffness and fatigue may be profound. Although primarily a disease of young and middle-aged women, rheumatoid arthritis strikes those of any age and men as well. Blood vessels, heart, lungs, spleen, and skin may be targets in addition to joints. In children the disease is known as juvenile rheumatoid arthritis. X-rays may show mild or severe joint destruction. A protein antibody called rheumatoid factor is found in the blood in 70–80% of patients with adult rheumatoid arthritis.

The concept that rheumatoid arthritis may be genetically transmitted has been supported by recent evidence that the histocompatibility antigen HL-A DW_4 is found in 48% of rheumatoid patients, compared with 16% of persons free of the disease. The HL-A antigens are part of a group of genetically inherited glycoproteins found on the surface membranes of every cell in the body. Several different varieties of HL-A antigens are known, and the variety of combinations in which they can be found make it improbable that any two persons will have identical sets. These antigens are responsible in part for determining the extent to which the body's immune system will recognize and reject foreign tissue.

The cause of rheumatoid arthritis is not known, but immunogenetic factors appear to predispose a person to the illness in the proper environmental setting. Perhaps triggered by a virus, another microorganism, trauma, or some other foreign agent (antigen), the body begins manufacturing antibody protein to defend itself. The antibody, having reacted with its antigen, becomes altered somehow so that it appears foreign to the immune system. Assisted by enzymatic proteins in the blood called complement, rheumatoid factor reacts with the altered antibody (which now acts as an antigen) to form insoluble immune complexes that deposit in the joint. The immune complexes are ingested by leukocytes (scavenging white blood cells) and trigger the release of mediators of inflammation including lysosomal enzymes that kindle the fires of arthritis.

Lysosomal enzymes also are quite capable of degrading proteoglycans, the major constituent of cartilage. Altered cartilage may become antigenic and thus

251

perpetuate the inflammatory process. Another cellular enzyme, collagenase, is released by cells of the synovium and breaks down another component of cartilage, collagen, causing erosion of the joint at the cartilage-synovium junction.

The key to successful management of rheumatoid arthritis is a comprehensive program calling not only for medication but also for physical therapy, occupational therapy, vocational rehabilitation, psychosocial counseling, education of the patient and family, and sometimes surgery. Aspirin and gold salts have been additional standbys in the treatment. Orally administered corticosteroids have fallen into disfavor except under certain circumstances. A host of nonsteroidal anti-inflammatory agents have been released by several pharmaceutical companies. While not curative in the usual sense, these drugs have been effective in reducing pain and inflammation in patients unresponsive to medication. Dozens of new nonsteroidal anti-inflammatory drugs are currently being investigated, and some should be released in coming years. Immunosuppressive (cytotoxic) drugs and antimetabolites, also used in the treatment of cancer, have been successful in some patients under controlled conditions but have not fulfilled expectations of their effectiveness.

Penicillamine, a drug available for the treatment of a rare metabolic disorder called Wilson's disease, also has been used experimentally against rheumatoid arthritis. It predictably lowers the blood rheumatoid factor in patients with rheumatoid arthritis and even produces remissions in some. Although it shows great promise, such side effects as skin rash and kidney disturbance are not rare. Levamisole is still another investigative drug that has produced remissions in some patients. A recent small-scale study offered some evidence that orally administered zinc sulfate, a common compound sometimes used to aid the healing of wounds, can help reduce swelling and facilitate body movement in patients with rheumatoid arthritis.

Many surgical restorative procedures are available for joints persistently inflamed or destroyed by rheumatoid arthritis. Their use must coordinate with the overall management program. Total hip replacement is now a standard operation with a good or excellent result in 95% of the patients. Finger joints, knees, elbows, shoulders, and ankles are being replaced with increasing frequency.

Rheumatoid arthritis still cannot be cured. A great deal can be done, however, to achieve short- and long-term goals for pain relief, improved function, personal and environmental adaptation, and prevention of further joint changes.

Ankylosing spondylitis. Ankylosing spondylitis is a chronic inflammatory disorder of the spine that usually begins in young male adults. Peripheral joints may be involved as well. Pain and stiffness may cause the

Courtesy, The Arthritis Foundation

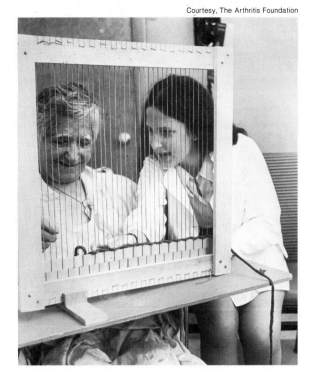

Physical therapy helps arthritis-stiffened fingers maintain maximum use and mobility.

victim to bend progressively forward unless a proper exercise program and anti-inflammatory drugs are introduced. The spine may ultimately fuse (poker spine). In some victims symptoms may be completely absent and in others quite severe. An occasional man is surprised to find late in life that the X-rays of his spine show extensive ankylosing spondylitis even though he felt nothing out of the ordinary.

The cause of ankylosing spondylitis is not known. This disease is now the prototype of those conditions associated with the histocompatibility antigen HL-A B27. Almost all patients with ankylosing spondylitis have this genetic factor on the surface of their blood cells. Some 4–5% of normal people exhibit HL-A B27 as well. These people are much more likely to develop ankylosing spondylitis than persons lacking the factor. The detection of HL-A B27 in the blood often helps to identify the disease when diagnosis has been difficult.

Systemic lupus erythematosus. Systemic lupus erythematosus (SLE) is a disease, usually of young women, in which joints and multiple organs of the body are inflamed. A butterfly-shaped rash over the nose and upper cheeks frequently erupts after exposure to sunlight. Victims may experience a variety of manifestations including joint pain, chest pain, kidney failure, neurologic abnormalities, and anemia. Complaints are often nonspecific and include fever, malaise, weakness, fatigability, weight loss, and irritability. A variety of autoimmunologic phenomena are exhibited, the most significant being antinuclear antibodies in the blood and an abnormal white blood cell called the LE cell. Antinuclear antibodies react with the nuclear constituents of the victim's own cells; the LE cell is produced following reactions involving one of a family of these antibodies.

Research into systemic lupus erythematosus has intensified within the past few decades. Immunologic mechanisms are now known to be clearly involved in the production of lupus lesions, and it is quite likely that both genetic and viral factors are also important considerations. SLE affects primarily women; it appears to be hereditary in some cases and has occurred in identical twins, but otherwise no clear-cut genetic pattern has yet been established.

Survival of lupus patients has improved greatly in recent years; the number of patients alive five years from onset of the disease exceeds 90%. Whether the improved survival rate in this heretofore invariably fatal disease has been due to better overall management such as control of infection or to corticosteroids and immunosuppressive drugs is still a moot point. The most severe aspect of SLE is a kidney involvement; kidney dialysis and transplantation have saved many lives.

Other connective tissue disorders. Although SLE is the prototype of acquired connective tissue disease, polymyositis (inflammation of muscles), scleroderma (hardening of the skin and internal organs), and vasculitis (inflammation of blood vessels) also are seen occasionally. Their protean manifestations, their often bizarre variable course, and their tendency to overlap one another sometimes confuse not only the patient but also the physician. Even those organs without connective tissue may be involved. Acquired connective tissue diseases are to be differentiated from those of a hereditary nature, most of which are quite rare.

In recent years a specific "mixed connective tissue disease syndrome" has been described. Victims of this disorder have features of polymyositis, scleroderma, rheumatoid arthritis, and vasculitis. They experience joint inflammation, diffusely swollen hands, Raynaud's phenomenon (decreased finger circulation upon exposure to cold), esophageal dysfunction, muscle weakness, lymph node enlargement, and high concentrations of globulins in the blood. All patients show a positive antinuclear antibody test with a peculiar speckled pattern. An unusual factor called "antibody to extractable nuclear antigen" (ENA) has been demonstrated. The condition is usually benign, often self-limiting, and quite responsive to corticosteroids.

A newly recognized connective tissue disease called diffuse fascitis with eosinophilia has been reported. Initially it appears either as scleroderma or polymyositis, but distinctive features allow it to be clearly separated from other acquired disorders of connective tissue. The legs, arms, and at times the trunk become diffusely involved, with puckering of the skin, sclerosis of the underlying tissues, and joint contractures. Elevated levels in the blood of particular white blood cells called eosinophils (eosinophilia) is an early feature. The natural history of this condition is not yet known, but corticosteroids seem to exert a favorable effect.

Waging war on arthritis

Arthritis with its variants represents one of the most prevalent diseases, striking more than one person in ten and claiming 600,000 new victims each year in the U.S. It is estimated that 3½ million Americans are disabled at any one time.

Arthritis is an expensive disease. More than $4 billion is spent annually in the U.S. on doctor bills, hospital care, drugs, quackery, and federal or private programs

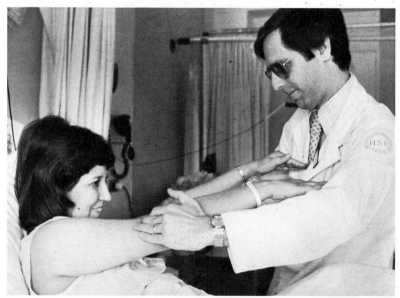

A lupus erythematosus patient is examined for possible inflammation of the joints. Great progress has been made in treating and controlling the disease, although its causes have not yet been discovered.

for arthritis. Indirect costs add up to more than $14 billion in lost wages, homemakers' services, ungenerated income taxes, disability support payments, and other types of compensation.

The Arthritis Foundation is a national organization with chapters throughout the U.S. Its professional wings are the American Rheumatism Association, consisting of physicians and scientists, and the American Society of Allied Health Professions, composed of physical therapists, occupational therapists, nurses, social workers, psychologists, and other medical support personnel. Arthritis Foundation programs include support for scientific and clinical research into the causes and treatment of arthritis, training of arthritis specialists, public information, public education, and services for arthritis sufferers and their families. The foundation fosters arthritis clinics, physician referral lists, home care programs, rehabilitation services, and mobile consultant units.

On Jan. 4, 1975, the National Arthritis Act was signed by Pres. Gerald R. Ford. It called for (1) an 18-member National Commission on Arthritis and Related Musculoskeletal Diseases; (2) a governmental interagency arthritis-coordinating committee; (3) grants for community demonstration projects; (4) an arthritis data bank for data useful in screening, prevention, and detection of arthritis; (5) development of widely distributed arthritis centers for arthritis research, diagnosis, treatment, rehabilitation, education, and related activities; and (6) expansion of the authority of the National Institute of Arthritis, Metabolism, and Digestive Diseases. As of early 1978, however, only a small amount of the money authorized by Congress had been appropriated. Several states have also organized programs to expand the arthritis cause.

Muscle diseases

Myopathies are those diseases that directly affect skeletal (voluntary) muscles. Muscular diseases may be congenital or acquired. They may be caused by or be associated with a variety of illnesses that include dystrophies, endocrine disturbances, metabolic abnormalities, toxins, electrolyte disturbances, infection, connective tissue diseases, and even cancer. Most myopathies cause weakness, usually of the proximal muscles (muscles located nearest the trunk). The weakness may vary in intensity and sometimes depends upon activity. It may be so subtle that it escapes the patient's attention, yet an observer may notice, for example, that the subject arises from a chair with difficulty. Some myopathies are painful, although most are painless.

Physical examination of myopathy victims may show tenderness, atrophy, and sometimes swelling. Blood tests may reveal increased levels of enzymes, reflecting breakdown of muscle. Urine, too, may reflect muscle destruction with increased levels of myoglobin and creatine. The electromyograph, a device that measures electrical impulses in muscle, in some cases can pinpoint the specific disease; in most instances it indicates the presence or absence of a myopathy. Muscle biopsies are often definitive in providing a diagnosis and should be considered in almost all patients who have a myopathy. Some of the important myopathies are considered below.

Muscular dystrophy. Muscular dystrophy refers to several hereditary disorders of muscle, some becoming evident early in childhood, others in adulthood. The extent of disability depends upon type, of which there are many. During the usual course of these disorders, muscle fibers degenerate, regenerate to some extent, and eventually become replaced by scar tissue and fat.

Duchenne type of muscular dystrophy, which affects primarily young male children, is usually severe and rapidly fatal. It progresses through childhood, resulting in inability to walk by early adolescence and in death usually before age 30. No satisfactory treatment yet exists for any of the muscular dystrophies.

Polymyositis and dermatomyositis. Polymyositis is a connective tissue disease in which the proximal extremities and trunk become progressively weaker because of muscle inflammation. When polymyositis is associated with an inflammatory skin rash, it is referred to as dermatomyositis. The cause is unknown, but it seems to be an autoimmune disease. Lymphocyte-mediated toxicity to the muscles has been noted in some patients with polymyositis. The disease may disappear spontaneously but not before several years have elapsed. Polymyositis patients have a greater chance of developing a malignancy. Corticosteroids are the drugs of choice and usually quite effective.

Infectious myositis. Although inflammation of the muscles secondary to bacterial infection is unusual, most people who have had influenza know that viral infections can cause painful muscles (myalgias). Whether viruses cause distinct inflammation of the muscles is still a moot point.

Trichinosis is a widespread form of myositis, caused by the parasitic roundworm *Trichinella spiralis*. The infestation is usually traced to infested pork that has not been thoroughly cooked. The parasite makes its way from the patient's intestinal tract to muscle tissue. Muscle pain, weakness, and fever result. The disease usually responds to special drugs.

Toxoplasmosis is another parasitic disease that is more common than previously believed. It may involve muscles, lymph nodes, liver, spleen, and the skin. *Toxoplasma gondii* is the causative agent sometimes carried by cats and birds. Toxoplasma antibodies may be found in the blood. The symptoms may resemble those of infectious mononucleosis, including fever, malaise, and changes in the lymph nodes.

Muscle diseases of nerve transmission. Myasthenia gravis, Eaton-Lambert syndrome, botulism, and the so-called restless legs syndrome are examples of disturbances at the neuromuscular junction. These neuromuscular syndromes are associated with inability of nerve endings at the meeting sites between nerve and muscle (synapses) to communicate chemically with muscle fibers for proper transmission of nervous impulses. Characteristically, repetitive use of muscles results in progressive weakness.

As many as half of all myasthenic patients have antibodies in their blood serum that react with muscles and other tissue components. Experimentally, myasthenia can be passively transferred via transplants of lymph node cells to normal animals from diseased animals. However, the disease does not develop in animals from whom the thymus has been removed, thus eliminating the source of thymus-derived lymphocytes (which function in the normal immune response). Treatment with drugs is usually effective for myasthenia gravis. Removal of the thymus is sometimes performed. A treatment called plasmapheresis, which has already been employed against several other diseases having immunologic involvement, recently has been used successfully on a small number of myasthenic patients. In this procedure the patient's blood is gradually withdrawn, cleansed of the antibodies believed to be involved in the disease, and then replaced.

—Warren A. Katz, M.D.

Kidney Diseases

Nephrology is the subspecialty of internal medicine that deals with the diseases of the kidneys. These organs play a vital role in the excretion of soluble waste products derived from the diet or from the body's metabolism. In addition, the kidney, under the influence of a number of hormones, regulates the body content of many substances in such a way that an excess of these substances obtained from the intake of food is excreted in the urine. These include water, sodium, potassium, chloride, magnesium, calcium, phosphorus, and other elements. The kidney also has the important function of excreting acids normally generated by metabolism.

Effective renal function can be only partially provided by dialysis with the artificial kidney. In part, the reason for this is that the kidney is also an endocrine organ in its own right, producing a number of vital substances, such as erythropoietin, a hormone that plays an indirect role in the formation of red blood cells; the enzyme renin, which affects the regulation of blood pressure and salt excretion; prostaglandins, hormonelike substances that have a variety of effects on blood vessels and on renal function; and active forms of vitamin D, which are required for calcium absorption and bone formation.

The basic renal unit is the nephron, of which each

kidney contains about one million. Each nephron consists of a filter, called the glomerulus (a structure composed of coils of blood vessels), which is connected to a tubule from which urine drains into the collecting tubules, the ureter, and eventually the bladder. Although the kidneys constitute only 0.4% of the body weight, they receive approximately 25% of the total output of blood from the heart. This extensive blood supply passes into the glomeruli, where about one-fifth of the plasma is filtered off in the form of a fluid that contains a virtually protein-free acellular ultrafiltrate of the blood. This fluid passes into the tubule, where a large number of regulatory processes take place as the result of hormonal action, local metabolism, and the effect of the constituents of the urine itself. In a healthy individual, these processes of secretions, reabsorption, and diffusion ensure that the volume and composition of all body fluids are maintained within limits best suited to the needs of the body.

Types of kidney diseases

Renal diseases may affect any part of the complex anatomical structure of the kidney: (1) the major renal blood vessels and their branches; (2) the glomeruli; (3) the tubules and supporting tissue; or (4) the calices (a series of cavities) and the pelvis of the kidney, the tunnel-shaped juncture of the kidney and ureter. Any of these parts may be affected by congenital, inflammatory, metabolic, and other illnesses.

The most important disease affecting the small blood vessels of the kidney is hypertension, or high blood pressure, which represents the major preventable cause of renal failure. In general, the more severe the hypertension, the greater the likelihood of renal damage. Often when a previous history is unavailable, it is difficult for the physician to ascertain whether the hypertension is primary or the result of preexisting disease in other renal structures. There are other diseases that affect the large and small renal blood vessels, but most of these are part of systemic disorders that also affect other organs such as the lungs, skin, heart, and brain.

The most frequently observed diseases of the kidneys, collectively known as glomerulonephritis, affect the glomeruli. There are many types of glomerular injury, but most result from abnormalities of immune mechanisms. In some types the predominant symptom is inflammation. Others cause selective damage to the basement membrane or progressive scarring. In one type of glomerulonephritis, which accounts for about 5% of the cases, antibodies react with the antigen of the glomerular basement membrane. In another group, which accounts for about 75% of all cases of glomerulonephritis, antibodies react with antigens from various sources in the blood to form immune complexes that deposit in the glomerulus. The accumulation of such immune complexes or of antibodies directed against the glomerular basement membrane can cause damage directly or by involving other cells and the participation of chemically active substances. The latter include a group of substances in the blood, collectively called "complement," which appears to attract neutrophils (a type of white blood cell) to the sites at which antibodies are deposited. The neutrophils then release substances that damage the glomerulus. In addition, other substances may be released in the formation of complement. One such substance, histamine, increases the permeability of the capillaries and allows more complexes to be deposited in the glomerulus, thus increasing the damage. The activation of the complement system also affects the blood platelets, which release destructive enzymes and increase capillary permeability. There may also be local clotting of the blood, which can be a factor in the eventual scarring of the glomerulus. The net result of these processes is inflammation, obstruction, or destruction of the glomerulus. A variety of substances may act as antigens initiating the disease, among them substances found in the microorganisms called streptococci, which are important causes of sore throat and of skin infection. Other bacteria, viruses, parasites, and drugs may also stimulate the production of antigens. In addition to damage to the glomeruli, tubular and interstitial damage may occur.

Another category of kidney diseases includes those that involve the tubules. Acute renal failure following shock, severe traumatic injury, ingestion of certain poisons, or the use of drugs that damage the kidneys is often called acute tubular necrosis. However, the principal functional effect of this condition is to decrease the filtering ability of the glomeruli. Other tubular disorders may be congenital, associated with systemic diseases, or may result from the use of drugs, especially large quantities of analgesics (pain killers). Radiation, bacterial infection, or excess of blood calcium or uric acid can also damage the tubules.

The calices and pelvis of the kidney receive the modified glomerular filtrate after its passage through the tubules. The urine then travels down the ureter into the bladder before it is passed. The most common problem of the calices or pelvis is obstruction, which can have a variety of causes including renal stones, enlarged prostate, tumors, or blood clots. Infection, called pyelonephritis, may occur in conjunction with obstruction or, more rarely and less seriously, without. Infection of the bladder or urethra is a common cause of discomfort but rarely causes significant kidney damage unless there are other problems.

Diagnosis

The clinical presentation of kidney diseases is often insidious, and significant loss of renal function can occur without complaint. There are certain symptoms that can be of diagnostic value, including frequency of uri-

nation during the day and at night, swelling of the ankles or other areas, pain over the kidneys, and an abnormal appearance of the urine, particularly the presence of blood or infection. The physician may make a diagnosis by taking a careful history or physical examination, by finding swelling of the extremities, hypertension, evidence of urinary tract obstruction, or signs of systemic diseases known to damage the kidney. Chemical analysis and microscopic examination of the urine may reveal the presence of protein, red and white blood cells, or casts of the renal tubule.

Renal function tests, which involve collection of blood and timed specimens of urine and measurement of the ability of the kidney to excrete substances, are also useful. X-rays following the injection of radiopaque dyes show the internal structure of the kidneys and ureters. The use of radioisotopic techniques to determine various aspects of renal structure and function is progressing rapidly, as is the application of ultrasound. Renal biopsy is the most specific diagnostic technique. Usually a small amount of tissue is removed by means of a special needle. The tissue is then examined by three different procedures: light microscopy, transmission electron microscopy, and immunofluorescent microscopy, which allows the detection of fluorescent labeled antibodies in the glomerular basement membrane. Another technique, scanning electron microscopy, allows the external appearance of the tissue to be observed.

The severity of renal disease is measured primarily by the degree of impairment of renal function and by the amount of protein that leaks into the urine. In mild renal disease there may be little impairment of renal function: with increasing severity, the number of functioning glomeruli is markedly reduced and, as a consequence, toxic substances normally excreted in the urine remain in the blood and the patient begins to experience symptoms. Renal failure exists when only a tiny fraction of glomeruli remain functioning. If a great deal of protein has leaked through the glomeruli to the urine, the plasma becomes depleted of protein and decreases in volume. Obvious swelling of the body results from retention of water and salt to compensate for the reduction of plasma volume. This process is called the "nephrotic syndrome." In some types of renal disorders the disease may abate for a time, or renal function may worsen very gradually; in others progression to full renal failure is rapid. In older patients decline of renal function is often accompanied by an increase in the blood pressure, which in turn may further aggravate the impairment and hasten the onset of renal failure.

Treatment

Many of the diseases affecting the kidneys have no specific treatment because the precipitating immunological abnormalities are not well understood. Cortisone derivatives and other groups of drugs having effects on the immune system are frequently used in these illnesses, sometimes with success. A new development in treatment is plasmapheresis, a process in which circulating immune complexes are removed from the bloodstream. Antibiotics, diuretics (drugs that increase the excretion of salt and water from the body), drugs for the treatment of hypertension, and those affecting calcium and uric acid deposition in the kidney all have a place in the management of certain renal disorders. Administration of substances such as calcium, potassium, sodium, and bicarbonate is occasionally required. Surgery plays an important role when obstruction to any part of the urinary tract is present. When renal failure occurs, dietary modification becomes important. Hemodialysis or kidney transplantation become necessary when less than 5% of function remains and all reversible causes have been excluded; these treatments are very expensive, as well as physically and emotionally traumatic. Thus prevention of renal disease, rather than treatment of the end-stage situation, is a major focus of current research.

(*See also* Urinary and Genital Disorders.)

— *Nathan W. Levin, M.D.*

Lung Diseases

Pneumococcal pneumonia, caused by *Streptococcus pneumoniae* (pneumococcus), still ranks as a major cause of death—25,000 a year in the U.S.—despite the availability of effective antimicrobial drugs. Of the 83 types of pneumococci, 14 are known to cause at least 80% of the serious pneumococcal infections in the U.S. The Food and Drug Administration recently licensed for manufacture and distribution a polyvalent vaccine, combining antigens effective against these 14 types. The vaccine became available to physicians in February 1978.

The vaccine induces formation of antibodies in recipients over the age of two years, and immunization is recommended for those at special risk for pneumococcal disease (the elderly, particularly in closed populations; those with chronic lung, liver, heart, or kidney dysfunction, diabetes, or sickle-cell anemia; those who have had surgical removal of the spleen). Studies show that the vaccine confers long-term immunity without booster injections, with few local effects (brief swelling and pain at the injection site), and with no serious complications to date.

Further research is directed toward making an even more polyvalent vaccine protecting against greater than 80% of pneumococcal strains, as well as a vaccine to be effective in the infant age group. The emergence of pneumococcus strains that have developed resistance to antibiotics emphasizes the value of vaccine prophylaxis. Of interest and importance is the experience thus far that the pneumococcus infections that are prevented by vaccine are not replaced by infections due to other bacterial pathogens. (*See also* Infectious Diseases.)

Influenza

Influenza is the only disease in man that occurs simultaneously in populations throughout the world. Patterns of epidemics are influenced by a tendency of the influenza A virus to change its antigenic and virulence characteristics through genetic recombination at intervals of about a decade and to resurface in forms to which people are no longer immune. The annual visits of these uncontrolled viruses may lead to mild sporadic

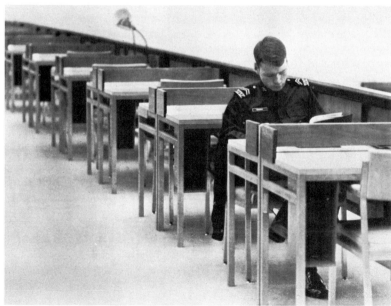

Epidemics of "Russian flu" early in 1978 struck especially hard at susceptible young people under the age of 25; the U.S. military academies were all hard hit, as this empty library evidences, as were colleges and military bases.

Wide World

epidemics or to global devastation. Thirty percent of people exposed to a new strain of influenza will be affected by it; it is estimated that influenza and its complications represent 25% of the economic costs of all respiratory illnesses.

Effective vaccines have been in use against influenza for over 20 years, but the immunity conferred is specific to a single strain and lasts only briefly (as opposed to the prolonged protection following an influenza infection). The vaccines require repeated modification as virus mutations appear. Furthermore, the degree of efficacy of these vaccines and the severity of reactions following their use are unpredictable. For these reasons the vaccines have not been widely accepted or used, and the annual winter menace has become a public, professional, and political concern. Despite the severity of the problem, national influenza policy has often been guided by little more than guesswork.

Early in the 1977–78 winter season an epidemic developed in the contiguous 48 United States, Hawaii, and Puerto Rico. Analysis of the infecting virus strains suggested that one-quarter resembled A/Victoria and three-quarters A/Texas. The Center for Disease Control in Atlanta, Ga., soon determined that deaths from these influenza strains exceeded the "epidemic threshold." Appropriate immunization, available from the 1976–77 winter, was recommended. In November the World Health Organization (WHO) international surveillance program identified other strains (epidemic in the Middle East and Far East) that resembled viruses not seen for more than 20 years. One strain, A/U.S.S.R., spread to the U.S. before a new specific vaccine could be developed. Initially sporadic, the infection soon became epidemic, mainly among students and personnel based at schools, military bases, and the United States service academies at Colorado Springs, Colo., West Point, N.Y., and Annapolis, Md. Because young people under 25 had no protective antibodies from outbreaks earlier in the century, they were the hardest hit. Despite the fact that the disease was capable of becoming epidemic, the second wave of A/U.S.S.R. influenza resulted in mild disease without mortality. Under the assumption that this strain—also called the "Russian flu"—will again arise during the 1978–79 winter, the virus was distributed for the development of a vaccine to be ready for testing by spring 1978.

Aside from the nonoutbreak of swine flu and the vaccine controversies of 1976, it is generally agreed that policy recommendations of the U.S. Public Health Service for handling influenza outbreaks have been sound and have resulted in reduced influenza morbidity and mortality. Unchanging consensus holds that (1) vaccination each autumn is wise for the elderly and for others with major chronic illnesses that are known to be at high risk for developing potentially fatal complica-

tions; (2) hospitalization for uncomplicated influenza is discouraged since it exposes the patient to hospital-acquired infections (which are more severe and resistant to therapy than those acquired elsewhere) and spreads influenza to the hospital's other patients; (3) the patient must inevitably endure three to ten days of influenza misery (which responds to measures no more complex than those advised in aspirin advertising), followed by an interval of fatigue and reduced resistance to secondary infections; and (4) the influenza patient who insists on further medical treatment often receives an injection of penicillin, a useless, expensive, and potentially harmful step, since penicillin is ineffective against viruses.

Current medical thinking recommends that the first available Russian flu vaccine go to people under the age of 25 who have medical disabilities that put them at high risk of serious harm from influenza. The first priority for a vaccine is usually given to those over 65 with chronic medical conditions, but this group is assumed to have had former exposure to this flu strain and thus is at least partially protected. Others argue that the fact that something closely resembling the Russian virus was present about two decades ago suggests that its immediate future circulation might be brief. Further complicating the issue is the view of other experts who expect a different virus to emerge and become the dominant type of influenza A throughout the world in 1979; an extraordinary feature of the natural history of an influenza virus is that the arrival of a new subtype appears to annihilate the old. It appears that only one variant exists at a time, while other noninfluenza viruses have subtypes and variants that continue to exist side by side.

In an effort to break the pattern of governmental stumbling from one flu crisis to another, on Feb. 23, 1978, Joseph A. Califano, Jr., secretary of health, education, and welfare, announced the first long-term national policy. Its goal is to aid state and local immunization programs, beginning in the fall of 1978, when trivalent vaccine will be available to protect against the Russian flu, A/Texas and the closely related A/Victoria, and B/Hong Kong. Pointing out the statistical safety of the vaccine—that one death occurs for every two million vaccinations while 20 die for each million cases of flu, and ten times that number from complicating pneumonia—federal planners hope to avoid the problems with liability for injury that marred the swine flu program. Questions of liability will be worked out between the states and the vaccine manufacturers, which is the current practice in state childhood immunization programs.

Studying the behavior of the flu epidemic in Houston, Texas, the Influenza Research Center reported in March 1978 that initial attack rates were highest in young children and that from this school group, the disease disseminated to the children's homes and to the adult population. Accordingly, the center recommended a new strategy for epidemic control emphasizing mass immunization of healthy children once surveillance has indicated that a virus has made a local appearance. Preschool children who have never been infected would seem to be a logical group to watch for the appearance of flu; this assumption, however, would require corroboration.

Another vital strategy would be the use of the antiviral drug amantadine during the immediate two weeks after immunization before full antibody protection has developed. Amantadine has not been widely used or recommended for the prophylaxis against or treatment of influenza. Research has shown, however, that the drug prevents virus uptake into human cells and is 50–70% effective in preventing clinical influenza. Given as therapy within the first two days of the illness, the agent can shorten illness and diminish the severity of symptoms. Effective prophylactic use would require continuous administration of amantadine throughout the entire season of potential exposure to influenza viruses, which would be far more expensive than alternate control measures. Amantadine holds the advantages of having effect against all existing and newly emerging influenza strains and of being available during the inevitable lags while new commercial vaccines are produced. Its safety for mass use, however, has not been established. (*See also* Infectious Diseases Special Report: Antiviral Drugs.)

Lung cancer

The first successful removal of an entire lung for cancer was performed by Evarts Graham in 1933, shortly before the case rate for lung cancer began its explosive rise. During the following four decades the incidence of lung cancer has increased far more than that of any other malignant tumor, the age-adjusted death rate per 100,000 population rising 106% in men and 70% in women. Lung cancer is now the most common malignancy (excluding skin) in men, and for the two sexes combined no tumor has a higher mortality rate. Although still up to six times more frequent in men, a sharply increased incidence of lung cancer in women during the past decade is alarming and is not fully explained by the unusual incidence of cigarette smoking in women.

A growing number of carcinogenic substances—asbestos, arsenic, chromate, nickel, uranium, bis(chloromethyl)ether, benzpyrene, cadmium—are being identified as hazards not only for those who are exposed through their occupations but as atmospheric contaminants of industrialized cities. The greatest risk, however, results from the personal air pollution of inhaled cigarette smoke; even the notorious tenfold higher incidence of lung cancer among asbestos workers requires the synergistic contribution of cigarette smoking —the combination of the two contaminants produces

results much more severe than the sum of the two taken separately.

Although surgery remains the best available form of therapy for lung cancer, only a third of patients qualifying for "curative resection" survive five years, and less than 10% of all patients with established lung cancer are alive five years after diagnosis. It is estimated that in 1978 nearly 90,000 people will die of lung cancer in the United States.

How can the grim trend be checked? Fortunately, the apathetic view that *symptomatic* lung cancer means already advanced disease (and that surgery is pointless) is being opposed by a more aggressive attack on the disease through earlier diagnosis and more effective regimens of therapy.

Earlier diagnosis. Categories of high-risk individuals have been defined, and screening programs attempt to follow such candidates from the healthy and asymptomatic state. Earlier diagnosis of lung cancer is now possible through several current techniques.

1. The flexible fiberoptic bronchoscope is thinner than the traditional rigid instrument. With the patient comfortably seated, it is easily maneuvered into small and distant airways, allowing visualization of the inner recesses of the lungs as well as collection of tumor tissue, brushings, and washings (noninvasive biopsies). Even tumors invisible on chest X-rays can be located by the fiberoptic bronchoscope.

2. Refinements in obtaining or inducing sputum and in examination of expectorated lung cells allow identification of cancers and in most instances the exact tissue type of cancer. (*See also* Cancer.)

3. Hormones and hormone precursors may be abnormally produced by lung cancers and detected by radioimmunoassay in the circulating blood. Combined with other information, these findings enhance the likelihood of proper diagnosis.

4. Noninvasive computerized axial tomography (CAT-scanning) represents the most important innovative development in diagnostic radiology since the introduction of image amplification. One of its major roles is in locating tumors of the lungs. The resolution of X-ray beams with the aid of a computer, obtained within a scanning time of seconds (eliminating the distortions caused by respiratory motion), detects in contrast image elements too small to be discerned by conventional X-ray techniques. It can help distinguish benign from malignant tumors and tumors from inflammation or collections of fluid, and it can look into traditionally "silent" recesses of the lungs.

Regimens for therapy. Treatment of lung cancer includes surgery, radiation, and chemotherapy, used individually or in combination. The combined approach has been refined and in given situations and with recent innovations is showing encouraging clinical results.

1. Total pneumonectomy, or surgical removal of an

Courtesy, Johns-Manville Corporation; photograph, *Medical World News*

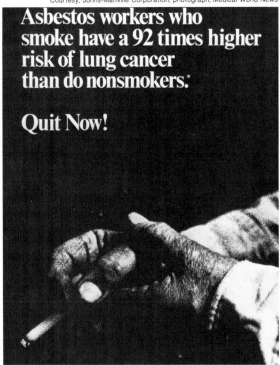

Asbestos workers who smoke have a 92 times higher risk of lung cancer than do nonsmokers.*

Quit Now!

The Johns-Manville Corporation banned smoking in all of its U.S. and Canadian asbestos plants after a poster campaign warning workers of the dangerous synergistic health threat they faced.

entire lung, for all "resectable" cancers is no longer considered essential. The trend toward removal of a single lobe of a lung, or in chosen cases individual segments of a lobe, has led to equivalent survivals along with a better quality of life for those whose pulmonary function has already been compromised by smoking or occupational damage. In cases of small tumors in peripheral locations that are detected early and removed promptly, the patients appear to do well, with a high cure rate and minimal loss of ventilating tissue.

2. Investigations hold promise that within special guidelines some patients may be spared postoperative radiation ("to kill the last remaining cancer cell") and its added pulmonary damage. For example, if a radioimmunoassay shows that an elevated level of abnormal hormonal or other secretion has cleared from circulating blood after surgery, it seems possible that resection has been curative since it is known that local and distant metastatic deposits secrete the same substances as the parent tumor.

3. Small cell (oat cell) carcinoma of the lung, which accounts for about 20% of all lung cancers, is almost never able to be cured by surgery because of its early spread to distant sites. Studies now in progress indicate that a bold regimen using chemotherapy (generally three drugs given sequentially) simultaneous with radiation of the primary tumor and brain (whether or not cerebral metastases are apparent) leads to complete or partial response in up to 75% of patients and over one year disease-free survival in one-third of patients. Toxicity from the combined treatments is no greater than that expected from each component given separately.

4. Pancoast's tumor, one filling the upper portion of the lung cavity of one side of the chest and frequently involving contiguous bone, is now treated with radiotherapy before radical surgery is undertaken, and one-third of such patients have survived five years.

5. Promising therapeutic innovations still under trial include: (a) routine elective radiotherapy of high-risk organs (liver, brain, bone) to destroy possible early metastases, or proliferating cancerous growths; (b) radiosensitization of the tumor by enriching its oxygenation or by hyperthermia (high body or tumor temperature), thus augmenting the effectiveness of the X-ray therapy; (c) the use, in addition to conventional X-rays and gamma rays, of high-energy subatomic nuclear particles, which, although more hazardous and expensive, are more powerfully destructive of tumor cells; (d) implantation of radioactive material into the tumor mass itself; and (e) enhancement of the patient's own biologic defenses by activating the body's immune system to attack the invading cancer cells while other therapeutic measures are being undertaken.

Tuberculosis

Because tuberculosis can now be managed with medication, an emphasis on the diminished overall importance of the disease overlooks the tenacity of the problem among several special groups: the alcoholic and skid-row derelict, the drug addict, residents of overcrowded ghettos, and people with personality disorders. A common denominator among all these groups is noncompliance with a prolonged therapy program—it is simply very difficult to get such patients to follow doctors' orders. Throughout the United States sanatoriums have been closed and tuberculosis patients rechanneled to private physicians, general hospitals, and clinics for early ambulatory care. The incidence of new infections in inner-city areas has failed to show an appreciable decline over a ten-year period, whereas the rest of the country has shown a 60% drop. In the South End of Boston, in New Jersey's Newark, and in Maryland's Baltimore at least one new case of tuberculosis is discovered every week. About half of these patients attend follow-up clinics only erratically despite adequate retrieval efforts by departments of public health. The routine case of tuberculosis can be successfully managed on a voluntary outpatient basis with intermittent or short-course drug regimens. However, under some circumstances it may be necessary, for the public good, to temporarily detain patients capable of spreading the infection. Many clinics employ skilled and strongly motivated teams resourceful at tracking down the recidivist patient, but even then the patient cannot be forced to continue treatment after the tubercle bacillus is no longer present in his sputum (although risk of relapse is still high). Irresponsible persons may thus maintain in the community a reservoir of contagion that is very difficult to eradicate.

In order to diminish this public health problem and to achieve a faster rate of decline in tuberculosis incidence than the current 5% per year, many public health officials favor stronger legal means for imposing, when necessary, fully supervised chemotherapy during six-month hospital confinement. Hospitalization would thereby be mandatory until the patient is disease-free and no longer a danger to the community.

Among compliant individuals the rationale for ambulatory treatment with an early return to family and employment rests on the finding that following a few days to three weeks of effective chemotherapy (at least two drugs taken daily) the infected individual is no longer contagious, although tubercle bacilli may remain in his sputum for weeks or months. Clearly, the risk of transmission applies to those exposed to the patient before the disease has been diagnosed. Therapy rapidly biologically attenuates the tubercle bacillus so that it is no longer strong enough to cause infection; this occurs long before the organism is totally killed and eliminated from the lungs.

Years of experience have now established that

Campaigns against spitting or smoking in public places have faced an uphill battle since the turn of the century.

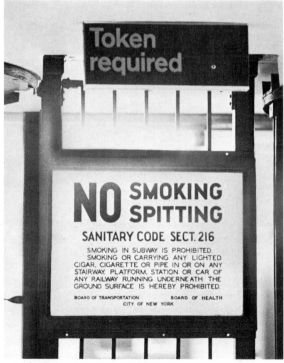

Wagner International Photos Inc.

among normal individuals without evidence of disease but at high risk of developing active tuberculosis (those who have reacted positively to tuberculin skin tests, particularly those known to have developed the reaction recently and who in addition have such debilitating conditions as diabetes, immunosuppression, silicosis, or a history of gastrectomy), the probability of future tuberculous illness becomes virtually nil following a regimen of oral isoniazid medication daily for one year. This program carries, in turn, its own risk of liver damage, which, however, is mild and reversible if recognized early. Further, liver damage is limited to only the 12 months of drug ingestion, while the threat of tuberculosis is life-long, and, in high-risk patients, liver damage is statistically less probable than developing tuberculosis. This is the only circumstance in which an antituberculous drug is used singly, and no drug other than isoniazid can be used.

Among the most welcome prospects in the treatment of tuberculosis is the probability of reducing the duration of therapy below the traditional 18 to 24 months. Studies, first in England and now in the United States, indicate that a mere six months of two or three drugs daily (in regimens including isoniazid or rifampin or both) achieves excellent results. Patients followed up for more than three years, however, are showing a small but unacceptable relapse rate. At this time it seems predictable that no more than 12 months of treatment will be necessary for optimal effect, and that nine or ten months may suffice.

Aspirin and pulmonary thromboembolism

The most common, serious, and potentially fatal postoperative pulmonary complication is embolization to the lungs of blood clots formed in deep veins. Using total hip replacement in people over 40 as an example of a surgical procedure at particularly high risk for postoperative thromboembolism, a group in Boston has demonstrated reduction of this complication from 45% in patients on placebo to 25% among those receiving 600 mg of aspirin (a standard dose) twice daily. An unanticipated and unexplained finding of the test was the relative lack of protection against thrombi in women (most of whom were postmenopausal and none on contraceptive medication).

The beneficial prophylactic effect of aspirin may result from its ability to interfere with the initial stages of blood clotting by reducing the tendency for circulating platelets to aggregate and to adhere to intravascular surfaces. Although for years clinicians have observed prolongation of bleeding time after ingestion of aspirin, the complex mechanisms by which this common household medication interferes with platelet function and acts as an antithrombotic (and anti-inflammatory) agent is not fully understood. (*See also* Heart and Blood Vessels.)

— L. Fred Ayvazian, M.D.

261

Special Report:

Update on Legionnaires' Disease

by L. Fred Ayvazian, M.D.

Had an earlier epidemic in Philadelphia gained notoriety, and had the puzzle then been solved, it might have been labeled "Odd Fellows' disease," and the hotel might have been closed in 1974. But two years later the explosive midsummer clustering of 182 pneumonias became a hot news item, and the syndrome was dubbed Legionnaires' disease even before scientists had a clue to its cause. Such is the power of the media: the hotel was soon shunned, and tourist lines disappeared from the Liberty Bell. Headlines reported first the grim series of 29 deaths and ultimately the emptying of the Bellevue-Stratford itself; the city's most distinguished hotel concealed an undetected and presumably uneradicated reservoir of the agent responsible for at least two outbreaks of a devastating respiratory condition.

An estimated 4,500 Legionnaires met in Philadelphia between July 21 and 24, 1976. On August 2 the Veterans Administration Clinic reported the first deaths from an acute febrile illness occurring among those who had attended the convention.

The nation had been warned to expect swine influenza, so the first reaction to the epidemic was that flu had struck the Pennsylvania American Legionnaires gathered at their 58th annual convention. The federal Center for Disease Control (CDC) in Atlanta, Ga., in what was to become the largest and perhaps most challenging investigation in its history, dispatched epidemiologists to work with local health officials in an attempt to confirm the exact nature of the illness. Within days the probability of influenza dimmed, and the greater magnitude of the problem became apparent.

The typical illness began seven days following the Legionnaire's arrival at the hotel and three days after he had returned home. First symptoms were malaise and headache and, within hours, high fever, often accompanied by chills. Cough, shortness of breath, pleurisy-like pain, and abdominal distress were common; about a fifth of those stricken became obtunded (showed some mental confusion). Attack rate increased with age and was higher in men than in women and among individuals with pre-existing chronic conditions such as emphysema and heart disease. As with a number of pulmonary afflictions, incidence was somewhat higher among smokers.

Nonspecific abnormalities were found in laboratory testing of blood and urine. Over 90% of chest X-rays showed infiltrations ranging from small patchy areas to widespread involvement of both lungs; some, additionally, showed fluid in the normally empty space between the lining of the lungs (pleura) and the chest wall, while others mimicked the patterns of relatively common viral and mycoplasma pneumonias, pulmonary edema (characterized by excess fluid within the pulmonary tissues), and even acute miliary tuberculosis. Many patients required treatment with oxygen or the support of mechanical ventilators; an alarming number developed irreversible shock. Improvement in most and death in 16% occurred usually at seven to ten days of illness. Outcome seemed favorably influenced by treatment with erythromycin or tetracycline but not with other antibiotic drugs. The intervals between probable time of exposure and onset of symptoms suggested an incubation period of two to ten days. The shape of the epidemic curve implied a common-source exposure (centering in the hotel lobby and extending to the sidewalk in front of the building), which began on July 22 and had ended by August 9.

Only primary illnesses were seen, with no secondary transmission to hotel roommates nor to members of the Legionnaires' families. This left open both the source of the etiologic agent and the question of vector: what mode, if not person-to-person? In the dramaturgy of collected data was the item that the entire supply of ice at the Bellevue-Stratford had been depleted within the first hour, but final interview and questionnaire analyses indicated no association between illness and use of ice, water, alcohol, or food, nor did facts implicate the air-conditioning system or contact with souvenirs, other fomites (inanimate objects such as clothing, dishes, books, etc. that may transmit infectious disease) pigeons, rodents, or insects.

To those closest to the investigation a cause other than infection seemed unlikely, but many features did not fit known patterns. Pus, the hallmark of acute pneumonia, was not expectorated; indeed, with most patients coughing was unproductive of sputum. The absence of bacteria in cultures and in diseased human lungs was distressing. Conventional tissue stains showed no bacteria in sick guinea pigs previously inoculated with human autopsy-lung preparations. Standard habits in culturing and histologic examination seemed not to apply. An etiologic participation by fungi or viruses, mycoplasmas, chlamydiae, and rickettsiae

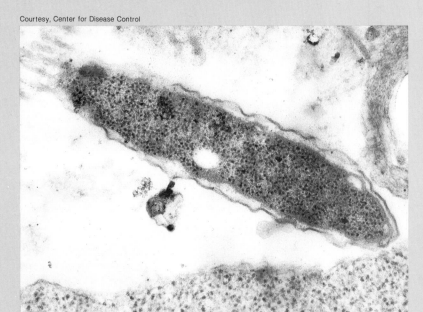

In 1977 the organism responsible for the outbreaks of Legionnaires' disease was isolated by researchers. Sporadic outbreaks have continued to occur.

(all parasitic microorganisms that can cause disease in man), even toxins, poisons, metals, and gases, could not be verified by traditional tests. Following months of study under the scrutiny of public concern and long after the outbreak had ended, little more than the clinical picture and the epidemic pattern were known. Many despaired that the problem would ever be solved.

The breakthrough came in December 1976 when a rickettsiologist (one of the Atlanta team of scientists), reviewing his slides, gave new attention to a small bacterium that had appeared with suspicious consistency in the tissues of guinea pigs inoculated with diseased human tissue four months earlier. This organism could not be cultivated and had been dismissed as an extraneous, inconsequential nonpathogen, such contaminants being frequently encountered in attempts to isolate rickettsiae. Desperate to follow all leads, however, the microbiologists used alternate and less orthodox methods in a renewed attempt to coax this organism's growth.

Among other ventures, spleen tissue from the suspect guinea pigs, stored at −70° C since initial collection, was thawed and inoculated into embryonated eggs. The embryos died within a week and were found to teem with bacteria, which agreed to grow on enriched media not normally used for primary bacterial culturing. The organism was a bacillus, which was negative on gram stain. The growth was slow, requiring more than the two-day interval following which preparations for bacterial diagnosis usually are discarded. The organism proved to be fastidious, preferring moisture, and flourishing optimally between the narrow pH range of 6.9 to 7.0.

Serum from patients convalescent from the disease was mixed with the organism found in the eggs, and a visible reaction indicated that antibodies specific for the agent were present in circulating blood. More telling was the finding that paired specimens drawn weeks apart showed the antigen-antibody reaction at higher dilution (fourfold or greater) in the second serum when compared with the first. This indicated that the individual with the positive serum reaction had recently recovered from the disease caused by the test organism; the reaction was also positive using serum from fatal cases. Over 90% of the Legionnaires' tests were positive; control samples from nonsuspect cases did not react. This indicated that the bacterium isolated from the eggs was in fact the etiologic agent of Legionnaires' disease. This remarkable organism, never before identified as a cause of human illness, and the disease it caused were finally officially christened "Legionnaires'" with the sanctioned agreement of the American Legion.

During this investigation the CDC learned of the earlier convention of the Independent Order of Odd Fellows at the Bellevue-Stratford Hotel in September 1974. A survey showed the former attack rate, incubation period, and clinical features were consistent with what was known as Legionnaires' disease, and of 392 Odd Fellows responding to a questionnaire 11 likely cases were identified. Serum from this group showed antibodies to the Legionnaires' bacterium, while 19 Odd Fellows who were not ill showed no seroconversion, or development of antibodies in response to the serum. Ultimately, 21 cases and three fatalities were identified, and it was also found that among Bellevue-Stratford personnel who were employed during both attacks a significant percentage showed elevated circulating concentrations of Legionnaires' antibody. Repeated testing showed no change in these levels, suggesting an old rather than a recent infection.

Other former epidemics of unexplained illness oc-

263

curred in July 1965 at St. Elizabeths Hospital in Washington, D.C. (94 cases, 16 deaths), and in July 1968 in Pontiac, Mich. (144 cases, no deaths). Blood samples from both of these outbreaks had been stored at the CDC and now, on thawing and testing, Legionnaires' seropositivity was demonstrated.

In July 1973, 252 vacationers from Scotland stayed at the same hotel in Benidorm, Spain; 10 developed what seemed to be pneumonia and, of these, 3 died. One blood specimen retained since that time was sent to the CDC in 1977 and proved to contain specific antibodies against the Legionnaires' bacillus. In 1977 another Scottish vacationer died of a pneumonia-like illness at the same hotel in Spain; tissue and serum sent to Atlanta again proved to be diagnostically positive for Legionnaires'.

In March 1977 patients were transferred into a new hospital building in Los Angeles before final construction had been completed, and during the next few months over 25 cases of pneumonia were shown to be due to the Legionnaires' organism. While pleurisy was a minor feature of the Philadelphia epidemic, almost half of the Los Angeles patients reported pleural pain, and of these two-thirds developed significant volumes of fluid around the lungs. Headache and muscle pain were common, and disorientation accompanied fevers over 105° F. Two untreated patients died; those treated with erythromycin showed dramatic improvement in two days or less.

New cases continued in patients and employees at this hospital into 1978. Among these were 6 of 11 patients who had undergone renal transplantation (and who were under immunosuppression therapy as a safeguard against organ rejection), and one of these six died. Because of this experience, the hospital announced in May 1978 that it was discontinuing its renal transplantation program until the risk of further infection had passed or a common source from which the patients could be isolated was found.

Also in 1977 small clusters of proven cases were identified in Tennessee, Vermont, Ohio, and Nottingham, England, and in Indiana in early 1978, with mortalities ranging from 10 to 26%. Apart from these epidemics, which tended to take place in the summer months, the Legionnaires' organism seems to have a low-level endemic capability throughout the year. It has a mortality of over 20% if the sporadic infection is not diagnosed early and treated promptly. Laboratory studies show that the organism is susceptible to treatment not only with erythromycin and tetracycline but also with rifampin, a drug used almost exclusively (and always with a "companion" drug) in the treatment of tuberculosis.

What, then, is the status of the Legionnaires' puzzle? In Philadelphia the epidemic was not a city-wide problem but limited to only one of the hotels used by the convention; this has remained a consistent pattern. Sporadic cases occur as isolated events and have not been responsible for secondary neighboring infections. The causative bacterium is unlike any previously encountered in medical bacteriology; DNA studies of its gene structure have not yet found a near relative. The organism has been around for a long time, and it is likely that its breeding place is in nature rather than in the human population.

While the reservoir for the bacillus may be in soil, excavation, construction, vigorous cleaning of carpeting and drapery, or heavy foot traffic may also be inciting activities. It is possible that no true "vector" exists but that infection is a factor of concentration and size of mobilized infective matter. The bacteria are probably airborne and inhaled. The lack of human-to-human transmission may reflect the pathology of the disease, which is characterized by pneumonia and not bronchitis; *i.e.*, organisms contained within monocytes and leukocytes (nucleated white blood cells) in the most peripheral alveolar sacs (smallest air spaces of the lungs) without free flow into the smaller or large airways. The cough, judging from tissue and sputum studies, does not dislodge bacteria and is contagion-free. One thing is certain: among untreated cases, the Legionnaires' fatality rate is high.

The question has been raised of whether a live attenuated Legionnaires' vaccine can be developed to protect the high-risk population from each year's potentially fatal respiratory illnesses that result from Legionnaires' infection, since etiological studies of routine respiratory problems, particularly during high-incidence seasons, are not done beyond conventional "sputum cultures for pathogens." However, it is known that two years following the Odd Fellows epidemic, the Philadelphia hotel employees showed stable levels of serum antibody, which apparently protected them against repeat infections. Judging further from the Michigan epidemic, a mild form of infection with the characteristics of bacterial attenuation (weakening) *can* occur. Such infections involve short incubation, no pneumonia, no deaths—characteristics of the low-virulent bacterial forms from which vaccines are commercially produced.

However, the most dramatic victim in this still-unfinished saga may be the hotel itself. The Bellevue-Stratford had been constructed in 1904 at a cost of $3 million; today, no amount of money could recruit artisans suitably skilled to refashion its style and majesty. It is reported that rehabilitation slated for the structure will be monitored by CDC epidemiologists. But should in the future pneumonia reappear on the premises, it will not escape publicity, and total razing of the historic structure might be the final result.

Medical Ethics

The continuing debate over abortion

Three U.S. Supreme Court decisions in June 1977 made it clear that the debate over the ethics of abortion was far from over. In 1973 the court ruled that a state could not override a woman's right, with qualifications, to an abortion; some thought that was the end of the abortion controversy. The more recent decisions reveal that the 1973 ruling only shifted the ground of the debate. In two recent decisions the court ruled that neither the Constitution nor federal law requires a state participating in Medicaid programs to pay for nontherapeutic abortions even if it pays for childbirth. The court also ruled that public hospitals are not required to perform abortions. Since these rulings about two-thirds of the states have decided not to pay for abortions through their Medicaid programs. The process of reassessing the public stance on abortion has led virtually every state legislature into complex political and ethical maneuvering; in addition, the budget for all of the Department of Health, Education, and Welfare was held up for two months at the end of 1977 over the controversy.

The argument from the critics of the new Supreme Court decisions is that the court has in effect denied the right to have an abortion to the woman who cannot afford to pay for the procedure even though she would have the right if she had the resources to get one. Stories of women being driven into illegal and unsafe back-alley abortion mills and of injury and death have appeared. On the other side opponents of abortion are claiming that they have a right not to have their taxes used for a procedure they consider immoral.

Three themes—all crucial for medical ethics at the end of the 1970s—emerge from the dispute. Does the individual right to privacy in choosing a course of action imply a right to claim the state's help in acquiring the resources needed if one chooses to act? Is a woman entitled to an abortion at state expense if she has the liberty to have an abortion without the state's actively interfering? Justice Lewis Powell, writing for the majority of the court in *Maher* v. *Roe*, claims that the 1973 decision gave a woman a qualified constitutionally protected right to make a decision to terminate her pregnancy. He claims that a state that does not pay for abortions "places no obstacles—absolute or otherwise—in the pregnant woman's path to an abortion. . . . she continues as before [Medicaid] to be dependent on private sources for the services she desires."

The older notion that a right is merely a liberty to be free from outside constraints, however, is currently being challenged by a newer notion that rights are really entitlements—that if citizens have a right to education or housing or food or medical services such as abortion, then someone has an obligation to provide the resources needed. The debate is much more basic to the definition of the obligations of society than the current controversy.

Second, the abortion decisions are forcing us to think more about what makes an action a medical procedure and whether it is important that it be called a medical procedure. The Supreme Court decisions emphasize that the state need not pay for abortions under Medicaid if the abortion is nontherapeutic, that is, if it is not "medically necessary" or "medically indicated." But some are asking why it is that medically indicated abortions get absolute priority over those that women need or want for other reasons. How necessary to the woman's health must the abortion be before it is covered? Considerations of these issues led to a five-month stalemate in Congress late in 1977. The House wanted to prohibit federal financing of abortion unless the woman's life was in danger, while the Senate favored a more liberal policy. Congress finally agreed that federal funds could be used in three circumstances: (1) when the mother's life would be endangered; (2) when severe and long-lasting physical damage, in the judgment of two physicians, would result from her giving birth; or (3) when such "medical procedures" were considered necessary for the victims of rape or incest, provided the crime had been reported promptly. The criteria are strikingly similar to those used in the 1960s to decide which abortions were legal. Today what was once considered a liberty has become an entitlement. This may once again lead women and physicians to claim either rape or risk of severe and long-lasting physical damage to health as a basis for getting abortions paid for by Medicaid. Both defenders and critics of abortion are still left with the question of why abortions for rape and risk to physical health require federal support, but not those for mental, social, or familial reasons. And why is abortion considered a medical intervention at all rather than a welfare support measure like housing or food subsidies? What is at stake is not merely the national abortion policy but our basic understanding of the meaning of health.

The third issue that is becoming increasingly clear is that the ethics of abortion is linked to the ethics of other procedures that generate controversy of their own. Genetic screening and prenatal diagnosis of genetic disease have come into their own in the last few years. It is now possible to detect the presence of dozens of genetic diseases in fetuses early in pregnancy. Once that diagnosis is made, however, for virtually all of these diseases the only intervention that is possible is abortion. A number of prenatal tests are available: blood tests of the pregnant woman, photographic examination of the fetus using sound waves, and amniocentesis (a procedure in which a sample of the fluid surrounding the fetus is withdrawn and studied). Amniocentesis was the subject of a study at the National Institutes of Health and was found, by their standards, to be safe.

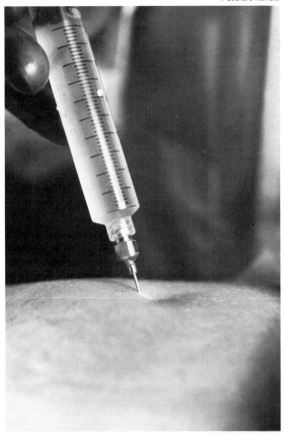

The ethical aspects of amniocentesis for genetic screening continue to be debated. In many cases of detected genetic disorders, abortion is the only alternative to the birth of a damaged child.

Some have challenged the ethics of these prenatal tests in spite of these findings. For one thing, some see the development of these techniques as unethical experimenting on human subjects. Even if the techniques were developed to the point that they were considered no longer experimental, some argue that interventions of this sort are inherently wrong—they are tampering with natural processes that ought to be left alone. Furthermore, safety is always a relative thing. Judgments about safety should depend not only on how serious the possible harms are likely to be but also on how advantageous the benefits are.

The most heated arguments surround the uses of the information gained by the prenatal diagnosis. If abortion is the only practical outcome, the ethics of prenatal diagnosis is contingent upon the ethics of abortion. Some argue that there are other real uses: a couple who are going to have a child with Down's syndrome may be able to prepare better for the change that will take place in their lives, even if they decide not to abort. The main use today of the information, however, is to plan an abortion during the time when abortion is legal and relatively safe.

Pressures have been exerted on the federal government and voluntary organizations such as the National Foundation-March of Dimes to withdraw their support from prenatal diagnosis in cases in which that diagnosis is linked to abortion. In some areas government agencies or private insurers are finding themselves in the strange position of paying for the rather expensive prenatal diagnoses (about $350 for an amniocentesis) but refusing to pay for the abortion that is the most common use of the information generated.

The cost-benefit quandary

The abortion controversies are tied in with a larger debate over the costs of health care. One reason for opposing Medicaid funding of abortion is the fear that the costs of the Medicaid program are getting out of hand. On the other hand, defenders claim that abortion and genetic screening programs are "cost-effective," *i.e.,* that they save more money than they cost. They save money in welfare costs and, at least in the cases of prenatal diagnosis, very expensive treatment regimens, sometimes requiring a lifetime.

But is it ethical to evaluate medical programs on the basis of costs? It seems crass to calculate the economic advantages of prenatal diagnosis and abortion. It is clear, however, that the cost of health care is becoming a major issue for society. The problems raised by these two interventions signal a much larger controversy over efforts to control health costs in general. We have just begun to explore the ethics of health planning and health cost containment efforts. A national conference was held recently in Washington, D.C., on value problems in policymaking in health resource allocation. Another conference sponsored by an agency of the federal government was devoted explicitly to ethical problems of the current cost containment effort.

While a few years ago the pressure was to increase the quality and accessibility of medical care, today the mood has shifted so that cost control is a major theme. Yet these efforts to control costs are raising serious ethical issues as well—they all require some judgment about how valuable a particular kind of medical care is. This requires not only medical facts but very subjective judgments about the value of alleviating depression in the psychiatric patient, "curing" pneumonia in a 90-year-old terminal cancer patient, eliminating the pain of childbirth with anesthesia, and treating lung cancer in those who choose to smoke. It also requires a determination of the costs or harms of such interventions. Is being unconscious when one's child is born a benefit or a harm? How much benefit is high-risk surgery if it cures some while making others more miserable? We are not even sure how to distinguish a benefit from a harm, much less a needed treatment from one that is merely desired or demanded. Yet as we move to the situation where more and more medical care is paid for by governmental or other third-party payers, we shall have to be able to make such distinctions.

Even if we can decide the relative benefits and harms of alternative health policies, it is not obvious that we should immediately choose the most efficient, the most cost-effective alternative. For one thing, the most efficient policy may not be the most fair. If it turns out that concentrating health resources on the poor and disenfranchised, the rural and urban groups who do not have adequate access to medical care, is also the most efficient way of improving national health statistics, then there may be little *ethical* conflict. (Political problems may still be great, of course.) In some cases, however, it may turn out that the most efficient ways of improving our national health statistics are also those that help groups who are relatively well-off. This will be true especially in cases where one emphasizes the economic benefits of keeping people healthy. Since a wealthy person loses more income when he is sick than a poor person, some of the calculations have led to the conclusion that it is economically more efficient to provide certain health interventions for those who are relatively well off. It is not at all clear, however, that that would be the most fair thing to do.

Another problem is the conflict between efficiency and freedom. The more we learn about what causes disease and what keeps people healthy, the more it becomes clear that life-style choices and voluntary behavior are crucial. When we did not know what caused lung cancer, it made sense to assume that the sick person was not responsible in any way for his illness. Now we are not so sure. Not only cancer but especially sports injuries, heart disease, medical problems related to being overweight and out of shape, and many other medical problems can be seen as having a voluntary component.

The easiest way to improve the national health statistics might be massive constraints on voluntary behavior. Within the past year government officials have considered plans to refuse to hire fire fighters who smoke. They proposed this on the grounds that these employees unfairly increase the cost of group health insurance. They are examining other ways to control behavior that increases health costs or to pass along the extra health costs to the individuals who engage in such behavior. Yet this efficient system would sacrifice the freedom we cherish. Many of the medical ethical questions once thought to be matters to be resolved between the doctor and his patient inherently intertwine with more social ethical questions of justice, freedom, efficiency, and social responsibility.

The decision to die

Another question that was once a very personal matter to be left to the physician, the patient, and his family is the decision about the stopping of medical treatment. At the beginning of 1977 California became the first state in the Union to pass a "natural death act." It

permitted individuals in that state to sign a document specifying that they would not want medical treatment under certain specified conditions. For treatment to be stopped the individual has to be terminally ill (death will inevitably result regardless of the application of life-sustaining procedures), and death has to be imminent. Even then the instructions to refuse treatment are not binding unless the person was terminally ill at least 14 days before the document was completed. Thus while some have criticized the legislation as the opening wedge toward tolerance of active mercy killing (euthanasia), others have argued that it permits nothing that was not already legal and, in fact, implies that a document written before one is terminally ill would not be binding on physicians. Since then a number of other states, including Idaho, Arkansas, New Mexico, Nevada, Oregon, Texas, and North Carolina, have passed similar legislation. None of the bills passed or actively under consideration would permit active mercy killing; none with a serious possibility of passage would give final authority to physicians to decide what ought to be done. The lesson of the Karen Quinlan case was that regardless of who should have final authority in the tragic cases where the patient cannot be his own agent, the physician cannot have complete authority.

In November 1977 the Massachusetts Supreme Court issued the most important opinion in this issue since Karen Quinlan's father was permitted to be her guardian for purposes of deciding whether to remove his daughter from a respirator. The Massachusetts court put in writing an affirmation of a lower court's 1976 recommendation that physicians could stop treatment on Joseph Saikewicz. Saikewicz, then 67, was a severely retarded, long-term resident of a state school who was suffering from incurable leukemia. The treatments being considered offered little hope and would be very disturbing to the man, who would not be able to understand their purpose. The high court, not unexpectedly, held that the cessation of treatment had been permissible. The controversial part of the case has turned out to be a statement in the opinion that the court should retain ultimate decision-making responsibility in such cases of incompetent patients. The court rejected the idea that attending physicians should have the final authority, much as the Quinlan decision did. It also ruled out leaving the matter in the hands of hospital "ethics committees." The controversial aspect of the Massachusetts decision is the claim that the patient's guardian and family should never be entrusted with the final decision about the course of treatment. Never before had there been any presumption that the court would have to review every decision and that the family could never play a decisive role. In fact, in Arkansas and New Mexico the family is given a definitive role by the laws that had been passed during the year. What remains unsettled is whether the courts in Massachusetts and elsewhere will really begin insisting on reviewing every such case and if so, how much weight they will give to the family and other potential guardians in deciding what the patient would want or what is fitting for patients who have never been able to make such decisions themselves.

A special instance of determining the right to refuse treatment occurred at the Los Angeles County-University of Southern California Medical Center burn unit. Bruce Zawacki, head of the burn unit, revealed that in a two-year period 24 patients were admitted to the burn unit who had been so severely burned that their survival would have been unprecedented—no other person with comparable burns had ever survived. These patients, who remained lucid and relatively pain-free for a few hours after their injury, were told of their situation in a compassionate but straightforward way. They were then given the choice of going ahead with the usual regimen of treatment or of receiving only pain medication and intravenous fluids until they died. Most patients chose the latter course; all ultimately died, including those who chose intensive treatment. In these instances the patients were fully rational and made a decision without the aid of relatives or other advisers.
— *Robert M. Veatch, Ph.D.*

Mental Health

Since the end of World War II biomedical knowledge has accumulated at a prodigious rate, and new, improved diagnostic and treatment procedures have resulted. Physicians can now cure, or at least control, human suffering and disabilities that were beyond their reach two decades ago. Frequently, however, technological innovations and modern breakthroughs, such as organ transplants, renal dialysis, open heart surgery, and vastly improved life-prolonging support systems, have prompted serious psychosocial responses and raised many ethical issues among the lay and medical populace alike. Consequently, physicians have had to face new therapeutic problems—particularly concern with a patient's mental health—that they have felt ill prepared to manage.

The biomedical knowledge explosion seemed to be leading modern medicine at an ever increasing rate toward a dehumanizing preoccupation with the specific parts of patients' bodies. Medical graduates recently completing their specialty training appear not to understand that patients are first and foremost human beings who also happen to have some incapacitating pathology. Thus over the last decade, in spite of the many improvements in the quality of medical care, patients have expressed a growing disenchantment with medical care that they have found to be very expensive, difficult to comprehend, inconveniently superspecialized, and highly impersonal. The social, cultural, and political changes of the 1960s as well as the various human rights movements were instrumental in

raising the health care consciousness of the patient/consumer. People began asking to be actively informed of and involved in the decision making about their health care. Patients, their families, and the community at large began to demand physicians who could deal not only with physical ailments but also with social, personal, economic, and human needs.

The changing medical curriculum

Traditionally the process of selecting applicants for medical school has favored those applicants with demonstrated competence and interest in the physical and biological sciences; those with a strong background in the humanities were very often screened out. Without downgrading the significance of the basic sciences in the medical curriculum, health care providers increasingly realized that students sorely needed to learn how to blend humanism with modern scientific health care. Medical school administrators and educators responded to these pressures by introducing into the medical curriculum occasional courses in the behavioral sciences, human sexuality, and medical ethics.

It was generally conceded that the long-lost skills of the "country doctor"—caring, understanding, and willingness to listen to the patient—had to be reintroduced into the current medical education. Fortunately there was now more scientific information on which to base the teaching of these revalued skills. In the previous two decades "soft data" scientists had begun to seriously investigate and accumulate information on the complex interrelations between life-style, incidence of illness, ability to maintain good health, and the general rhythms of the human cycle.

In 1970 the National Institute of Child Health and Human Development of the U.S. Department of Health, Education, and Welfare invited a distinguished group of medical educators, behavioral scientists, and medical students to meet in a series of four conferences to define what constitutes a "good doctor." The participants quickly realized that no consensus could be reached about what practicing physicians actually do, what they need to know, or how their performance could be judged. They concluded that medical schools had not clearly defined the type of medical practitioner they sought to graduate. Furthermore, it was pointed out that even if educational institutions clearly identified the essential areas of the behavioral sciences with which a physician should be thoroughly familiar, no one physician could be expected to cope with all facets of the behaviorally generated problems of modern medicine. To do so would require that the physician be, among other things, an expert diagnostician, therapist, case manager, technician, personal counselor, scientist, preventer of disease, economist, and politician. They concluded that the medical curriculum needed to be more personalized to help each student sort out relevant information as his or her career plans and

Leonard Kamsler—*Medical World News*

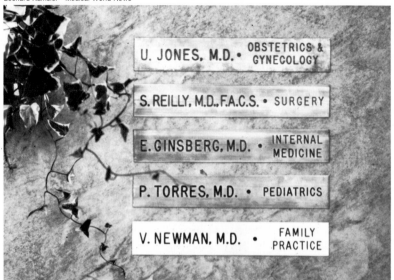

U. JONES, M.D. • OBSTETRICS & GYNECOLOGY

S. REILLY, M.D., F.A.C.S. • SURGERY

E. GINSBERG, M.D. • INTERNAL MEDICINE

P. TORRES, M.D. • PEDIATRICS

V. NEWMAN, M.D. • FAMILY PRACTICE

With medicine increasingly fragmented into specialties and subspecialties, concern is growing that medical students are not receiving the type of education that prepares them to deal with their patients' human and mental health needs as well as their medical problems.

interests begin to gel. There was unequivocal agreement both that the physician's training should extend to the behavioral sciences and that a discipline per se of behavioral sciences does not really exist. Rather, anthropologists, sociologists, psychologists, behavioral biologists, and economists as well as clinicians in every medical specialty can provide valuable help in identifying the educational requirements for producing a good doctor.

Defining exactly what is expected of a good doctor is very difficult. The criteria for this judgment may vary dramatically, depending upon whether one solicits the opinion of patients, fellow physicians, medical school faculty, or those responsible for the licensing and certifying examinations. Since the demand for health care service exceeds the supply, the market place as well fails to provide the necessary criteria. Research on the response of the patient to the type of medical care he is receiving as well as statistics on the actual efficiency of health care delivery are sorely needed to guide medical educators in planning the future medical curriculum. At present the minimal data that exist have had little impact on curriculum design or certifying and licensing examinations.

Nevertheless, there is now general agreement that the behavioral sciences should be an integral part of medical education. It is hoped that such a broadened curriculum would help the physician to view the human life cycle within a cultural context as well as from a biomedical standpoint and to deal with the individual patient first and foremost as a human being. This holistic approach to medicine would help sensitize the physician to cultural influences on the etiology and outcome of disease, thereby generally contributing to improved health care delivery. The curriculum would also teach techniques for improving communication in the doctor-patient relationship, for increasing patient acceptance of medical recommendation, and for improved teamwork among health care personnel. It is hoped as well that the physician would become concerned with the availability, accessibility, relevance, and cost of health care services.

The implementation of this new curriculum has varied enormously from school to school. Several medical schools, for example, have subscribed enthusiastically to the changing curriculum and required all their students to take a rigorous course in the behavioral sciences. The seminar listings are fairly comprehensive, treating such topics as the sociology of health and illness; pregnancy and birth; infancy, the toddler, and the preschool child; gender identity development; adolescence; the family in health and illness; human sexuality; middle years in women and men; aging; death and dying; psychosocial aspects of terminal and chronic illnesses; psychosocial aspects of drug abuse; and the professional's response to stress.

Many programs have attempted to systematically evaluate student response to the curriculum changes. The results have shown that while engulfed in attempting to absorb an overwhelming quantity of physical, chemical, and pathological information, students often underrate the significance of their behavioral science education and its relevance to the future of their medical practice. During their first two years of rigorous training in the basic sciences, most students view an additional course in the behavioral sciences as an irritant. However, by the end of two years of clinical education, they express definite appreciation for their work in the behavioral sciences and complain that it should have been expanded.

Human sexuality and the medical curriculum

Courses in human sexuality were also deemed to be an important addition to the medical curriculum. These

269

courses sought to further increase the human element in patient care and were met with enthusiasm by most students. The pioneers in the human sexuality courses soon recognized that a student's ability to absorb and comprehend sexual information was maximized once he or she had developed a more accepting attitude toward a traditionally taboo subject. It is therefore essential that medical students be made aware of the wide variety of sexual problems that exist, many of which may be presented to the physician.

The courses also sought to teach the student that sexuality and its expression are a fundamental part of one's total personality and that, unless physicians begin to understand their own sexual values, biases, and misconceptions, they will unwittingly be limited in their ability to provide optimal medical care. The student also learns that a physician needs more than his or her personal experiences and private opinions to help the patient and that in order to develop an empathic ear—without which a physician is professionally handicapped—it is essential to develop feelings of tolerance toward the values and life-styles of others.

Also explored in the sexuality courses are changing roles of men and women in contemporary society as well as the existence of a wide spectrum of human sexual behaviors. Students are also taught the accurate physiology of human sexuality, the physiology and psychology of sexual dysfunction, and the fact that physical and sexual health are interdependent and inseparable. Finally, students learn the therapeutic skills needed to develop sufficient rapport so that their patients feel comfortable in seeking information, reassurance, and therapy about sexual expectations or problems.

To attain these objectives the students are exposed to a markedly different educational strategy. When lectures are used, the speaker and the audiovisual aids focus on the attitude toward the subject matter being presented. Lectures may alternately be replaced by panel discussions of persons engaging in a particular life-style or experiencing the sexual problem under discussion. The content of these lectures or panel discussions covers the medical and, where appropriate, moral, ethical, religious, legal, economic, social, and psychological issues of topics such as contraception, planned and unplanned pregnancy, rape, homosexuality, myths and reality of male and female sexuality, sex and aging, sex and medical illness, sexual dysfunctions, and so forth.

Sexual attitude reassessment

Another format, unfamiliar to traditional medical education, has been termed sexual attitude reassessment (SAR). SAR programs are typically scheduled for two consecutive all-day sessions. In order to portray the wide range of sexual attitudes and behaviors that exist in our society, the SAR utilizes films, slides, tapes, panel presentations, nonverbal exercises, and small group meetings. Through the use of graphic audiovisual sexual materials, the participants view from one to several hours of explicit films, some of which are projected simultaneously. The commercially produced films are presented in a planned sequence that first introduces "hard core," explicit sexual activity, illustrating the broad variety of human sexuality behavior. This sequence of films is intended to desensitize the participants and render them less overreactive to explicit sexual stimuli. This phase is followed by the "resensitization" and "endorsement" sequence, which shows films specifically designed to present sexual activity between caring partners. The films are followed by small group discussions, focusing on what the material presented has evoked in each individual. Each small group has female and male leaders, and an attempt is made to have an equal number of men and women among the participants. Randomly included with the medical students are their spouses, partners, and other related health professionals. Such a mix is designed to facilitate the students' exposure to a broader range of opinions and expectations and thereby increases their opportunity for learning about themselves and other members in the group. As a result, this contributes greatly to cutting through the myths and mysteries of one's own feelings about sexuality.

Since physicians are required in the course of daily medical activity to make frequent physical contact with patients, they must learn to sort out the feelings they will experience. Hence, in order to augment the participants' awareness of their own bodies, trust exercises and body massages are also part of the SAR process. They learn about the distinctive meanings of touch (professional versus social, comforting versus sensual, and so forth) as well as the significance of nonverbal behavior.

In order to expose the students to a wide variety of persons, a panel on alternate life-styles is also included, providing panelists and participants with the opportunity to interact with one another as real people. The SAR process with its group discussions, films, body awareness exercises, and panels constitutes an intense 16-hour weekend experience. Students consider the SAR to be a very enlightening and useful, if somewhat anxiety-provoking, learning experience.

In summary, medical educators have begun to formally recognize the need to offer the medical students an opportunity to become more cognizant of their own attitudes and values and to become more sensitive to the feelings and expectations of their patients. The current direction in medical education indicates a healthy potential for growth for tomorrow's physicians and patients as well as the prospect for improved and humanized health care for everyone.

—*Francois E. Alouf, M.D., and*
Edward A. Tyler, M.D.

Special Report:

Health Care for Teenagers

by Derek H. Miller, M.D.

The Industrial Revolution of the mid-19th century left a vastly influential and complex legacy to the Western world. In addition to the sweeping economic and social changes wrought by the revolution, far subtler but equally far-reaching psychosocial effects were to be felt. Prior to the revolution the status of most individuals in the Western world was defined at birth. With the exception of a small elite, most individuals were born into clearly defined roles, growing up to be farmers, millers, laborers, and so forth as had their fathers before them. For these individuals the adolescent transition from childhood to adulthood was marked by no special developmental tasks. Only for the affluent, who had complicated decisions and choices to make as adults, did the onset of puberty announce the psychosocial moratorium of adolescence. Since the revolution, however, role definition at birth for many has yielded to vastly more complex adult life decisions for everyone. The individual is now faced with increasingly complicated societal demands—vocational, social, and sexual—and adolescence has acquired a new definition as a highly stressful period of development associated with the psychosocial reactions to puberty.

The need for specialized adolescent health care

Adolescent psychology has been studied since the beginning of this century, but with some notable exceptions the special problems and needs of the adolescent were not recognized by organized medicine or psychiatry until after World War II. As late as 1960 the British Ministry of Health was classifying hospital patients as either children—those younger than 16—or adults. Epidemiological figures for the incidence of adolescent disease in that country were very difficult to distinguish. It was not until the early 1960s that the classic work on adolescent physical development, *Growth at Adolescence* by J. M. Tanner, was produced.

Apart from some boarding schools with special therapeutic programs, inpatient psychiatric treatment for disturbed adolescents was almost impossible to obtain until the middle of the 1950s. Adolescents who suffered from major mental illnesses were sometimes hospitalized, but no particular effort was made to provide for their special educational and emotional needs. Children and adolescents were generally placed in state or private hospitals alongside adults and usually responded poorly to the empty psychosocial programs in these hospitals. Very often adolescents spent an excessive amount of time in isolation, in restraint, or under sedation. Or often they were prematurely discharged.

In many hospitals today physically ill adolescents younger than 16 are still placed in children's wards, while those over 16 are cared for as adults. Given the psychology of adolescence, this classification may cause major problems in the giving of adequate care. The emotional needs of the adolescent patient are not met, and physical recovery may be impeded.

The adolescent's response to a stressful and difficult time of change may be a withdrawal from a situation he cannot cope with; he may wish that he could return to an earlier, more secure stage of his life.

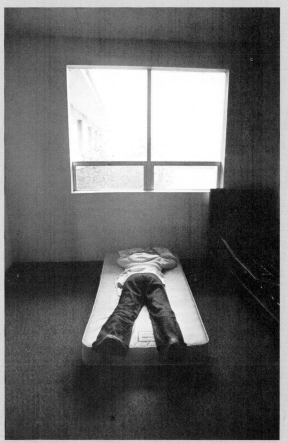

Thomas S. England

Adolescents are commonly seen by staff in general hospitals as difficult to treat either because they slump into passivity or become rebellious when given medical instruction and treatment.

For physical and psychological problems not requiring hospitalization, teenagers often see the pediatricians who have looked after them since they were infants, visiting the physicians at their parents' urging. But adolescents may resent the pediatrician, who is perceived both as an agent of the parents and as the representative of the adolescent's own unacceptable childish wishes. Similarly, psychotherapists who treat smaller children may find it difficult to be sufficiently flexible in their attitudes and manner to cope with the vagaries of adolescent communication.

Physicians who treat adults are generally accustomed to patients' either conforming to their wishes or, alternately, consulting another doctor. Hence, these physicians may not take kindly to the adolescent reluctant to accept a medical recommendation. A further difficulty arises in treating adolescents along with older patients, as the former may perceive the diseases of the middle-aged and the elderly as a threat to their own bodily integrity and sense of immortality (a usual concept in adolescence).

Adolescents are difficult to treat in both psychiatry and general medicine because the physical changes that they are undergoing, although gratifying in some ways, reinforce their disturbing feelings of helplessness. When anyone feels helpless, whether actually or potentially, the behavior of others is easily misconstrued as critical, tormenting, or persecutory. This in turn reinforces the feeling of helplessness because there is a confusion about the accuracy of the perception. Furthermore, physical or emotional illness beyond the individual's control is again likely to reinforce the feeling of helplessness. In response to these feelings, the adolescent attempts to gain a sense of mastery or control.

Often the physically or emotionally disturbed adolescent's efforts to gain a sense of control cause difficulty to the medical personnel caring for him or her. When suffering stress, young people tend to behave in ways that the adult world often finds unacceptable but that in fact may subtly increase the adolescent's sense of control. When the young person does not respond to an adult's attempt to help, the latter then tends to become angry, frustrated, and intolerant. Thus a convoluted sense of mastery is gained by the adolescent, who, feeling adults to be critical and persecutory, actually provokes them to behave in this way.

Another adolescent response to stress is to abandon striving toward mature growth, falling back instead on childish behavior patterns. Thus psychologically disturbed adolescents may refuse to care for themselves physically, use drugs, be as negativistic as a two-year-old, or refuse to follow medical recommendations.

They may retreat to bed and seemingly abandon all attempts at recovery. Sometimes they may be either physically or verbally aggressive and occasionally behave in sexually provocative ways; at other times they become unnecessarily angry with other patients.

Adolescent psychiatry

These issues and others—among them the most distressing being the rapidly growing suicide rate among troubled 15- to 24-year-olds, which has more than doubled in the past decade—have led to attempts first in psychiatry and then in general medicine to create special services for adolescents. However, some branches of medicine, namely orthopedic and rehabilitation medicine, both of which provide care to large numbers of adolescents, are still reluctant to accept the greater effectiveness of treatment programs uniquely designed for adolescents. In addition, nursing students are still inadequately trained to recognize the specific needs of the adolescent patient, and thus nursing care of adolescents is often ineffective.

In the U.S. the first reported inpatient psychiatric care facilities for adolescents were developed at Bellevue Hospital Center in New York City prior to World War II, but unfortunately they did not survive the war. After the war Great Britain followed suit with the creation of a special program at the Maudsley Hospital in London. But in the U.S. for a number of years there remained, with the exception of certain residential schools, no programs specially designed for psychologically disturbed adolescents. Child psychiatry, which had been born in the mid-1920s, began to flourish in this period, but typically most inpatient facilities refused to admit adolescents older than 13 because they were thought to be excessively difficult patients. The available outpatient psychiatric treatment for adolescents frequently proved unsatisfactory as well, since adolescents generally seek help in times of crisis and were frustrated by the inevitable wait of days or weeks prior to an appointment. In the interim the crisis would resolve itself in some fashion—even an unsatisfactory one—and by the time the adolescent's appointment had arrived, the adolescent often refused any help. Further problems arose from the lack of consensus among child psychiatrists in that period as to what the relationship should be between the needs of the parents and those of the adolescent.

Since psychiatric services were not then generally provided for adolescents aged 13 or 14, the notion developed in the postwar years that adolescents could not really be helped by psychiatry. It was thought that some adolescents would grow out of their difficulties or that they would be helped when they reached adulthood. And in fact the number of adolescents over the age of 18 being treated in psychiatric clinics was burgeoning. However, many poor and minority-group adolescents whose psychological difficulties showed

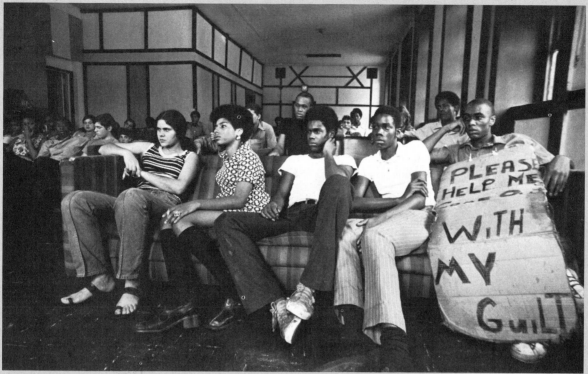

A number of U.S. hospitals established adolescent health care programs as a response to the drug culture widespread in the 1960s and 1970s.

in their disturbed behavior ended up in the penal system, a practice that still continues and serves as an excuse not to provide them with adequate psychological care.

In the mid-1950s, in response to the spreading of the drug culture to middle-class adolescents and the lack of help available to them, a number of hospitals in the U.S. began to create adolescent health care programs. Adolescent patients between the ages of 13 and 18 were first admitted to the Menninger Clinic in Topeka, Kan., in 1955. Similar programs were started at the same time at the Payne Whitney Psychiatric Clinic in New York City, at Michael Reese Hospital and Medical Center in Chicago, and at the University Hospital in Ann Arbor, Mich. Gradually a substantial body of literature about the psychiatric treatment of emotionally disturbed adolescents began to grow, and toward the end of the decade the classic works of Peter Blos and Erik Erikson on adolescent psychological development were published.

Prior to this time excellent residential schools had been developed in the United States. Some, such as the Hawthorne Cedar Knolls School in New York City, run by the Jewish Board of Guardians since 1890, had provided long-term treatment for adolescents for many years. Other schools of note were the Orthogenic School in Chicago and Bellefaire in Cleveland, Ohio, which were run, respectively, by the European-born professionals Bruno Bettelheim and Fritz Meyer and

provided further models for the new hospital-based programs.

There were no parallel psychiatric programs in Great Britain, however, where most disturbed adolescents were contained within the educational system. In 1944 Parliament had passed an educational act making it the responsibility of the educational system to educate children according to their needs. So-called maladjusted children were placed in the private school system upon medical recommendation or were alternately sent to specially developed schools for maladjusted children which were generally run by nonmedical educators. The first British outpatient program especially designed to diagnose and treat psychologically disturbed adolescents was created at the Tavistock Clinic in London in 1959–60. It was not until the mid-1960s that special psychiatric centers for emotionally disturbed adolescents were created in England.

In the early 1960s a number of attempts were made in various parts of the U.S. to create special programs for adolescents needing residential care in the psychiatric system. Very often these programs did not survive, however, because the cost of caring for adolescents in psychiatric hospitals is inevitably greater than that of caring for adults. These higher costs are due in part to the need for adolescent care programs to provide not only medical staff but also specially trained therapeutic personnel in the fields of education, recreation, and career counseling.

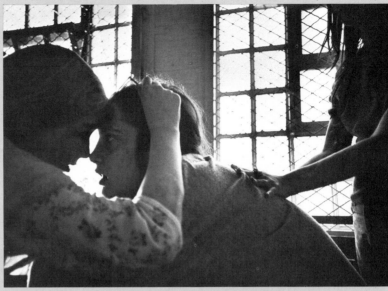

Adolescents institutionalized for mental and emotional disorders were formerly either classed as children or treated no differently from adults. It is now well recognized that a different approach is needed to define adolescents' problems and present an attainable means for their solution.

Another reason for the demise in the U.S. of many adolescent programs was the fact that most hospitals dealt with them administratively as part of child psychiatry. Consequently child-adolescent programs were developed in many hospitals throughout the country, and separate adolescent psychiatric programs began to disappear. A substantial number of residential programs for adolescents closed, and the pressure not to provide residential care for adolescents still continues. The current trend toward community psychiatry has encouraged the idea that placing adolescents in any type of institution is an unsatisfactory solution, an idea based in part on the fact that most institutions for adolescents have indeed been unsatisfactory.

In 1957 a group of psychiatrists interested in working with adolescents met in New York City and later that year formed the Society for Adolescent Psychiatry of New York. With the assistance of this group similar organizations were formed in Philadelphia (1962), Los Angeles (1963), and Chicago (1964). In 1965 the four societies began to plan the formation of a national organization, and two years later the American Society for Adolescent Psychiatry came into being. Since these early strides the number of psychiatrists involved in the specialized care and treatment of adolescents has continued to grow significantly, and at present there are 18 constituent societies in adolescent psychiatry with over 1,600 members as well as numerous committees on adolescent health care in other related medical organizations. The problems of adolescent psychiatry and health care have been the subject of numerous national and international conferences, which are reported on, along with other developments in the field, in the annual volume *Adolescent Psychiatry,* founded in 1971. The interest in this field had grown so great that in 1978 the U.S. President's Commission on Mental Health set up a special task force to review the needs of adolescents insofar as health care was concerned.

Expanded research in adolescent psychiatry has produced much significant data, among them studies on the effects of drugs on adolescent personality development. Other recent findings of note include increasing evidence of success with drug therapy to treat certain types of violent behavior and the discovery that depression in adolescents is frequently masked and difficult to detect—unlike in younger or older persons—requiring the development of special diagnostic skills. Additionally, there are indications that continuous, rather than intermittent, care for adolescents, whether in a hospital or outpatient clinic, leads to an improved prognosis in the case of some mental illnesses. Finally, it is now recognized that certain major illnesses such as manic-depressive psychosis occur in adolescents as well as in other segments of the population.

Adolescent medicine

The development of adolescent medicine made significant progress in the early 1950s. In 1951 the first medical program for adolescents in the world was started at Children's Hospital Medical Center in Boston by J. Roswell Gallagher, an internist and former school doctor of Phillips Exeter Academy in Exeter, N.H. Other programs began in the late 1950s and early 1960s, notably at Children's Hospital of the District of Columbia in Washington, D.C., Childrens Hospital of Los Angeles, Cincinnati General Hospital and Columbus Children's Hospital, both in Ohio, and Montefiore Hospital and Medical Center in New York City.

Felix Heald, who had developed the adolescent program in Children's Hospital in Washington, D.C., in 1962, received a special grant in 1964 from the Department of Health, Education, and Welfare to train physicians and other medical personnel in adolescent medi-

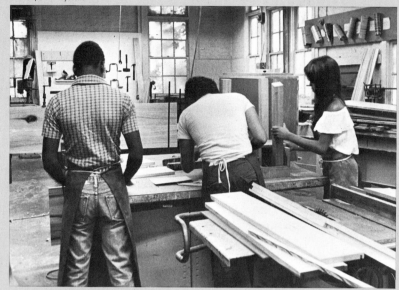

At Hawthorne Cedar Knolls School, maintained by the Jewish Board of Guardians in New York, emotionally disturbed young people can learn woodworking; participating in a creative process may be an effective form of therapy.

cine. The postgraduate minitraining program, which Heald instituted, convened for its first annual session in March 1965, with seminars on such topics as adolescent gynecology, endocrinology, nutrition, the response of the adolescent to chronic illness, and the issues of death and dying.

The goal of these seminars was to interest and teach a small number of deeply committed physicians who might then become leaders in service programs, teaching, and research. Eventually some 30 physicians who had participated in the seminars joined forces to create a more formal organization, and the Society for Adolescent Medicine was begun in April 1968. Now, ten years later, the roster boasts more than 550 members in the United States whose primary specialty is adolescent medicine.

The relationship between adolescent medicine and adolescent psychiatry has probably been at least as close as the relationship between child psychiatry and pediatrics. Liaison medicine is of particular significance when dealing with adolescents because psychologically disturbed adolescents commonly have covert physical ailments, and physically ill adolescents almost always suffer from serious psychological problems. This syndrome is particularly prevalent among adolescents who suffer from chronic ailments such as diabetes and epilepsy. Another new focus of adolescent liaison medicine is the college campus, where the stresses of competitive academic life and career decisions combine to trigger emotional and physical problems. More and more students are seeking help nowadays, and the mental health center is an integral fixture of the college campus.

The major problem in health care delivery for both adolescent medicine and adolescent psychiatry is that these subspecialties are not always accepted as being of value by the medical profession or by society at large. To some extent the presence of such programs is a threat to the existing organized systems of medical care. In general hospitals that do have programs in adolescent medicine there may be no one physician in charge of a unit. Thus the program tends to be disrupted from time to time by the psychological upsets of the patients. The fact that the physicians in teaching hospitals are always changing means that it is inordinately difficult for the adolescent patient to get the continuous care necessary for improvement.

Unfortunately, a number of programs in adolescent psychiatry have been terminated because the institutions are unaware of what is required to provide adequate infrastructural support for this subspecialty. Nevertheless, both adolescent medicine and adolescent psychiatry remain highly significant and growing subspecialties dedicated to the care of an age group in which physical, psychological, and social changes all occur at the same time.

Of particular interest is that the principles of geriatric care are remarkably similar in many ways to those of adolescent care. Old age is likewise a time of life in which physical, social, and psychological changes converge, creating tremendous stress on the individual. Geriatric studies thus potentially promise further insight into adolescent development. Meanwhile, the increasing understanding of adolescent psychology has begun to be integrated into the currently developing picture of the individual's continuous emotional growth throughout life, laying to rest the original concept that personality development stops in childhood.

Neurologic Disorders

Multiple sclerosis (MS) is an incurable crippling disease of the brain and central nervous system. Most victims die after many years of chronic disabling symptoms that may affect speech, muscle control, ability to walk, and other neurological functions. MS affects both men and women, and the peak incidence of the disease is in the individual's most productive years, between 20 and 40 years of age. While it is known that there are 500,000 victims of the disease in the United States alone, these figures may reflect only a fraction of the real number of cases, since the symptoms of the disease are often fleeting and difficult to diagnose in the early stages.

Of particular interest to the scientist is the geographical distribution of the cases. As one goes north from the Equator, the number of recorded cases increases, reaching a maximum in the northern European and Scandinavian countries and in the northern United States. For reasons that are not clear, certain areas of the world have an extremely high incidence, such as the Orkney and Shetland Islands in the North Sea off Scotland. This distribution suggests that susceptibility to MS may be closely related to a gene pool common to northern European Caucasians. Indeed, the disease is much rarer in blacks in any part of the world. As always in medicine, there are certain exceptions to this rule, notably the relatively low incidence of the disease in northern Japan at approximately the same latitude as northern Europe and a decreased incidence in native-born white South Africans.

For some time physicians have also known that multiple sclerosis tends to run in families. Most statistics indicate a 5–10% greater chance of contracting the disease than if there were no multiple sclerosis in the family. This genetic inheritance does not, however, follow classic autosomal recessive patterns, since it appears quite commonly in individuals with no previous evidence of the disease in the family. All that can be said at the present time in this regard is that there seems to be a greater susceptibility to the disease in certain families.

The genetic component

The renewed interest in a possible genetic factor in MS stems from observations in laboratory animals that an immune response to any foreign substance is genetically based. For example, one mouse strain responds to a particular virus or foreign substance, while another is incapable of doing so.

These observations in inbred strains of mice led immediately to similar studies in humans. As is common in medicine, the test systems employed were actually developed for a different purpose. During the early stages of kidney transplantation research it was noted that kidneys obtained from closely related individuals were not rejected by the recipient's immune system, while organs from unrelated individuals frequently were. Tests were undertaken using blood serum obtained from women who had given birth to several children. It is known that multiple pregnancies cause women to produce small amounts of antibodies directed against those antigens in the fetus that were inherited from the father. In these tests researchers were able to detect antigens on the surface of leucocytes (white blood cells). The test was relatively simple to perform. Antiserum was obtained from these women and mixed with the leucocytes from the individual to be tested along with a standard amount of complement—a group of proteins present in blood that have a role in the immune reaction. If the antiserum contained antibodies that were directed against those antigens on the cell, the interaction of the antibody with the cell in the presence of the catalyst complement resulted in the death of the cell. Careful and often tedious experiments with blood serum determined that these antigens were inherited from the parents, two major antigens from each parent. These antigens were called human leukocyte antigens (HL-A) and formed the foundation of the human histocompatibility complex, which is now the cornerstone of many immunological studies and concepts. This finding was immediately put to clinical use; if patients were to have successful kidney transplants, their antigens had to closely match those on the surface of the donors' cells. The unexpected dividend from these transplant findings was the observation of the genetic inheritance of these antigens and its relationship to the immune response to certain antigens and, by analogy, to certain disease states.

With this in mind, multiple sclerosis researchers used the same type of test to determine whether victims of the disease had similar genetic backgrounds. It now appears that MS individuals do have genetic markers on the surface of their cells that are present in a much greater percentage of MS individuals than in nonsusceptible individuals. With the present state of knowledge, it cannot be said absolutely that these markers automatically predispose to the disease. For example, at least a third of the population carry these markers and are not affected. However, the findings at least point the way to the strong possibility that there is a genetic predisposition to the disease. Studies in Scotland strongly emphasize this point, since it was found that a very high percentage of MS individuals in the Caithness area did indeed have these markers, compared with nonaffected individuals from the same area.

Searching for the cause of MS

The cause of MS is unknown; there are vast numbers of possible causative agents, but a number of investigators now believe that a virus is the cause of multiple sclerosis. Backing for this hypothesis once again comes from animal studies, notably, a disease of sheep called scrapie. The agent is a presumed virus that replicates in young sheep. Neurological symptoms somewhat similar to MS eventually appear after a long incubation period. In man there are also several examples of a virus that lies dormant for a number of years only to appear and reappear at intervals. The most notable example of this is the common "cold sore," which often appears on the corners of the mouth after exposure to sunlight or cold and which is caused by a herpesvirus. This infection clears, only to reappear a year to two later. During its quiet period it can be demonstrated that the virus is present in the nerve cells supplying the affected area of skin but is in a dormant state. Why it flares up and causes the acute sore at specific times is unknown. Another example is found in New Guinea, where a neurological disease called kuru, transmitted by a presumed virus, is passed from human to human because of the cannibalistic practices of some of the inhabitants.

One theory of the etiology of MS holds that the common measles virus or a variant of it is involved in the disease process. The arguments are as follows: people with multiple sclerosis appear to have higher amounts of measles antibodies both in the serum and, more strikingly, in the spinal fluid than do unaffected individuals. The white blood cells (cells involved in the reaction to foreign substances) obtained from venipuncture appear not to recognize measles virus yet react to all other substances normally. However, it must be emphasized that all these findings are controversial and not accepted by all researchers. For example, other viral antibodies have been found in the serum and spinal fluid of multiple sclerosis patients. In fact, careful work by a group of Scandinavian investigators has shown that only 10–20% of the antibodies detected in the spinal fluid of MS patients have measles specificity. The specificity of the remaining 90% of these antibodies is really unknown. Does this mean there is more than one agent involved, or is the test only a reflection of something else abnormal? While the measles theory is attractive, it is quite possible that a completely unrelated virus is at work, or it may be one that acts and looks like measles virus. These findings may indeed be clues to some other underlying and as yet not understood disease process in multiple sclerosis. Whether or not they are reflections of the actual agent or disease mechanism remains unanswered.

Another theory holds that MS is an autoimmune disease, caused by a malfunction of the body's immune defense system. This states that for unknown reasons multiple sclerosis individuals react to their own nervous tissue as if it were foreign tissue. Simply put, the process could proceed as follows: a common virus or agent—like measles—enters the central nervous system during the usual childhood infection. Because of a defect in the immune response to this agent (presumably genetically based), certain particles of virus are not eliminated from the brain and remain dormant for a number of years in the central nervous tissues. Under conditions not entirely understood (stress, trauma, hormonal imbalances, etc.), the virus reactivates and causes brain tissue damage in localized areas. These "altered" brain tissue antigens are recognized as foreign and call forth groups of cells in the host called lymphocytes and macrophages and antibodies, all designed to eliminate foreign substances from the body. These "autoantibodies" are so named because they are directed against the body's own tissues and not against foreign substances. The ensuing "battle" results in further destruction of the surrounding tissue, resulting in a scarred area called a plaque. If the virus is intermittently activated, the plaques will appear over a number of years, giving rise to the intermittent nature of the clinical symptoms (periods of quiescence are called remissions, and times of activity are called exacerbations). The stimulation that causes autodestruction of brain tissue may come from sources other than viruses; in any event, the prime defect resides in the host, permitting the formation of antibodies or cells directed against the host's tissues.

Support for this theory comes from an animal model called "experimental allergic encephalitis," or EAE. Here injection of foreign brain tissue into animals caused a progressive neurological disease that is mediated by the production of cellular immunity that is directed against the host's nervous tissue. The disease can be transmitted to nonimmunized animals by lymphocytes (without antigen) obtained from diseased animals. While this seems a fruitful source of MS research, EAE in general does not look or act like MS. However, this does not necessarily mean the two diseases are unrelated, since it is always possible that members of different species react in different ways to the same immunological stimulus.

A third theory advanced by a number of investigators is the concept that there is an inherent defect in the tissues of multiple sclerosis patients. This theory states that the tissues of patients with the disease contain lower amounts of unsaturated fatty acids than do tissues of nonaffected individuals. As a result of this defect, myelin (the covering material of nerves) is imperfectly formed in the body and will break down under the stress of numerous environmental factors. The end result is the disease.

Treatments

It must be remembered that it is entirely possible that none of these theories is correct and that MS arises from a totally different cause. For the time being, though, the current prevailing theories form the basis of most of the known methods of treatment of MS. If the theory that the immune systems of multiple sclerosis individuals are unable to recognize certain viruses is true, then treatment programs designed to enhance the immune response to these agents are indicated. A part of such therapy is the administration of an agent called "transfer factor," which, for reasons not well understood, transfers immunity to a given antigen without the recipient's having ever been exposed to the foreign substance. Clinical results in the U.S. and in Scandinavia have been ambiguous. The use of transfer factor has not resulted in any clear-cut benefit even when given in monthly injections for a considerable period of time.

A second therapeutic approach has been to assume that MS is a disease in which increased reactivity to one's own tissues is the primary cause of the symptoms. Agents selected for their ability to depress the immune response are used. A number of clinical trials have been or are being conducted, and all of the evidence is not in as yet. However, while the use of certain immunosuppressive (or anti-inflammatory) agents such as steroids appears to decrease the time course of acute symptoms, these agents do not appear to alter the course of the disease significantly. Furthermore, they have many unpleasant side effects if administered over a long period of time.

Another option is the therapy that maintains that increasing the levels of unsaturated fatty acids in the blood may eliminate the disease's symptoms. This has resulted in the famous "sunflower seed" diet (high in unsaturated fatty acids), which has been tried in many countries including the United Kingdom. There still is a controversy concerning the pros and cons of these studies, with no striking results having been produced.

Studies to find the cause and develop a cure for multiple sclerosis are continuing, but the process is time-consuming, laborious, and difficult. Efforts to find an effective treatment must of necessity be tried with human patients, since animal models are not accurate indications of the disease. Early in 1978 it was revealed that the U.S. Food and Drug Administration had approved for experimental use myelin basic protein, a drug, as treatment for MS. The drug was being tested under the auspices of the Salk Institute in La Jolla, Calif., as a possible method of stopping the progress of the disease. The course of testing hoped in addition to verify the theory that the disease was of autoallergic origin rather than of another form of causation.

—*John B. Zabriskie, M.D.*

Occupational and Environmental Health

Our health is now seen as inseparable from the total environment, which includes home and workplace. Our homes can become contaminated with toxic substances from a variety of sources, such as cleaning materials, adhesives, paints and strippers used in arts and crafts and home repairs, some forms of insulation, cigarette smoke, and contaminants on work clothes. At

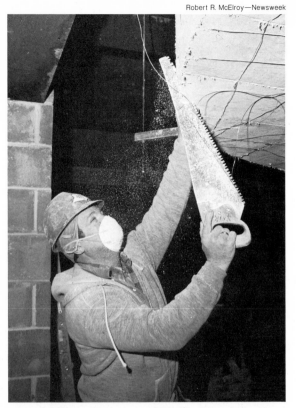

In April 1978 the Department of Health, Education, and Welfare launched a major effort to inform past and present workers with asbestos of the dangers they and their families face from this carcinogenic material.

work constant surveillance is necessary to ensure that adverse health effects do not go unnoticed among workers who change jobs or do not realize that an illness may result from exposure to physical and chemical hazards.

Setting standards

It is evident that in our personal lives we choose to accept certain risks, *e.g.,* the food we eat, the speed at which we drive automobiles, the number of cigarettes we smoke. As individuals we each make personal judgments weighing these risks. For contaminants in the environment and in the workplace, there is usually far less opportunity for the individual to assess the risk or to avoid the hazard when it is viewed as unacceptable. The regulatory agencies of the federal government are now far more active on behalf of the public, a trend that is in part a reflection of the consumer movement of the 1970s. The Environmental Protection Agency (EPA), the Occupational Safety and Health Administration (OSHA), the Consumer Product Safety Commission (CPSC), and the Food and Drug Administration (FDA) are all responsible for the setting of standards to ensure that food, water, air, therapeutic drugs, and articles and substances we use in our homes and at work do not cause harm.

The EPA is responsible for implementing the Toxic Substances Control Act of 1976, and the first phase is the development of an inventory of more than 70,000 chemicals in commercial production. It is expected that each year an additional 400 to 1,000 substances will be proposed for production. When the inventory is completed in 1979, manufacturers of new chemicals may be required to submit data that provide information on tests for carcinogenicity (ability of a substance to produce cancer), mutagenicity (capacity to produce gene mutations), and teratogenicity (capacity to produce severe malformations in fetuses), as well as tests for effects on the environment.

Large-scale epidemiologic studies, which are essential for the evaluation of environmental effects on health, are very expensive and may need to be maintained for 20 years or more to ensure that enough reliable information is collected. An additional difficulty is that recent federal legislation has imposed more stringent requirements on investigators to protect everyone's right to privacy. The private citizen has also become more sensitive about sharing personal information with scientific investigators, and, as a result, new epidemiologic information for the public good is now very difficult to obtain, particularly in areas of reproductive research.

The *Atlas of Cancer Mortality for U.S. Counties*, published a few years ago, showed the geographic distribution of cancer prevalence throughout the U.S. in the white population. Recently a second atlas showing the geographic distribution of cancer in the nonwhite population has confirmed the conclusions of the first volume—that concentrations of cancer deaths exist in industrialized areas, particularly New Jersey, where the state legislature has called for more extensive and detailed studies. In time, understanding cancer mortality rates should lead to more precise standards for controlling the environment. Collaborative studies of workers in particular industries are currently being done, with management providing employment and exposure records, unions ensuring the cooperation of their members for clinical examination and history taking, and universities doing the data analysis and epidemiologic interpretation. For example, the United Rubber Workers International Union negotiated in its master contract with the "big six" rubber companies (Armstrong, Firestone, General Tire, B. F. Goodrich, Goodyear, and Uniroyal) in 1970 for a half cent per hour per worker for studies on the morbidity and mortality of rubber workers by the Schools of Public Health at Harvard University and the University of North Carolina. In 1976 the amount for participating in such collaborative studies was raised to one cent per hour per worker.

Workers' rights

Since passage of the Occupational Safety and Health Act in 1970, unions have given considerable attention to enforcement of the law and to reduction of hazards in the workplace by encouraging the formation of safety committees and use of the grievance system. Under the act a worker has the right to report a hazard to OSHA without fear of discrimination or loss of job. Workers have also become more aware of the dangers of contaminating other family members when showers and a place to change clothing are not available. Lead, asbestos, beryllium, and other chemicals have been found to have adverse effects on the workers' family when contaminated clothing is laundered and when dust accumulates in the house itself.

Many of the actions being taken by regulatory agencies have been forced by suits brought by consumer and environmental activist groups and labor unions on behalf of their members or the public; *e.g.,* the Environmental Defense Fund, the Oil, Chemical, and Atomic Workers International Union. Where legal action has failed, labor unions are using collective bargaining as a means to improve the health and safety of their work environment. Unions have also negotiated for the workers' right to know what dangers are in the workplace. The use of trade or code names for chemicals frequently prevents workers from knowing the extent of the danger, although exposure to a chemical that can cause cancer or other equally serious illness may be part of their daily work. For example, toxic substances are frequently found on the shop floor in containers without an identifying label to describe the contents. A number or some letters will be used as a simple code, with no indication of the dangers if the substance is spilled, inhaled, or comes in contact with the skin or eyes.

The National Labor Relations Board recently supervised an agreement between the Oil, Chemical, and Atomic Workers Local 6-258 and Consolidated Printing Ink of St. Paul, Minn., which set a precedent under collective bargaining. An unfair labor practice charge had been filed because the company had refused to provide lists of chemicals and their toxicity, as well as monitoring and medical data. The National Labor Relations Act states that the employer must bargain in good faith, so that information necessary to allow the union to bargain intelligently and effectively about working conditions must be supplied upon request. The local union won the right to know the generic names of all chemicals used by workers at Consolidated Printing Ink and all monitoring results. The need for more trained toxicologists, epidemiologists, and biostatisticians is now becoming acute as this kind of worker protection becomes more common.

In many cities and states active groups of workers with support from unions and health professionals have been more aggressive in independently identifying hazardous work conditions in particular work settings. They have adopted a common identifying nomenclature, CACOSH (Chicago Area Committee on

Occupational and environmental health

Occupational Safety and Health), PHILAPOSH (Philadelphia Project on Occupational Safety and Health), MASSCOSH (Massachusetts), NYCOSH (New York), NCOSH (North Carolina), and RICOSH (Rhode Island), and have all been quite effective in bringing the problem of worker hazards to a wider audience. The view has developed only very recently that workers have a right to know that they are working with dangerous chemicals.

Radiation exposure

Extensive investigation by the U.S. Departments of Defense and Energy has now begun to evaluate the effects of past exposure to ionizing radiation among federal workers who do not come within the jurisdiction of OSHA. The diagnosis of leukemia in some soldiers who participated in field exercises immediately following nuclear weapons tests 20 years ago has lead to congressional hearings and initiation of epidemiologic studies by the Center for Disease Control (CDC) of the United States Department of Health, Education, and Welfare. Similar studies have begun of U.S. shipyard workers who have built and refitted nuclear submarines. In contrast to exposure to chemicals, where the individual's dose is usually impossible to assess, radiation exposure can be measured accurately by means of a film badge attached to a person's body. Extensive efforts are now being made to reconstruct the range of radiation doses experienced in the nuclear tests and in shipyard work in order to continue the examination of biological effects of ionizing radiation. Such studies have been going on for over 50 years, much longer than for most chemical hazards. In the case of the shipyard workers, the radiation exposure has usually been within the allowable occupational limits, but there must be close surveillance over long periods of time to be sure that current standards for occupational exposure provide full protection.

Treating Kepone poisoning

Kepone is a pesticide that provoked a stir of publicity a few years ago when it was discovered that the substance had caused serious illness to plant workers and their families. Though Kepone is no longer manufactured, it can affect people who had no direct contact with it. Discharges from the manufacturing plant in Hopewell, Va., ended up in the James River and in fish as far away as the Atlantic coast off New Jersey.

Kepone poisoning has now been successfully treated by cholestyramine, a therapeutic drug already in use for the reduction of blood cholesterol levels. Treatment of 22 workers at the Medical College of Virginia with cholestyramine resulted in rapid excretion of Kepone, which appears to become bound to the resin in the drug. In addition to reduced blood levels of Kepone, adipose (fatty) tissue concentrations were also reduced. The severe neurological symptoms of tremor,

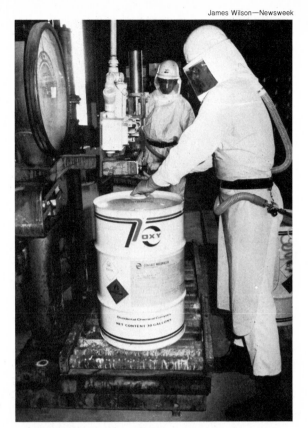

Several manufacturers of DBCP, an agricultural pesticide, ceased production of the chemical when it became known that, despite protective measures, the chemical was causing sterility in factory workers.

stuttering, and muscle dysfunction abated, and in those who had experienced marked or complete reduction in sperm count, regeneration occurred. Cholestyramine is being investigated further for possible treatment of individuals with bodily burdens of other pesticides and those who have experienced polybrominated biphenyl (PBB) contamination in Michigan.

Animal studies in determining carcinogens

The Delaney amendment specifically prohibits addition to food of any substance that causes cancer in animals; the controversy concerning extrapolation of animal data to human beings has implications for environmental and occupational health as well. OSHA's policy for identification of carcinogens strongly emphasizes the importance of animal experiments, which are justified on the basis of the scientific methodology developed over many years of biological research.

Acrylonitrile, used in the manufacture of plastic and synthetic rubber and fibers, has been identified by OSHA as a suspect human carcinogen associated with an excess risk of lung and colon cancer in workers in an E. I. du Pont de Nemours and Co. plant. Although the human experience does not provide definite proof of cancer, exposure of mice to the same compound

280

has definitely caused tumors. OSHA estimated in February 1978 that 125,000 workers could be in contact with acrylonitrile and issued an emergency order to reduce worker exposure to the lowest practical level. There is to be a tenfold reduction of the previous standard of 20 parts per million averaged over eight hours using improved work practices, engineering controls, and, if necessary, respiratory protective equipment.

The controversy surrounding OSHA's new carcinogen policy restricting worker contact with substances based on animal findings involves on the one hand a view that a "safe" or "acceptable" level should be established for exposure to carcinogens and on the other hand OSHA's position that a safe level is impossible to determine. OSHA has also issued an order to reduce to the lowest feasible level worker exposure to benzene, which is known to cause leukemia in human beings. In contrast to almost all other known human carcinogens, benzene has *not* been found to cause cancer in animals. Public hearings and court rulings can be expected in the future to establish the acceptance or rejection of these OSHA procedures. The arguments will be primarily concerned with the issues of proof that a substance can cause cancer in human beings and the issue of how much risk is acceptable.

Occupational hazards and human reproduction

Human reproduction is now of more interest to workers exposed to pesticides, organic solvents, and other toxic substances. The 1970 census showed that 43% of the total female population of the U.S. was working. Subsequent studies by the National Center for Health Statistics showed that during a one-year period, 1972–73, there were 88 pregnancies ending in live birth for every 1,000 women in the labor force, ages 15 to 44, which was 41.5% of all live births in the country during that time. The total number of babies born each year who accompany their mothers *in utero* into the work environment can be estimated at approximately 1,250,000.

Very few epidemiologic studies have ever been done in the United States that included women workers, so it was surprising to find that women who worked in hospital operating rooms, where they were exposed to anesthetic gases, showed a far more adverse reproductive experience than was the case for women working in other parts of the hospital. Further investigations, which included male dentists who also use anesthetic gases, showed that their wives experienced spontaneous abortions and gave birth to children with congenital abnormalities related to the gases, though not to the same degree as the women workers themselves.

Exposure to lead has long been known to result in adverse reproductive experience for women leadworkers and wives of male leadworkers. Public attention has also been focused on pesticide workers exposed to dibromochloropropane (DBCP) at Occidental

Chemical Co. in Lathrop, Calif. A group of nine workers talking during their lunch hour realized that none of their wives had borne children for several years. Medical examination of each man showed either no sperm production or a seriously diminished number of sperm. Further studies on other men working with the same chemical elsewhere in the United States showed the same effect. These observations highlighted the severe lack of scientific knowledge concerning the effects of toxic substances on male reproduction.

There is now an increased concern that the reproductive systems of both men and women must be protected. However, there has been more attention directed to women workers by management, particularly concerning suspension from the job, dismissal, or initial job discrimination, resulting in conflict with the equal employment opportunity laws. Unions (particularly the United Auto Workers) have worked intensively to prevent a disparate effect on women workers in the case of lead exposure, where some women went so far as to be sterilized in order to retain their jobs where there was high exposure to lead. There has been a marked increase in studies of the effects of toxic substances on reproduction, including epidemiologic studies of

In late 1977 a ban was called for on a component of permanent hair dyes, 2,4-diaminoanisole sulfate, that has suspected carcinogenic properties; hairdressers repeatedly exposed to the dye are at risk.

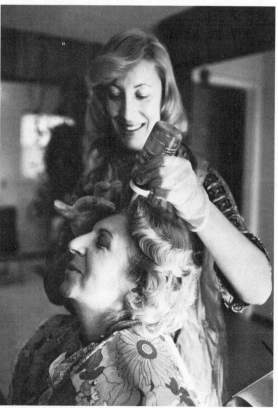

L. L. T. Rhodes—Taurus Photos

men and women exposed to hazardous chemicals at work, though it will be some time before as much definitive information as we see for cancer-causing substances becomes available. In the meantime, a conservative view should be taken in protecting men and women of childbearing capacity from exposure to toxic substances with known and suspected effects on the reproductive system in animals or human beings. (*See also* Pregnancy and Birth.)

Workers' compensation

The recognition of many more work-associated diseases may soon lead to a reevaluation of workers' compensation, a federally mandated, state-administered program going back to the early years of the century. Workers' compensation hearing boards are operated by states, and generally there has been little acknowledgement of the new understanding of occupational disease. Many workers' claims, particularly if the disease does not appear on the state list of compensable diseases, are challenged and the compensation denied. For example, only a very few workers of the thousands suffering from byssinosis ("brown lung"), a respiratory disease associated with cotton dust exposure, have been awarded compensation.

The state listings of awards do not nearly match the known number of job-related injuries and illnesses, now more accurately recorded because of National Institute for Occupational Safety and Health (NIOSH) studies and OSHA enforcement procedures. A study in the state of Washington of illness in workers showed over one-third to be job related, yet a check of the state workers' compensation statistics included only 3% of these same workers. Whereas an industrial accident is likely to be obviously related to the work activity, diseases such as chronic respiratory disease and cancer, with their long periods of latency, may become clinically evident long after exposure to the causative agent, so that proof of the relationship may be impossible to establish. The workers' compensation program is underwritten by private insurance companies and can cover the cost of workers' medical and hospital care and compensation for physical impairment. Weekly benefits may continue indefinitely.

One group of workers—coal miners disabled by black-lung disease (anthracosis)—have been paid benefits by the Social Security Administration, a federal program. The passage of the Coal Mine Health and Safety Act in 1969 assured financial support for disabled miners and their dependents. The enormous debt of illness and death in the coal industry can be perceived in part by the extent of Social Security payments made, amounting to over $65 million per month by 1975, with an overall cost to the federal government of $1 billion annually for the black-lung compensation program. The Black Lung Benefits Revenue Act was passed in February 1978 and now sets an excise tax on coal to pay for benefits, shifting the burden of benefit payments to the coal industry. The new Black Lung Disability Trust Fund is administered by the secretary of the treasury, who collects an excise tax of 50 cents per ton on underground-mined coal and 25 cents per ton on surface-mined coal. However, the amount of the tax can be no more than 2% of the coal's selling price. No other occupationally related disease has yet been seen to require such a massive long-term financial commitment of money as recompense for the generations of illness suffered, although federal compensation for asbestos workers who have contracted lung cancer or asbestosis is being discussed by the U.S. Congress.

Compensation to the victims of environmental disasters for impairment of health and loss of livelihood—as in the episodes of PBB contamination in Michigan and Kepone contamination of the James River in Virginia—is also under consideration in the U.S. Congress, with public hearings being held by the House Commerce Subcommittee on Consumer Protection and Finance.

A concern for quality of life

Public policy decisions based on scientific data—the responsibility of the public and elected officials—must take into account public health, environmental protection, and economic cost. But risks and benefits are extremely difficult to quantify. Because ionizing radiation has been one of the most intensively studied hazards, it has been possible to establish the risk of cancer from a *specific dose* of radiation whether used for diagnostic or therapeutic purposes in medical care, in the industrial setting, or for power generation. The risk for fatal malignancies per rad (radiation absorbed dose) is estimated to be one in 10,000. Such estimates have not yet been possible for toxic substances such as pesticides, organic solvents, and heavy metals, though it is known that cancer risks are much higher for some, *e.g.,* asbestos.

It is important to keep in mind that the intense concern with ionizing radiation in comparison with other environmental hazards comes from the extensive worldwide monitoring of water, air, food, animals, and people over a 25-year period. Current concerns for the safe containment of toxic substances must start from a base of comparative ignorance; *e.g.,* Kepone and polychlorinated biphenyls (PCB's). Similarly, the data on cancer have been more directly available from death records in contrast to the paucity of information on reproductive effects, neurological effects, and heart, lung, liver, and kidney dysfunction due to toxic substances. Many illnesses due to occupational and environmental hazards result in shortened lives and impaired quality of life but have been accorded far less public attention than they deserve.

(*See also* Cancer.)

—*Vilma R. Hunt, B.D.S.*

Special Report:

Stress on the Job

by Harold M. Visotsky, M.D.

Hans Selye has defined stress as "the non-specific response of the body to any demand made upon it." In his work over the last 40 years Selye has tried to convince the professions that any kind of stimulus or any type of normal action, *e.g.*, the organism's fight against a specific disease, could provoke a stereotypical response in the human body. The individual reacts to a specific stimulus with the appropriate response: sweating when it's hot, laughter when something is funny, tears in a sad situation. But superimposed, as well as underlying, each of these specific responses is the general adaptive response, or the adaptation syndrome, which helps all of us respond to stimuli in the world around us.

There are three scientists whose ideas in the area of stress research stand out. One is Hans Selye, who borrowed the word *stress* from physics to describe the body's response to everything from infection and reactions to heat to levels of emotion stemming from anger or passion. Adaptation, the concept that as organisms become more independent of their surroundings they develop more complex capacities in stabilizing their internal environment to counterchanges in external circumstances, was first defined by French physiologist Claude Bernard about 100 years ago. The third person, who worked out the complex adjustments of the neuroendocrine system in its attempt to preserve the internal environment, was Walter Cannon, who expanded Bernard's theory into the concept of homeostasis, or balance. Over a period of 30 years Cannon showed that the sympathoadrenal system is responsible for coordinating all of the "fight or flight" responses that are orchestrated to meet an external challenge. These three men are responsible for the current efforts in understanding stress and man's adaptation to his environment and to his co-occupants of this world.

Stress and adaptation

There is a definite pattern or rhythm to the human organism's stress response, which may vary from person to person but is known as "the general adaptation syndrome." Stage 1 is the "alarm stage," which consists of two phases. At first, the body's resistance is lowered (the shock phase), and then the resistance is raised as the physiological defenses are mobilized (the counter-shock phase). The symptoms are: pounding heart, racing pulse, and dryness of the mouth.

Stage 2 is the "resistance stage," during which maximum adaptation occurs. The earlier symptoms of excitability in the alarm stage will have diminished. But the adrenal glands are enlarged, and the body is prepared to function with major organ systems at peak output. Should the state of stress persist until reserves are depleted, a final stage (the exhaustion stage) will be entered.

René Dubos, in his book *Man Adapting* (1965), warns that repeated stimulation of the endocrine glands leads to irreversible body wear and tear. Persistent stimuli such as fear, anxiety, overcrowding, loud noises, and exposure to new situations all combine to overtax the adaptive reaction. Stress and adaptation, then, go hand in hand.

Recent research has attempted to elucidate the specific circuits or routes for the neurophysiological and neuroendocrine aspects of the stress responses. It was believed at one time that the body and the mind were aroused together from a state of equilibrium, or tranquility, to one of readiness for action in the face of stressful stimulation. But as more sophisticated physiological and psychological studies and measures were elaborated, it became clear that the disassociation of arousal occurs. Essentially, the thinking circuits may be on a high output, while the autonomic—*i.e.*, the automatic "fight or flight" response—are on a low output. Or this may be reversed. Obviously, understanding these mechanisms has great relevance to the management of stress reactions.

Frank Ochberg, in a psychiatric study of the handling of terrorists, applies this theoretical understanding to dealing with terrorists. The besieged authorities may feel that their attempts to manipulate food, water, light, and heat or even to administer sedatives in food will bring a hostage holder to the stage of physiological exhaustion. But, in fact, they may be diminishing the terrorist's capacity for rational thought by reducing the central nervous system arousal while activating the visceral and autonomic systems. The result may be a finely tuned animal—unfettered by reason, dangerously coiled, and ready to spring.

Measuring occupational stress

Stress reactions are primarily defensive in nature and, depending on whether they are insufficient or excessive, may in themselves produce diseases related to

Michael D. Sullivan

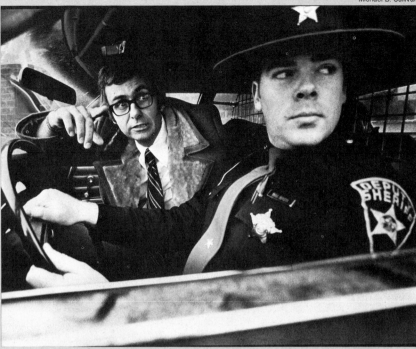

It may come as a surprise to learn which occupations have been found to create high levels of stress. It may seem obvious that a law enforcement officer faces great stress, but studies have shown that musicians are also among the most highly stressed workers.

our adaptation. In every aspect of our life we are confronted with "stressors" (stimuli) and stressful situations. Not all of these stressors and stressful situations are negative or of painful content. Many stressful situations result from the response to good news, to promotions, to successful emotional activities.

The stimulus may be brief, measured in seconds or even milliseconds, or extend over the length of a working day, week, or month. Because work occupies a significant portion of all of our lives, we frequently see work as a determinant in defining our levels of satisfaction and success with life. Since work is an integral part of most adults' lives, it affects attitudes—at work, at home, and in leisure activities. We have learned to accept prevalent concepts that state that work—and particularly, executive work—is highly stressful and produces a variety of psychosomatic illnesses: the "executive ulcer," hypertension, etc. But studies have shown that stresses related to jobs and work are fairly pervasive and are related both to the attitudes and to the personalities of the workers. The match between the job, the personality, the attitude, the coping capacity of the individual, as well as his relationship to co-workers and family, all are determinants as to whether there is a high concentration of job-related stress.

In a recent study of job-related stress and job-related emotional disorders, workers such as quality-control inspectors, musicians, public-relations representatives, dishwashers, and warehousemen were listed as holding the top ten occupations producing the most damaging emotional stress. This is not to ignore those highly stressful jobs held by air-traffic controllers, assembly-line workers, and policemen. But they were

ranked in a lower order based on a scale created by the National Institute for Occupational Safety and Health (NIOSH) in a study on all job classifications.

Those jobs that have been traditionally thought of as highly stressful—such as news editor, doctor, principal, or teacher—were surprisingly low in the ranking. This is not to suggest that they are not stressful occupations, but in those jobs a certain measure of autonomy or power or control helped to alleviate the severe effects of the stress by increasing the individual's self-esteem and, therefore, his coping capacity.

Other occupations that are "public-contact related" and involve situations over which the workers have little control usually run the highest risk of being affected by the job-related stress. For example, in the health professions, nurses aides and other health technicians working around patients who are demanding, who are suffering, and who are in great need of reassurance are caught between the demands of the patient and the doctor's orders. One can see extensions of this in terms of other public-related jobs: waitresses, sales clerks, etc. In situations where management has rigid control over policy but the employees are responsible for doing the job without having the authority to modify it, extreme stresses can be built up.

Individual response to stress

In a Canadian symposium on psychological stress in the mid-1960s a number of experts explored what was known about stress and its relation to illness, maladaptation, and human dysfunction. Mortimer Appley and Richard Trumbull summarized some of the findings.

1. "Stress is probably best conceived as a state of

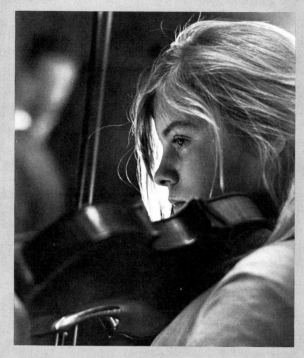

the total organism under extenuating circumstances, rather than as an event in the environment."

The ability of the individual to respond to a particular stressor is related to the individual's personality, coping capacity, state of previous learned responses (experiential pattern), and self-esteem.

2. "A great variety of different environmental conditions is capable of producing a stress state."

Essentially, "One man's meat is another's poison." Individuals not only respond to a variety of environmental stressors but may react with exaggerated symptoms to particular stimuli.

3. "Different individuals respond to the same conditions in different ways. Some enter rapidly into the stress state; others show increased alertness and apparently improved performance; and still others appear to be 'immune' to the stress-producing qualities of the environmental conditions."

Meyer Friedman and Ray Rosenman have written extensively about "Type A" and "Type B" personalities, which were correlated with clinical observations of socioeconomic stress and emotional strains. Meyer and Rosenman correlated personality types with physical disorders such as cardiovascular illnesses. While not everyone is a "racehorse" or a "turtle," being a racehorse is not necessarily harmful, provided one has good coping and homeostatic mechanisms. The value of gratification and self-esteem derived from job or other life situations, as well as methods of handling excesses of anxiety or stress, must be related to the question of whether a high stress occupation causes illness. Thus it is not so stressful being a racehorse as it is being a turtle who wants to be a racehorse and consequently acts like a racehorse, not like a turtle.

4. "The same individual may enter into a stress state in response to one presumably stressful condition and not to another."

5. "Consistent intraindividual but varied interindividual psychobiological response patterns occur in stress situations. The notion of a common stress reaction needs to be reassessed."

Each individual has a specific and unique spectrum of stressors. These are related to past experiences, value systems, and the social context in which he lives. They are further related to such variables as age, education, state of health, personality, sex, and feelings about the one's social class. For example, a highly educated woman holding a boring, menial job but having inhibited feelings about expressing anger may have a significant amount of stress—represented as frustration or even as physical symptoms.

6. "The behaviors resulting from operations intended to induce stress may be the same or different, depending on the context of the situation of its induction."

It is not the specific and identifiable stress components of a person's occupation or life situation that cause stress problems; rather, it is how the person perceives the stresses in his job or life. For example, a policeman may not be stressed as much by life-threatening situations such as disarming a hold-up man or even intervening in family fights as by being treated discourteously in court by being made to wait around all day after just having come off duty.

7. "The intensity and the extent of the stress state and the associated behaviors may not be readily predicted from a knowledge of the stimulus conditions alone but require an analysis of the underlying motivational patterns and the context in which the stressor is applied."

Thomas Holmes and Richard Rahe developed a method for measuring life changes and ranking them in terms of magnitude and impact. They ranked life events such as the death of a spouse or parent, divorce, marital separation, illness, injury, promotion, marriage, loss of job, etc., and assigned a life-change unit value to each event. By correlating life-change scores with the health and medical history, Holmes and Rahe postulated that changes in life-style that require a great deal of coping and adjustment correlate with illness. The higher the number and degree of life changes an individual undergoes, the higher the risk of subsequent severe illness.

Executives live stressful lives both at their jobs and in their personal lives. What this observation indicates for all is that when a work-related crisis of major proportion happens to coincide with a major personal crisis, it could create grave problems. The impact of a job transfer, or even promotion, can create unmanageable stress at times when related to events at home such as a spouse's going back to school or work, children's

285

leaving or having left home, a major illness or death in the family or among close friends.

While much is said about the negative destructive aspects of stress, stress is necessary for well-being. Stress and stressors are all around—at work, at home, and in the general environment. They are not likely to abate or disappear. Rather, the identification of the stress pattern, the variant styles of coping with stress, and the mechanisms for studying stress comprehensively are becoming more available.

8. "Temporal factors may determine the significance of a given stressor and thus the intensity and the extent of the stress state, and the optimum measure of effect."

Acute stress may be directly related to the temporal factors; however, it may lay down patterns for repeated reactions that respond automatically to stressful stimuli. It requires a relearning, desensitizing regimen to correct such a mechanism. Chronic stress patterns may be due to the length of time the stressor is in operation, leading to a breakdown of the homeostatic mechanisms and even physical illness, or a repeated pattern of automatic responses.

Extreme difficulty in a job may be a source of stress, but workers like this laundry attendant may suffer from the lack of stimulation present in a more repetitive and undemanding occupation.

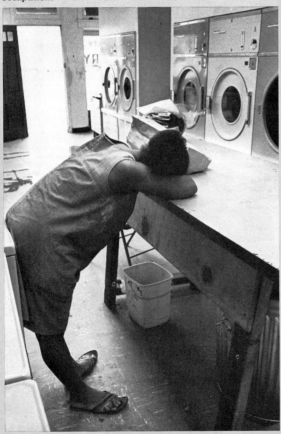

Michael D. Sullivan

What makes a job stressful?

There are many factors that contribute to job stress. They may relate to the work organization, which may provoke conflicts and misunderstandings that lead to stress, or the job itself may be the source of the stress. It may be so demanding that it does not allow the individual to recoup, or it may be so boring that it creates a stress from lack of stimulus to attention.

Role conflict. One of the major sources of job stress is role conflict. When incompatible demands are made by two or more persons on one individual, the compliance with one demand makes it more difficult, if not impossible, to comply with another. Role conflicts within a job may also relate to areas of position and role within a home situation. Two examples are (1) a conflicting status involving position within the family ("low" man at home; "high" man at work), or (2) the role within the job may be so demanding as to raise conflict and guilt from denying time and attention to the family. Overtime and extensive take-home work will frequently raise conflicts. Almost half of all American workers in a recent national sample felt caught in the middle between two conflicting persons or factions on the job. This leads to low job satisfaction, low morale, low confidence, low loyalty, and, usually, high tension.

Ambiguity. Another element of job stress is ambiguity. Even astronauts, who are assumed to live in high states of danger and of stress, have surprisingly lower levels of stress than expected. This has to do with the fact that astronauts have a clear-cut mission and a precise set of directions in a highly oriented series of predetermined operations. However, the ground controllers, who have the ultimate responsibility for all contingencies and who are confronted with ambiguities, problem solving, and emergencies, show the greatest amount of emotional distress and conflict. Studies have shown that one-third or more individuals in the United States felt their job descriptions were vague and ambiguous. They felt they did not have enough information to perform their job adequately and were often unclear about the scope of their responsibilities.

Boundary crossings. Another form of job-related stress has to do with those individuals who work inside and outside the organization at the same time. Jobs fitting this category are those of salesmen, truckers, labor negotiators, and certain types of repair and service technicians. As stated earlier, certain types of health personnel, such as nursing staff and paramedical workers who take orders from doctors but fulfill requests from patients, are also related to the boundary-crossing area. Such individuals tend to feel caught between the demands of the clients with whom they must deal and the requirements of their own management systems. Policies and directions may be in conflict or so rigidly defined they cannot be interpreted as circumstance dictates. Corporate pressures and politics are responsible for escalating stress among service-oriented employees who serve other departments in a large organization. Personnel who are never required to cross company or departmental boundaries report that they have less tension than the boundary crossers.

Overwork. Another aspect of organizational and occupational stress is overwork. The amount of overwork is related to the individual and to the type of work that is done. There are quantitative overloads as well as qualitative overloads. Administrators in large corporations usually complain about quantitative overloads. They may complain about not being able to become extensively involved with one problem because of the necessity of solving a large number of problems. In universities the quantitative aspects are not as pressuring, but the qualitative aspects become an issue. Robert Conn at the University of Michigan has stated that in our culture the problem in dealing with overwork is a common belief that being busy means being productive. Many individuals organize their activities so that they are constantly busy and rushed, and they have the constant feeling of being overworked. This occurs because of poor scheduling, poor delegation, and poor organization.

Promotions. Promotions are another source of organizational stress. Although on the surface promotion is a form of recognition for activities and work well done, it can create a variety of problems. Lack of promotion is, of course, a situation in which the process of not being recognized and not being properly rewarded is a job-related stress. However, receiving a promotion can affect an individual by a change in status involving the learning of new jobs and skills, relating to new individuals, and functioning at different levels of responsibility. Even changing one's own task orientation and moving to an entirely different level of activity can be stressful. An example is moving from an assembly line, where a worker enjoys working with his hands and feels productive, to a supervisory role where he must instruct and monitor other workers. Promotion, or over-promotion, is a critical problem when a worker is promoted beyond the scope of his level of competent activity.

Boredom. Boredom is another job-related stress. Many jobs are boring, monotonous, repetitious, and meaningless in terms of the totality of the operation. We frequently think of factory jobs as repetitive and monotonous, but many office jobs are also monotonous and repetitious. Somewhere between 10 and 15% of workers are dissatisfied with their jobs because the jobs are boring. Most workers deal with dull jobs through absenteeism, extended sick-benefit usage, and inattention to detail. They move around frequently, creating extensive costs for the industry in which they are working.

Job loss. Job loss is the most conflict-laden, the most traumatic experience in assessing job-related stress. It creates economic problems through the loss of income in addition to loss of self-esteem and prestige and a sense of doubt about competence. Unemployment is equated with failure in our society and is looked on with disfavor. During periods of unemployment the worker may tend to project feelings of failure onto the company. Or he may manifest his feelings in illness. The employee then assumes a sick role rather than an unemployed role. In times of high unemployment with job layoffs, visits to physicians increase. It is as if this is a rationalization to explain unemployment; *i.e.,* a sense of not feeling well or being ill as an explanation for the fact that the individual is not at work.

In recent years the impact of civil rights litigation and legislation leading to affirmative action programs has made a great impact on job opportunities and job-related stress. Women and minorities find themselves in previously unavailable jobs. While this represents a real gain in equalizing their status, it does lead to building of pervasive tensions and stresses. The solitary woman on a corporate board not only is in a lonely position but often feels that she is constantly on stage. The same is true of other members of minority groups who must work through their feelings of being token representatives. Even when workers can resolve such problems, the adjustment activities of new surroundings, cultural assimilations, and alienated feelings place heavy demands on their coping capacities. Such changes, in turn, stress the old guard elements of top and middle management. By the very nature of having change imposed from without, pressure is also imposed on those who may be passed over or treated in ways other than those expected from the old system.

Corporations and industry have begun to invest heavily in training their staffs in life-adjustment and coping techniques. Many support training seminars and symposia and employ behavioral scientists as consultants for their employees and management personnel.

Individuals are also taking steps to reduce stress in their lives; they are meditating, taking courses in self-assertion, jogging, running marathons, and doing body-building exercises. Whether one engages in meditation or vigorous exercises is not the prime factor. What is important is that people are involving themselves in techniques that relieve tension and stress and make them healthier.

We know now that there are alternatives for coping with job stress. These range from analyzing the stressful work schedules to changing skills, even to changing jobs. What is essential is to identify and clarify the elements of stress in each area of functioning and relate them to the individual's particular method of reacting. Stress can be useful in stimulating our bodies and minds to tolerable work and life activity limits. Too much is destructive; too little deprives us of stimulation and, in the end, is also harmful.

Pediatrics

Contributions from the many subspecialties of pediatrics—neonatal medicine (that dealing with the newborn), perinatal medicine (dealing with the periods before and after birth), infectious disease, immunology, genetics, hematology, neurology, nephrology, cardiology, radiology, pediatric surgery, child psychiatry, and so forth—have accounted for a great surge of progress in the prevention and treatment of disorders of childhood. More important than each individual advance, perhaps, is the interdisciplinary team approach best exemplified by pediatric and neonatal intensive care units, where the skills of the subspecialists merge in the care of a single patient with multiple problems.

New clinical syndromes

Kawasaki disease, or mucocutaneous lymph node syndrome, is an acute febrile disease of prepubertal children. Although it had been described in Japan in the 1960s, the first case was not recognized in the United States until April 1971. As of December 1977 nearly 200 cases had been described in the United States, adding to those documented in Canada, Australia, Europe, and the Middle East.

The clinical picture includes prolonged fever unresponsive to antibiotics; conjunctival inflammation; dry lips with fissures, and inflammation of the mouth and throat, including a "strawberry tongue"; redness and edema of the palms of the hands and soles of the feet, followed by peeling of the skin at the tips of the fingers and toes; skin rash; swollen, painful lymph nodes in the neck; and the absence of other established disease states such as scarlet fever. Cardiovascular complications are primarily responsible for the mortality rate of about 1–2%. Aseptic (viral) meningitis, arthritis, and inflammation of the liver and kidneys also have been reported.

Rickettsia microorganisms and viruses have been implicated in the etiology of this disorder, but the evidence has been inconclusive. Infection is thought to be the most likely cause. Parenthetically, *Leptospira* spirochetes have been incriminated as a cause of disease in a group of children with symptoms comparable to those of Kawasaki disease. Corroboration of this observation is needed to establish the relationship.

Infantile hypotonia, often called the floppy baby syndrome, previously had been attributed to a variety of neurologic, metabolic, and muscle disorders. A significant percentage of cases, however, were of unknown origin. A recently recognized cause of this syndrome is infant botulism. Almost 80 cases have been identified, and several hundred others are likely to have occurred.

The first recognized case occurred in California, and subsequently the majority of patients have been reported from the same area; more recently, cases have been documented in 17 other states. England was the first country outside the United States to report a case. Presumably, the intensive surveillance and educational efforts in California that have made physicians aware of the syndrome may explain the geographic distribution of cases.

Patients with infant botulism generally are constipated and then become lethargic and listless. Usually over the following one to seven days these symptoms are followed by slow feeding, a feeble cry, droopy eyelids, poor head control, and general weakness. Gag and pupillary light reflexes are reduced. Signs of illness may be mild, and not all babies are noticeably floppy. An electromyogram (which records minute amounts of electrical activity associated with muscle function) may show a pattern of brief, small, abundant electrical waves that is characteristic of the disease.

Infant botulism is quite different from traditional food-borne botulism. Babies become ill with botulism because the bacterium *Clostridium botulinum* infects

Tomisaku Kawasaki, of Tokyo's Japan Red Cross Medical Center, has been credited with identifying an acute febrile disease of young children. Kawasaki disease, or mucocutaneous lymph node syndrome, can result in cardiovascular damage and even death.

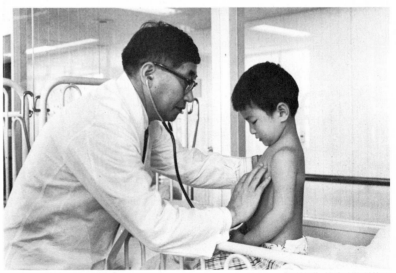

the infant gut and produces its neurotoxin inside the patient's intestines. Adults and older children are resistant to this type of infection for unknown reasons, and they get botulism only by eating botulinal toxin contained in an improperly preserved food. Unlike food-borne botulism, infant botulism has a fatality rate under 3% and a quite favorable prognosis. Present treatment consists of meticulous supportive care, with feeding and breathing assistance in some cases.

The delineation of this disease has been an extraordinary achievement. Much remains to be learned about its range of severity (it appears to be one cause of crib death), the source of the bacteria, the mode of transmission, the variations in host susceptibility, the global geographical distribution, improving treatment, and, most importantly, its prevention.

Recently the group B β-hemolytic streptococcus (GBBS) has displaced the gram-negative class of bacteria as the single most important cause of infection in the newborn. This change is a microbiological and epidemiological enigma.

Although the infection with group B may range from the simple presence of the bacteria in the blood without other symptoms to involvement of the bones, joints, and other systems, there are two distinct forms (early onset and late onset) of GBBS infection that have become apparent clinically and epidemiologically. The early onset form first appears as an acute respiratory illness, with the infection generalized through the body; shock is a result. Onset of the illness is in the first week of life, frequently within 24 hours of delivery. In the majority of cases obstetric complications such as prolonged rupture of membranes, maternal fever, and premature onset of labor are present. This suggests that the infection is acquired during delivery. In full-term infants mild respiratory distress with rapid, shallow breathing is followed by the rapid development of shock, cessation of breathing, and death. However, as many as two-thirds of affected infants are premature, and a significant number of them will have bluish skin and grunting respiration, mimicking the respiratory distress syndrome (RDS), which is frequently seen in premature infants. X-ray examination of the chest of the newborn shows either a bronchopneumonia or the characteristic abnormal pattern associated with RDS. Early onset disease, therefore, is acquired before delivery or during passage through the birth canal of a mother who is a carrier of the organism. All three types (I, II, III) of GBBS have been correlated with this pattern of disease.

Diagnosis is confirmed by the isolation of the organism from blood or other body fluids or tissue. A regimen of penicillin G or ampicillin, with or without an aminoglycoside, is begun as soon as the infection is identified. Outcome is dependent on factors such as age, weight, complications before or at delivery, status of the infant at time of diagnosis, and judicious use of antibiotics. The mortality rate may be 50% or higher.

The second major category of infection, late onset disease, usually occurs after the first week of life, with the predominant manifestation being purulent meningitis, inflammation of the coverings of the brain and spinal cord with the formation of pus. In contrast to the early onset form, there is no evidence that the mother is the carrier of the bacteria: the predominant strain is type III, which may be isolated from environmental sources. The disease is less sudden and severe and the mortality rate is lower (about 20%), although the consequences for the central nervous system may be graver. Therapy consists of the same antibiotics indicated for early onset disease, continued for two weeks after the bacteria are no longer present in the cerebrospinal fluid.

Efforts to prevent GBBS infection are receiving increasing attention. The development of a vaccine that could protect the newborn would be invaluable. Bacteriologic surveillance of the pregnant mother and father may identify the carrier state, but this would be of only limited help since infection occurs in only one of 200 infants in whom the bacteria are present. Similarly, antibiotics administered to the pregnant mother to eradicate the organism have not permanently eliminated GBBS. At the time of birth a variety of regimens have been used in umbilical cord care as another means of preventing the growth of GBBS, and some have been of benefit.

Until recently inclusion blennorrhea had been considered a mild conjunctivitis, or infection of the mucous membranes of the eyelids, occurring within the first few days of birth; it was not felt to be a serious threat to the infant. *Chlamydia trachomatis,* a bacterium commonly present in the genital tract of the pregnant female, had been recognized as the cause. Antibiotic therapy has ameliorated this persistent infectious process. Clinically, its major importance had been in differentiating it from the more serious gonococcal conjunctivitis, an ocular infection occurring during the first few days after birth, caused by the gonorrhea microorganism.

Knowledge of the spectrum of infection with *Chlamydia* has now been broadened. New evidence indicates that *Chlamydia* is a cause of a low-grade, feverless, prolonged pneumonia of early infancy and is a significant cause of acute pelvic inflammatory disease in female babies and idiopathic epididymitis in males. Another member of this group (*Chlamydia psittaci*) is responsible for the pneumonia acquired from birds, especially parrots and parakeets.

The new observations on *Chlamydia* were made in a group of 20 infants, 4 to 24 weeks of age (mean age of 6 weeks). They had rapid respiration and spells of a staccato cough—similar to that of whooping cough but without the "whoop." Vomiting and cyanosis (bluish tint of the skin) were sometimes present. The patients did not seem very ill, but the symptoms lingered for longer than a month. Listening to the sounds of the lungs revealed persistent, fine, crackling noises. Chest X-rays confirmed the clinical findings of diffuse, patchy infiltrates (pneumonia) throughout the lungs. Interestingly, less than half of the patients had a history of a preceeding conjunctivitis.

Alterations in blood chemistry were found upon laboratory examination of the patients' blood. In a small but significant number of cases, other viruses such as cytomegalovirus, respiratory syncytial virus, rhinovirus, and adenovirus were also cultured, but the significance of their presence is unclear. Antibody response to *Chlamydia* was significantly elevated. Chlamydial pneumonia is treated with either sulfisoxazole or erythromycin, administered orally or by injection for a two-week period.

Immunization update

Diphtheria, whooping cough (pertussis), tetanus, poliomyelitis, measles, German measles (rubella), and mumps are major infectious diseases preventable by the administration of available vaccines. However, the number of cases of measles has increased dramatically from 24,500 in 1975 to an estimated 65,000 in 1977. Three outbreaks of whooping cough were reported in the U.S., in Maine, Florida, and Georgia. Parents seem to be failing to immunize their children either because of a general lack of sufficient health care or because these childhood diseases are no longer seen as a real threat to health. Persistence of the infectious agents in the community is fostered by a relatively low level (60–70%) of immunity in the general population.

A major effort to achieve a 90% immunization rate involves enforcement of state laws requiring immunization upon entry into the school system. Data from Alaska, Detroit, Mich., and Cincinnati, Ohio, confirm the feasibility and success of this approach.

Medical therapy of the ductus arteriosus

In the fetus the ductus arteriosus is a large blood vessel connecting the main pulmonary artery to the descending aorta. During *in utero* life it allows blood to bypass the nonfunctioning lungs and provides a channel crucial for the passage of unoxygenated blood to the placenta, where oxygenation of the fetal blood can occur. As a result, the amount of blood returning from the lungs is small, an aid in reducing the workload of the fetal heart. After birth, when breathing begins and blood no longer circulates through the placenta, the ductus arteriosus closes. This usually occurs within the first 12 to 24 hours after birth. If it does not close, the overtaxed heart of the infant fails. When the ductus remains open, or patent, surgery must be performed to close it.

The mechanism of closure of the ductus arteriosus has been related to the higher blood oxygen concentrations of the delivered newborn and to his gestational age at the time of birth. More recently the prostaglandins, a group of potent agents affecting the tone and caliber of blood vessels, have been shown to affect the tone of the ductus, causing it to stay open after birth. Prostaglandins are known to cause abortions and are clinically used for that purpose, but they also are normally present in the body in small amounts.

It has been discovered that nonsteroidal anti-inflammatory agents such as aspirin and indomethacin may inhibit the synthesis of prostaglandins in the body. Two still experimental uses of prostaglandins and of one of these inhibitors have been investigated. Severe congenital heart disease can exist in which the surgery necessary for closure of the ductus would be life-threatening. If the patent ductus allows adequate systemic blood flow or passage of blood through the lungs, infusion of prostaglandin E results in dilation of the ductus. This allows the newborn to survive until the surgical procedure can be performed in a controlled rather than an emergency fashion.

On the other hand, small babies with severe respiratory distress syndrome frequently have a patent ductus arteriosus as a complicating feature of their pulmonary problem. The use of a prostaglandin inhibitor, indomethacin, may effect closure of the ductus arteriosus by pharmacological means alone, averting the need for surgical closure.

Infant development

Technological advances in neonatal intensive care units have allowed the survival of small, sick infants previously doomed to death or to severe mental handicaps. At the same time, interest in the behavior of the newborn has intensified.

The neonate no longer is considered passive or neurologically incomplete but responsive and interactive from birth. Visual, auditory, tactile, and olfactory sensations elicit predictable responses from the healthy newborn who has regained a state of equilibrium and is in an alert state of consciousness. The newborn is able to respond to facial expression and to the spoken voice. In fact, the newborn is able to distinguish the odor of his own mother's milk from that of a wet nurse. More surprisingly, at two or three weeks of age the baby has been observed to imitate facial and manual gestures, a response involving cognitive function.

A behavioral assessment scale for the newborn has been constructed in which an infant's capacity to integrate external and internal stimuli and to interact with the environment is measured. The state of consciousness (alertness) is recorded, and the infant's best response to a variety of stimuli forms the basis of this evaluation. Testing the ability of the newborn to interact with his examiners and demonstrate that he has adapted his behavior to sensory stimuli is coupled with a modified neurologic examination. Infants who exhibit

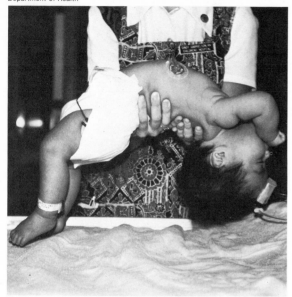

A child with infantile hypotonia, or "floppy baby syndrome," exhibits the characteristic lack of muscle tone that gives the disease its name; it was recently discovered that the cause is an infection by Clostridium botulinum.

a narrow range of states during their first months make it difficult for their caregivers to distinguish what their needs are, which may be placing the infants at risk of compromised later development.

The phenomenon of bonding (attachment), a process by which the infant and parents attach to one another to form a secure, loving relationship, has begun to be studied systematically. Impetus for the current scientific inquiry into the bonding process was provided by efforts to determine causes for the diseases of presumed nonattachment as seen in infants who have failed to grow (a condition sometimes called failure to thrive), neglected and battered children, and adults who seem to lack the capacity to form human bonds. Researchers have supported clinical findings that indicate that separation of pre-term, sick, and even full-term infants from their mothers may result in an alteration of attitudes and behavior that can persist for months or years after birth. The role of the father in the neonatal period has been studied less extensively than that of the mother, but recent research has challenged the exclusiveness of the mother-infant relationship and has helped open hospital nurseries to less restrictive family visiting. (*See also* Pregnancy and Birth Special Report: Midwifery, Prepared Childbirth, and Home Birth.)

Breast-feeding and nutrition

New evidence has supported the renaissance of breast-feeding as the desirable form of nourishment during infancy. Human milk, with its lowered protein concentration, has been found to be qualitatively different from milk from artificial sources. This is of greatest importance to the premature infant who is biochemically immature in contrast to a full-term baby. The amino acid concentrations in human milk are quite different from those in the milk of cows or other mammals and are more appropriate for the needs of the infant metabolism.

Information on the anti-infective properties of human milk has been resurrected. In one U.S. study nursing infants had fewer gastrointestinal and respiratory infections than infants fed artificial formulas. Human milk contains a luxuriant amount of white blood cells (especially macrophages and mononuclear cells) and in addition has a wide array of substances that contribute to the "host resistance factors" that operate in the body's antigen-producing response to invading disease-causing bacteria. Presumably they help account for the decreased number of infections in breast-fed babies.

Although iron concentrations are similar in human milk and cow's milk, iron is absorbed much better by the infant feeding on breast milk and protects the suckling baby from iron-deficiency anemia. Zinc, a trace element now under intensive investigation because of the recognition that its deficiency causes severe disorders, also is absorbed better. In the Middle East, especially in Iran and Egypt, growth failure, lack of development of the genitalia, and enlargement of the liver and spleen have been seen in vegetarians who also exhibit geophagia (the habit of eating clay or earth). These abnormalities have been correlated with zinc deficiency. Dietary zinc supplements seemed to have corrected the disorders.

Acrodermatitis enteropathica is a severe disease of early childhood that has been related to a disturbance in the physiology of zinc. This inherited disorder is characterized by severe diarrhea, dermatitis, loss of hair, growth failure, underdeveloped genitalia, and increased susceptibility to infection. Dietary zinc supplementation, presumably overcoming a defect in absorption of zinc, results in a rapid recovery. Modest therapeutic success in treating this disease was formerly achieved by feeding the patients human milk, which contains a zinc-binding factor that allows for increased gastrointestinal absorption of zinc.

(*See also* Genetic Disorders; Pregnancy and Birth; Urinary and Genital Disorders.)

— *David Ingall, M.D.*

Physical Fitness and Sports Medicine

Interest in sports medicine has been accelerating rapidly in the United States. Health professionals are joining sports-related organizations; scientific meetings discussing sports medicine are being held; and clinics treating sports-related injuries are being planned and opened. Increasing public participation in all forms of

Sports participation for all

People of all ages are becoming involved in long-distance running. Nearly 200 marathon runs (26 mi, 385 yd) were held in the U.S. in 1977, the largest, the renowned Boston Marathon, involving nearly 3,000 participants. The number of runs over six miles, excluding regular collegiate competition, was well over 1,000. In response to the huge volume of new customers, many new styles of running shoes have been introduced. Along with the number of runners, injuries have increased proportionately. (See Physical Fitness and Sports Medicine Special Report: Jogging Injuries.)

The United States Olympic Committee opened training centers for amateur athletes in Squaw Valley, Calif., at the site of the VIII Olympic Winter Games of 1960, and at Colorado Springs, Colo. These centers began to receive sports teams sent by various national sports federations for limited periods of testing and training. Nearby sports facilities are used for practice since the centers have not yet acquired their own equipment. Although first priority was being given to the training of the elite athletes who expect to participate in the Pan American Games of 1979 and the Winter and Summer Olympic Games of 1980, eventually the training centers will be open to other young athletes as well.

Reports of training methods from Eastern Europe stimulated demonstrations and trials of monitoring athletes' training and performance by microanalysis of blood urea nitrogen, lactic acid, and pH, with computerized instant feedback. The purpose of these studies is to schedule training programs to take maximum advantage of an athlete's improvement, to prevent overtraining, and to forecast maximum potential. These training methods are most applicable to events such as swimming and running over stated distances for time, both of which produce directly measurable results.

The United States Association for Blind Athletes (USABA) was established in November 1976 as a permanent organization to sponsor competitions for blind athletes. It formulated national rules for participation of visually handicapped athletes in wrestling, swimming, track and field, and goal ball. The first national USABA championships were held for four days in March–April 1977 at Western Illinois University, in Macomb, Ill. USABA participants, both male and female, are classified according to degree of visual acuity. The organization is enabling them to compete within the U.S. and abroad with sighted as well as blind athletes.

Sports hazards

In 1977 the Amateur Hockey Association of the United States made the wearing of face masks mandatory for all players under its jurisdiction. It also established a Hockey Equipment Certification Council, which developed standards for the certification of face masks for ice hockey.

Rebound tumbling apparatuses (such as the trampoline) are used for the training of gymnasts and divers as well as in physical education programs to develop body awareness, balance, and coordination. This equipment came under increasing attack in 1977, when civil suits for liability amounting to millions of dollars were brought against manufacturers, program sponsors, and individuals. Thirty-four cases of paralysis and three deaths have been reported. Many schools locked up their rebound apparatuses when they were unable to obtain liability insurance covering their use. Meanwhile, the United States Gymnastic Safety Association has developed improvements in teaching methods for the use of this type of apparatus, which are incorporated in its new *Gymnastics Safety Manual*, and has implemented a trampoline instructor certification program. The Consumer Product Safety Commission has issued a fact sheet outlining construction features and safety procedures for users based on performance standards developed by the American Society for Testing and Materials.

A judgment was rendered in 1977 against a ski slope operator in Vermont for injuries that resulted in permanent disability to a skier who was tripped by underbrush concealed beneath the snow. This ruling has increased insurance rates for slope operators in general and has caused some to terminate their operations. It seems unlikely that even the most careful grooming of ski slopes can guarantee freedom from all possible hazards that might trip a skier—or from liability claims that might allege injuries from such hazards.

Skateboarding proved to be a hazardous form of recreation. The Consumer Product Safety Commission reported in 1978 that 25 teenagers had been killed in skateboarding accidents in the previous two years, either as a result of head injuries from falls or by being struck by automobiles. In addition, thousands of fractures were reported, usually in novice riders.

An increase in violent behavior by athletes and spectators, particularly at professional sports events, was apparent in 1977. Baseball, football, ice hockey, and basketball each provided its share of incidents. Athletes were fined and suspended from play; suits were brought for liability; and both spectators and athletes were seriously injured. A variety of theories accounting for the manifestation of these behaviors were brought forward, but the only solutions attempted were an increase in the penalties levied against offending athletes by the professional clubs. Measures to control drinking of alcohol by spectators, which appeared to be a principal cause of rowdy behavior, were conspicuous by their absence. Sports promoters and players alike were alarmed that the violence might culminate in players' being killed by an out-of-control audience.

—Allan J. Ryan, M.D.

Physical Fitness and Sports Medicine

Special Report:

Jogging Injuries

by Alan J. Ryan, M.D.

In the past few years jogging and running have become extremely popular activities among Americans. Estimates of the number of people who run range from 10 million (nearly 5% of the population) to as many as 25 million. Some of these people undoubtedly jog or run on an irregular basis, but a very large number, of all ages, participate regularly in self-imposed running and jogging programs or as members of physical fitness or running clubs.

Certainly for many people the attractiveness of jogging and running stems largely from their well-publicized physical benefits. For people living sedentary, affluent lives the most important benefits are probably the positive effects on the cardiovascular and respiratory systems. A well-designed running program increases the efficiency of the heart and lungs. By efficiency is meant simply that the heart and lungs and their related organs are able to perform their functions better and with less work. And a healthier heart and healthier lungs reduce the susceptibility to diseases such as heart attack, stroke, and emphysema and also promote better general health.

Running and jogging also have other "secondary" beneficial effects. Many people are undoubtedly attracted to running as an effective way to develop better muscle tone and to lose weight. Many runners claim important psychological benefits, particularly a reduction of tension and anxiety, problems that cause other complaints such as tiredness and insomnia. But runners are also prone to injuries, particularly injuries of the feet, ankles, legs, and knees. Proper footwear and conditioning, along with other precautionary measures, can help prevent these injuries. Proper care for them can in most cases prevent serious complications. It is important, however, to understand these injuries and why they occur.

Based on the length of the stride and on the position in which the foot meets the ground, a theoretical distinction can be made between running and jogging. In practice, however, there are so many individual differences in strides and foot positions that it is reasonable to define jogging simply as slow running. Both joggers and runners may suffer injuries, but because they run harder and usually run farther and more frequently, runners are likely to have more frequent and more serious injuries than are joggers. Overuse is a principal factor in such injuries.

Common injuries

The most common injuries of both joggers and runners occur in the lower extremities. Some injuries are caused by running itself or by the circumstances under which it is done. Other injuries are the effects of human anatomy or of abnormal conditions in runners. All of the injuries are brought on by the greater force (up to three or four times the body weight) with which the runner's feet strike the ground and by the number of times this contact is made.

The feet and ankles. Hemorrhages that sometimes occur beneath the toenails may lead to the loss of the nails. This problem occurs when the toes are driven down into the toe of the shoe. Hemorrhaging can usually be prevented by the wearing of shoes that have about an inch of space (a thumb's width) between the largest toe and the tip. Properly fitting shoes may also help to prevent the hard corns that sometimes form when the toes are squeezed together too tightly. A shoe that is either too narrow or that does not provide

"You think we should run in place? In place of what?"

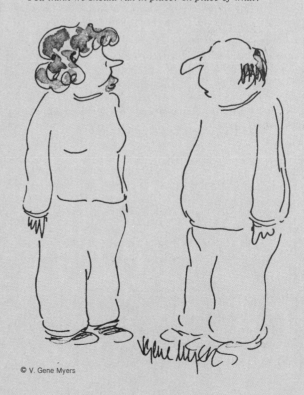

© V. Gene Myers

proper support for the toes can create problems for runners.

Bruises sometimes occur where the first metatarsal bone joins the big toe. This problem may develop in anyone, but running increases the likelihood of such bruises. Blisters on the soles of the feet are caused by rotational stress on the skin. Runners may prevent these by wearing shoes that fit properly, by wearing socks that fit the foot snugly, and by lubricating the skin with petroleum jelly. Thick calluses may crack and become painful. Shaving down calluses will prevent such complications.

Because the runner pushes off from his big toe and the head of his first metatarsal bone, several problems can arise in this area of the foot. The simplest injury is a painful and disabling sprain of the joint, which may require support for treatment. The two small sesamoid bones under the metatarsal head may also become painful and tender and may even fracture. Persons who have a short and movable first metatarsal head, with the sesamoids behind rather than under it, often develop a painful callus over the head of the second metatarsal. Runners affected by this condition often rotate the foot excessively and produce a strain on the longitudinal arch.

Strains on both the transverse and the longitudinal arches occur in the middle of the foot in runners who rotate their feet excessively and whose heels are tilted inwards. These problems can be treated and prevented by the use of orthotics, plastic casts made from the runner's foot with built-in corrections. Orthotics help the foot hit the ground in the correct position and help the runner make a normal transitional movement from impact to the push-off as the foot leaves the ground.

Stress fractures may affect any of the metatarsal bones, but the second, third, and fourth, in that order, are the most frequently injured. Fractures seem to occur most commonly in runners with delicate bone structures and with a tendency to excessive rotation of the foot. A fracture at the base of the fifth metatarsal may occur as the result of the pull of a tendon that attaches there.

In the rear of the foot a common complaint is pain just in front of the heel. This is usually due to inflammation of the plantar fascia, the fibrous layer on the sole of the foot, which attaches to the heel at that point. Calcium deposits in this attachment are sometimes visible on X-rays and are usually called "bone spurs." Stretching the plantar fascia and cushioning the heel are effective treatment.

If sensory nerves that come into the side of the foot are compressed, they produce a painful neuritis. The problem is corrected by relieving the pressure. Painful bumps over the back of the heel are due to bursitis caused by rubbing of the shoe or by poor positioning of the heel. They can often be corrected by the use of an orthotic.

The point at which the Achilles tendon attaches to the heel bone is frequently a site of inflammation in runners. The inflammation may result from overuse, pressure of an improperly fitted heel counter, or inward rotation of the heel and may become chronic. A bursa, a water-filled sac, between the tendon and heel bone may also become inflamed. Because of repeated strain, ruptures of some of the fibers of the tendon may occur. A complete rupture usually occurs in a tendon already weakened by minor strains and is more common in older runners.

Runners most often sprain their ankles from stepping into depressions or off of curbs. An inversion

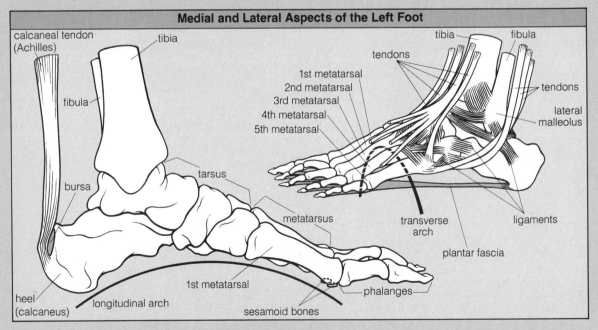

Medial and Lateral Aspects of the Left Foot

calcaneal tendon (Achilles)
tibia
fibula
bursa
tarsus
metatarsus
heel (calcaneus)
longitudinal arch
1st metatarsal
sesamoid bones
phalanges

tibia
fibula
tendons
1st metatarsal
2nd metatarsal
3rd metatarsal
4th metatarsal
5th metatarsal
tendons
lateral malleolus
transverse arch
ligaments
plantar fascia

sprain, in which the ligaments on the outside are more seriously injured, is the most common type. Ankles that are sprained are easily sprained again if they are not properly treated by support or, occasionally, by surgical repair. Another injury of running is the dislocation of the tendons in front of the lateral malleolus (the ankle bone). The injury occurs when the connective tissue that holds the tendon in place is torn.

The legs. Ruptures of fibers in the calf muscle sometimes occur as the result of landing off balance on the foot. These ruptures are painful and disabling but heal in time with support. Pain down the outer side of the leg can be more troublesome. It is due either to pressure on the peroneal nerve or to sciatic pain arising from a problem in the lower spine or hip.

Pains in the muscles of the leg, especially in the front and rear tibials, are known as "shin splints." In Great Britain they are sometimes called "fresher legs" because they commonly occur in the untrained person who is beginning to run. A number of factors appear to be involved, including inadequate warm-up, improper footwear, too great an oblique angle from the hip to the knee, and running on hard surfaces.

If such pain persists for more than a week, the possibility of a stress fracture should be investigated. A stress fracture may occur in either the tibia or fibula, producing tenderness and swelling and eventually a

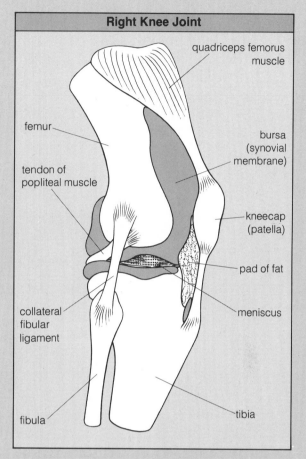

Right Knee Joint

quadriceps femorus muscle

femur

bursa (synovial membrane)

tendon of popliteal muscle

kneecap (patella)

pad of fat

collateral fibular ligament

meniscus

fibula

tibia

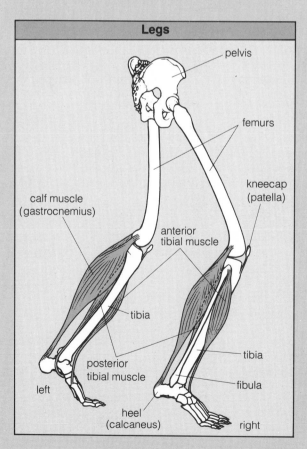

Legs

pelvis

femurs

calf muscle (gastrocnemius)

kneecap (patella)

anterior tibial muscle

tibia

tibia

posterior tibial muscle

fibula

left

heel (calcaneus)

right

stress line across the bone. Pain that occurs only after a few minutes of running and that subsides completely on rest is indicative of a "compartment syndrome." The pain, accompanied by swelling and tenderness of muscles in the leg, is due to the swelling of muscle surrounded by tight connective tissue, which compresses the nerves and cuts off the blood supply.

The knees. Pains around the knee may originate in the kneecap (patella), ligaments, cartilage, or the tibia. In some persons the patella may be partially or completely dislocated. Repeated dislocation wears away cartilage and bone on the back of the kneecap (a condition called chondromalacia patellae), which causes pain, swelling, and sometimes disability.

Painful swelling and tenderness over the growth center of the tibia just below the knee occur in young runners. This center does not usually unite firmly with the shaft of the knee until around age 18.

Pain, and even calcification, may occur in the ligaments of runners' knees, especially on the outer side. This may result from improper balance or alignment of the foot and leg. Injury to one of the internal cartilages of the knee may occur from landing too heavily with the knee fully extended. Pain, swelling, and disability result, and sometimes the cartilage in the runner's knee may need to be removed surgically.

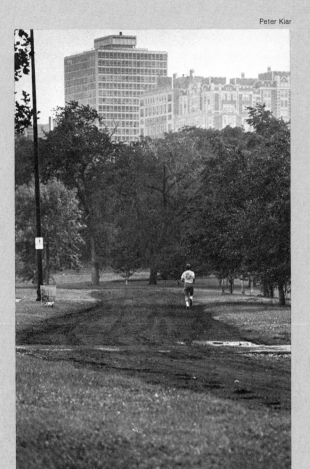

While the runner tones up his heart and respiratory system, he must take care with proper warm-up exercises and shoes not to damage his musculoskeletal system.

Runners, especially sprinters, sometimes strain the rear thigh muscles (hamstrings). This injury is usually due to muscles that are too tight. Pulled hamstrings can, however, be caused by postural faults that allow a forward tipping of the pelvis, which produces imbalance between the two thighs and between the quadriceps on the front of the thighs and the hamstrings. Especially in young runners, severe stress on the thigh muscles may actually pull off portions of the femur or pelvis to which they are attached. Bursitis and stress fractures sometimes occur on the femur itself.

A forward curvature of the spine (lordosis) may cause back pain in runners. Problems with the vertebrae such as a forward slipping of one vertebra over another may cause not only low back pain but also sciatic radiation of pain down the back of the leg.

If one leg is shorter than the other, the unequal length produces a tilt of the pelvis and lateral curvature (scoliosis) in the spine. This condition may cause only discomfort in walking but will usually cause recurring low back pain on running. Placing a lift on the heel or inside the heel of the shoe will ordinarily relieve this kind of pain.

Other injuries. Frostbite of the penis may result from the combined effects of cold synthetic shorts and reduced circulation due to compression by an athletic supporter. Irritation of the nipples occurs in both male and female joggers because of friction from a shirt or bra. Joggers can prevent this irritation by applying petroleum jelly before running or by covering the nipples with gauze and adhesive tape.

Microscopic or even visible amounts of blood and protein tissue sometimes appear in the urine after a hard run. Called athletic pseudonephritis, the condition is commonly found in athletes competing in other sports as well. The problem appears to be associated with dehydration, the diversion of blood away from the kidneys to the muscles, and constriction of capillaries in the kidneys. This constriction allows protein and red blood cells to pass more freely through the kidneys' filtering membrane. It is not thought to cause permanent damage to the kidneys.

Preventing injuries

Running shoes that fit the foot properly, have a strong shank and firm heel counter, and cushion the heel and sole well are helpful in avoiding many injuries of joggers and runners. An even surface that yields is better for running than is a hard surface. Beginning runners should not attempt too much too soon and should be careful not to increase their speed or the distance covered too rapidly. A warm-up of ten minutes that includes loosening-up exercise and a cool-down of about the same time that includes stretching exercise will help to prevent injuries.

When running in high temperatures and humidity, runners should be careful to keep well hydrated in order to avoid heat exhaustion. In very cold weather runners should wear warm, loose-fitting clothing. Woolen socks, gloves, and a hat that covers the ears help to prevent hypothermia and frostbite. The intake of cold air is ordinarily not troublesome unless the runner is susceptible to anginal pain.

Pregnancy and Birth

In recent years the pregnancy rate has declined dramatically in the United States. Regardless of the reasons for the decline, it has been made possible by the development of completely effective contraceptives and readily available early termination of pregnancy. The medical care required for pregnancy and childbirth is becoming increasingly expensive and is one of the few areas of medical care that remains incompletely covered by most insurance plans.

The declining pregnancy rate, which of course results in fewer children per family, has stimulated an increasing emphasis on the importance of delivering a strong, unblemished infant with high intellectual potential. New attention has thus been focused on those areas that adversely affect the health of the developing fetus and the newborn infant.

The study of teratogens

At one time it was felt that the developing fetus was well protected by the uterus and the placenta (afterbirth). We now know many substances cross the placenta and adversely affect the fetus, particularly at an early stage in the development of the heart, brain, bone, and other organs. The fetus may well be damaged by drugs or other outside influences that are perfectly harmless to the mother.

Medical science includes an area of study known as teratology. Etymologically this is defined as "the study of monsters"; the term is also used to include the study of abnormal development. Drugs or other outside influences that produce abnormal development of the fetus are referred to as teratogens. Most substances that produce abnormal development have their effect in the early stages of organ development. In the human fetus development of most organ systems is relatively complete by the end of the third month. Exceptions to this rule include the central nervous system and the skeletal system, which continue to develop over many years.

A number of problems exist in the study of teratogens. Frequently a woman uses a drug or another substance for a very short period of time and in some cases uses the substance even before she knows that she is pregnant. Experiments with animals frequently show results that do not hold true for humans. A hereditary predisposition must exist before some drugs will have an adverse effect on the fetus. In addition, almost all teratogens must be given at a very specific time in the pregnancy in order to have a demonstrated effect.

Drugs are not the only cause of abnormal development. In a recent summary of causes of defects it was found that only 2–3% of fetal defects are related to drugs and chemicals. Another 2–3% are felt to be related to infection in pregnancy. The largest group—as much as 70%—falls into the category of unknown origin. Current research is aimed at reducing the number of conditions in the unknown category, so that they may be avoided or counteracted.

Fetal alcohol syndrome

One of the most recently recognized substances that produce abnormal development is alcohol. In 1973 the pregnancies of a number of mothers known to be heavy drinkers were followed, and their infants were studied. At the time of birth it was noted that babies were small in terms of length and weighed less than other babies. The babies had a high incidence of small heads, defective joints in their hands and feet, cleft palate, and heart abnormalities. The researchers studying these infants termed their abnormalities "fetal alcohol syndrome." Some of the babies were so severely affected that they died after birth, and when their brains were studied they were found to be poorly developed; some portions were actually missing. The infants that survived showed impaired intellectual development as well as decreased ability to use certain muscles. It is believed that the fetal alcohol syndrome is not a rare occurrence. It may exist in many degrees of severity, but its most common manifestation is mental impairment.

Opinion is varied in regard to what a pregnant woman should do about the use of alcohol. Some scientists

An infant exhibits the characteristic facial appearance of the fetal alcohol syndrome, caused by the mother's heavy intake of alcohol during pregnancy. A number of physical and mental abnormalities can be present.

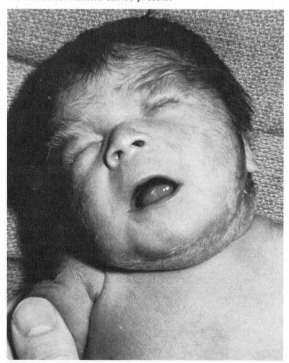

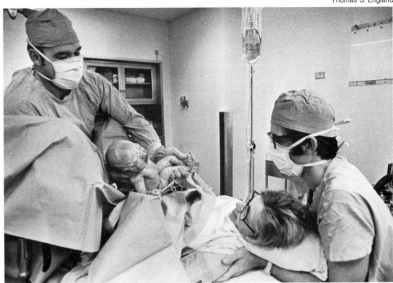

Both father and mother delight in the first sight of their newborn child. Some hospitals now allow men to participate in the labor and childbirth processes.

feel that it should be totally avoided because of the possibility that the fetus may be affected by even very low or infrequent doses; others feel that one or two drinks a day may be safe. Until complete information is available, it is prudent that the pregnant woman totally abstain from all alcoholic beverages. (*See also* Alcoholism and Drug Abuse.)

Drugs and pregnancy

The number of drugs used by women is astounding—one study showed that the average number of medications taken by pregnant women is ten, and other investigators found as high as 40% of all pregnant women taking four or more medications. Little is known about the effect of every drug on the developing fetus. Physicians and pregnant women alike are being advised to avoid any medications that are not strongly required.

Occupational hazards

Working women are becoming increasingly aware of occupational hazards. The American College of Obstetricians and Gynecologists recently published medical guidelines for working women during pregnancy. Some of the findings include the following:

1. Pregnant workers should be protected against undue risk of exposure to infections. For example, it might be unwise for a pregnant woman to be employed in a contagious unit of a hospital or in a medical laboratory.

2. Increased number of miscarriages and stillbirths among female workers exposed to excessive lead levels are a recognized risk. Some studies have also shown chromosome breaks and increased fetal death in wives of vinyl chloride workers.

3. The usually allowable concentrated chemicals in the air should be reduced for the pregnant worker, since pregnancy brings an increased respiratory rate and breathing volume.

4. Exposure to anesthetic gases used in hospital operating rooms is associated with an increased rate of congenital abnormalities. Attention is now being directed to better design of anesthesia equipment.

The same study also discussed the risk in employment if a pregnant woman has a preexisting health problem or a problem pregnancy. The study offered the following suggestions:

1. When poor fetal growth is diagnosed, a woman should limit her activity, should not perform strenuous physical tasks, and should probably be discouraged from working after the sixth month of pregnancy.

2. Women with high blood pressure may require decreased activity, rest at home, or hospitalization. They may undertake nonstrenuous work in the first six months with surveillance on an outpatient basis.

3. Women pregnant with twins should limit their activity, should not perform strenuous tasks, and should probably be discouraged from working after the sixth month. (*See also* Occupational and Environmental Health.)

Advances in childbirth

Many changes are taking place in the care of pregnant women as well as in the management of labor and delivery. In 1942 Grantly Dick-Read suggested that those pregnant women who were properly conditioned and educated underwent much more comfortable labors and deliveries, requiring little pain medication and minimal anesthesia. Read's early work has spawned a number of activities aimed at education and conditioning—psychoprophylaxis, prepared childbirth, childbirth education, and Lamaze training. Many of these systems now make use of the father. (*See* Pregnancy and Birth Special Report: Midwifery, Prepared Childbirth, and Home Birth.)

— *Robert Rogers, M.D.*

298

Special Report:

Midwifery, Prepared Childbirth, and Home Birth

by Albert W. Isenman

As recently as a generation ago the attitudes of young parents and prospective parents toward childbirth were quite different from what they are today. There was considerable concern about the possible death of the mother or infant. The childbearing process was cloaked in myth and mystery, and the pregnant woman was isolated from the child's father during the birth. The technology of the hospital was viewed as offering the means of victory over pain and risk.

A number of social and technological trends provide a different picture of the childbearing experience today. Young parents are often well informed about their own bodies and the physiology of pregnancy, labor, and delivery. The common use of contraceptives has made reproduction a matter of choice. Improvements in antibiotics, in delivery techniques, and in the general health and nutrition of the population at large have helped to reduce the risks of childbirth, and nowadays the key question is not merely survival but rather the quality of life.

Progress in obstetrics is most apparent as a technological phenomenon, with delivery rooms and newborn nurseries now equipped with devices, surgical techniques, and electronic monitors unheard of only a few years ago. "Perinatology"—the subspecialty in medicine that studies as a unit the mother, fetus, and events surrounding the delivery—has led to greater use of these devices and surgical interventions.

Ironically, the current trend among prospective parents toward "natural" childbirth gains momentum amid an ever increasing array of technological innovations in medical care. The juxtaposition of these two phenomena has triggered some fundamental conflicts as well as some changes in obstetrical thought and practice. The public has displayed a steadily growing distrust of hospitals and physicians with an alarming rise in malpractice lawsuits. At the same time, health care personnel have recently begun to lend a more sensitive ear to public entreaties for "humanizing" maternity care, and of late attention has been focused on alternatives to the conventional, sterile, and costly procedure of giving birth in a hospital. Among these alternative childbearing experiences are midwifery, home birth, prepared childbirth, and what is known as family-centered maternity care.

Midwifery

Until the middle of this century, attendance at childbirth by midwives was common, particularly in rural and isolated areas of the United States. Where physicians were few or altogether unavailable, people relied on a knowledgeable "granny," a woman who customarily assisted women during delivery. Usually the midwife had no special qualifications beyond simple experience, and indeed none was demanded. Nor are any demanded for the uncomplicated delivery. Services provided by these midwives were limited. Prenatal care was virtually nonexistent. Midwives were usually able to allay some fears in an uncomplicated delivery by advising mothers of what to expect. They provided succor in pain and sympathy in tragedy. Technical services amounted to assisting the mother in bearing down, severing the umbilical cord, helping her to expel the placenta, and providing for the general cleanliness and comfort of the mother and child.

Problems associated with childbirth in this setting were common. Infant mortality was high and injuries frequent. Maternal deaths were always a very real possibility, and subsequent problems related to infection and damage to the woman's reproductive system were frequent. Owing to the isolated nature of midwife activity, midwives could not share information with one another or obtain help in emergencies.

Midwifery, along with quackery, hucksterism, and patent medicine, was subject to the organized and concerted attack of the health professions in the early part of the 20th century, falling into popular disfavor as more formally trained physicians were available and more community hospitals were built. Even though several thousand midwives still practiced in the United States by the 1950s, the very word *midwife* had by then acquired a quaint and archaic ring. At that time the practice of midwifery had been reduced to the traditional lay midwife who still flourished in isolated areas and to the registered nurse who provided midwifery services in concert with rural physicians. Midwives in the latter category are exemplified by the Frontier Nursing Service, which provided maternity services in rural areas of Kentucky for many years and which was linked to a few physicians for emergency backup. Against tremendous cultural and sanitary odds, the professional training of these nurses-turned-midwives, coupled with emergency physician support, pared down the rate of death and injury to mothers and infants. These professional nurse-midwives formed their own specialty association, the American College of Nurse-Midwives, to establish common standards for training and to encourage public confidence in their qualifications. As late as 1960, however, there were still fewer than 400 such nurse-midwives, almost all practicing in rural and occasionally inner-city areas.

In the late 1960s, however, the health profession began to take a new look at nurse-midwives for several reasons. First, the birthrate had been exponentially increasing for several years, and demographers began to predict an unprecedented population explosion as the large group of post-World War II babies reached adulthood and began their own families. Second, the number of physicians specializing in obstetrics seemed to be leveling off, while the number of general practitioners who provided obstetrical services actually fell. Third, by this time childbirth for healthy women was commonly considered a much less risky event than in the past. Clearly, some way to provide services to huge numbers of new parents was needed, and nurse-midwifery seemed to provide a ready answer. In 1970 the American College of Obstetricians and Gynecologists (ACOG), the Nurses Association of ACOG, and the American College of Nurse-Midwives endorsed a joint policy statement that approved nurse-midwives' acceptance of responsibility for the complete care, when working in concert with an obstetrician, of uncomplicated maternity patients. In practice this generally meant that nurse-midwives could manage maternity cases as long as the birth was proceeding normally and as long as physician backup was readily available.

This gave the practice of nurse-midwifery a tremendous boost. The number of training programs for nurse-midwives began to expand, and state laws forbidding maternity services by nonphysicians began to be modified to provide for the practice of nurse-midwives.

There are now a number of recognized academic programs across the country that prepare registered nurses to become Certified Nurse-Midwives (CNM's). Several are two-year programs that award a concurrent master's degree in nursing. Other briefer programs award only the certificate. All have common academic and practical requirements as established by the American College of Nurse-Midwives and build upon previous training for the basic RN degree and experience in obstetric nursing.

A key feature of the nurse-midwifery philosophy is the notion of the team approach to maternity care—the assumption that obstetricians, nurse-midwives, nurses, and others organize to support one another in caring for maternity patients, each bringing certain special skills to the situation. This suggests that the boundary between the services of obstetrician and nurse-midwife is the division between the "normal" and the "complicated" birth. In practice the ability or inability of patients to pay for care also seems to be operative. Of the more than 1,600 CNM's in the United States, nearly half are practicing in hospitals, largely in public clinic settings. The remainder are about equally divided among working or teaching in nurse-midwife programs, working as obstetric nurses, or being without work. Only a small number of CNM's are employed in situations where they care for private as well as clinic patients.

The explanation, of course, is that the expected

For many years the Frontier Nursing Service provided Kentucky women with trained midwife services in an area where physicians were scarce. The movement toward the use of midwives with physician backup is growing today in urban as well as rural areas.

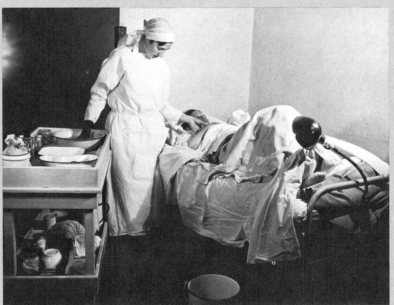

Courtesy, Frontier Nursing Service; photographs, Gabrielle Beasley

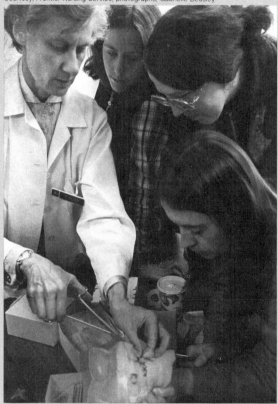
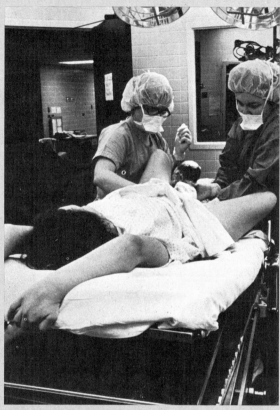

(Left) Students of midwifery at the Frontier Nursing Service receive training in suturing. (Right) A midwife delivers a newborn in a hospital, with standby help available in emergency situations.

population boom and attendant need for vast numbers of nonphysician health personnel did not take place. There was instead a precipitous drop in the birthrate in the 1970s. Young adults now have a tendency to delay beginning their families and, as a rule, they are also having smaller families than their parents had. There also seem to be small gains being made in the number of physicians specializing in obstetrics. So the employment market for CNM's has centered in settings that do not attract physicians.

Yet several signs point to a bright future for nurse-midwives. One is the continuing pressure for cost containment in health services. Because personnel costs account for most of the cost of health services, and because most deliveries are uncomplicated and hence within the abilities of the nurse-midwife, greater utilization of nurse-midwives can be expected in the institutional setting.

It is also quite possible that nurse-midwives will begin to be used more in the private office setting as more obstetricians recognize the economically advantageous opportunity of expanding services without adding another physician to the payroll. Finally, as demand for family-centered and prepared childbirth increases, nurse-midwives and obstetrical nurses will be increasingly relied upon because of the greater individual at-

tention and emotional support that they can provide for the low-risk patients who choose these alternative forms of childbirth.

Prepared childbirth

As the childbirth experience was moved from the home to the hospital, it became more and more of a controlled experience. Public trust in the sciences generally and in hospitals in particular had grown concurrently with the quest for a safe and painless way to give birth. General anesthesia was commonly used in the delivery room, and strict sterile conditions were maintained. "Confinement" was once the common word used to describe labor and delivery, and hospitalization for childbirth had many of the same characteristics as hospitalization for illness: restricted visiting privileges, isolation, and physician control.

Some authors questioned this approach in the 1930s and 1940s, notably Grantly Dick-Read in England and Fernand Lamaze in France. These obstetricians pioneered the concepts of prepared childbirth—or "natural" childbirth, as it is popularly called—concepts that are beginning to be in wide use in the United States today.

Birth preparation classes are now available in many communities through a variety of sponsoring agencies.

301

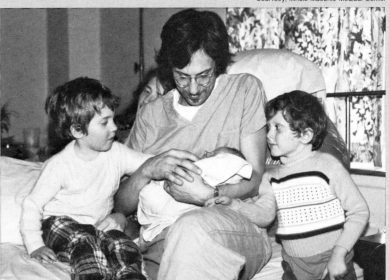

In a homelike atmosphere at an "Alternative Birthing Center" at Chicago's Illinois Masonic Medical Center, the whole family can take part in the birth of a new member. Older children can greet the new arrival within minutes after birth, and friends and family can be present to offer help, encouragement, and support.

Often the hospital where a woman plans to deliver will hold such classes or will be able to make a referral to an acceptable agency.

Women learn special breathing and relaxation exercises that can be used during labor and delivery to alleviate pain and anxiety and to help the birth process. Emphasis is also given to the role of the father in childbirth, including his helping the mother to breathe and relax during labor, timing of contractions, assisting with personal hygiene and comfort, and psychological support. The delivery itself is not necessarily conducted without an anesthetic. Usually local anesthetics and some analgesia may be employed for comfort. But because the emphasis is on conscious, active participation by the parents, general anesthesia, tranquilizers, and sedatives are usually avoided.

Even with prepared parents, however, it was still uncommon even in the early 1970s to find hospitals that allowed fathers to accompany mothers to the delivery room. Those hospitals with progressive policies still placed strict limits on access, often permitting the father's role to amount to little more than that of observer and hand holder.

Researchers studying childbirth continued to explore the ramifications of the hospital delivery. Human and animal studies by Marshall Klaus and by Niles Newton developed the concept of parent-child "bonding," or the emergence of psychological attachments and identification between the parents and the newborn. Much of the literature on the subject of bonding suggests that the relative cold, stress, and light of a conventional delivery room may serve to interfere with this attachment process.

This viewpoint did not attract much attention until some parents began to advocate childbirth at home to avoid the impersonal, technology-laden hospital experience. This stimulated the health establishment to take a closer look at some of the alternatives to conventional delivery. The ACOG, while reaffirming its belief in the safety of the hospital environment, urged that hospitals try to create a more personal and attractive setting for childbirth. The American Medical Association recently issued a statement supporting the humanization of the birth experience; it urged hospital medical staffs to review their policies on delivery to help support the birth and nurturing process.

The most innovative approach is epitomized in institutions that have special "birthing rooms" for couples electing participatory childbirth. With this concept the traditional labor room, delivery room, and postpartum room are combined into one small suite. Usually the room is attractively decorated with homey furniture, music, and reading materials and is made more comfortable with relaxed visiting rules. The medical instrumentation is either reduced, disguised, or removed. The mother progresses in labor and is not moved to a different place for delivery or recovery. Great emphasis is placed on participation by the father, even in helping deliver the infant and in severing the umbilical cord. The infant is immediately given to the parents for holding and fondling in an effort to facilitate bonding and to allow it to develop eye contact and to begin nursing. Once the mother and her infant have stabilized medically, plans are made for early discharge, often within a day, and consequently the hospital bill is generally considerably lower than it would be with conventional procedures.

Reports from the small number of hospitals that have instituted alternative birth facilities are generally quite positive. Feedback from parents who have used the facilities indicates that they have found them effective in promoting relaxation, privacy, and participation. Yet the risk of an emergency is reduced by having conventional hospital facilities and services only a step away, should mother or infant require intensive care. Contented users of such facilities report no disruption or interference with hospital services. Neither have such facilities led to any increase in patient infection or in readmission following early discharge.

Parents considering participating in similar family-centered maternity services should anticipate a number of special requirements. First, most institutions with birthing centers require a high degree of preparation by the parents, including childbirth education classes and familiarity with labor and delivery as well as with possible deviations from the "normal" birth. Often parents must agree to transfer to conventional labor and delivery if the need arises. Only low-risk parents are eligible to participate in the experience. Mothers with previous obstetric problems, preexisting diseases, signs of labor complications, or anticipated high-risk infants may generally expect a more conventional experience.

Alternative birth facilities in the hospital setting are expected to proliferate in the future. These family-centered maternity care facilities provide the only real compromise wherein the medical profession's concern for safety and preparedness is maintained while allowing for individual participation by parents in a homelike environment.

Home birth

In the mid-1930s fewer than 40% of births in the United States occurred in hospitals, and there were about 60 maternal deaths for every 10,000 live births. Today about 99% of mothers give birth in hospitals, with fewer than 3 deaths per 10,000 live births. An important claim of the medical profession is that improvements in surgical technique, instrumentation, and sanitary conditions provided in the hospital directly contributed to the reductions in both maternal and infant mortality and morbidity rates.

There has been little popular disagreement with this claim until recently. But changes in the public attitude toward the health establishment, the individual's desire for personal participation in health care, and other cultural trends have stimulated a small but vocal minority to call for childbirth to be returned to the home. Some persons estimated that about 35,000 births would take place outside the hospital setting in 1978 in the United States. This represents 1 to 1½% of the total births. Although this is a relatively small number, the enthusiasm of home-birth advocates has led some writers to refer to the phenomenon as a "movement." Probably no other phenomenon in obstetrics and gynecology has received as much popular attention since the introduction of oral contraceptives.

Observers of the home-birth situation report that most couples who choose this route do so in an attempt to regain control of the childbirth experience from the impersonal and technologically oriented hospital; they also apparently wish to revive a sense of family and community participation that existed in previous generations. Rarely are economic reasons given for advocating home birth.

The point of contention between advocates and opponents of home birth is on the question of safety. The most enthusiastic of home-birth advocates claim that this approach is even safer than childbirth in the institution since it reduces the possibility of surgical intervention in the birth and exposure to drugs, anesthetics, and infection from other hospital patients and personnel. The most critical opponents of home birth state equally strenuously that even the most apparently normal pregnancy can momentarily precipitate into a disastrous event that only a hospital is prepared to handle and that to attempt home delivery is tantamount to infanticide.

A few attempts to compare results scientifically have been made. One widely quoted study reported on a series of about a thousand home deliveries compared to a matched population of hospital deliveries; it concluded that outcome in terms of mortality and morbidity was comparable. Another study by a medical association traced birth certificates through the health departments of most states and concluded that the risk of infant death was two to five times greater in the home delivery than in the hospital. Case studies of home and hospital delivery are also quite common, with stories of success and of tragedy being cited to support or refute each position.

The fact is that the definitive scientific study on the home delivery question has not yet been done, since several methodological weaknesses prevail in the research outlined above. Some studies of home delivery are said to understate bad outcomes because obstetrical emergencies are often transferred to hospitals and are thus recorded as hospital, not home, deliveries. Tracing birth certificates is difficult because of wide variation in accuracy from state to state. And case studies, though rich in detail, give no clue as to proportions and rates across large population bases.

Thus any couple entertaining thoughts of a delivery at home must consider the risks and benefits in light of several important factors: their relative health, history, and knowledge of the childbirth process; whether or not the home birth is to be attended by a professional; whether backup equipment for problems can be present; whether rapid transportation to a medical facility is ready. They must also consider the very real though infrequent possibility of a bona fide emergency and the speed with which this can occur—the death of a mother through hemorrhage or the death of an infant by respiratory distress are phenomena of minutes and are often not predictable before delivery.

The vocal minority of home delivery advocates maintains that the experience is worth the risk. In the health establishment, concern for the safety of this view is changing the face of the hospital maternity service.

Skin Conditions

In the field of dermatology new knowledge and new methods are being added to the medical capabilities at an awe-inspiring rate. Almost daily new understanding and new techniques are being applied to the diagnosis and treatment of skin diseases.

Prevalence of skin diseases

Until 1977 it was difficult to get a reliable estimate of the prevalence of skin diseases in the United States. There were many indicators pointing to their important effect on the health of the population and their enormous economic and military impact. Several surveys among general physicians showed that in both rural and city practices about one patient in ten to one patient in seven (10 to 14%) saw a doctor for some complaint related to his skin or its appendages (hair and nails). Figures from states such as California, in which occupational and industrial dermatoses are reported, show that skin diseases constitute 50 to 70% of all occupational diseases.

It has long been recognized that skin diseases in the armed forces produce an enormous handicap to military operations. For example, in the Mekong Delta in Vietnam, skin diseases—particularly fungal infections of the feet and legs associated with wetness and severe prickly heat—during the rainy seasons (June through October) in 1966–67 accounted for 70% of all man-days lost in U.S. military operations.

While these figures suggest the magnitude of the disability and cost attributable to skin diseases among Americans, they do not permit a sufficiently accurate estimate of their prevalence in the population at large. A much more accurate estimate was made possible by the findings of the Health and Nutrition Examination Survey (HANES) of 1971–74, published by the National Center for Health Statistics in January 1977. A total of 20,749 persons from 65 preselected different locations thoughout the U.S. were examined by qualified dermatologists. The results of these examinations indicated that in the U.S. population between the ages of one and 74 years (an estimated 194 million) significant skin diseases—that is, those conditions requiring some form of treatment—probably affect nearly one-third (31.2%), a total of 60.6 million persons. Of these, 2.1 million are likely to have some form of dermatologic disability that is severe enough to be a handicap to gainful employment or housework.

While these estimates show the huge burden skin disease places upon the health of the people, they do not give a complete picture of suffering and economic loss. Many skin diseases disfigure and cause emotional disturbances far beyond their physical gravity. And many skin diseases incapacitate during the years of maximal productivity and sensitivity, peaking during the formative and energetic years between 15 and 25.

Acne

Numerous publications and observations indicate that acne is one of the most common of human ills. The above-mentioned HANES survey indicates that in the population of one- to 74-year-olds, 13,913,000 have acne requiring treatment. This figure must be modified by two facts: first, almost all of these are between 12 and 25 years old—that is, precisely those years when appearance can be critical to self-confidence and to emotional adjustment to life's stresses; second, acne lasts for many years, not just a few days like the common cold or a fever blister. Considering these facts and figures, it is not astonishing that millions of adolescents seek relief and cures of these blemishes, spending over $100 million per year on a wide range of over-the-counter remedies and thronging into skin specialists' offices.

To meet these needs, dermatologists and other scientists have devoted money, time, and thought to the understanding of acne and to improvement in its management. As a result, acne patients coming to the skin specialist or to skin clinics in medical schools and hospitals today have a better chance of receiving effective treatment than they did 15 to 20 years ago. The administration of suitable antibiotics, such as tetracycline, by mouth is probably the most common medical treatment. Careful evaluations have shown that this treatment is safe, has little or no adverse effects in the majority of acne patients, and that relatively small doses are effective in many cases. Even the small risks of systemic treatment with antibiotics now can be avoided by the use of tetracycline, erythromycin, or other antibiotics in external applications instead of by mouth. Topical lotions containing tetracycline have recently been approved by the Food and Drug Administration for the treatment of acne. Several studies by dermatologists have shown this local application to be about as effective as oral tetracycline in most cases—although perhaps somewhat slower in reaching its maximum therapeutic effect. Two other forms of external treatment of acne have established their usefulness—namely, the local application of vitamin A acid (retinoic acid), introduced by A. M. Kligman, J. E. Fulton, and G. Plewig in 1969, and of preparations containing benzoyl peroxide, introduced by Samuel Peck and Louis Chargin in the 1930s but not in wide use until recently.

Most recently it has been reported by reliable authorities (Gerd Michaëlsson, Lennart Juhlin, and Anders Vahlquist), that giving small amounts of zinc by mouth is about as effective as tetracycline by mouth and is less expensive and still safer than the systemic antibiotic. Despite favorable results reported in carefully controlled studies, other studies have not shown zinc therapy to be as effective as tetracycline. Zinc administration carries some risk of toxicity and should be given under the supervision of a physician.

These approaches to the management of acne must be seen in the light of the following limiting factors:

1. Under the best circumstances, they are not curative but will serve to keep the condition under control and the patient looking presentable while the disease is running its course. They must, therefore, be continued until the acne cures itself in its due time, as most cases do.

2. In order to have the best chance to succeed, all these treatments must be individually selected, carefully fitted, adjusted, and repeatedly readjusted to suit the type, state, and reactions of the individual patient.

For these reasons, acne is best treated by experienced practicing physicians such as dermatologists or in dermatologic clinics of hospitals and university medical schools. There are many medical schools with specialty clinics or sessions set aside for acne treatment.

Acne clinics that advertise

In recent years, dozens of commercial and advertising acne clinics not connected with universities or medical schools have sprung up in many parts of the U.S. There has been considerable criticism of these clinics, particularly by the medical establishment. Before going to an advertising clinic the acne sufferer should examine it critically and do some "comparative shopping" to get answers to the following questions:

1. Will the personal attention of an experienced, qualified physician be greater, more individualized, and more precisely fitted to the patient's particular problem in the advertising clinic than in a dermatologist's office or university skin clinic? Or will more of the management in the advertising clinic be left to assistants giving nonindividualized, cut-and-dried routines and regimens?

2. Is the management offered by the advertising clinic actually more modern, more up-to-date, and more effective than that in a board-certified dermatologist's office or in a university dermatology clinic, or are the advertised claims of superiority unfounded?

3. Are the sanitary conditions and cleanliness in the advertising clinic as good as in the physician's office or university clinic?

4. Is the cost of visits, medication, and other treatment modalities offered by the advertising clinic less or more than that in the dermatologist's office or in the university clinic?

Unfortunately, there are advertising acne clinics in which costs are higher, treatment is less individualized, and personal physician attention to the particular patient is less than that in the average physician's office. In addition, the advertised claims of newer methods and better results are exaggerated by some of these clinics, and in some, cleanliness and hygiene are not at a desirable level. The above statements are based on the appraisals of certain of the advertising acne clinics by trustworthy authorities in dermatology. However, their criticisms do not necessarily apply to all advertising acne clinics.

In accordance with the principles of free speech and free enterprise, advertising is permitted to physician members of the American Medical Association. But solicitation and false and misleading claims and fraudulent and deceptive advertising are not permitted. One fundamental question is: who will review the published advertisements and decide the truth or falsity of their statements and claims? Physicians have always conscientiously attempted to maintain the high standards of American medicine by prohibiting false and misleading claims by members of their profession. Medical societies are generally in a better position to ascertain the correctness of claims made in advertisements for acne clinics than other agencies, including those of government.

Zinc

In recent years it has been observed that zinc is related to many skin conditions. A notable example is a deficiency of the trace metal zinc that occurs in a rare but serious, sometimes fatal, disease of infants, acrodermatitis enteropathica; administration of small amounts of zinc can cure the trouble (E. J. Moynahan and P. M. Barnes, 1973). (See Pediatrics.)

Zinc is needed in the human body for the functioning of more than 40 different biologically important enzymes. And zinc is apparently particularly important for healthy skin, hair, and connective tissue. Kenneth H. Neldner has reported that the list of conditions in which the correction of zinc deficiency or the administration of small doses of zinc by mouth may be beneficial is growing and includes wound healing and leg ulcers in addition to acrodermatitis enteropathica and acne.

Griseofulvin and fungal infections: a question of cancer

While there are many antibiotics that are effective against bacterial infections, there is only one—Griseofulvin—that is useful in fungal infections of the skin, hair, and nails. In 1958 this antibiotic was introduced in human therapy, first by Harvey Blank of Miami, Fla., and then by David Williams, Robert Marten, and Imrich Sarkany of London, following demonstration of its effectiveness in experimental animals. The administration of Griseofulvin has revolutionized the management of many common fungal infections of skin, hair, and nails. It has turned previously ravaging, widespread occurrences of scalp infections of children, endemic to certain areas of the world, particularly Arab countries, from a difficult therapeutic problem into a relatively easily controlled condition. Griseofulvin given by mouth has proved not only effective in many superficial fungal skin infections but also eminently safe as far as short-term ill effects are concerned.

But the possibility has now appeared that the administration of this sole effective systemic agent against these exceedingly common infections may have to be prohibited by law. For it has now been shown that large doses (50 to 100 times the effective human dose) of Griseofulvin given to newborn rats aid in the production of cancer by known cancer-producing agents. Agents with this adjuvant action are called cocarcinogens.

The question arises: should mankind be deprived of the single effective systemic drug against a host of disfiguring, discomforting, and sometimes incapacitating skin and hair infections because huge doses injected in the newborn of another species have acted as a cocarcinogen? This is a most difficult question to answer. To date no case of cancer in any way attributable to Griseofulvin has been reported in the tens of thousands of patients who have received the antibiotic. But it is not altogether unusual for cancers to appear as late as 20, 30, or more years after exposure to carcinogenic agents. Since the first administration of Griseofulvin to man was less than 20 years ago, and the antibiotic has been given steadily ever since, the mean elapsed time since first exposure of the entire exposed population probably is less than 10 years. There is, therefore, a remote possibility that some cancers in whose production Griseofulvin played a cocarcinogenic role may still turn up.

Herpes simplex, warts, and cancer

Herpes simplex and warts are among the most common infections that plague mankind. Some years ago herpes simplex (familiarly known as fever blister or cold sore) was shown to be due to two different viruses—herpes simplex type 1, usually causing skin eruptions above the waist, and herpes simplex type 2, producing eruptions mainly below the waist. And now there is evidence that herpes simplex type 2 infection of the female genitals may play a role in the causation of cancer of the cervix.

Until very recently, the common but different-looking types of human warts were thought all to be due to one and the same virus. Common or vulgar warts, plantar warts on the soles, and the cauliflower-like large papillomatous warts in the ano-genital regions were thought to owe their differing appearances solely to the different regions of the body in which they grew. Now investigations in France and Poland, and in the U.S. by Franklin Pass, Keerti Shah, and others, have shown that some of the different types of warts are each due to slightly different variants of what is known as human papillomavirus. Moreover, it now appears likely that certain of these wart viruses—notably the one causing the large cauliflower-like warts of the ano-genital region, the one causing plantar warts, and the one causing a familial, rare, generalized warty disease known as epidermodysplasia verruciformis—are capable of pro-

ducing skin cancers. But in light of the millions of ano-genital and plantar warts physicians and dermatologists see, the relative incidence of skin cancers arising from these lesions is exceedingly low.

It is certainly of more than passing interest and significance that the two viruses that have been incriminated in the production of solid malignant growths (cancers) in humans are those that are associated with quite banal, commonplace skin lesions that affect most people at one time or another. For example, antibodies indicating previous exposure to herpes simplex are found in the blood of over 90% of city dwellers. And the fact that a great many children and many adults have had skin warts is so well known that it requires no statistical proof.

—*Marion B. Sulzberger, M.D.*

Surgery

Like other medical specialties, surgery has advanced dramatically in the past decade, influenced by new social imperatives, technological developments, and escalating costs. With ever increasing specialization the discipline has become greatly diversified.

In discussing advances in surgical techniques, it is tempting to focus on those developments that are widely treated by the media; for example, the rebuilding of deformed skulls, the reattachment of severed limbs, and the successful transplantation of major organs. More important, however, are the less spectacular, more common surgical procedures. Since nearly every person will, at some time in his lifetime, undergo some kind of surgery, it follows that familiarity with some of the intricacies of these activities is not only necessary but advisable. The purposes of this short review, then, are to summarize some of the factors that have contributed to recent advances in surgical techniques, to present some of the allied disciplines that are involved in the practice of surgery, and to review some important issues in contemporary surgery.

Contributions of technology

Technological developments, stemming largely from military and industrial research, have had a far-reaching impact on the practice of surgery. Applications of computer technology, the development of synthetic materials, and revolutions in electronics are only a few examples of such developments, which have contributed significantly to improved surgical outcomes.

In the continuing quest for improvements in the maintenance of sterility, the avoidance of infection, and the facilitation of healing incisions, contemporary technology has produced a wide range of disposable surgical equipment—sutures, drains, drapes, injectables, and caps, masks, gloves, and other operating attire. Although this aspect of contemporary surgery is taken for granted, the ready availability and widespread use of such products have improved and advanced the state of the art. Another equally important improvement in the surgical setting has resulted from the increasing use of visual aids in the form of high intensity fiberoptic lights worn and directed by the surgeon in conjunction with magnifying lenses. Taken together, these improvements assure a sterile, well-isolated, and illuminated operative field. Used with special instruments and sutures, they allow exquisite technical maneuvers in an optimal setting.

As surgical procedures have become more invasive and more complex, monitoring equipment has likewise become more refined and sophisticated. The evolution of small portable or fixed units to monitor vital signs and physiological measurements before, during, and after surgery continues. In nearly every surgical suite there are instruments that continuously and accurately display data on such important variables as heart rhythm, arterial pressure, brain waves, and body temperature. Other portable units worn by patients in and out of hospitals allow the electrocardiogram to be recorded continuously and even telemetered. The large computer is giving way to the small microprocessor, thus making complex calculations available in the operating and recovery rooms where they are needed. Most recently, hand-held calculators have been programmed to give surgeons and physicians immediate information on blood volume, the amount of blood pumped by the heart, the resistance against which the heart pumps, the amount of blood passing through the

Swift transport of accident victims to specialized trauma treatment and surgical centers has resulted in an increased survival rate.

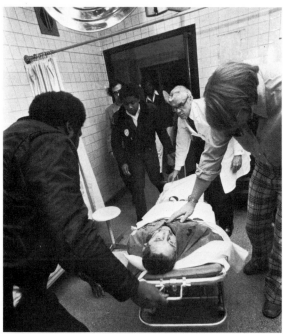

Ted Cavagnaro

lungs, the resistance across the lungs, and the time required for blood to cross the lungs. Monitoring equipment has also contributed to the refining of anesthetic administration.

Another development of recent years is the growing use of rapid transport methods, including helicopter services, to facilitate the transfer of patients from sites of injury or catastrophe to facilities equipped to deal with major trauma or specific emergencies. Members of surgical teams are often assigned to mobile facilities, and resuscitative measures are initiated earlier than was previously possible. These new methods are often critical in affecting the ultimate outcome of treatment.

Increasingly sophisticated blood banking techniques are another aspect of contemporary surgery whose importance cannot be overemphasized. Patients are rapidly typed and crossmatched, essential clotting factors assessed, and major resources mobilized within minutes or hours. Special blood products can be airlifted across the country within hours, and it is not uncommon for a severely injured patient to receive, in very short order, 50 to 100 units of blood and blood products within a 6–12 hour period. And the availability of these services is not limited to major medical centers. A number of blood substitutes can be used prior to the availability of vital constituents. Massive blood and specific clotting factor replacements have contributed to the management of traumatic injuries, hemorrhagic shock, and patients undergoing open-heart surgery.

New diagnostic methods, largely a result of applied computer technology, have been of considerable benefit to surgeons. The evolution of complex computer systems coupled with specialized X-ray and nuclear medicine techniques now allows the visualization of internal organs with a precision unknown until quite recently. Computerized axial tomography (CAT) scanning of the head has changed the practice of neuroradiology and neurosurgery. Head injuries can be scanned noninvasively for specific lesions requiring urgent surgery, and diagnostic pneumoencephalography has been made obsolete. Similarly, the heart can be serially monitored by noninvasive means before, during, and after surgery, and increasingly, other organs are being examined with these techniques or variations thereof. Sonography, a diagnostic method that uses sound waves, had its basis in physical principles developed in antisubmarine warfare during World War II. Sonographic techniques have produced a means of noninvasive diagnosis in which size, configuration, motion, and deformities of vital organs can be determined with great accuracy.

Contributions of medicine

Recent developments in medicine—such as new drugs and further understanding of basic physiological processes—have also contributed toward improved surgical conditions and results. Among the areas so affected are treatment of infection, replacement of fluids and nutrients, and management of shock.

Increasing attention to the avoidance and treatment of surgical infections has resulted in an impressive record of achievements. It is now possible to isolate and rapidly test offending microorganisms and to treat their effects with specific antimicrobials. Natural and synthetic antibiotics and specific bactericidal agents are widely available; for instance, the aminoglycosides for suspected gram-negative infections. Moreover, ever increasing understanding of the metabolism of microbes and their toxic products has permitted the development of specific, selective-acting agents. The contributions of infectious disease experts in the care of surgical patients continue to be a cornerstone of the discipline.

It is no longer expected that the debilitated surgical patient will continue to lose weight or suffer decreased ability to combat infection or capability to heal an incision. There are now available a wide variety of plastic indwelling catheters that can be inserted into a peripheral artery or vein and, if necessary, further advanced into the circulatory system. The catheters are attached to filters, some of which have elements to remove air bubbles and to allow for the infusion and measurement of a number of physiological solutions. Fluid electrolytes, such as potassium and sodium, and trace elements, such as magnesium and zinc, can be added in appropriate amounts. And nutrients can be provided in the form of high glucose concentrations and specific amino acid supplements. New concepts, promulgated within the area called *hyperalimentation* (Hyper-A), have altered the course of and metabolic response to all major surgery.

The diagnosis and treatment of shock and metabolic disorders associated with surgery continue to occupy the attention of surgical investigators. Shock has come under increasing scrutiny, and the description of the hyperdynamic shock state that exists in the presence of normal, or oftentimes increased, amounts of blood ejected from the heart remains a problem that is not completely understood. Glucose, insulin, and potassium solutions are being used, and total nutrition by means of injected glucose and amino acid preparations has become a cornerstone of adjunctive surgical therapy. The posttraumatic hypermetabolic state, in which the severely injured surgical patient undergoes a spontaneous increase in metabolic rate, is thought by some to be mediated by the release of specific hormones; *e.g.,* catecholamines and prostaglandins. True understanding of these complex phenomena remains a major goal of current surgical research.

Ear, nose, and throat surgery

Tonsillectomy and adenoidectomy, performed individually or simultaneously, still constitute the most common operations in the United States. In 1975, 786,-000 procedures of this nature were performed. This, however, represented a decline from previous years, possibly attributable to decreasing birthrates. Sixty percent of these procedures were performed on children under the age of six. However, acute ear and upper respiratory tract infections spontaneously decrease after the age of six, and the efficacy of these procedures for treating some conditions remains uncertain. For certain indications, *e.g.,* difficulty in swallowing and upper airway obstruction, the results are excellent.

Cardiovascular surgery

In excess of 100,000 open-heart operations are being performed in the United States each year. A large proportion are undertaken for the ravages of coronary artery disease, and an entire discipline within cardiac surgery has evolved for the diagnostic and surgical management of these patients. A major advance within heart surgery has been the use of improved methods to protect the heart during reparative procedures, with considerable attention being directed toward the use of chemical solutions that suspend myocardial contractions. These cardioplegic solutions are infused into the isolated heart during surgery while circulation is supported by a heart-lung machine.

New synthetic graft replacements for diseased arteries, such as PTFE (expanded polytetrafluoroethylene, or Teflon) and filamentous Dacron, are promising new additions to vascular surgery. Especially outstanding are those substances of particular applicability for arterial reconstructions in the lower extremities. The human umbilical cord is also used for grafts.

Equally deserving of mention are the continuing improvements in implantable cardiac pacemaker technology. The newer units are smaller, lighter, and longer-lived and have programmable capabilities to vary rate, pulse contour, voltage output, and pacing modes. (*See also* Heart and Blood Vessels.)

Cancer surgery

Remarkable advances have been made in the diagnosis and treatment of cancerous growths. For example, tumor markers, which are measurable products in body fluids, can now be used to identify subclinical cancer and provide a means of assessing the patient for localized or possibly curable tumors. Liver cancer produces a measurable protein constituent (alpha-fetoprotein); certain uterine and testicular cancers produce human chorionic gonadotropin (HCG); carcinoembryonic antigen (CEA) has a substantial applicability in predicting the recurrence of cancer of the large intestine; and serum thyrocalcitonin levels or thyroglobulin immunoassays can be used to detect thyroid cancer. In addition, serum acid phosphatase isoenzymes have been found to be elevated in instances of prostatic cancer, and an immunological test of white cell (lym-

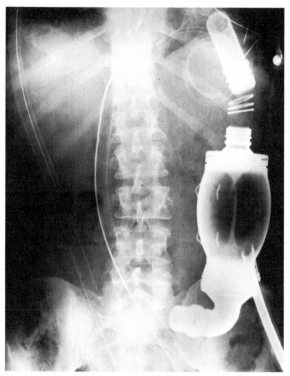

A temporary mechanical heart, the ALVAD, sustains the life of a heart-transplant patient until surgery is possible. Several successful trials of the device have been reported.

phocyte) adherence to glass surfaces may be used to detect the presence of metastatic breast cancer. Radiation and chemotherapy treatments continue to offer improved results, often in conjunction with surgery. In general, however, experts agree that major advances in transplantation biology must precede any enlargement of the scope of cancer surgery.

Transplantation

Understanding of the basic mechanisms controlling the immunologic responses to transplantation continues to increase. In the area of kidney transplantation, chemical pretreatment of the donor kidney has resulted in a 72% three-year survival rate of the grafted kidney. Renal preservation methods have improved, and it is now possible for a donor kidney to be transported from one center to virtually any other in the United States for implantation. Similar capabilities for preservation of donor hearts are being developed.

Liver cells are being transplanted on an experimental basis into the abdomen and into the veins draining into the liver; interest continues in experimental methods of transplanting islet cells, which produce insulin, a procedure that has potential value for treating diabetics. And, for the first time, mechanical partial artificial heart implantation has been used to sustain a patient with irreparable heart damage while a suitable donor heart was sought. The single-chamber mechanical

heart substitute, called an ALVAD (abdominal left ventricular assist device), is joined to the apex of the left ventricle and to the abdominal aorta. To date it has been used successfully to extend the lives of several heart surgery patients.

Contemporary issues

New social imperatives, patient and public advocates, and escalating costs continue to confront surgery. The economics of surgery has emerged as a complex, problematic, and multifaceted area of overall concern, deserving of continued analysis, scrutiny, and revision. Other current concerns involve social and ethical issues. For example, it has been alleged that poor patients are operated upon too frequently; that the rich are treated differently and more frequently, to their benefit; that enormously successful surgeons enjoy life-styles in excess of services delivered; and that unnecessary surgery abounds. Each of these allegations is being carefully examined. Following widespread controversy about unnecessary surgery in welfare patients, the Department of Health, Education, and Welfare recently announced a program designed to curb such abuses. Under the program, the government would pay for a second medical opinion for Medicare patients facing elective surgery.

There has also been much recent attention in the lay press devoted to questioning the efficacy and expense of coronary artery bypass surgery, perhaps the most common major heart operation performed today. There is widespread agreement that this type of surgery is, indeed, beneficial, lifesaving in certain instances, and effective in relieving symptoms of angina pectoris. Whether or not it prolongs life remains open to question.

—John C. Norman, M.D.

Teeth and Gums

Since the early 1900s varying degrees of attention have been given to the significance of dental infection for the well-being of the entire body. At present dental infection as a source of the spread of microorganisms to other critical sites in the body is considered to be a serious threat to the health of certain high-risk patients. The spread of oral microorganisms, mainly bacteria, to other diseased sites in the body can produce life-threatening, often fatal, disease. As a consequence of the complex medical management of some disease processes and conditions, some patients suffer an extreme liability to infection. The mouth, particularly the tissue immediately adjacent to the teeth, is overwhelmingly the most common site of chronic infection in human beings and is also the most likely site of entry of microorganisms into the bloodstream, allowing them to circulate to sites distant from the mouth—a condition known as bacteremia.

The impact of oral infection on health

Following the discovery of the world of microflora in the latter part of the 19th century, it was discovered that the mouth contains a rich population of bacteria and, less commonly, some fungi and even some protozoans. Under the conditions of the common inflammatory dental diseases, the bacterial population can become very heavy—a condition called oral sepsis. While oral sepsis or infection was considered to be unfavorable to the mouth itself, the general consequences of oral sepsis were not widely appreciated until about the turn of the century. It was noted that some patients showed improvement in infections in other parts of the body when oral infections were eradicated. It then came to be known that even patients without a specific disease in a particular site had an improved general well-being when oral infections were eradicated. Such improvements in health led to a general view that the mouth was an important source of the difficulties found in other remote parts of the body. It came to be that many vague complaints without a specific diagnostic determination or well-understood biological basis were blamed on bad teeth. Tooth extraction was seen as a remedy for rheumatism, for example. By the 1930s the understanding and treatment of dental diseases had improved considerably. The technique of treating the pulp inside the tooth became refined and more widely used; because a carious lesion had penetrated to the inside of the tooth, the tooth was not necessarily lost. In addition, the significance of periodontal disease was more widely understood, and new treatment methods were devised. Alarmed by the tendency to extract salvageable teeth, often for vague and ill-defined reasons, dentists undertook a campaign of public education.

It soon became established, however, that a specific problem, rheumatic heart disease with damaged heart valves, could be subject to blood-borne infectious agents arising from oral infection. Many years passed before a more complete understanding of the method of spread of this infection and appreciation of its great importance came to be known. In the interim some care was taken in the removal of teeth in patients having a history of rheumatic heart disease—antibiotics were administered during the extraction. At that time antibiotics had recently been discovered and developed. One of the major threats to a person having damaged heart valves consequent to rheumatic heart disease is the development of subacute bacterial endocarditis (SBE), an inflammation and infection of the inside lining of the heart chambers. SBE is a serious disabling disease that, despite vigorous medical management, often results in death. It was noted that often, but not always, such patients developed SBE following dental extractions or other dental treatments.

In the early 1950s eye surgeons noticed that eye infections often subsided following the eradication of oral infections, a significant observation, since eye infections can be very stubborn, chronic infections resistant to treatment. At this time intensive efforts of investigation were being directed to studying rheumatic heart disease, particularly the local phenomena around damaged heart valves. It was found that in the original infection of rheumatic heart disease the infecting bacteria, β-hemolytic streptococcus, provoked a sensitivity reaction in connective tissue, particularly the connective tissue in the mitral valve of the heart. After this inflammation of the valve subsided the valve was left altered by scarring. The alterations varied in degree but very often prevented the valve from effectively closing and separating the heart chambers, with consequent regurgitation of blood backward through the valve during the heart muscle contraction. It was also found that instead of a usual smooth laminar flow of blood past the valve structure, there were disturbances in blood flow such as swirling whirlpools around the valve. Any bacteria in the bloodstream then would not just flow past the valve but could be trapped in these whirlpools and held in the area along with deposits of fibrin, which would protect the bacteria from attacks by leukocytes. In addition, the scarred tissue provided an attraction for certain bacteria, particularly α-streptococcus, a very common inhabitant of the mouth and throat. Strep throat was known to be related to the primary infection in rheumatic heart disease caused by β-hemolytic streptococcus. It now became apparent that strep throats caused by α-streptococcus were a common cause of reinfection. Thus, dentists and physicians directed more attention to the relationship between dental infections and rheumatic heart disease, and a specific regime of antibiotic coverage for dental extractions was more widely used.

In the mid-1960s two important medical developments caused additional concern in relation to chronic dental infection. The medical management of hematologic neoplasms made great strides in the use of chemotherapy, producing remissions in many leukemias and lengthening life expectancy. At the same time, sophisticated medical and surgical techniques had evolved that allowed for the transplantation of major organs such as the kidney and the heart. The success of such transplants depended upon immunosuppressive therapy, preventing rejection of the transplanted tissue by the recipient's defense mechanisms. While chemotherapy and immunosuppressive therapy are great advances, they produce some liabilities, the most dangerous of which is a blanket destruction of the patient's biological defense capabilities. Infection could threaten the life of the patient or cause a resistant local infection to develop that could cause considerable damage because of destruction of tissue. The latter is most directly seen in the mouth, where a small common dental abscess that would be easily contained by most people could, in patients with liability, cause extensive destruction of the jawbones, with possible loss of many teeth, possible facial deformity, and, in the case of the upper jaw, perforation through to the nasal sinuses.

Another group of susceptible patients are those who have had a prosthetic implant such as an artificial hip. Prosthetic implant devices are made of materials selected to produce as little tissue reaction in the recipient as possible; however, in most cases some tissue reaction takes place even if it is only to accommodate the tissue to the presence of the prosthetic device. Part of this reaction is the formation of granulation tissue. The presence of a prosthetic device seems to provide an attraction for microorganisms circulating in the bloodstream, and the granulation tissue provides a filterlike network that seems to entrap circulating microorganisms. If a blood-borne infection is established around a prosthetic device, the only recourse is to remove the prosthetic device, an obvious disability for the patient.

Patients who have suffered serious kidney disease, with either failure of function of the kidneys or removal of kidneys, are also at risk. In order to sustain life these patients must undergo frequent dialysis, the circulation of the patient's blood through a machine that acts like a kidney in removing the waste products that are the result of normal metabolism. In order to facilitate the connection of the patient's bloodstream to the dialysis machine, shunts are implanted in the patient's vessels, allowing for a quick and less traumatic connection to the dialysis machine. Bacteria in the bloodstream are attracted to these shunts just as they are to implanted artificial prosthetic devices, and inflammatory reaction can cause the loss of the shunt. While a new shunt can be placed in another site, there are only a few suitable locations, and the loss of a shunt site because of infection is not a trivial matter for a patient already carrying a difficult biological burden.

Clinical infections are found far more often in the mouth than any other area of the body. However, it is not merely the presence of infection in the mouth that makes the presence of viable bacteria in the blood so likely but infection combined with certain unique features of oral physiology. The inflammatory response to chronic infection is called granulomatous inflammation, or granulation tissue. A fundamental feature of this type of inflammation is a rich network of thin-walled vascular channels, forming a tissue that is easily compressible and acts like a sponge. Eating causes movement of the teeth, and in the contiguous tissues the intermittent application and release of biting force, in effect, acts as a pump, compressing and releasing the granulation tissue. Bacteria are thus pumped into the bloodstream. It has been experimentally demonstrated that persons with even minimal gingivitis will have a measurable bacteremia after eating only one slice of bread. Such bacteremias were found to be of slight degree, and lasted only for a short time. Studies of patients who had moderate or severe gingivitis or actual periodontal disease with separation between the tooth and bone exhibited a far more severe degree of bacteremia that lasted for much longer periods of time. The source of the bacteria is the sulcus, or periodontal, pocket around the tooth, a space that contains oral debris and bacteria. It should be remembered, however, that teeth are moved not only during eating. Many people clench their teeth or rub their teeth together; still others grind their teeth together while sleeping—a phenomenon called bruxism. At all of these times the possibility of producing bacteremia is present. Dental caries, or tooth decay, may penetrate the pulp of the tooth and cause necrosis of the pulp. Consequently, bacteria from the mouth have a route in the inside of the tooth through the pulp canal to the end of the root of the tooth, buried deep in the bone. Here the body responds with the granulomatous inflammatory reaction. Testing for the presence of bacteria in granulation tissue from dental and periodontal patients has resulted in a finding that only about 20% of this type of granulation tissue contains bacteria. This leads to the conclusion that dental diseases provoking a granulomatous inflammatory response are probably not important sources of bacteremia. But this conclusion overlooks the fact that granulation tissue can have a very dynamic circulation, and bacteria entering the lumen of these vascular channels are quickly carried away. The major repository of the bacteria population is just inside the pulp canal of the tooth. When the tooth is moved, the resulting pressures cause bacteria to enter the granulation tissue.

Dental treatments that produce intermittent manipulation of teeth, such as extractions and the cleaning of teeth, particularly below the gingival level, must be considered hazardous, tending to produce bacteremia. In high-risk patients a precise regime of antibiotic administration is utilized to prevent survival of the bacteria pumped into the bloodstream. In addition, efforts are made to minimize the amount of intermittent manipulation by the dental treatment, although such a restriction appreciably prolongs treatment times.

The ease with which bacteremia can be created by manipulation of the teeth and gingiva produces a dilemma. Brushing of the teeth is desirable because the almost exclusive cause of gingivitis is the accumulation of debris around the teeth. On the other hand, brushing could be considered a producer of the pumping action sending bacteria into the bloodstream. Actually, if performed correctly, the brushing of teeth is more of a sweeping motion rather than a back and forth movement. In addition, if the teeth are kept clean, the chronic inflammatory granulation tissue is not present, and the consequent possibility of bacteremia caused by brushing is slight. The benefits of proper tooth brushing far outweigh the risks. However, other types of cleaning techniques for teeth may present a significant risk. A water-flushing device for dental hygiene uses very rapid pulsations in a stream of water that is quite effective in removing debris from around teeth, but it has been reported that the rapid pulsations of the water stream are far more likely to cause bacteremia than brushing the teeth. Another technique for cleaning the teeth and strengthening the gingiva is the use of intradental stimulators, rubber devices that are inserted between the teeth to massage the gums. Thus the pulsating water-stream cleaning technique and intradental gingiva stimulators may be a cause of bacteremia in some patients and may be a serious and important hazard for those patients who have liabilities to bacteremia.

Changing faces

The arts of maxillofacial prosthetics, oral surgery, orthodontics, and plastic surgery have evolved to a point of remarkable accomplishment. The reasons for facial surgery are about equally divided between functional requirements and aesthetic requirements. However, the dramatic impact is usually concerned with the aesthetic alteration, and this is too often mistakenly thought to be the only reason for facial change. The face and its supporting structures have a complex physiology, but equally important to the patient is the social and psychological value of having a satisfactory facial appearance.

Orthognathic surgery is the manipulation of jawbones or parts of jawbones into more favorable relationships for functional and aesthetic purposes. The indications of malfunction and the guides for correction are usually found in an analysis of the teeth. Hence, orthognathic surgery is often a combination of oral surgery and orthodontics. Obvious examples of functional and aesthetic problems are an overdeveloped or underdeveloped lower or upper jaw; abnormal use of facial or tongue muscles, causing dental and jaw deformities; facial disability caused by the treatment of tumors in the oral-facial area; and congenital deformities. In the past some of these difficulties, particularly those of lesser degree, were successfully managed through orthodontic treatment, which, however, was slow and tedious; sometimes, after a long period of treatment, reversion occurred. Orthodontics manipulated the teeth into favorable functional relationships, and the associated alteration in the bone usually resulted in giving a more desirable aesthetic value to the face. However, orthodontic treatment usually could not cope with gross alterations in the relationship between the upper and the lower jaws. At present the improved knowledge of vascular and nerve supply of the jaw and facial areas, combined with refined surgical techniques, has allowed for appreciable surgical alteration of the human face. This involves removal of portions of jawbone or transfer of portions of jawbones to other

sites or taking a bone graft from other body sites to the jaws. In the lower jaw the ramus area—the back part of the lower jaw—gives the most opportunity for surgical manipulation. Thus, if the lower jaw is too protrusive, the correction is usually made in the back part of the jaw rather than removing the front protrusive part of the jaw. The success of these procedures depends heavily on the stabilization produced by the interdigitation of the upper and lower teeth. A careful analysis of the jaw structure and the teeth must be made. In preparing for such surgery, detailed studies are made of the facial bones and teeth, and replica plaster casts are made of the teeth and dental arches. Mock surgery is performed by cutting and realigning X-ray films and cutting and realigning the plaster casts in order to determine the best ways to accomplish the desired result and to determine the chances for a successful result. This is all done before a patient is advised that surgery is feasible. While the time of actual surgery is relatively short, orthodontic appliances are usually employed for a considerable time following surgery. These act as a splint to maintain the newly established favorable relationships and to prevent reversion. While the surgical alteration of jawbone relationships is a difficult and trying ordeal for a patient, the social benefits derived from an improved aesthetic value of the face are of great benefit.

Maxillofacial prosthetics fulfills a role that cannot be accomplished through biologic manipulation: the results of surgery may fall far short of the desired goal, or surgical alteration may be entirely impossible. In that case the creation of artifical prosthetic devices is invaluable. For example, as a consequence of treatment of facial tumors, patients are often left with large holes in their faces that defy surgical correction. A patient with such a problem may become a prisoner in his home, afraid to expose to public view such a noticeable facial disability. The creation of an artificial nose, eye orbit, or ear can open the door to the everyday social activities that most people take for granted.

Remarkable progress has been made in the development of materials, techniques of fabrication, and skills of the maxillofacial prosthodontists in designing and applying such devices. The devices are not easily detectable except under close scrutiny; the presence of the device is certainly preferable to the marked distraction that would be caused by the unhidden facial defect. While the amelioration of a facial defect by an artificial device is the most dramatic result of the prosthetic appliance, it should be remembered that function may have also been enhanced. For example, persons who have communication in the hard palate between the mouth and nasal passages have extraordinary difficulty in speaking, eating, and drinking. The closure of such a hole with a prosthetic device immediately allows for almost normal speech and ingestion.

—Robert A. Goepp, D.D.S., Ph.D.

Trends in Medicine and Health Care

When a speaker addressing the American Osteopathic Association remarked that "many people are allergic to the 20th century," his seemingly facetious statement was based on the fact that the stresses of a highly industrialized society are increasingly seen as a major factor in the health of the citizenry. Whether these stresses are physical—air and water pollution, hazardous occupations, high noise levels—or psychological—overcrowding, alienation, anxiety—their effects on health are as pronounced and undeniable as the great plagues of infectious disease were on the health of earlier eras. In addition, the life-styles and diets adopted in a relatively affluent and urbanized society tend to profoundly affect health and well-being. Indeed, as new medical discoveries are made, it becomes apparent that health is not determined solely by an isolated "medical" aspect of life; health is an intricate and complex entity but one over which the individual has a great deal of control. Contemporary medicine, then, must be flexible and adaptable, utilizing any means, traditional or innovative, to strengthen health and cure disease.

Life's pressures

It has long been recognized that single traumatic events—experiencing the death of a loved and needed person, an accident, financial ruin, the breakup of a marriage—can be sources of malignant stress, causing debilitation, malaise, and even death. What behaviorists are now learning is that the ongoing stress of a life-style that compels an individual to act in a manner contrary to his needs can also lead to physical and mental disease and a decreased life-span.

Male and female roles. Life-styles generated by the traditional societal roles of men and women are a prime example of this phenomenon. Some researchers believe that men do not live as long as women because the behaviors expected of or accepted in men are dangerous or even life threatening. Men traditionally are expected to be aggressive, fearless, ambitious, and well in control of their emotions. They work at physically demanding jobs in hazardous surroundings and participate in active, high-risk sports. They consume more alcohol and tobacco (and more illicit drugs) and are more likely to handle firearms. And the male death rate from coronary disease, for example, far exceeds that of women. Furthermore, the differential is increasing: in the 1920s women lived on the average two years longer than men; in the 1970s they are living an average of eight years longer.

On the other hand, women who break out of the traditional role of homemaker find other sources of stress. Austrian researcher Maximiliane Sinovacz reported in 1978 to a U.S. women's group on the "weekend stress syndrome"—a condition discovered in a study of 1,370 Austrian married women who had sought work outside the home. These women felt that they were still responsible for maintaining the home and doing the housework as well as for their paid work and resented using their weekend days to do household chores. Even when husbands and families shared the housework, the women still felt the stress of responsibilities.

Suburbia. Edward A. Wynne, a University of Illinois education professor, charged in his book *Growing Up Suburban* that suburbs are hardly havens of space, quiet, and fresh air but rather sources of isolation and alienation. Wynne found that suburbs can be so removed from the diversity of the working world of adults and from interaction with people of many educational, economic, and social backgrounds that suburban-raised children are ill equipped to deal with the adult world. He cites the growing suicide rate for teenage white males—3.7 per 100,000 deaths in 1950 and 11.9 per 100,000 deaths in 1974—and the growing suburban drug problem as support for his claims.

Suburban isolation was also named as a factor in the cases of housebound women caught in an unending round of depression, passive television watching,

A recent study showed that children born to women living in the high-noise airplane flight paths of the Los Angeles International Airport showed a higher than normal incidence of birth defects.

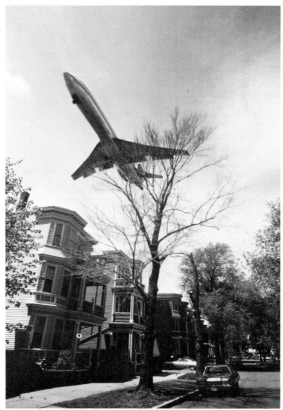

EPA—Documerica

snacking, and obesity. Jessie Bernard of Pennsylvania State University suggested that in these women nutritional habits were directly linked to their mental state, a problem exacerbated by television's tempting food commercials and day-long presentation of emotionally charged soap opera programming.

Physical effects. The physical malaise generated by stress can be as severe as the psychological. Researchers in Rochester, N.Y., found that a high percentage of children with juvenile rheumatoid arthritis came from broken homes and had experienced the stress of going through a divorce. It was found that children born to women living near the high-noise areas of Los Angeles International Airport showed a higher than average incidence of birth defects. A World Health Organization meeting in Geneva, Switz., found that as nations develop industrially, the incidence of hypertension in the population increases. A change in diet and increased stress are both implicated as causes. Micronesians, for instance, develop hypertension when they migrate to New Zealand. Hypertension is rare, even with advancing age, in rural Africa but more common in urban Africa.

Life-style choices that affect health

There is perhaps no more far-reaching principle in the field of public health than the realization that life-style and personal habits have a profound effect on the standards of health of a nation. The promotion of preventive medicine, in the sense of a healthful life-style, is a major goal of the Federal Bureau of Health Education. Billions of dollars in insurance costs, not to mention the toll in lost work time and shortened lives, could be saved if the following lifelong habits were established in the U.S. population.

1. Eat three meals a day at regular times; avoid snacks.

2. Eat breakfast every day.

3. Engage in moderate exercise at least three times a week.

4. Sleep seven or eight hours a night.

5. Don't smoke.

6. Maintain weight at or slightly below "ideal" levels.

7. Drink alcohol sparingly, if at all.

A man of 45 who practices six or seven of these habits will live on the average more than ten years longer than a man who practices three or fewer. The statistics hammer home the message: 40% of all Americans are 20 or more pounds overweight; smokers have a 70% greater chance of developing coronary heart disease than do nonsmokers; cirrhosis of the liver—nearly always due to excessive alcohol intake—is still a major cause of death in the U.S.; 76% of all deaths in the U.S. are due to conditions that can be avoided, ameliorated, or even cured by proper attention to diet, exercise, controlled alcohol and tobacco consumption, and control of stress. Some physicians go so far as to state that modern medicine is reaching a plateau beyond which it cannot significantly affect the health of large numbers of people; life-style choices are now the means by which the statistics of health in the U.S. can be improved.

It is important to remember that each of the seven points listed above involves a conscious choice by the individual in an aspect of life over which he has control. His good health is then not founded on accident or arbitrary circumstance or on any imposed paternalistic regulation. In 1978 the Department of Health, Education, and Welfare (HEW) launched an all-out campaign to curb smoking in the U.S. but could not force the public to stop smoking by banning the manufacture or sale of cigarettes or probably even by ending government support of tobacco growers. The state of Tennessee required parents of small children to equip

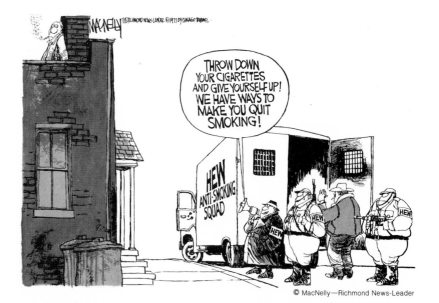

© MacNelly—Richmond News-Leader

Peter Kiar

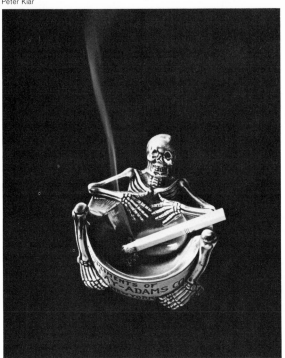

Despite the warnings and grim reminders, cigarette use in the U.S. continues to grow, a clear-cut case of an individual's choosing an unhealthy life-style with full knowledge of the consequences.

family automobiles with approved restraint systems for children too small to use seat belts but could not realistically enforce their use.

Acceptance of unconventional therapies

There are few facets of life that cannot be involved in the maintenance of health or the curing of disease. Nontraditional modes of therapy that might have been scoffed at a few years ago or practiced only in ethnic enclaves are finding a place in the medical mainstream.

Holistic medicine. At an April 1978 conference, Holistic Health: A Public Policy, sponsored in part by several branches of HEW, participants included acupuncturists, evangelists, yoga practitioners, advocates of alternatives in childbirth, insurance executives, psychiatrists, dance therapists, and Senate staff members, as well as government officials with a responsibility for national health care. Holistic health emphasizes the prevention of disease and places responsibility with the individual as "self-healer"; any means may be used to achieve this end. Although mainstream Western medical practices are not ignored, they are seen as only one part of the available therapy and by no means as the only effective one.

Biofeedback. After an initial flurry of publicity on biofeedback as a tool of pop psychology, this technique is being studied carefully and used to treat dis-

orders ranging from learning disabilities to asthma to colonic disorders. Biofeedback seeks to give the individual full control over his body by making him aware of and in command of his bodily functions, some once thought to be involuntary and uncontrollable. Biofeedback has shown dramatic effects in dealing with migraine or tension headaches, and with stress due to tension. Biofeedback techniques are being applied to sufferers of hypertension, stroke-induced paralysis, fecal incontinence, phobias, and epilepsy. Many times it is tried as a last resort when medication or physical therapy has proved ineffective. The New Hampshire Lung Association has used biofeedback in an attempt to help teenagers stop cigarette smoking—evidence of growing acceptance by the medical establishment.

Pet therapy. An Ohio State University project utilized "pet therapy" to deal with emotional disorders. It was theorized that the warm, unquestioning affection shown by pets could help bring out withdrawn patients who recoiled from human contact and refused to interact with therapists. Once the patient had responded to the companionship of the pet, he could begin to care for the pet's needs, further leaving his withdrawn state. When the ice had been broken in this way, the therapist could help the patient discuss his problem. Further contact with the pet provides a secure source of affection and reinforces the therapeutic process. The researchers also found that many pet owners expressed their own psychological problems through their pets, and sometimes induced similar problems in the animals. Discussion of an animal's problem was a way to lead into a discussion of the owner's problem.

Computers and health. The applications of electronic communication to medicine are many and varied. The Chicago Medical Society has established a library of 150 tape recordings of health messages; topics one to six are Vasectomy, What Is a "Normal" Bowel?, Can Medicine in the Home Poison Your Child?, Hemorrhoids, Early Prenatal Care, Breast Cancer. A person wishing to know more about a listed topic simply dials the "Tel-Med" number and tells the operator the number of the tape he wants to hear. Leaflets describing the service and listing the topics are distributed by Blue Cross and Blue Shield. New York City has a similar service.

At the University of Wisconsin Center for Health Sciences, a computer asks a patient some 70 multiple-choice questions and provides an almost instant estimate of his chances of living a long and healthy life. Using statistical data, the computer calculates the individual's odds, taking into account the family medical history and present habits. Suggestions for improving the odds are also given. The computer's developers see the system as an inexpensive alternative to yearly examinations for low-risk patients. And as an educational tool, the benefits are obvious.

—*Anita K. Wolff*

Special Report:

Medicine and Health on TV

by Ellen Bernstein

Public interest in medicine, health, and fitness is greater than ever before. Newspapers, books, and magazines are reflecting this trend—giving more and more space to coverage of medicine for the lay reader. Most newspapers have medical and science reporters and carry question-and-answer columns by physicians, psychologists, psychiatrists, and even sports medicine specialists. Women's magazines have long recognized the reader's interest in her body, but now nearly every general interest periodical addresses health issues. *Esquire Fortnightly*, "for the *man* who wants more out of life," carries a regular health column entitled "The Body." Further evidence of this interest is the advent of health book clubs. Indeed, there is such a plethora of books published on medicine and health—on subjects as diverse as holistic medicine, how to lose weight fast, facing midlife crises, and freedom from stress—that such clubs can offer a wide selection of new books each month. Radio, too, reports on health. A Chicago all-news station covers health issues 30 times a week—almost as often as it covers movies and entertainment.

Since television is a constant companion of most Americans, it is not surprising that medicine and health are becoming an increasingly important area of coverage for this medium, too. Though TV is most often viewed as bad for our health—among other things it is blamed for causing aggression in children and declining reading scores in school-agers and for making us a nation of sheep, ready to buy any product we are told we should have—the fact remains that for many American adults it is the chief source of news and vital information. It is estimated that children watch an average of 25 hours a week; that means by the age of 18 a youngster has viewed two full years of TV. That many producers and broadcast executives are now making a commitment to presenting nonfiction health and medical programming is in many ways a welcome phenomenon; TV, long thought of as making us ill, is now showing an interest in keeping us well.

From Dr. Kildare to Dr. Ulene

In the late 1960s and early 1970s medical dramas featuring such heroic healers as Ben Casey, Dr. Kildare, and Marcus Welby, M.D., were among the most watched of television's offerings. So convincing were many of these programs that the good Dr. Welby received thousands of letters requesting medical advice. Since everyone is likely to get sick and hope for some saving miracle, these medical soap operas have a ready-made audience. (Paradoxically, one of the most enduring and popular of the dramas is "M*A*S*H," which portrays medicine at its most unheroic.) In 1956 the American Medical Association (AMA) established the Physicians' Advisory Committee on Television, Radio, and Motion Pictures to aid imaginative scriptwriters with technicalities in medical scenarios. The committee now reviews some 300 scripts a year for accuracy and appropriateness.

Though there are still several dramas on the air that appeal to morbid curiosity about disease, TV today is responding to the public's interest in health by taking a more serious approach to medicine. Local news broadcasts have health and science reporters. Renaissance-type doctors are a special draw on morning talk shows: Arthur Ulene is the "family doctor" on the popular "Today" show, and Timothy Johnson makes regular appearances on "Good Morning America." There are also prime-time specials on health and medicine, short public service spots, public broadcasting shows on a variety of medical science-related subjects, and magazine-format programs that have major segments devoted to health.

The medical beat. Many local news broadcasts now have a medical "beat." Though most common in large metropolitan areas, this kind of journalism seems to be a growing phenomenon. Some stations employ physicians with reporting skills; others have nonphysician reporters who can cut through complicated medical jargon and interpret information for viewers. In the fall of 1977 a two-day conference in Chicago drew TV medical journalists from all over the U.S. to share information and sources and to raise questions about what types of medical stories ought to be covered on the air.

In addition to covering national and local medical news, local reporters can help viewers sort out information cued to other news stories. In response to a U.S. Senate report on nutrition, one Chicago news show devised a five-part, week-long quiz to enable viewers to evaluate their own nutritional habits. Reporters also direct viewers to local medical facilities—for example, clinics that do free diabetes screenings; they explain how a new device works, how reliable it is, and where to get it—an example is a do-it-yourself preg-

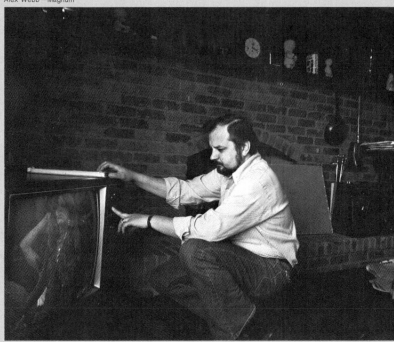

Television coverage helps fill the nationwide demand for information about health and medical matters. Medical coverage was once limited to highly unrealistic dramas in hospital settings, but the trend today is toward factual, informative programming.

nancy test, which became available in 1977; and sometimes they advise when it's okay to be your own doctor and when it's best to consult a physician. If there is a local flu outbreak, medical reporters can keep viewers abreast of symptoms and treatments.

Art Ulene, who has a regular segment on a local news broadcast in Los Angeles as well as his "Today" spot, has developed self-instructional materials that he shows on the air. When he described a brochure on breast self-examination, viewer response was phenomenal: 100,000 women wrote to request copies. William Rader, a Los Angeles-based psychiatrist, doesn't do therapy on the air but uses time on an evening news broadcast to profile people who have had mental health problems and conquered them, thus inspiring others and destigmatizing psychiatric problems.

Specials. Prime-time health specials are becoming a significant part of national network programming. In January 1978 NBC presented one of the most ambitious programs, "Medicine in America—Life, Death, and Dollars," which looked at some of the most explosive issues of the day: unnecessary surgery, second opinions, radical versus modified-radical mastectomy, competition among hospitals, "CAT fever" (the expensive and questionable purchases by many hospitals of computerized axial tomography machines), Health Maintenance Organizations (prepaid health plans), and superspecialists. The show addressed the complexities of the health care system—a system that affects everyone—and emphasized the absence of any quick solutions to problems. Money, politics, new trends, and preventive medicine were handled in a particularly animated way. The dynamic possibilities for conveying

information over the air are endless—a key reason for the medium's tremendous popularity. In "Medicine in America" the soaring health care cost phenomenon was simplified so that the average viewer could begin to understand the issues. This three-hour special, which took 11 months to prepare, drew an estimated 8 million to 12 million viewers. While it, like any other special on TV, was subject to criticism for oversimplifying, not presenting all sides of an issue, and being dictated to by advertisers, the sheer numbers that tuned in to "Medicine in America" cannot be ignored, and the fact that people probably learned more that night than they had known about issues that vitally affect them says quite a bit about the potential of television as a healthful medium.

In the 1977–78 season CBS presented three specials that were part of "The Body Human" series: "The Miracle Months" (on pregnancy and birth), "The Red River" (on the circulatory system), and "The Vital Connection" (on the brain). These one-hour programs focused on the latest advances in medicine and utilized the dramatic possibilities of probing photography. Some truly extraordinary vignettes showed life and death crises of actual people. As dramatic as "Marcus Welby," this series allowed the viewer to enter the surgical arena; among the delicate operations shown were open-heart surgery and brain surgery that was directed by a courageous, fully awake patient. However, "The Body Human" series has also been criticized, particularly for placing too heavy an emphasis on "miracles."

Other recent specials have treated such topics as mental illness, drugs and adolescents, and chemical food additives. There have also been special reports, prepared in response to news of the day; for example, a half-hour report on Legionnaires' disease was shown in the midst of the enigmatic outbreak that caused great panic following the Legionnaires' convention in Philadelphia in 1976.

News magazine shows. Another format for exploring medicine and health on the air is the so-called news magazine show. About 10% of the programming on the highly regarded "60 Minutes" is devoted to health-related subjects. In one recent season the range of stories spanned a bogus health spa that attracts desperate cancer patients, a clinic that treats phobias, therapists who sexually exploit women, sugar consumption in the U.S., hair dyes and cancer, Valium addiction, conventional treatments for heart disease, and a nurse who works with dying patients. The latter segment, entitled "A Dose of Reality," showed a woman who was dying of leukemia talking candidly about her fears. This kind of honesty on camera clearly had the potential of demystifying and humanizing dying by bringing it into the living rooms of millions of viewers.

NBC's monthly "Weekend" program has also devoted many of its segments to health issues—recently, for example, it addressed the economic and political issues of the existence of too many hospitals and the use of dialysis for treating schizophrenia.

Public television. Public television has taken the possibilites of educating about medicine and health many steps further than network television and has had some truly innovative programming. "Nova" devotes about one-quarter of its one-hour, documentary-format shows to medicine- and health-related subjects. Recent topics covered in depth have included deafness, smallpox eradication, vitamin C and Linus Pauling, transplants, antibiotics, contraception, sleep and dreams, and the controversial issues of human experimentation and genetic engineering.

"Over Easy," a lively show begun in the fall of 1977 that runs five nights a week, focuses on issues of importance to the elderly. The variety-format show covers life-style, nursing homes, nutrition, medicine, Social Security, psychiatry, food stamps, hearing aids, eyeglasses, and numerous other topics that affect senior citizens, who are generally not addressed by programs on network TV or local commercial stations.

"Daniel Foster, M.D.," is an award-winning weekly program that focuses on medical topics of wide public concern. Host Foster interviews prominent specialists, who discuss the latest medical advances.

Public television prepared a particularly unusual six-part series entitled "Feeling Free," which ran first in the spring of 1978 and was scheduled to be repeated. A cast of handicapped children show what it is like to live with handicaps—the aim of which is to bridge the gap between themselves and other children.

Public service messages. In the fall of 1977, when immunization levels of U.S. children were discovered to be deplorably low, the AMA aired a series of creative public service spots urging parents to have their children immunized against common, preventable childhood illnesses. The U.S. Department of Health, Education, and Welfare later joined in the drive to boost immunization among children with a series of messages that appealed to children themselves, using popular characters from the movie *Star Wars.*

Timothy Johnson, a Boston-based physician, has developed a series of 90-second informative health messages—news inserts called "Update on Health"—which are sold to local television stations around the U.S. The subjects range from nutrition to breast cancer; the spots aim at telling viewers how to stay healthy.

The Architectural and Transportation Barriers Compliance Board is using television spots to publicize the "Access America" campaign—to raise American consciousness about stairs, curbs, hard-to-open doors, and other obstacles that prevent large numbers of handicapped but otherwise able citizens from using public buildings.

Medical societies utilize air time to practice preventive medicine: when the American Lung Association began doing antismoking messages on television in 1968, cigarette consumption declined dramatically. However, in 1971, when cigarette ads were banned from TV, antismoking spots were also cut back, and smoking rates increased. Now the Lung Association receives approximately $6 million in free public service air time to educate and inform about air pollution, nonsmokers' rights, emphysema, chronic bronchitis, and asthma. It is unfortunate that few of these spots—or those of the American Heart Association, the American Cancer Society, and many others—are aired during prime-time broadcast, because there is evidence that such efforts *do* motivate viewers.

Healthy potential

There are obviously many potential benefits from the coverage of medicine and health stories on television, no matter what the format. Vital health information can be disseminated to the largest possible numbers in the broadest way. The possibilities for effective preventive medicine are particularly great. When New York City medical reporter Frank Field demonstrated on the air the Heimlich maneuver to dislodge food in a choking victim, more than a thousand viewers contacted him later to report they had been able to save lives. Most reporters who cover medicine and health see their jobs as getting accurate messages across quickly, in a balanced and understandable way; that they can sometimes save lives is a particularly gratifying bonus.

Twenty-five million Americans have high blood pressure, and half don't know they have it. There are also huge numbers of people who are obese or alcoholic or have diabetes or other chronic life-threatening conditions and don't know the seriousness of their problems. Television, more than any other medium, has the capability of reaching them. Though Art Ulene cannot prescribe medicine for his millions of "Today" viewers, he can show how other people have been helped, alert people to the fact that they may have diseases such as hypertension, and point out what that may mean for their health in the long run. If people are told about a problem and directed to sources of help, lives can be saved.

We are daily bombarded with reports of new discoveries, the rising costs of health care, and cancer-causing chemicals in the foods we eat; television can help interpret this barrage of information and can aid the consumer in deciding what to believe and what not to believe. A straightforward presentation, whether by a physician or a reporter, can help break down barriers of public fear and misunderstanding.

An ABC documentary on women's health several years ago examined a kind of intrauterine contraceptive device used by some two million women—the Dalkon Shield—that had caused many deaths, septic abortions, and uterine infections but that remained on the market. The show was instrumental in getting the manufacturer to withdraw the device and stop producing it because it reached and alarmed so many people at once and mobilized effective forces to action. Women now are spared serious risks of that particular contraceptive device.

Implicit dangers

But medical reporting can be tricky, and television as a medium has many pitfalls. There are many dangers in attempting to disseminate medical information over the air. For one thing, TV reporting in general has a tendency to be sensational—for the most part an inappropriate way to address health and medicine. Reporting on breakthroughs and new developments can have the effect of creating highly unrealistic levels of expectation and threatening the doctor-patient relationship. Many lay viewers have heard of some new drug that was being used on only a very small-scale, experimental basis, have gone to their physicians requesting it, and when it could not be provided, the patients have lost faith. A few years ago reports of the so-called curative powers of laetrile—a drug dispensed in Mexico—led many desperate cancer victims to abandon traditional treatments they were receiving in the U.S. and to squander thousands of dollars, and worse, precious time, on a highly suspect, unproved remedy.

Another snare is TV's inevitable short time structure. Should a subject as complex as hyperactivity in children be discussed if a reporter has only 75 seconds to do it? Is it better not to report on a subject at all than to cover it in a cursory way? Sometimes too little information tends to misinform and cause undue alarm.

Describing some of the symptoms of hyperactivity may lead parents who don't have the full story to jump to the conclusion that a perfectly normal but rambunctious child is ill.

Several years ago a segment on "60 Minutes" called "Deadly Medicine" addressed the subject of thyroid cancer in people who had received X-ray treatments to the head and neck area more than a decade earlier. This had been a common practice for such conditions as enlargement of tonsils, acne, and sinusitis. Many critics feel that the presentation made the risk of developing tumors sound much greater than it actually is and that the number of people who were unnecessarily alarmed by the report outweighed the benefits to the very small percentage who may have discovered tumors as a result.

Yet another drawback to excellence in television medical coverage is censorship, particularly since the subject is the human body. Phil Donahue's syndicated day-time interview program prepared a special feature on natural childbirth that was banned in many cities because it was "too graphic."

But short segments that don't give all the facts and misleading, overglamorized stories probably are not the greatest obstacles to television's realizing its potential to provide information; rather, much of the good information that can be and is conveyed is counteracted by advertisers. Recently commercials for sugared cereals have come under attack. Nutritionist Jean Mayer has said that TV is a vending machine that creates nutritional illiterates and that its most impressionable audience—young children—is manipulated to desire foods, particularly sugared cereals, that indeed may be harmful. It follows that before TV can truly realize its potential as an effective medium for conveying vital health information, it is urgent that the government and the Federal Communications Commission (FCC) take strong measures to control the contents of advertisements.

The future

There is a quiet revolution going on in health care and the way it is going to be delivered in the next decade. Schools, government, society, the family, the individual, and the media all share responsibility for health care. The media are just beginning to realize their potential roles. TV in particular has barely scratched the surface. We need more and better medical programming and health and science reporting. Prevention needs to be emphasized. The AMA is enthusiastic about the trend but warns that doctors should not engage in solicitation during TV appearances.

The interest people are showing in health and medicine may mean doom for Marcus Welby. But NBC has created a new prime-time series—"Lifeline"—hour-long shows devoted to examining the professional and personal lives of real life medical specialists.

Urinary and Genital Disorders

Within the past five years a new awareness of the male component as a cause of infertility has emerged. This interest is based on an improved understanding of the biochemical, hormonal, and developmental aspects of sperm formation and maturation. In addition, an atmosphere of increased sexual awareness in society has prompted many men to seek medical evaluation and treatment in childless relationships.

Male fertility failure: types and treatment

Three major categories of male infertility are currently recognized. The first group comprises primary causes, which include failure of testicular formation during embryonic development, failure of the testes to contain the primary cells necessary to produce sperm, and a failure of the developing sperm cells to mature normally into sperm. In addition, failure to produce normal sperm (*i.e.,* in number, shape, size, and motility) may be associated with testes that have not descended into the scrotum and even with those placed in the scrotum through corrective surgery. Secondary causes, the second group, include those factors associated with infection or trauma—mumps with testicular involvement as a young adult; infection of the ducts directing sperm to the vas deferens secondary to gonorrhea or other bacterial infections; and blockage of the vas deferens from surgery (vasectomy), trauma, or congenital development failure. The final group includes those situations of infertility in which normal sperm formation, motility, shape, and numbers are present, yet the sperm are not capable of fertilization. This last group represents a significant number of the infertile male population.

Urological assessment of an infertile male involves appraisal of general health and identification of the cause of infertility. Such problems as the absence of testicles or of sperm-producing cells are presently unsolvable situations. Failure of sperm cells to mature may be treated in certain situations by endocrine (hormonal) drug administration, but the results are poor at best. Such obstructive lesions as ductal blockage may frequently be improved by surgical bypass procedures designed to establish a continuous route for sperm transport.

Patients in the final group show no anatomic or hormonal disturbance upon examination. All evaluation criteria show normal results. This represents a large segment of the populace in which the potential for fertility obviously exists. Immunologic factors have been suggested as the cause but have yet to be documented. Rest, carefully regulated application of heat to the scrotum, diet, and hormone administration have contributed in certain cases to fertility.

In general, evaluation of the male as a cause of infertility in a childless relationship can categorize the type of fertility failure. Surgical treatment or hormonal or dietary therapy may be helpful in a few situations. In others, despite the present lack of success in restoring fertility, continuing research offers a promise for the future.

Bench kidney surgery

The concept of "bench surgery" implies removing an organ from the body, keeping it viable, performing the indicated surgery, and then placing the organ back into the patient. Bench surgery of the kidney has recently become a distinct surgical technique because of advances made through kidney preservation and transplant surgery. During its time outside the body the kidney is maintained by a preservation machine which pumps a solution through the renal blood vessels, keeping the organ cool, moist, and alive.

Application of this surgical technique is reserved for a few selected types of kidney problems. Narrowing (stenosis) or dilatation (aneurysms) of the renal blood vessels may be selected for bench surgery. Kidney tumor surgery may be approached in this fashion, particularly if there is an indicated need to preserve a portion of the diseased kidney.

Bed-wetting

Enuresis, commonly called bed-wetting, is defined as urination while sleeping. It is recognized as a developmental retardation but without any reflection on intelligence. It is found in both sexes frequently associated with a typical sound and sometimes very deep sleep pattern. Voiding may occur once or several times while the child is asleep. Left untreated, nearly all children will stop by age 16. Continued occurrence through puberty and into adulthood creates family anxiety, interpersonal conflict, fear, and trepidation.

Enuresis alone does not signify any overt anatomical defect or disease. It is frequently found in families in which parents or grandparents had enuresis, suggesting a hereditary predisposition. An important point to remember is that the victim does not wet because of hostility or vindictive motives; it is not voluntarily controlled. The primary problem appears to be related to the enuretic's deep level of sleep, which essentially eliminates subconscious control over the bladder.

Enuresis does not require medical intervention unless it persists beyond age ten. Urological assessment occasionally is encouraged by the amount of familial or patient anxiety and concern that it provokes. Medical evaluation may simply include a history and physical exam and a urine analysis. There may be indication to suggest a kidney and bladder X-ray to exclude hidden obstruction of the kidney, bladder, or ducts (ureters) connecting them.

Treatment of the enuretic may be simple or somewhat involved. Primary treatment in the child should include encouragement and parental warmth and understanding. Fluids should be restricted at the last meal and essentially none allowed until the next morning. The bladder must be fully emptied before sleep.

Further treatment may require drugs that alter sleep level and quiet the bladder. Two such drugs are Tofranil and Tofranil-PM; these agents are reported to be 40–80% effective in controlling or curing the enuretic child. But drug therapy should be restricted to persons at least 8–10 years old. Tofranil-PM is highly effective for the individual who has multiple episodes of wetting during sleep.

Auxiliary methods of sleep modification include the simple bell and pad device, which is designed to wake the person when he or she wets. The concept is that wetting appears to occur at approximately the same time each night. By awakening at that time, a mechanism of arousal anticipation occurs. This arousal changes sleep from an extremely deep level to one of subconscious awareness, where urinary inhibition occurs. In standard trials of the bell and pad device results of 60–70% success have been reported. The only effective and acceptable version of this device is battery powered, costs $20–$40, and is usually available from retail catalog suppliers. Children who fail to respond to these techniques are considered too immature and require a 6–12 month interval before receiving another round of treatment.

— *Casimir F. Firlit, M.D., Ph.D.*

World Medical News

Resurgence of several serious infectious illnesses in various parts of the world and evidence of overconfidence in the ability to control disease offered grim reminders in recent months that most major afflictions of mankind were far from conquered. In Europe reports of growing heroin addiction were becoming a matter of serious concern. India continued to grapple with its overpopulation problems, albeit in a new way, while some African nations experienced difficulty with the opposite phenomenon, that of infertility.

Immunization programs

There were continuing signs in the developed countries of a relaxation of vigilance against once common infectious diseases. The percentage of children in these nations receiving protective immunizations of all kinds declined, in part because of publicity given the adverse side effects of some vaccines and in part because of a false sense of security generated by years of successful disease control. In late 1977 the British secretary of state for health reported that in the U.K. the proportion of children vaccinated against polio, tetanus, and diphtheria had slipped from 80 to 75% in recent years and that vaccinations against whooping cough had plunged from 78 to 39%. In the past quarter of a century polio vaccination had reduced incidence of

the disease in England and Wales to less than five cases per year, but in the first ten months of 1977 about three times that number were reported.

Several less developed countries formulated plans for new or expanded immunization programs. As part of a country health programming exercise Burma developed an immunization campaign against five common childhood diseases, establishing a target date of 1982 for major reductions in incidence of polio, diphtheria, whooping cough, and tetanus of the newborn and in the annual risk of infection with organisms causing tuberculosis.

Cameroon followed evaluation of its first nine months of an immunization program—which included dispensing vaccines against diphtheria, tetanus, whooping cough, tuberculosis, measles, polio, and smallpox to 22,000 children—by stepping up its publicity campaign and developing more efficient methods of processing children through vaccination stations. Indonesia put forward a multistage immunization expansion plan that involved vaccination of selected population groups against diphtheria, whooping cough, tetanus, and tuberculosis, with expectations of significant drops in mortality associated with these diseases. By 1979 an additional 1,100 health centers were to have been added to the approximately 2,300 existing in that country at the end of 1976.

Infectious diseases

Malaria. Despite several decades of eradication programs, malaria was staging a comeback in Asia, Africa, and Latin America, and late-1977 estimates placed the number of cases of the disease worldwide at about 120 million. Malaria resurgence seemed most dramatic in India, where reported cases skyrocketed from 40,000 in 1966 to nearly six million 11 years later. Sri Lanka, Pakistan, some African countries south of the Sahara, Guatemala, Honduras, El Salvador, and Nicaragua were other nations especially hard hit.

Growing resistance of mosquitoes, which transmit the malaria blood parasite from person to person, to DDT and other conventional insecticides was cited as a primary cause of increased disease incidence. In Central America some medical experts blamed reduced government interest in increasingly expensive insecticide-spray programs and use of DDT by cotton growers, a practice that promoted development of DDT-resistant strains of mosquitoes in cotton-growing areas. Recent rises of malaria in India were also attributed to early monsoon rains and a shortage of drugs and insecticides. It was suggested that a return to pre-DDT approaches—draining mosquito breeding areas and continuously checking water supplies—together with use of protective drugs would be necessary until an effective vaccine, still perhaps ten years in the future, could be developed against the disease.

Sleeping sickness. A UN-sponsored seminar in

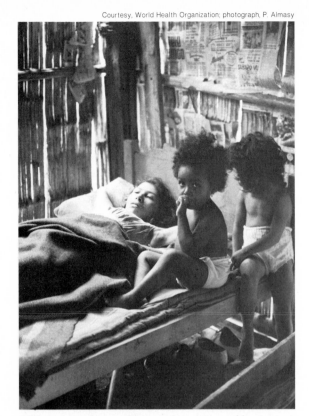

Malaria is proving a stubborn and recurring problem in most countries of Asia, Africa, and Latin America, despite the eradication efforts of national and international health agencies.

Kenya in September 1977 on tsetse-fly control heard warnings of growing tsetse infestation over vast regions of Africa where wars were interfering with fly-control campaigns. The director of the UN Food and Agriculture Organization's tsetse surveillance effort stated that political instability and revolutionary movements were making the necessary monitoring difficult, and other seminar participants testified to the impossibility of continuing insecticide-spray programs in the midst of clashing armies and guerrilla actions. The tsetse fly, whose parasite-transmitting bite causes sleeping sickness (also known as Chagas' disease or trypanosomiasis) in man, which can result in death, and a similar disease in livestock, was reported to be reinvading Rhodesia, where a previously successful eradication program had been virtually halted because of guerrilla activity. The fly was also reemerging in southern Angola, a battleground between rebels and government forces, and in the lowlands of Ethiopia, where clashing Somalis and Ethiopians had caused internationally sponsored tsetse-control campaigns to be suspended.

Russian flu. A new influenza virus closely resembling a strain in worldwide circulation between 1947 and 1957 made its appearance in the U.S.S.R., Hong Kong, and China in late 1977. By the end of the year

it had struck about 15%, or 40 million, of the Soviet population and was reported to have caused widespread absenteeism in Hong Kong schools. Officially called A/USSR/77 and dubbed the Russian flu virus, the organism produced comparatively mild symptoms lasting three to five days and tended to infect children and young adults under the age of 20, who were not old enough to have developed any immunity from exposure to the virus's close relative of the late 1940s and the 1950s. Epidemiological laboratories in various parts of the world received samples of the virus for evaluation and possible vaccine development. By early 1978, however, although Russian flu had been reported in several other countries including Finland and the U.S., it had given little evidence of becoming a serious problem anywhere.

Cholera. A major cholera epidemic struck the Middle East in mid-1977, claiming several thousand victims in Syria, Jordan, Lebanon, Egypt, Saudi Arabia, and Israel by the end of September. Cases were also suspected in Iran, Iraq, and Turkey. Initially local health ministries, fearing loss of tourist revenues, were reported to have delayed revealing the true nature of the disease, attributing outbreaks of illness to food poisoning or some other less serious problem. In Syria, where the epidemic hit hardest, the government banned sales of street-vended fruits, vegetables, and ices and closed swimming pools, public beaches, and open-air cafes in an attempt to stem the spread of the cholera bacterium, which infects the human gut and is transmitted by food and water contaminated with fecal matter. The Egyptian health ministry launched a campaign to vaccinate 13 million Egyptian citizens and ordered the burning of garbage piles in Cairo and Alexandria. Several cases of cholera were reported in Great Britain, Italy, West Germany, and The Netherlands, all brought in by persons returning from Middle Eastern trips.

A cholera epidemic battered Tanzania in late 1977, with more than 5,000 cases reported during a five-month period beginning in October. The Tanzanian government responded with a program that included construction of emergency sanitary facilities, an intensive poster campaign, quarantine of large areas of the country, and a ban on transport of fruits and vegetables from infected regions. Neighboring Kenya had reported 117 cases of the disease by March 1978, and Somalia took protective steps to prevent the spread of the disease into that country.

Rabies. Rabies continued and even accelerated its relentless spread among European wildlife, moving across the Alps into northern Italy and from France into Switzerland. The epidemic was believed to stem from a tremendous increase in the highly rabies-susceptible fox population of Europe in the years following World War II, due to a decline of its natural predators and an increase in prey. In France figures released for a recent 12-month period revealed that more than 2,000 rabid

322

foxes had been killed or found dead and that rabies had been detected in scores of dogs, cats, cattle, and horses. Systematic gassing of fox dens with phosgene gas, financial support to hunting organizations, and bounties on fox tails ranked high on France's list of rabies-control measures. Through gassing, Denmark was maintaining itself in a rabies-free condition, and Great Britain was protecting itself by means of a mandatory six-month quarantine for all animals brought into the country. Rabies was also a problem in the U.S., where the disease held a stronghold in the wild skunk population.

Some medical authorities felt that the best approach to rabies control would be to immunize the wild population of susceptible animals; in the U.S., for example, investigators were exploring ways of encapsulating vaccine in sugar pellets that could be hidden in bait. A new rabies vaccine for humans—made from virus grown in human cell culture and requiring only six injections for immunity instead of the normal course of 14 to 21—gained approval for use in several countries. The improved vaccine was developed at the Wistar Institute in Philadelphia and successfully passed clinical trials at the World Health Organization's rabies research center in Teheran, Iran.

Heroin addiction

Reports from drug officials in the U.S. and Europe indicated a soaring use of heroin by Western Europeans, the result of a shift in Asian drug traffic from Southeast Asia to Europe following American troop pullouts at the close of the Vietnam War. The area bounded by Austria, England, Italy, and Norway was cited as containing the fastest growing population of addicts in the world. In a five-year period the number of identified heroin addicts in this region rose almost tenfold, from 9,000 to 88,000, whereas annual heroin seizures over the same period jumped from 25 lb to 1,500 lb.

A heavily attended conference of European and Middle Eastern narcotics specialists meeting in Amsterdam in October 1977 to discuss drug traffic control reflected the growing concern of Europeans over hard drug addiction, which had once been considered primarily a U.S. problem. Some European officials also blamed rising heroin use on American users touring Europe and on increased travel by European youths to Asian countries.

Surgery and transplants

In late December 1977 an international team of surgeons announced the first successful use in a human being of a total artificial heart; *i.e.,* one that supplies both chambers, or ventricles, of the heart with blood. Working at Zurich Hospital in Switzerland, the team used tubing to connect the external device to the heart of a woman who had suffered severe heart failure following cardiac surgery. The mechanical pump, devel-

oped by an Italian bioengineer, maintained the patient's life until her natural heart could function well enough on its own. Related experiments in the U.S. had involved animals and used a device that supplied only one of the heart ventricles.

Heart transplant surgery remained a quiet but active field of research, notably at Stanford University, where Norman Shumway had pioneered the surgical techniques of the heart transplant operation in animals, and in South Africa, where Christiaan Barnard had performed the first successful such operation on a human being in 1967. In the decade following Barnard's milestone more than 350 heart transplant operations had been done by several dozen surgical teams worldwide; as of early 1978 about one-fourth of the transplant recipients were still alive, most of them patients of Shumway. Because of low patient survival rates and the difficulty in obtaining donor organs when needed, by the late 1970s most heart transplant teams had stopped their operations. Shumway's group at Stanford remained an exception, however, and their patient survival rates were reported to be improving steadily.

In October 1977 Barnard and a team of surgeons in Cape Town transplanted the heart of a chimpanzee into a male patient to supplement the patient's own rapidly failing organ. This "piggyback" style of transplant had been performed several times using human hearts; Barnard had used this technique once in June with a baboon's heart, which failed under the circulatory load in four hours. The chimpanzee heart transplant was intended as a temporary measure until a human heart became available, but the patient survived only 3½ days.

In the face of a shortage of voluntary organ donors, France put into force in April 1978 a law that abolished donor authorization before death as a prerequisite to removal of organs for transplant surgery. The right of the decedent's family to forbid organ removal for such purposes was also taken away. Instead, persons who did not wish to donate organs were required to register themselves on a special list, which would be consulted by surgeons before proceeding with a transplant. The new law excluded minors and the mentally handicapped, for whom donor authorization was still required from parents or guardians. One part of the legislation dealt crucially with determination of the moment of death and hence with the moment transplant operations could begin; in essence it left the question to the two major medical bodies in France, both of which currently held that the determining factor in defining death is the presence of cerebral death.

Population control

Under the new leadership of Prime Minister Morarji R. Desai, India experienced a sharp shift from the coercive birth-control policies of Indira Gandhi that were intended to stem the country's rapid population growth of about 35,000 per day. Just prior to Gandhi's electoral defeat in March 1977 public-health clinics were performing nearly a million sterilization operations a month. By contrast, in the first four months of the Desai regime the monthly average was 50,000, and the number of women who received intrauterine devices fell to a third of its former level.

Inability of an abnormally large number of couples in the central African nations to have children was the subject of a special report recently issued by the London-based International Planned Parenthood Federation. The report cited surveys that delineated large regions of central Africa in which infertility afflicted 30% of couples. The spread of gonorrhea was reported as the primary cause of infertility; when the disease goes untreated in women, it frequently results in fallopian tube blockage, which prevents travel of eggs from the ovaries to the uterus. Hypothyroidism and infection after childbirth in women and a mosquito-borne disease that makes men sterile were also implicated. The report stated that the problem was leading to divorce and child theft in countries where progeny are "insurance policy, entertainment, old-age pension and welfare assistance rolled into one."

Mental health

A resolution condemning the Soviet practice of employing compulsory psychiatric treatment for political purposes was narrowly approved by secret ballot at a meeting in August 1977 of the World Psychiatric Association in Honolulu. The move capped several months of public disclosures by Soviet emigrants citing hundreds of cases in which psychiatric diagnoses had been made allegedly to silence mentally healthy dissidents. One particular diagnosis that came under severe criticism at the conference was "sluggish schizophrenia," a malady often ascribed to Soviet citizens who took issue with their government's policies. According to one U.S. psychiatrist at the conference, "Even if one should accept the diagnosis of sluggish schizophrenia . . . one must wonder why a disease without delusions, hallucinations, or agitated behavior should require injections of chlorpromazine [an antipsychotic drug and tranquilizer] for its treatment." U.S. delegates also made it clear that their criticism was not limited to the Soviet Union but extended "to all other countries where such conditions exist."

Two Canadian investigators reported in late 1977 that certain areas of the brains of victims of schizophrenia contain about double the normal number of receptors for dopamine, a chemical that transmits nervous impulses from one nerve cell to another. Calling the discovery the "first direct understanding" of schizophrenic symptoms, they suggested that the overabundance of dopamine receptors, which are carried on the surface membranes of nerve cells, make schizophrenics oversensitive to their own brain signals, resulting in a flood of bizarre thoughts, delusions, and hallucinations.

The two scientists examined brain tissue taken from 20 schizophrenics who had died and found extra dopamine receptors concentrated in two anatomical regions: the limbic system, a collection of brain structures that together regulate emotion, and the caudate nucleus, a mass of nerve cells that helps mediate body movements. Other researchers investigating dopamine receptors in the brain, however, remained skeptical, finding in their own research no clear-cut distinction in this regard between normal and schizophrenic brains. Nevertheless, some kind of link between schizophrenia and dopamine did seem reasonable; for instance, amphetamine drugs, which can produce schizophrenic symptoms, were known to trigger the release of dopamine in the brain.

Smoking

Great Britain experienced a disappointing consumer reaction in a recent drive to promote a less hazardous cigarette. As part of a coordinated campaign costing more than $100 million in development and publicity, tobacco companies chose mid-1977 to introduce various brands of cigarettes containing 25–40% cellulose, a wood-pulp product that yields no nicotine and substantially less carbon monoxide and tar when smoked. Early sales, however, proved much less brisk than expected, with smokers' comments ranging from "too mild" and "too dry" to wry remarks about contracting "artificial cancer" and "Dutch elm disease." A major reason for poor acceptance was thought to be the decision of the British Treasury to tax cellulose content as if it were tobacco, making the price of the new cigarettes no cheaper than conventional brands. An earlier, single-brand marketing approach in Switzerland and West Germany had also failed to interest smokers in such "safe" cigarettes.

In Japan, where per capita consumption of cigarettes—seven per day per person—was the highest in the world, antismoking efforts were beginning to produce results. In part because of increasing awareness of the health hazards of smoking, sales of tobacco in 1976 fell for the first time. Despite lucrative returns the government-monopolized cigarette-sales business in Japan recently began a campaign stressing tidiness in smoking to counter an enormous countrywide refuse problem, and voluntarily limited the amount of television and newspaper advertising for cigarettes. Efforts to curb smoking went back to 1970, when Tokyo subway stations promoted a "no-smoking time" on jammed train platforms during morning rush hours. In 1978 the Japanese Parliament addressed the subject for the first time, and one government official promised to make no-smoking areas of the lobbies in the country's hospitals and clinics.

—Charles M. Cegielski

Health Education Units

The following section contains the third in a series of instructive articles on important medical topics and health-related concerns. It is largely through general health education that individuals can maintain and enhance their physical well-being. While the units emphasize the activation of the layperson's sense of responsibility for his or her own health, their purpose is to inform, not to prescribe.

Contributors

Charles M. Cegielski
Saving Money on Prescription Drugs; Beware of Mixing Drugs.
Associate Editor, Britannica yearbooks, Encyclopædia Britannica, Inc., Chicago.

Lester L. Coleman, M.D.
Emphysema; Fear; Peptic Ulcers; Alcoholism; Cosmetic Surgery; Glaucoma and Cataracts.
Nationally syndicated health columnist, King Features Syndicate;
Assistant Clinical Professor, Albert Einstein College of Medicine of Yeshiva University, New York City;
and Attending Surgeon, Otolaryngology, The New York Hospital
and Manhattan Eye, Ear, and Throat Hospital, New York City.

Alvin N. Eden, M.D.
Overweight Children; Juvenile Diabetes; The Importance of Fathering;
Measles and German Measles; Chickenpox, Shingles, and Smallpox; Hyperactive Children.
Pediatric columnist; Director of Pediatrics, Wyckoff Heights Hospital, Brooklyn, New York;
and Associate Clinical Professor of Pediatrics, New York University School of Medicine, New York City.

Robert McHenry
Quizzes: *Are You What You Eat?; Shouldn't You Be Jogging?;*
How Do You Rate as a Patient?; What Do You Know About Sex?
Senior Editor, G. & C. Merriam Co., Springfield, Mass.

Christine Timmons
Contraception: The Choices (in part); *Living Wills and Organ Donation.*
Free-lance writer and editor, Chicago.

Louise B. Tyrer, M.D.
Contraception: The Choices (in part).
Vice-President for Medical Affairs, Planned Parenthood Federation of America, New York City.

Cartoons by John Everds

Contents

Saving Money on Prescription Drugs

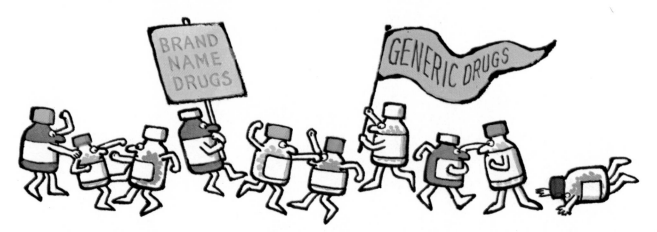

More than nine out of ten people who consult a doctor for some illness or complaint that does not require hospitalization come away from the visit with at least one prescription. Other than exercising their freedom to do business at the pharmacy of their choice, many of these patients regard themselves merely as messengers who dutifully transport the communication "expensive medicine," encoded in scribbles on the prescription blank, between physician and pharmacist. Such questions as what can influence drug prices, what exactly the doctor prescribed, how he or she came to this decision, and whether the pharmacist has any options in interpreting the doctor's instructions are usually not asked; yet it is these factors that sometimes profoundly affect the cost of a drug to the consumer. With some awareness of certain facts regarding the marketing, prescribing, and dispensing of drugs, the consumer often can obtain prescription drugs for substantially less money. Moreover, recent legislation in many U.S. states is making drug overpricing by the manufacturer less profitable than it once was.

Generic versus brand-name drugs

Essential to an understanding of why some drugs can be bought less expensively is a knowledge of the distinction between "generic" and "brand-name" drugs. In general every drug acquires three names at some time in its career. The first and most basic is its chemical name, which describes to the chemist who is concerned with isolating or synthesizing the drug its exact molecular structure. During its development by the drug company the drug is also assigned an official, nonproprietary name, commonly called its generic name; it is by this name that it becomes known to pharmacologists and medical research scientists. Finally, just before it appears on the market, the drug

receives a brand name, one that is usually shorter and easier to remember than its generic name and is sometimes suggestive of the drug's effects. For example, one very commonly prescribed drug would be unrecognizable to most people by its chemical name, $(+)$- α-4-(dimethylamino)-3-methyl-1,2-diphenyl-2-butanol propionate hydrochloride; its generic name, propoxyphene hydrochloride, might be more meaningful, but the great majority of patients who have taken the drug to relieve pain know it by its most popular brand name, Darvon.

Every new drug, along with its manufacturing process, is protected under U.S. patent law for 17 years, during which time the original developer has exclusive right to make and market it and to set prices without concern for competition. After this time the patent on the drug expires, and the drug enters the public domain; any other manufacturer is then free to make and sell the drug as long as it does not use the original brand name, which is protected by trademark law.

As an illustration, the tranquilizing agent known generically as chlordiazepoxide hydrochloride was patented by Hoffmann-La Roche Inc., who sold it for 17 years in vast quantities under the brand name Librium. The drug entered the public domain in 1976 and since then has been made and offered for sale by several other companies. Some of these firms have given the drug such new brand names as A-poxide (Abbott Laboratories) and SK-Lygen (Smith Kline & French Laboratories); others have used only the generic term. On the other hand, Valium, another extremely popular tranquilizer made by Hoffmann-La Roche, is protected until 1985 from being sold by any other company either under the drug's generic name, diazepam, or under another brand name. Hence diazepam can be bought from only one source. (The accompanying list shows

Frequently Prescribed Brand-Name Drugs
Available Generically or Under Other Brand Names

brand name	generic name	brand name	generic name
Achromycin V	tetracycline HCl	Doriden	glutethimide
Alpen	ampicillin	Doxinate	dioctyl sodium sulfosuccinate
Amcill	ampicillin	Doxychel	doxycycline hyclate
Aminodur	aminophylline	Dramamine	dimenhydrinate
Amphojel	aluminum hydroxide gel	Dulcolax	bisacodyl
Amytal	amobarbital	Duotrate	pentaerythritol tetranitrate
Android	methyltestosterone	Dyspas	dicyclomine HCl
Anspor	cephradine	Ekko	diphenylhydantoin
Antivert	meclizine	Elavil	amitriptyline HCl
Antora	pentaerythritol tetranitrate	Elixophyllin	theophylline
Apresoline	hydralazine	E-Mycin	erythromycin
Aquachloral	chloral hydrate	Endep	amitriptyline HCl
Aquatag	benzthiazide	Equanil	meprobamate
Aralen Phosphate	chloroquine phosphate	Erypar	erythromycin
Aristocort	triamcinolone	Erythrocin	erythromycin
Armour Thyroid	thyroid	Esidrix	hydrochlorothiazide
Artane	trihexyphenidyl HCl	Eskabarb	phenobarbital
Azo Gantrisin	sulfisoxazole with phenazopyridine	Eskalith	lithium carbonate
		Ethril	erythromycin
Azo-Stat	phenazopyridine	Exna	benzthiazide
Bacarate	phendimetrazine tartrate	Fastin	phentermine
Benadryl	diphenhydramine	Felsules	chloral hydrate
Bendopa	levodopa	Feosol	ferrous sulfate
Benemid	probenecid	Fer-In-Sol	ferrous sulfate
Bentyl	dicyclomine HCl	Fero-Gradumet	ferrous sulfate
Benzedrine Sulfate	amphetamine sulfate	Fiorinal	butalbital compound
Betapar	prednisone	Formtone-HC	hydrocortisone with iodochlorhydroxyquin
Betapen-VK	penicillin VK		
Bicol	bisacodyl	Fulvicin-U/F	griseofulvin
Bonine	meclizine HCl	Furadantin	nitrofurantoin
Bontril PDM	phendimetrazine tartrate	Gammacorten	dexamethasone
Bristamycin	erythromycin	Gantanol	sulfamethoxazole
Bronkolixir	theophylline, ephedrine, phenobarbital, guaifenesin	Gantrisin	sulfisoxazole
		Grifulvin V	griseofulvin
Bu-Lax	dioctyl sodium sulfosuccinate	Grisactin	griseofulvin
Butazolidin	phenylbutazone	Hexadrol	dexamethasone
Butibel	butabarbital sodium with belladonna	Histaspan	chlorpheniramine maleate
		Hydrodiuril	hydrochlorothiazide
Buticaps	butabarbital sodium	Hydropres	hydrochlorothiazide with reserpine
Butisol Sodium	butabarbital sodium		
Cafergot	ergotamine with caffeine	Hytone	hydrocortisone
Cerespan	papaverine	Ilosone	erythromycin
Cetacort	hydrocortisone	Ionamin	phentermine
Chloromycetin	chloramphenicol	Isordil	Isosorbide dinitrate
Chlor-PZ	chlorpromazine	Janimine	imipramine HCl
Chlor-Trimeton	chlorpheniramine maleate	Kaon	potassium gluconate
Choloxin	sodium dextrothyroxine	Kenacort	triamcinolone
Colace	dioctyl sodium sulfosuccinate	Kesso-Bamate	meprobamate
ColBENEMID	probenecid with colchicine	Kessodanten	diphenylhydantoin
Comfolax	dioctyl sodium sulfosuccinate	Kessodrate	chloral hydrate
Compocillin-VK	penicillin VK	Kesso-Mycin	erythromycin
Cort-Dome	hydrocortisone	Kesso-Pen	penicillin G
Cortef	hydrocortisone	Kesso-Pen-VK	penicillin VK
Cyantin	nitrofurantoin	Kesso-Tetra	tetracycline
Cyclopar	tetracycline	Kudrox	magnesia and alumina
Cyclospasmol	cyclandelate	Lanoxin	digoxin
Cytomel	liothyronine	Larodopa	levodopa
Darvon	propoxyphene HCl	Larotid	amoxicillin
Decadron	dexamethasone	Ledercillin VK	penicillin VK
Delta-Cortef	prednisolone	Letter	sodium levothyroxine
Delta-Dome	prednisone	Libritabs	chlordiazepoxide
Deltasone	prednisone	Librium	chlordiazepoxide
Demerol-HCl	meperidine HCl	Lithane	lithium carbonate
Dermacort	hydrocortisone	Lithonate	lithium carbonate
Deronil	dexamethasone	Luminal	phenobarbital
Dexedrine	dextroamphetamine sulfate	Maalox	magnesia and alumina
D-Feda Gyrocaps	pseudoephedrine HCl	Macrodantin	nitrofurantoin
Dilantin	diphenylhydantoin	Mandelamine	methenamine mandelate
Dimetane	brompheniramine maleate	Melfiat	phendimetrazine tartrate
Diodoquin	diiodohydroxyquin	Meprotabs	meprobamate
Dolene	propoxyphene HCl	Metahydrin	trichlormethiazide
Domeboro	aluminum sulfate, calcium acetate	Metandren	methyltestosterone
		Meticortelone	prednisolone
Donnatal	belladonna, phenobarbital	Meticorten	prednisone
Dopar	levodopa	Miltown	meprobamate

continued on next page

brand name	generic name	brand name	generic name
Mol-Iron	ferrous sulfate	Rexamycin	tetracycline
Mylanta	magnesia, alumina, simethicone	Robicillin VK	penicillin VK
		Robimycin	erythromycin
Naqua	trichlormethiazide	Robitet	tetracycline
Nebralin	pentobarbital	Seco-8	secobarbital
Nembutal	pentobarbital	Seconal	secobarbital
Neo-Corovas	pentaerythritol tetranitrate	Ser-Ap-Es	hydralazine, hydrochlorothiazide, reserpine
Neosporin	bacitracin, neomycin, polymyxin		
Neo-Synephrine	phenylephrine HCl	Serpasil	reserpine
Nico-400	nicotinic acid (niacin)	Serpasil-Esidrix	hydrochlorothiazide, reserpine
Nicobid	nicotinic acid (niacin)	SK-65	propoxyphene HCl
Nicocap	nicotinic acid (niacin)	SK-Ampicillin	ampicillin
Nitro-Bid	nitroglycerin	SK-Bamate	meprobamate
Nitroglyn	nitroglycerin	SK-Erythromycin	erythromycin
Nitrong	nitroglycerin	SK-Lygen	chlordiazepoxide HCl
Nitro-SA	nitroglycerin	SK-Penicillin VK	penicillin VK
Nitrospan	nitroglycerin	SK-Petn	pentaerythritol tetranitrate
Noctec	chloral hydrate	SK-Pramine	imipramine HCl
Orasone	prednisone	SK-Soxazole	sulfisoxazole
Oretic	hydrochlorothiazide	SK-Tetracycline	tetracycline
Oreton Methyl	methyltestosterone	Somophyllin	aminophylline
Orinase	tolbutamide	Sorbitrate	isosorbide dinitrate
Oxy-Kesso-Tetra	oxytetracycline	Soxomide	sulfisoxazole
Panmycin	tetracycline	Spaz	belladonna, phenobarbital
Pavabid	papaverine HCl	S-P-T	thyroid
Pediamycin	erythromycin	Statobex	phendimetrazine tartrate
Pen A	ampicillin	Stental	phenobarbital
Penapar VK	penicillin VK	Sudafed	pseudoephedrine HCl
Pensyn	ampicillin	Sumycin	tetracycline
Pentids	penicillin G	Supen	ampicillin
Pentritol	pentaerythritol tetranitrate	Sustaverine	papaverine HCl
Pen-Vee K	penicillin VK	Synthroid	sodium levothyroxine
Peri-Colace	dioctyl sodium sulfosuccinate with casanthranol	Tandearil	oxyphenbutazone
		Tanorex	phendimetrazine tartrate
Peritrate	pentaerythritol tetranitrate	Tedral	theophylline, ephedrine, phenobarbital
Pfizer-E	erythromycin		
Pfizerpen G	penicillin G	Tempra	acetaminophen
Pfizerpen VK	penicillin VK	Tenuate	diethylpropion HCl
Phenergan	promethazine	Terramycin	oxytetracycline
Pil-Digis	digitalis	Tet-Cy	tetracycline
Pipanol	trihexyphenidyl HCl	Tetrachel	tetracycline
Plegine	phendimetrazine	Tetracyn	tetracycline
Polymox	amoxicillin	Theobid	theophylline
Premarin	estrogens, conjugated	Thorazine	chlorpromazine
Principen	ampicillin	Tofranil	imipramine HCl
Priscoline	tolazoline	Totacillin	ampicillin
Pro-Banthine	propantheline bromide	Trantoin	nitrofurantoin
Probital	propantheline bromide with phenobarbital	Tremin	trihexyphenidyl HCl
		Trimox	amoxicillin
Progesic	propoxyphene HCl	Tuinal	secobarbital and amobarbital
Proloid	thyroglobulin	Tylenol	acetaminophen
Pyribenzamine	tripelennamine HCl	Uri-Tet	oxytetracycline
Pyridium	phenazopyridine	Uticillin VK	penicillin VK
Quadrinal	theophylline, ephedrine, phenobarbital	Vasospan	papaverine HCl
		V-Cillin K	penicillin VK
Quibron	theophylline with guaifenesin	Veetids	penicillin VK
Quinidex	quinidine sulfate	Velosef	cephradine
Quinora	quinidine sulfate	Vibramycin	doxycycline hyclate
Raudixin	rauwolfia serpentina	Vioform-Hydrocortisone	hydrocortisone with iodochlorhydroxyquin
Rau-Sed	reserpine		
Remsed	promethazine	WinGel	magnesia and alumina

brand-name drugs that are available generically.)

The prices that manufacturers charge for a drug and consequently the price that the consumer pays (allowing a certain markup by the pharmacist) are materially influenced by the drug's patent status. For a drug still under patent, like diazepam, a price monopoly exists, and the consumer has little choice but to pay high prices for that drug, whether it be prescribed generically or by brand name. For a drug in the public domain, however, there usually exists a range of prices. In the late 1970s, for example, the typical price to the chain-store pharmacist of 500 ten-milligram capsules of chlordiazepoxide hydrochloride ranged from more than $40 (for Librium) to less than $15 (for one of the generic brands). Generics are usually made by smaller companies, who charge lower prices, but this is not a fast rule. Sometimes a brand-name drug will undersell its generically labeled equivalent.

329

How the doctor and druggist determine drug prices

In states that currently do not have effective generic drug legislation (and in most states prior to the upswing in interest concerning such legislation), the pharmacist is required by law to dispense exactly what is written on the prescription blank. If a brand-name drug is called for, be it cheap or expensive, no other brand-name or generic equivalent can be substituted. In order to allow the pharmacist some freedom in choosing among the various available chemical equivalents, the doctor must prescribe the drug only by its generic name.

Despite this power that the physician has to select drugs that will entail the least expense for the patient, historically the most expensive drugs have outsold their counterparts and still continue to do so. An obvious reason, of course, is the 17-year lead time the developing company has to habituate the physician into thinking only in terms of the brand name. Then, too, as was mentioned above, the proprietary name is designed to be much easier to remember than the generic one. Another important factor is the effect of the tremendously expensive advertising campaigns of the large drug companies, who bombard the physician with promotional literature, exhibit their products in the pages of medical journals, and send company representatives, called detail men, to distribute samples and convince the physician of the superior quality of their company's drugs.

This last concern regarding quality often comes up when a patient questions why his or her physician does not prescribe generically, and underlying it are years of bitter confrontation between the large drug suppliers and their supporters and the promoters of generic prescribing. The former group asserts that all drug equivalents are necessarily not the same, and particularly that attention to freshness, good quality control, and judicious use of compounding materials (like binders and disintegration agents), which do not interfere with drug action, are more likely to be attributes of large drug companies than of small ones. The latter group points out that about half of all drugs recalled in the U.S. because of substandard quality or mislabeling are products of large drug companies, that large companies often sell both brand-name and generic equivalents of the same drug at different prices, and that many drugs supplied under a high-priced brand name by one company and under a low-priced generic name by another company are in fact identical products purchased from a third company. Whereas this controversy presently shows little sign of abating, it does not seem to have produced any good reasons to expect significant differences in quality between chemically equivalent generic and brand-name drugs on the U.S. market.

Even if one is able to convince the doctor to think generically, this accomplishment in itself is not neces-sarily sufficient to save money, for except in the relatively few states that have rigorous mandatory generic-drug laws, the pharmacist generally is under no obligation to fill prescriptions with low-priced brands or even moderately priced ones. Sometimes the pharmacy markup is based on a formula that involves a percentage of the drug's cost to the pharmacist; in such cases it is to the druggist's advantage to select a more expensive product. In addition, some pharmacies do not have the room or turnover rate to stock multiple varieties of every drug; instead they stock the most popular brands, which are usually also the most expensive. Again, the power to overcome these obstacles to saving money lies in the hands of the doctor, who can specify on the prescription the manufacturer of choice or, more practically, the cheapest version of the drug that the pharmacist stocks.

Checklist for saving money

Once in possession of a few facts concerning prescription drugs, the person who needs to visit the local druggist has a good chance of saving money. The suggestions given below should be of help.

1. Ask the doctor exactly what drug is being prescribed and what it is supposed to do.

2. Determine from the doctor (who actually may not know) or from an appropriate list (*see* list) if the drug is a brand name and if it is in the public domain (*i.e.,* if it is available under its generic name or other brand names).

3. Ask the doctor to prescribe generic drugs whenever possible and to specify the cheapest version stocked by the pharmacist. Remember that the permissive substitution laws on the books of many states do not require the pharmacist to dispense generic or low-cost brand-name drugs. If the doctor refuses to write generic prescriptions, try to find out if he or she has a sensible reason.

4. If the prescribed drug is to be taken for a long period of time (*e.g.,* blood-pressure medicine), have the doctor request enough of the drug for that duration. The cost per dose drops as the purchased quantity of drug increases.

5. Compare the prices asked by different pharmacies for filling the same prescription. Cost of a drug to the pharmacist and the pharmacist's markup can vary significantly. Some large chain-store pharmacies keep a price list of common drugs at the counter for customer inspection.

6. Determine if a generic-drug law exists in your state. Many such laws require that the customer be informed of a substitution, and some in effect give the customer a chance to veto the pharmacist's decision in favor of another brand.

—Charles M. Cegielski

Are You What You Eat?

"Know thyself," said the philosopher, so perhaps you ought to examine what you know about what you eat. That stuff in the refrigerator today may be the you of tomorrow.

1. Meat contains certain vital amino acids not found in vegetable matter—true or false?

2. Natural vitamins and synthetic vitamins are exactly the same and are of equal value to the body—true or false?

3. Eating carrots will improve your ability to see at night—true or false?

4. Vitamins as a class are distinguished from other chemical compounds required in the diet by (a) the amount required, (b) their complex structure, (c) their solubility in fatty acids, (d) the way in which they are utilized by the body.

5. Which of the following elements is not required for the health of the human body? (a) zinc, (b) copper, (c) cobalt, (d) antimony, (e) phosphorus, (f) molybdenum.

6. If you could maintain your adult body at complete rest for 24 hours, your caloric expenditure for that period would be approximately (a) 0, (b) 500, (c) 1,000, (d) 1,500, (e) 2,000.

7. An average man in a sedentary occupation who is not notably active in his free time will use over and above the basic caloric requirement about (a) 400, (b) 800, (c) 1,200, (d) 1,500, (e) 2,000 calories.

8. Which of these diseases does not result from a deficiency of some dietary requirement? (a) rickets, (b) kwashiorkor, (c) dengue, (d) sprue, (e) scurvy, (f) marasmus.

9. Kwashiorkor results from a deficiency of (a) vitamin B_6, (b) biotin, (c) manganese, (d) protein, (e) starch, (f) chloride.

10. The normal adult requires about (a) 100, (b) 50, (c) 10, (d) 1, (e) 0 grams of sugar in the daily diet.

11. Fats of certain sorts are required in the normal diet—true or false?

12. Milk is a perfect food—true or false?

13. Fiber is thought to be important in the diet because it (a) speeds the movement of food through the intestines, (b) is easily digested, (c) prevents the

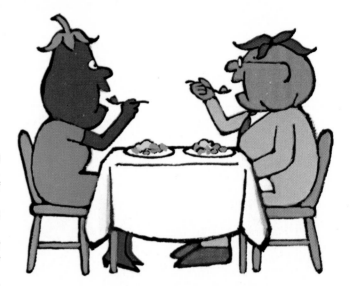

growth of bacteria in the intestines, (d) promotes the mixing of digestive enzymes with food.

14. A breakfast of four ounces of orange juice, two scrambled eggs, two strips of bacon, a slice of white toast with butter and jelly, and an eight-ounce glass of milk provides the body with about (a) 100, (b) 300, (c) 500, (d) 700, (e) 900 calories.

15. Alcoholic beverages contain no nutrients—true or false?

16. Cholesterol has been causally linked to heart disease and atherosclerosis—true or false?

17. If you were to avoid all foods containing cholesterol, you would still have a measurable serum cholesterol level—true or false?

18. Fats contain the most calories per unit weight, followed by carbohydrates and then proteins—true or false?

19. Large doses of certain vitamins beyond dietary requirements can be of particular value in preventing disease and promoting general health and vigor—true or false?

20. The commonest nutritional disorder in the United States is (a) iron-deficiency anemia, (b) goiter, (c) protein deficiency, (d) overweight, (e) alcoholism, (f) diabetes.

21. Beyond simple reduction of caloric intake, special diets such as those requiring periodic fasting, the consumption of large amounts of water, or the nearly exclusive eating of citrus fruits can be especially effective for weight loss in certain persons—true or false?

22. It is possible to eat too much protein—true or false?

Answers

1. False. All the amino acids needed by the body for protein synthesis can be obtained from a well-chosen combination of vegetables.

2. True. They are chemically and physiologically indistinguishable.

3. True. Night (or dim-light) vision depends on the presence in the retina of the eye of a pigment called rhodopsin, or "visual purple." The body manufactures this pigment and requires vitamin A to do so. Carrots contain no vitamin A (no vegetable does), but they do contain large amounts of a pigment called beta carotene, which the body can convert to vitamin A. So, if you are suffering from impaired night vision due to vitamin A deficiency, carrots can cure you.

4. (a). Vitamins are required in amounts on the order of a thousand to ten thousand times smaller than those required of other substances such as the amino acids.

5. (d).

6. (d). It would take that much energy to keep you breathing, your heart beating, your organs functioning, your cells metabolizing, and your muscles in their normal state of slight contraction. Any voluntary movement would add to that basic minimum.

7. (b). It doesn't leave much leeway for those rich desserts, does it?

8. (c).

9. (d).

10. (e). There is no dietary requirement at all for sugar. Sugar is a pure source of calories, which can be obtained from virtually any food, and contains no other nutritive value.

11. True. Fats are broken down in digestion into their constituent fatty acids. These acids play various roles in the body's metabolism, many of them not yet well understood. Fatty acids also help transport the fat-soluble vitamins (A, D, E, and K) through the body. The essential fatty acids are derived principally from the unsaturated fats of vegetable rather than animal origin.

12. False. If by "perfect" is meant that milk alone can sustain life. It does contain large amounts of several vitamins and minerals but by no means all that are necessary. Moreover, for some adults drinking milk can produce discomfort, indigestion, and, in those with particular sensitivity, even severe illness.

13. (a). The theory, yet unproved, rests on the observations that certain population groups who suffer practically no bowel cancer or related diseases have diets high in fiber and that food passes through their alimentary tracts nearly twice as fast as it does in populations with diets like that of the United States.

14. (d). The caloric intake is 55 for the juice, 220 eggs, 100 bacon, 60 bread plus 50 butter and 55 jelly, and 160 milk.

15. False. Beer, for example, contains a small amount of protein, calcium, phosphorus, riboflavin, and niacin and traces of other nutrients in addition to the caloric value of carbohydrate and alcohol. Wines are of similar composition. Distilled spirits, on the other hand, contain only calories.

16. False. High levels of cholesterol circulating in blood serum have been associated statistically with those conditions, but no causal link has been established. Some recent studies have suggested that even the statistical correlation is properly to the ratio of various types of lipoproteins, which are substances that link chemically with cholesterol to allow it to circulate.

17. True. Cholesterol is synthesized in minute quantities in all body cells and in significant quantities by the liver. The less cholesterol taken in from the diet, the more is produced in the liver.

18. False. Fats are first, at an average of 9.3 calories per gram but protein (5.4) actually outheats carbohydrates (4.1). These are "heats of combustion" as measured in a calorimeter. The caloric values actually available to the body are approximately 9, 4, and 4.

19. Unknown. Such claims have been made, as by Linus Pauling for vitamin C and by others for vitamin E, but the evidence that has been offered in support is disputed or ambiguous. In particular, vitamin E, while apparently a dietary necessity, has not yet been associated with any deficiency disease or condition; little is known of its action in normal quantities.

20. (d).

21. False. Keeping down the calories is the essential task, closely followed by exercise to use them up. Bizarre and faddish diets are likely to fall short in supplying other essential nutrients.

22. True. Excess protein, above what the body actually requires at the moment, cannot be stored and thus must be excreted. The nitrogen in protein is the main problem and can tax the ability of the kidneys to filter it out of the blood. Persons with potential kidney problems are especially susceptible to trouble. Moreover, in the average American diet protein is more often than not accompanied by fat, as in meats and dairy products, and too much of the one thus means too much of the other as well. Nutritionists recommend that protein comprise only 10 or 15% of the daily caloric allowance.

— Robert McHenry

Overweight Children

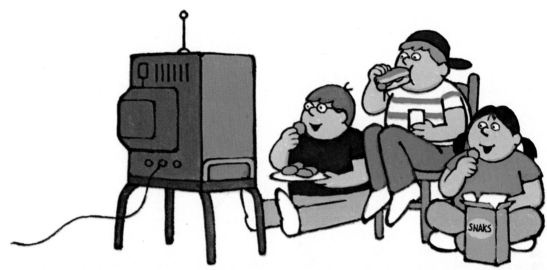

Obesity in the United States has reached epidemic proportions. It is estimated that well over 20% of our population—over 70 million people—are overweight. According to the National Center for Health Statistics the prevalence of obesity continues to increase. Sen. Edward Kennedy, speaking before the Senate Select Committee on Nutrition and Human Needs, called obesity "America's number one health defect." Said Kennedy, "While children of West Africa melt away from starvation, America stands in ironic contrast as a land of overindulged and excessively fat. In many ways, the well-being of the overfed is as threatened as that of the undernourished."

Adult obesity: a problem that begins in childhood

Most practicing pediatricians can vouch for the fact that the problem of obesity begins early in life: too many of our infants and children are being overfed and underexercised and started on the road to a lifetime of fighting obesity and its many dangers. It is safe to say that at least 20% of all the children in the U.S. are overweight. What's more, the great majority of these obese children grow up and remain fat all their lives. Further, it is clear that the longer a child stays fat, the greater the risk of his remaining obese.

Early-onset obesity (the obesity that begins in childhood) is much more difficult to treat than late-onset obesity (the obesity that starts in adulthood). In addition to the problem of the tremendous increase in the numbers of fat cells, the obese child faces the psychologically damaging problems of distortion of body image, devaluation of self, and impaired interpersonal adjustment. Persons with late-onset obesity have not been shown to manifest this combination of traits.

The treatment of adult obesity is extremely difficult and, too frequently, unsuccessful. Moreover, the relapse rate in overweight adults who *are* successful in reducing is well over 90%. According to C. S. Chlouverakis, director of the Obesity and Lipid Abnormalities Service at the E. J. Meyer Memorial Hospital in Buffalo, N.Y., "Only 25% of grossly overweight persons are able to lose as much as 25 pounds and 5%, 40 pounds." Routine treatment for 100 obese patients in the Buffalo obesity clinic was even less successful: only 12% were able to lose 20 pounds, and only one patient lost 40 pounds. Two years later only two patients had maintained their weight loss.

Such dismal statistics make it clear that the best solution to the obesity problem is to start with our children—to ensure that they are thin from the beginning so that they will have a good chance of remaining thin the rest of their lives.

What's so bad about being fat? As far as adults are concerned the answer is obvious: obesity shortens life, and it leads to a much higher incidence of such serious problems as heart attacks, high blood pressure, strokes, kidney disorders, diabetes, and arthritis. In addition, the adult who is markedly obese has a greater incidence of cirrhosis of the liver and of serious orthopedic problems.

Special complications of childhood obesity

As far as childhood obesity is concerned, many parents and grandparents and some professionals still

333

mistakenly believe that fat babies are healthier, but just the opposite is true. There is an extremely high correlation between childhood obesity and the incidence of many medical problems. Children who are markedly overweight suffer more consistently from respiratory illnesses than thin children. It has been shown that overweight children have a higher incidence of high blood pressure than thin children. Because fat children are more likely to consume large amounts of sugary snack foods, they are excellent candidates for tooth and gum problems. Studies have shown that the fat child also suffers more accidents. The reason is not too hard to see when one considers that they make larger targets, are less coordinated, and simply can't move as fast as their thinner peers. In school athletic programs the fat child has a higher incidence of injuries.

The dangers of childhood obesity do not end with physical problems. The psychological and social difficulties of the obese schoolager and adolescent are obvious. Fat youngsters are rarely popular with their peers; they are viewed as "different." And frequently their behavior sets them apart because they can't keep up with more active and athletic playmates. Too, obese children manifest personality traits very similar to those of minorities and other groups subjected to prejudice. These traits include withdrawal, depression, and being overly concerned about status. The overweight adolescent is especially vulnerable. At the time when he or she should be building self-confidence and self-es-

teem—when the body is changing, emotions are in turmoil, and both boys and girls are highly conscious of the opposite sex—to be overweight is often a tragedy.

It is an unfortunate but certain fact that society discriminates against the fat. A study showed that prejudice against the obese cuts the chance of college acceptance in half. Finally, there are economic hazards associated with obesity. For any employment, all other things being equal, a thin person will almost always be chosen over a heavy person, because most people associate fatness with ill-health, lack of self-discipline, and even lack of ability.

The greatest single danger of childhood obesity is that it is a precursor of adult obesity. The intractable nature of childhood obesity, combined with the very serious physical and psychological problems that are associated with it, make it clear that *prevention* is the best answer.

Preventing obesity

A child becomes fat due to a number of different factors, usually in combination. Before the 1950s obesity was thought to be caused in most instances by an endocrine disorder. We now know that childhood obesity is rarely due to a hormonal imbalance. The so-called sluggish metabolism or sluggish thyroid that was blamed for the extra pounds has now been shown to be almost nonexistent. In the experience of most pediatricians who treat childhood obesity, endocrine

The overweight child is more vulnerable to both physical and psychological ills. The best solution to the problems of obesity is prevention— to ensure that children are thin from the beginning so that they have a good chance of being thin for the rest of their lives.

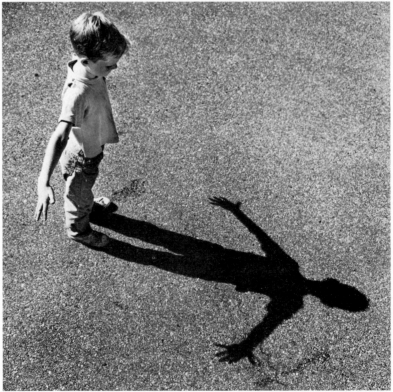

dysfunction is rarely seen. A parent can be almost 100% certain that obesity is *not* the result of an endocrine disorder if a child is overweight but of a normal height for his or her age.

The consensus at the present time is that there are four main factors leading to obesity in children: (1) heredity, (2) increased numbers of fat cells, (3) improper eating patterns, and (4) lack of exercise.

We cannot do anything about our genes, but we certainly can attack the problems of fat cell multiplication, improper eating habits, and lack of exercise. The successful treatment of childhood obesity must be based on establishing proper nutritional habits in our youngsters and creating a climate for increased exercise and activity.

Heredity. It has been known for many years that fat runs in families. Studies have demonstrated that 80% of the children born of two obese parents will become fat. When both parents are thin, there is only a 10% chance of that child's having a problem with extra pounds. These statistics demonstrate that a family history of obesity places some children at increased risk of becoming overweight. Thus if such children eat too much of the wrong foods and exercise too little, they are more likely to get fat.

Although statistics concerning familial obesity are rather cut and dried, we do not know what produces this tendency. One theory is that the regulatory center for appetite located in the hypothalamus of the brain may be genetically set higher or lower in different people. Genes may determine the way in which a person absorbs, digests, and excretes food. Body build passed down from parent to child also plays a part in determining whether a child will be fat or thin or inbetween. A small group of the population are *ectomorphs*—people who have relatively small bodies, long legs and arms, and long tapered fingers. Those in this group usually have small appetites, and no matter how much they eat they are not likely to have a weight problem. On the other side of the scale are *endomorphs*, who generally appear to be shorter, rounder, and softer, with shorter arms and legs, and often have considerable difficulty in maintaining normal weight. A *mesomorph* falls in between. Jules Hirsch, a pioneer in the field of childhood obesity, has found that the ectomorphic infant is relatively protected against obesity. But in our society, given the quantity of foods and constant barrage of eating stimuli, a certain percentage of endomorphs and mesomorphs become obese.

While inherited tendencies to be overweight are certainly important, no child must become fat. Even a confirmed endomorph with two fat parents and a hearty appetite need not be overweight. If that child's parents are aware of the inheritance factor right from the start, and if they concentrate earlier and harder on the problem of prevention, the child will have an excellent chance of growing up thin and healthy.

Fat cells. It has been demonstrated that the longer a growing child is fat, the greater the number of fat cells that child accumulates. There are critical periods when the too-rapid multiplication of fat cells occurs—during the first two years of life and during the adolescent stage of rapid growth. It has been shown that the total number of fat cells can never be reduced. After growth has been completed, a person can reduce his fat cells in size by losing weight but can never reduce them in number. However, we do not know why increased numbers of fat cells predispose a person to obesity. Whatever the reason, the results are clear. An individual who has been fat throughout childhood ends up with tremendous numbers of extra fat cells, and this individual finds it much more difficult to maintain normal weight. With these facts in mind, parents must make every effort to raise a thin child who will not accumulate extra numbers of fat cells. If the child is already fat, the earlier the child's weight is reduced, the fewer fat cells he will end up with as an adult.

Eating habits. Though the issue of infant nutrition is a complicated one, subject to great debate, there is evidence that breast-fed babies are less likely to develop into obese children than bottle-fed babies. This may be because breast-feeding mothers are less frantic than bottle-feeding mothers about introducing solid foods, which add calories that are not required nutritionally. Also, bottle-feeding mothers tend to be more concerned about amounts, *i.e.,* making sure the infant consumes a certain number of ounces of formula, while breast-feeding mothers do not measure the amount of milk a child takes in but rather stop feeding when the baby seems satisfied, a more natural situation. For these and other reasons breast-feeding is considered the ideal way to feed an infant.

Whether breast- or bottle-fed, it is important that the child not be started on cow's milk, which has too much salt and protein, until at least six months of age. This measure, too, seems to help prevent obesity. The Committee on Nutrition of the American Academy of Pediatrics recommends that a child stay on breast milk or formula for the first year of life.

Far too many of our children grow up never having learned how to eat properly. Overstuffed from the moment they are born, they not only get fat but are often poorly nourished despite the large amounts of food they consume. Added to the modern habit of eating too much for our energy needs is the growing emphasis on the wrong foods. So-called junk foods seem to be the order of the day; *i.e.,* high calorie, nonnutritious foods. This trend is aided and abetted by the advertising industry, whose commercials during children's television programs promote junk foods. A nutritionist monitored 29 hours of network children's television programs for a week and found that 82% of the commercials featured "antinutrition" foods. On the other hand, it is

335

quite rare to see commercials for apples or carrots.

Unfortunately, because we lead busy lives, it is becoming more difficult for families to eat meals together. Many of us grab a quick breakfast, high in sugar content, such as a doughnut or Danish. Lunches are grabbed at school or work or are often skipped altogether or replaced by a series of snacks. Dinners may be eaten as a family, but even these meals are becoming rare events in many households. What is more, they too often consist of convenience foods with dubious nutritional values. In between these so-called mealtimes, there is continuous snacking. It has been estimated that between 30 and 50% of all the calories we consume are taken as snack foods.

Since prevention of childhood obesity rests with the parents, it is crucial that a child be taught proper nutrition, despite outside pressures. Junk foods must be eliminated from the house, and the child must be served three well-balanced, nutritious meals each day. Fruits and vegetables should take the place of candy and soda. Children learn by example, so parents must take the lead.

Exercise. There is no question that lack of exercise is one of the main reasons for the epidemic of obesity in our children. Food *does* put on pounds but only if the calories taken in are not expended in activity. There must be a balance of calorie intake and energy output to keep weight stable. If a child eats more food than he requires to keep his body going, he will gain weight, and if he eats less, he will lose. Nutritionist Jean Mayer has stated that "probably no single factor is more frequently responsible for the development of obesity than lack of physical exercise." Studies have shown that the majority of fat adolescents actually eat less than the average nonobese adolescent of the same sex. The inactivity easily accounts for the calories that permit excessive fat deposition. Hilde Bruch has studied overweight children extensively and noted that out of 160 obese youngsters studied, 76% of boys and 88% of girls were almost totally inactive. Ruth L. Huenemann, of the University of California School of Public Health, says, "The problem is not eating too much, rather, it is eating too much for the energy expended. The generally low level of physical activity that appears to be characteristic of American youth and the consequent low caloric need make increased activity an essential part of the regimen in our obesity prevention and control."

The problem of inactivity versus weight gain begins early in life. In our society, from the time babies are born they are protected from exertion—pushed around in strollers, confined in playpens, and driven around in cars. With increasingly overcrowded urban areas, growing street traffic, fewer play areas, and less open space, parents often must make "appointments" for their children to play with each other. This "play" too often consists of sitting in front of the television set munching cookies and pretzels.

Parents must make every effort to encourage exercise and physical activity. Children must be taught to participate in athletics from an early age because exercise habits, like eating habits, are hard to change. A child who does not move much will undoubtedly turn into an inactive adolescent and then a sedentary adult. Making exercise a family affair right from the beginning is extremely useful. Bicycle riding, ice skating, skiing, bowling, hiking, and swimming are all excellent activities for the entire family. Children should be encouraged to become proficient at a sport, because once they do, they are more likely to enjoy and continue the activity. Thus sports that can be continued all one's life are excellent. While team sports such as football, hockey, and baseball are all fine exercise, it is not always easy to organize a team. Sports that don't require great numbers, such as bicycle riding, swimming, Ping-Pong, and tennis, have obvious advantages.

Losing weight

While "fat proofing" is the key to preventing childhood obesity, what if a child is *already* overweight? The earlier an overweight youngster's weight is brought down to normal, the better off he or she will be. Appetite suppressants, injections, and hormones such as thyroid can be dangerous and contraindicated in children; besides, they generally do not work. Crash or fad diets should never be used. It is dangerous for a growing child to lose weight too rapidly. The overweight youngster and the parents should see a physician in order to map out a plan to slowly get rid of the extra fat. The doctor will probably provide a specific diet. Meals must be tailored to meet the individual needs of each child; for example, a growing adolescent requires more calories than a two-year old. However, certain guidelines may be followed for all overweight children over two years of age. These are: (1) cutting down on rich desserts, (2) using skim milk, (3) reducing starches, (4) serving poultry, veal, and fish more often than the red meats, and (5) eliminating added sugar to foods such as cereals and beverages.

With rare exceptions a child should never lose more than one to two pounds per week. Dieting should be a slow and steady process. A little simple arithmetic will demonstrate how easy it is to lose one pound each week: 3,500 calories equals one pound of fat. Therefore, a 500-calorie reduction each day will do the trick ($500 \times 7 = 3,500$). The 500 eliminated calories per day may be handled by eating 250 fewer calories and burning up 250 extra calories by exercise. Simply by eliminating five chocolate chip cookies a day and riding a bicycle for 30 minutes, a child can lose a pound in a week. By eliminating the available junk foods in the house and by encouraging increased, daily physical activity, the child can readily achieve the goal.

—*Alvin N. Eden, M.D.*

Juvenile Diabetes

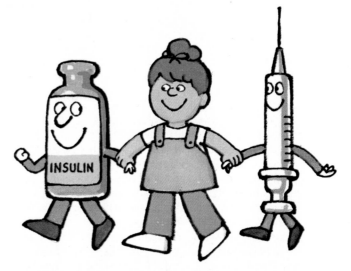

Juvenile diabetes mellitus is the most common endocrine disease of children. It is estimated that between 100,000 and 150,000 children in the United States are diabetics. Put another way, one out of every 1,000 to 2,000 school-age children has this illness. Out of the entire population suffering from diabetes mellitus, 5% are children; 4% of all diabetics experience onset before 15 years of age. A child can develop diabetes at any age, although rarely seen during infancy, it most commonly affects children 10 to 12 years of age.

Characteristics of juvenile diabetes

Diabetes is a chronic disorder of energy metabolism resulting from a deficiency or total lack of insulin. Insulin, a hormone manufactured by the beta cells of the pancreas, primarily affects carbohydrate metabolism. Its main action is to keep blood sugar levels within the normal range. Without enough insulin production in the pancreas, the diabetic's blood sugar rises to dangerously high levels, interfering with proper biochemical functions in the body.

The cause of juvenile diabetes mellitus is unknown. Whereas maturity or adult-onset diabetes often is related to obesity, this is not the case in children. There is a genetic factor involved, but most children with diabetes do not have a family history of the illness. Identical-twin studies do point to some genetic component to the condition, since it has been shown that if one identical twin has diabetes, there is a 50–70% chance that the other identical twin will also become a diabetic, whereas the incidence of diabetes in fraternal twins is only 2%.

Diabetes usually involves four stages of development: (1) prediabetes; (2) suspected diabetes; (3) chemical, or latent, diabetes; (4) overt diabetes. This classification is useful in managing maturity-onset, or adult, diabetes, but in children the progression through these four stages is so rapid that for all practical purposes the diagnosis is made and treatment begun in the fourth stage, the stage of actual or overt diabetes.

The onset of juvenile diabetes mellitus is rapid and abrupt. The symptoms usually last just a few days or at most a few weeks before the child reaches the state of a diabetic coma. The most important signs and symptoms are polyuria (frequent urination) and polydipsia (excessive thirst).

Polyuria is frequently the symptom that first is noticed and brought to a physician's attention. The child starts to urinate much more frequently than before, and is often brought to the doctor because of enuresis, or bedwetting, which suddenly starts after he has previously been dry at night. Others signs of diabetes are weight loss, weakness, and irritability. If the disease is not diagnosed and if treatment is not begun during this phase, the diabetic child rapidly goes into diabetic acidosis. Diabetic acidosis is characterized by abdominal pain, vomiting, rapid and deep breathing, and signs of dehydration. The child's eyes become sunken and the skin becomes very dry. There is a sweet-smelling acetone odor to the breath, and if immediate treatment is not instituted, the child lapses into unconsciousness and coma. Unfortunately, too many children are not diagnosed until they are rushed to the hospital in a diabetic coma. Most commonly affected are children under two years of age.

The presence of juvenile diabetes mellitus should be suspected when a child shows the symptoms just described. A definite diagnosis can easily be established by an examination of the urine and the blood. The urine will contain large amounts of sugar and acetone, and the blood sugar level will be very high.

Treatment and management

Once the diagnosis of diabetes is made, most authorities believe that it is best to hospitalize the child for treatment and for educational purposes. If the illness is managed properly and there is sufficient cooperation between the physician, parents, and child, this should be the only hospitalization the child will ever require for the illness. The treatment of juvenile diabetes must be aimed at the day-to-day prevention and control of symptoms and at the prevention, if possible, of later vascular complications, the major cause of difficulty for the diabetic. The three major areas of treatment are: insulin, diet, and patient and parent education.

Insulin. Before the discovery of insulin just over 50 years ago, there was no effective treatment for the diabetic child. However, with the advent of insulin, the treatment and prognosis have been dramatically improved. All children with diabetes require the use of insulin given by injection. The diabetic child must take an insulin injection every day for the rest of his life. The oral hypoglycemic agents (drugs used to lower the blood sugar) that are useful for the treatment of diabetes in some adults are not effective in the management of juvenile diabetes. Further, the adult diabetic can at times be treated by diet alone, but this does not hold true for the child. The juvenile diabetic requires the use of insulin, which acts to lower his blood sugar level and which controls and prevents the effects of the disease. There are several types of insulin, some of which are short acting and others longer acting in controlling the blood sugar level. The child's physician will determine which type of insulin or insulins is most effective and will also calculate the proper dose. The sites of the daily injections should be rotated. The older child can easily be taught to administer his own injections, while the very young diabetic needs to be given the insulin shots by a parent.

The daily dose of insulin must be adjusted, depending on the amount of sugar that the child excretes in his urine. It is therefore important that urine specimens are routinely checked for sugar four times each day. This should be done before breakfast, before lunch, before dinner, and before bedtime. A school-age child can easily be taught to check his own urine by means of a sugar dipstick. Parents must remember that infection raises the sugar levels and will require increased amounts of insulin. If a child who previously has been well regulated with a specific number of units of insulin suddenly starts excreting large amounts of sugar in his urine, it is likely that he is coming down with some sort of infection, and his physician should be notified.

The main complication of administering insulin is the possible development of hypoglycemia (a low blood sugar level). If the child is given too large an amount of insulin, his blood sugar level will be lowered too much and he will enter a hypoglycemic state. It is most important for parents and the child to be taught to recognize this possibility. The main symptoms of a hypoglycemic reaction are increased sweating, dizziness, weakness, blurred vision, and rapid breathing. If this is allowed to progress too far, the child may become disoriented, have seizures, and lapse into a coma. When the diabetic child begins to show the early signs of hypoglycemia, he should simply consume some readily assimilated sugar—drink a glass of sweetened orange juice or eat a piece of candy—and his symptoms will immediately be relieved.

Diet. There are many schools of thought concerning the precise diet for the juvenile diabetic. A well-balanced, nutritious diet that maintains normal growth and prevents obesity is what is required. This diet, tailored to meet the individual needs of the child, should consist of three meals plus two snacks, one snack after school and the other before bed. It is obviously important to restrict cake, candy, and other sources of excess sugar. It is also wise to follow a "prudent" diet, one that is low in saturated fats and cholesterol: skim milk, no more than three to four eggs per week, and fish, fowl, and veal more often than red meats. "Diabetic" foods should be avoided except for occasional low-calorie soft drinks. A general rule that can be a useful starting point is a daily intake of 1,000 calories plus 100 calories per year of age; *i.e.,* a four-year-old diabetic can be

Special camps for diabetic children allow youngsters to participate in this important childhood experience. Diet and medication are carefully controlled, and the child learns that despite his disease, he can live a normal life. Here a child maintains the daily check of his urine for sugar content.

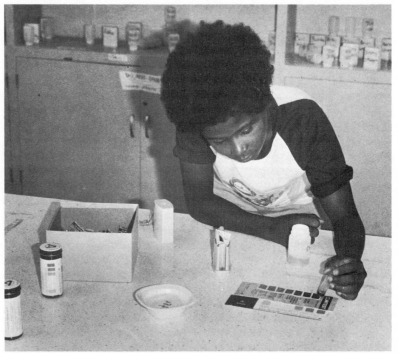

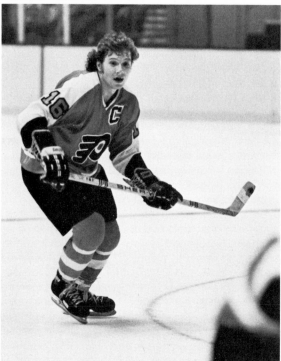

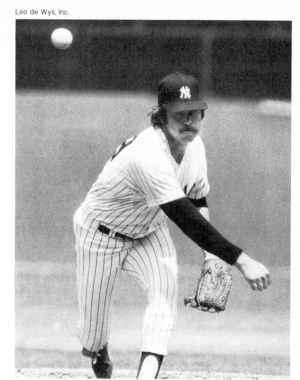

The diagnosis of juvenile diabetes need not restrict a child's activities. Bobby Clarke (left) and Catfish Hunter are diabetics who have reached the top ranks of major-league sports.

put on a 1,400-calorie-a-day diet. However, as mentioned previously the diet must be altered for each child. A diet that is carefully calculated but that results in the child's always being hungry and likely to cheat on what he eats is obviously not serving its intended purpose and must be adjusted.

Patient and parent education. Education is an extremely important part of the overall management of juvenile diabetes. Both the parents and the older child must be stimulated to learn more about diabetes through reading and through group teaching conferences. The child must be motivated to follow the program his physician has mapped out. Fears concerning the disease must be allayed, and emotional support must be provided.

After the diagnosis is made, the parents and the child often are shocked, bewildered, depressed, and frightened. The biggest task to be faced is to be able to accept the condition and with it the fact that it will require lifelong care. It is important to try to create a positive, optimistic attitude. Most diabetic children will accept the few limitations imposed on their lives once they realize that they will feel healthy and will be able to continue their previous activities. Unfortunately, many parents do not react with such equanimity. Often extra strain is put on the family structure, with one parent blaming the other for refusing to take on some of the responsibilities for the child's care.

It has been shown that emotions can affect the blood sugar level and that severe emotional trauma can trigger an attack of diabetic acidosis. "Problem" diabetic children who require repeated hospital admissions because of poor control are usually those who have not been able to adjust to the realities of their disease. It is essential for the well-being of the child that the physician help the parents make the adjustment by compassion and understanding as well as through education.

Living with diabetes

The diabetic child should not be restricted in any way as far as his physical activity is concerned. On the contrary, he or she must be encouraged to participate in all manner of sports and athletics. Adequate physical exercise is helpful not only in terms of psychological implications but because insufficient exercise is one of the factors that raises blood sugar levels and alters insulin requirements. Diabetics have become famous and successful athletes—hockey player Bobby Clarke and pitcher Catfish Hunter are two examples—and children with diabetes should be told about them.

There is one situation that tends to separate the diabetic child from his nondiabetic friends: summer camp programs. Unfortunately, most ordinary children's camps will not enroll diabetic children, declining to take responsibility for special diets, insulin injections, and possible hypoglycemic reactions. To fill this need special camps for diabetic children have been established in both the United States and Canada. The benefits of the camping experience are many. Association with other diabetic children, exposure to good medical and dietary care, the opportunity to learn more about the illness, and the chance to become more self-sufficient are all important reasons for a child to attend one of these camps. Camps are well supervised by competent nurses, physicians, and dietitians. They are listed with both the American and Canadian diabetic associations.

The prognosis of juvenile diabetes mellitus is related primarily to the major complication of this disease—vascular disease. Good control of the blood sugar level is said to improve the long-term prognosis, probably slowing the development of blood vessel complications. The consensus among diabetic specialists is that good blood sugar control is important for overall prognosis. The small blood vessels throughout the body are gradually affected by diabetes, especially the vessels of the eyes and the kidneys. It takes from 15 to 20 years after the onset of diabetes for these changes to begin to develop. Another vascular complication of diabetes is arteriosclerosis (hardening of the arteries), which starts at an earlier age in the diabetic than in the general population. This is an additional reason for using a prudent, low-cholesterol, low-saturated-fat diet, which helps to slow down the arteriosclerotic progress. Although the average life expectancy of the juvenile diabetic is lower than the nondiabetic of the same age, there are many exceptions. Because of good medical management, more and more juvenile diabetics are now growing into adulthood without evidence of significant vascular damage. However, it is true that the earlier the child develops diabetes, the more time he will have to develop vascular complications; and so, on the average, the prognosis is less favorable than if diabetes had begun at a later age.

Until very recently there have been few basic changes in the management of juvenile diabetes. But in 1973 an experiment with inbred rats reported actually curing diabetes by means of transplantation of pancreatic material. Since then, other investigators using animals have confirmed this remarkable accomplishment. It is much too early to determine whether transplantation will be applicable to children. Tissue rejection is the big problem that must first be overcome in order to begin research with human patients, but if the pancreatic transplantation technique turns out to be successful, the whole field of diabetes medicine will be dramatically changed. Rather than just being able to control this illness by means of insulin and diet, it may become possible to actually cure diabetes, and, in so doing, to prevent the diabetic process from progressing to the late vascular complications. This hope for the future is yet another reason to keep the diabetic child as healthy as possible and to approach the problem of juvenile diabetes with hope and optimism.

There are many childhood diseases that are more serious and life-threatening than diabetes mellitus. With proper management, a child with diabetes should be able to achieve a full, productive, and satisfying life. If handled properly, the juvenile diabetic will be able to function as a perfectly normal child.

—*Alvin N. Eden, M.D.*

Emphysema

Emphysema can be a devastating disease that devitalizes its victims. The disease is particularly unfortunate because, in most instances, it is preventable. Only when emphysema is recognized early, however, is it treatable or reversible.

With a better understanding of the causes of emphysema and with a greater commitment to its prevention, the disease could be virtually eliminated. On the other hand, few diseases demand as much dedication by doctors and cooperation by patients for effective treatment.

The process of breathing

The functioning of every organ of the body and of every cell within each organ depends on a constant supply of oxygen. Without oxygen, cells fail, organs degenerate and stop functioning, and the body eventually dies.

The lungs are elastic organs that almost completely fill the chest cavity. From the moment of birth the lungs expand and contract like bellows to fill themselves with air. The diaphragm, which separates the chest cavity from the abdominal cavity, is a powerful muscle that keeps the lungs functioning. Other muscles of the chest wall are used during inspiration or expiration of air. When air is inhaled through the mouth and nose, it passes through the pharynx, larynx, trachea, and bronchial tubes to the lungs. The bronchial tree, so-called because it resembles an upside-down tree, branches into two large bronchial tubes. These tubes divide again and again, ending at their tips in millions of alveoli, or air sacs. In the walls of the alveoli are tiny capillaries, the smallest of all of the blood vessels, which extract oxygen from the inhaled air. Through the pumping action of the heart the oxygen is distributed through the arteries to every part of the body. At the same time, carbon dioxide, a waste product in the blood, is exchanged in the air sacs and exhaled through the lungs.

This life-giving process is repeated more than 5,000 times a day throughout life. That it continues without interruption is one of the wonders of the human body. It is estimated that the body needs about a pint of oxygen every minute throughout life for the organs to function normally.

With exercise the body's demand for oxygen increases enormously. If the lungs and the heart are in good health, there is enough reserve within them to furnish the additional oxygen that the body needs during activity. The heart beats more rapidly, the lungs expand more frequently, and the exchange of oxygen and carbon dioxide increases in the alveoli.

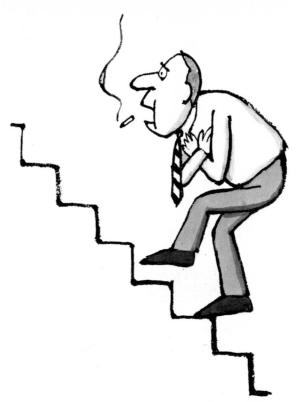

If the lungs are affected by disease that destroys the pulmonary reserve, the breathing process becomes impaired, and the supply of oxygen to the entire body is reduced. Severe pressure is imposed on the heart and other organs to compensate for the lungs' decreased ability to carry on their function.

The disease and its symptoms

Emphysema is a disease of the lungs that seriously affects the entire breathing process. The word is Greek in origin and means "overexpanded." One of the most serious effects of emphysema is the loss of the elasticity and the overinflation of the lungs. Even after taking a deep breath, a person with emphysema can only incompletely fill his lungs with fresh air and has difficulty emptying them of their accumulated carbon dioxide. The air sacs also become overinflated and lose their elasticity. These changes in the lungs interfere with the exchange of oxygen and carbon dioxide.

When air is trapped in the lungs, the chest fills out to become what is described as a "barrel chest." (For an as yet unexplained reason, with emphysema and other chronic lung diseases the nails of the fingers become clubbed, thickened, and markedly enlarged.) Shortness of breath, the inability to walk even a short distance without severe strain, and a bluish discoloration of the lips are other symptoms of respiratory distress caused by emphysema.

Causes of emphysema

Repeated bouts of bronchitis, pneumonia, asthma, and other respiratory infections—as well as inhalation of industrial fumes, polluted air, and tobacco smoke—are

341

the major causes of emphysema. Any persistent cough should have its origin determined. Neglecting such a cough increases the possibility of developing emphysema. When the cause of a cough is determined, it must be eradicated with intensive treatment. If emphysema is detected in its earliest stage, it can frequently be prevented from developing further.

Of all the controllable causes of emphysema, the greatest single factor is smoking. A person with bronchitis or any other lung or heart disorder who also smokes is greatly increasing the risk of destroying his health. Cigarette smoking, particularly, is associated with a shortened life expectancy. It is estimated that 300,000 Americans die prematurely each year from diseases, including emphysema, directly related to smoking.

Tobacco smoke contains chemicals, tars, nicotine, and carbon monoxide that create a particular burden on the air sacs of the lungs, where they interfere with the exchange of oxygen and carbon dioxide. The repeated inhalation of pollutants in the air, fumes from factories, and substances like silica, asbestos, and other irritants has much the same effect. Lungs already weakened by exposure to such irritants are more likely to develop emphysema.

Diagnosis of emphysema

If emphysema is suspected by a doctor, tests can be performed to substantiate the diagnosis. Pulmonary function departments in hospitals use complex electronic measuring equipment for such tests. Normal readings are compared with readings for patients with chronic bronchitis, asthma, and emphysema in order to give an accurate indication of the individual person's respiratory capability.

Pulmonary function tests can establish the resiliency and the elasticity of the lungs. Blood and breathing studies can determine how well oxygen and carbon dioxide are being exchanged in the alveoli. The respirometer determines how much oxygen the body needs at rest and during activity. The spirometer is used to determine the capacity of the lungs. A full assessment of the lungs' capacity and their limitations helps establish a treatment program for the patient.

Treatment of emphysema

The most important restriction for the person with emphysema is to refrain from smoking. The patient must also make an effort not to spend time in smoke-filled rooms and must guard against exposure to dust, fumes, and air pollutants.

There are additional methods of treatment for sufferers of emphysema. Antibiotics and medical detergent inhalations help to liquefy the thick mucus secretions that develop in the lungs. Oxygen can be administered to compensate for the oxygen deficit caused by the disease. Cortisone and bronchodilating drugs are sometimes effective. Postural and breathing exercises and postitive-pressure breathing techniques can alleviate some of the distress of emphysema and can help to reduce obstructions in the lungs caused by the accumulation of secretions.

Comprehensive programs for respiratory care and rehabilitation can also markedly improve the life of a person afflicted with emphysema. A positive program can help a person live at home and often return to his job, but the treatment program must often involve an entire family. Only when the family as well as the patient understand the disease, its cause, and its control can they learn to cope with the illness and to establish realistic goals toward recovery.

Rehabilitation teams offer comprehensive programs that include the services of doctors, nurses, respiratory therapists, physical therapists, vocational counselors, and psychiatric consultants. Such programs try to help the patient function in dignity within the limits of his capacity. The ultimate goal of rehabilitation teams is to restore the individual to the fullest possible physical, emotional, social, and economic potential.

Prevention of emphysema

As preventive medicine has become increasingly urgent, smoking has become a major health issue. Smoking is a serious hazard to health that causes a great deal of unnecessary disease. Not only is smoking a major cause of emphysema, bronchitis, and other respiratory disease but it also is a major contributing factor to heart disease and to cancer of the lungs, mouth, and bladder.

More effective ways to prevent people from starting to smoke must be developed. Likewise, more effective methods to help smokers stop the habit must be found. The government must make a firm commitment to controlling air pollution and to protecting the health of industrial workers. Through such preventive measures the incidence of many diseases, including emphysema, could be significantly reduced.

— Lester L. Coleman, M.D.

Contraception: The Choices

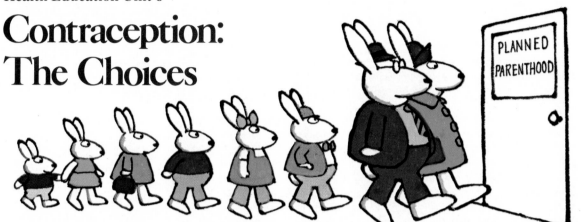

Much progress has been made in the last two decades in developing new and more effective forms of birth control, and current research promises even more efficient methods of contraception. The improvements of the last decade made in the Pill, the contraceptive "miracle" of the 1960s, have recently been somewhat offset by the growing evidence of the occasional serious, and even potentially fatal, side effects of Pill use. As these dangers become known, an increasing number of women are looking to other methods of contraception. This is presently seen in a revival of interest in the diaphragm but more strikingly in the growing number of men and women who are electing contraceptive sterilization.

Currently available methods of birth control, however, offer myriad effective choices that are briefly explored below. Ineffective or very unreliable methods of contraception, such as douching and withdrawal (coitus interruptus), have not been included. The failure rates for each method are reported in terms of the theoretical effectiveness rate (that achieved if the method is always used perfectly) and the use-effectiveness rate (the pregnancy rate occurring among an average population of users).

Sterilization

For many couples who are sure that they want no more children, sterilization offers a permanent method of contraception. Sterilization is a surgical procedure that can be performed on both men and women and a method of birth control that now rivals the use of birth control pills among married couples. A sure method of contraception, requiring no attention or effort prior to intercourse, sterilization procedures have become both easier and safer in recent years.

There are now several sterilization techniques for women, the most prevalent being the tubal ligation, or tying of the tubes. In a tubal ligation the fallopian tubes, where the ovum descending to the uterus is fertilized

by the sperm, are cut and tied back or cauterized to prevent the union of egg and sperm. The female continues to ovulate and menstruate, but the ovum is logistically prevented from uniting with the sperm. Current techniques include the laparoscopy and laparotomy, in which the tubes are tied through an abdominal incision, and the less frequent culdoscopy and colpotomy, in which the surgeon works through an incision in the back of the vagina.

Sterilization for men, called a vasectomy, involves the cutting and tying off of the ends of the vas deferens, the tubes through which sperm is carried from the testes to the penis. The production of sperm continues, but the sperm, blocked in the testes, are simply reabsorbed into the body. The man continues to ejaculate during intercourse, but the semen contains no sperm; thus impregnation is impossible. A simple, brief procedure usually done in a doctor's office or a clinic, a vasectomy must be followed up to test the man's sperm count. Until the sperm count is nil, another method of contraception must be used during intercourse to insure against pregnancy.

Neither sterilization operation affects hormone production, male or female characteristics, sex drive, or orgasm. There may be some temporary soreness or pain after the operation, and there is a slight chance of developing swelling, bleeding, or infection.

Couples should decide upon sterilization only after very careful consideration, as this method of birth control should be regarded as permanent. There has been, nonetheless, considerable progress in procedures to reverse sterilization. While these developments are encouraging, the choice of sterilization as a method of birth control should still be considered irreversible.

Failure rate. Method failures: less than 1 per 100 men or women a year. User failures: none.

Disadvantages. While reversals are not impossible, sterilization must be considered irreversible.

Advantages. Completely effective; no need to use

temporary methods of birth control (*except* for the brief period after vasectomy until semen no longer contains sperm).

Oral contraceptives—"the Pill"

Oral contraceptives, or birth control pills, are pills taken in a series that contain synthetic female hormones similar to the natural hormones that regulate a woman's menstrual cycle. The most widely used birth control pill, the "combination pill," combines the hormones estrogen and progestin (synthetic progesterone) and prevents pregnancy by suppressing ovulation. The progestin-only pill (also called the "mini-pill") does not affect ovulation but rather alters the uterine lining and cervical mucus and is hence not as reliable as the combination pill. While it is not entirely known how this progestin-only pill works, it is thought that the uterine and cervical changes tend to inhibit the sperm's entry into the uterus, its penetration of the egg, and, failing that, the implantation of the fertilized egg in the uterine wall. The sequential pill, which uses estrogen alone and consequently introduces many more risks and side effects than the other two types of pills, is far less effective and was recently ordered off the market by the Food and Drug Administration (FDA).

While the Pill is obviously a highly effective means of birth control, there is continuing controversy over the risks and side effects incurred by Pill users. The growing body of evidence shows that Pill users run increased risks of circulatory problems—among them, blood clots, stroke, and heart attack—and may run a higher risk than nonusers of certain types of cancer.

The recently released results of a nine-year study in Great Britain indicated that in general women who use oral contraceptives run a 40% higher chance of a Pill-related death than women who have never used the Pill. Among the particular findings, the study correlated increased risk of death with increased length of time on the Pill and with the increased age of the Pill user. As well, it was found that the Pill user who smokes is three times more likely to die from a heart attack than her nonsmoking counterpart.

The Pill's lesser side effects may include weight gain, nausea, swollen breasts, spotting, headaches, depression, and disposition to vaginitis and urinary tract infections. Often these problems disappear after a few months on the Pill. If they persist, a switch to a "low-dose" brand of pills (*i.e.,* with less estrogen) may be helpful. Adverse reactions such as severe headaches, loss of vision, sudden chest, arm, or leg pains, or shortness of breath should be reported to a doctor immediately. All women on the Pill should routinely have an annual physical examination with a Pap smear.

Because of the dangers associated with the Pill, some women should never use it. These include women with circulatory problems (excess blood clotting or a history of stroke or heart attack), hepatitis or other liver disease, cancer of the breast or other reproductive organs, cystic fibrosis, sickle-cell anemia, and those who are nursing infants or who are pregnant. Women with other health problems are cautioned against using the Pill; these include women with diabetes or prediabetes, epilepsy, asthma, high blood pressure or mild varicose veins, cardiac or renal disease, uterine fibromyomas, chloasma, sickle-cell trait, extreme weight problem, and those who are heavy smokers or who are over 35 years old.

Since the effects of long-term Pill use are not yet known, there is concern about the length of time a woman should take oral contraceptives. Some doctors recommend a three-month halt in Pill use every two to three years, while other physicians approve continuous Pill use for up to ten years.

There is no consensus about the effects of oral contraceptives on conception after Pill use is stopped. Most women are able to conceive normally, while others may be rendered temporarily or permanently infertile or may experience a high rate of miscarriages.

Failure rate. Method failures: less than 1 (combination) and 2 to 3 (mini-pill) per 100 women a year. User failures: 2 to 4 per 100 women a year.

Disadvantages. Not for use by women with certain health problems; entails increased risk of minor and major circulatory problems and may be related to certain types of cancer; may produce uncomfortable side effects such as weight gain, nausea, swollen breasts, headaches, and depression.

Advantages. The most effective temporary method of birth control; convenient to use; may reduce premenstrual cramps and tension as well as the menstrual flow itself; may reduce iron-deficiency anemia.

IUD (intrauterine device)

The IUD is a small piece of shaped material (generally plastic) that is inserted into the uterus; threads attached to the IUD extend through the cervix into the vagina to help in checking the placement of the device. While it is not known exactly how the IUD prevents pregnancy, the presence of a foreign body (the IUD) in the uterus seems to create a uterine condition unfavorable to pregnancy. After the woman's body adjusts to an IUD, she does not need to prepare for intercourse, although she is advised to use spermicidal foam or cream at midcycle to further increase protection. It is also recommended that she check monthly for the IUD's threads to ensure its correct positioning.

Insertion of the IUD by a physician may be painful, as the uterus must be stretched to accommodate the device. Cramping and bleeding during and after insertion are common, and the body may altogether expel the IUD. The discomfort encountered during insertion usually subsides within several days, but some women report consistently more pronounced premenstrual cramping and backaches.

Even if successfully inserted, the IUD may later be expelled by the body. This usually occurs in the first three months and often during menstrual flow, sometimes without the woman's knowledge. Hence, a frequent check for the IUD's strings is advisable. In rare instances the uterus or the abdominal wall may be perforated by the IUD, requiring surgical removal of the device.

Some women have difficulty using the IUD, particularly those who have never been pregnant. For these women the possibility of expelling the device is high, and new, smaller types of IUD's using copper wire and slowly released doses of the hormone progesterone have been developed to accommodate this problem. Some women should not use the IUD. Women who have any of the following conditions are included in this category: pregnancy, endometriosis, venereal disease, vaginal or uterine infection, an extremely small uterus, bleeding between periods, large fibroids, uterine deformities, use of anticoagulants, cardiac disease, anemia, or sickle-cell disease.

Once inserted, the IUD can be left in place for years, provided no complications arise. With the new copper and progesterone IUD's, more frequent replacement is necessary, the former requiring replacement about every five years and the latter every year.

While the IUD is a highly effective method of birth control, it is nonetheless possible to become pregnant —frequently a tubal pregnancy—while wearing an IUD. Miscarriage is very likely, but the fetus can be carried to term without harm from the IUD. It is nevertheless advisable that the IUD be removed, if possible, to reduce the possibility of miscarriage or infection.

Failure rate. Method failures: 2 to 4 per 100 women a year. User failures: none.

Disadvantages. Slightly increased risk of pelvic infection; risk of rare but possible perforation of the uterine or abdominal wall; may cause severe cramping upon insertion and continually severe monthly cramping with periods; expulsion rate high among women who have never been pregnant.

Advantages. No procedures required prior to intercourse; cannot be felt by either partner; is reversible.

Diaphragm

The diaphragm is a shallow rubber cup with a round rim that fits securely in the vagina to cover a woman's cervix, preventing access of the sperm to the cervical canal. The diaphragm must *always* be used with contraceptive cream or jelly. When properly positioned, a diaphragm blocks the entrance to the womb and the spermicidal cream inactivates any sperm that may slip past the rim of the diaphragm.

The diaphragm is an entirely safe and, if correctly and consistently used, generally reliable method of birth control. There are no side effects from the use of the diaphragm, although a particular brand of spermi-

cidal jelly or cream may prove irritating to the woman or her partner. In this case a simple change of brands can eliminate the problem.

Women with a severely displaced uterus, whose bladder protrudes through the vaginal wall, or with other openings (fistulas) in the vagina are unable to use the diaphragm. For those who can use this form of birth control, a pelvic examination is required to determine the correct diaphragm size for each woman. When getting fitted for the diaphragm for the first time, a woman should ask her physician for complete instructions on how to properly prepare and insert the diaphragm. After childbirth, abortion, pelvic surgery, or after a weight gain or loss of 15 lb, the diaphragm size will need to be changed.

In general a diaphragm, properly cleaned after use, should last for several years. Nonetheless, the diaphragm should be periodically checked for tears by holding it up to the light and by filling it with water and watching for leaks.

The diaphragm can be put in up to six hours before intercourse, but each time sex is repeated, more jelly or cream must be inserted in the vagina (without removing the diaphragm). The diaphragm must be left in place for six hours after sex, and douching must be avoided during this time period.

Failure rate. Method failures: 2 to 4 per 100 women a year. User failures: 10 to 20 per 100 women a year.

Disadvantages. Requires insertion prior to intercourse; may become dislodged in woman-superior position or in women with a relaxed vagina resulting from childbirth; a new size is required if weight is gained or lost, or following pregnancy, abortion, or pelvic surgery; some women find the discharge of jelly unpleasant.

Advantages. No side effects; effective, if properly and consistently used; usually not felt by either partner.

Condom

The condom, the oldest of the barrier methods, is a sheath of thin rubber or animal tissue, shaped like the finger of a glove, that covers the man's penis during intercourse. At climax a man's semen is caught inside the condom so sperm cannot enter the woman's uterus. Because condoms act as barriers, they also offer considerable protection against sexually transmitted disease. A few men and women are allergic to rubber; switching to animal tissue sheaths may solve the problem. The latter also transmits heat better, which may help a man who feels that a condom dulls sensation.

Failure rate. Method failures: 2 to 4 per 100 women a year. User failures: 10 to 20 per 100 women a year.

Disadvantages. Requires putting on prior to climax; care is needed to prevent slipping off or tearing; sometimes criticized for decreasing sensation.

Advantages. Easily obtainable, inexpensive, convenient method of birth control; requires no medical supervision; offers protection against venereal disease.

Contraceptive foam, jellies, or suppositories

This barrier method of contraception, containing a sperm-killing chemical, is deposited in the vagina by means of a plunger applicator so that it covers the cervix. The contraceptive spreads into the vaginal and cervical crevices, forming a barrier to prevent sperm from entering the uterus. Contact with the chemical ingredient inactivates the sperm. The foam appears also to offer some protection against contracting venereal diseases.

One or two applications of foam are inserted very shortly before *each* intercourse. The foam must then be left in place for six to eight hours after intercourse, and douching must be avoided for this same period of time. Combining foam with use of the IUD, condom, or periodic abstinence increases effectiveness of these other methods.

Failure rate. Method failures: 2 to 4 per 100 women a year. User failures: 15 per 100 women a year.

Disadvantages. Must be applied prior to intercourse; leakage is sometimes a problem; may irritate vagina or penis; rare instances of allergic reactions.

Advantages. Does not require a medical examination or prescription; easy to insert; no side effects; may help to prevent contracting venereal disease.

Periodic abstinence — "natural" birth control

The "natural" method of birth control is a contraceptive system by which a woman abstains from intercourse just before, during, and after her period of ovulation, the time at which she is fertile and hence most likely to conceive. For women whose menstrual periods are very regular, the period of ovulation can be fairly readily determined: about 14 days before the start of the next expected period. For women whose periods are irregular or for those who are careless about keeping track of their menstrual cycles, this method is likely to be very unreliable.

For those who are committed to natural birth control, several systems can be used for keeping a careful record of the menstrual cycle. Two or all three systems used in combination are more effective than one used alone.

The calendar system consists of keeping records of the date each flow starts and the length of time between periods. Using the number of days in the shortest and longest cycles, a woman can calculate the earliest date and the latest date she is likely to be fertile in her next menstrual cycle.

The so-called temperature system is more reliable, but longer abstinence is required. A woman takes her body temperature (with a special thermometer) each morning before getting out of bed. A rather small but sharp rise occurs when the ovum is released. After three days at the higher temperature level, the unsafe period should be past.

Another method, the vaginal mucus system, is based on detecting the changes in a woman's vaginal moisture. Normally cloudy and tacky, mucus will become clear and slippery and stretch between the fingers when the ovum is released.

Failure rate. Method failures: 5 to 10 per 100 women a year. User failures: 20 to 30 per 100 women a year.

Disadvantages. Unreliable if periods are irregular; even regular periods and normal temperatures can be affected by fatigue, emotional stress, or just a cold; requires expert instruction and consistent care for success; the periodic abstinence may be frustrating.

Advantages. Acceptable to those whose convictions prohibit other methods of birth control.

Abortion

Abortion is the termination of a pregnancy by medical means. Although abortion is legal and safe in most of the world, there is considerable controversy surrounding the moral issues of abortion, and it is not always readily available. Abortion is generally not considered a preferable method of birth control; it should be considered an alternative for dealing with pregnancy rather than a means of preventing it.

For abortion within the first three months, vacuum aspiration is the best and most widespread method. For later abortions other techniques, such as saline or prostaglandin instillation or evacuation, are used. The risk of serious complications or death is very low for legal abortions performed within the first three months but rises slightly as the pregnancy advances. The mortality rate for legal abortion is approximately 1.5 deaths per 100,000 early (first trimester) abortions. Women should be carefully counseled about all options with regard to an unwanted pregnancy, and the final decision as to a course of action must be made by the woman. A medical history, a physical examination, and appropriate laboratory testing must be performed. This should include an Rh blood factor test so that women with Rh-negative blood may receive a gamma globulin solution to protect them against sensitization to this factor that could adversely affect the outcome of future pregnancies. The procedure in the first three months is often performed under local anesthesia, and the woman is able to go home within a few hours. Abortions in the second trimester usually require a hospital stay. There are no data that prove whether multiple abortions have an adverse effect on future fertility. But women who have an abortion are usually highly motivated to adopt an effective method of birth control.

— Christine Timmons and
Louise B. Tyrer, M.D.

Shouldn't You Be Jogging?

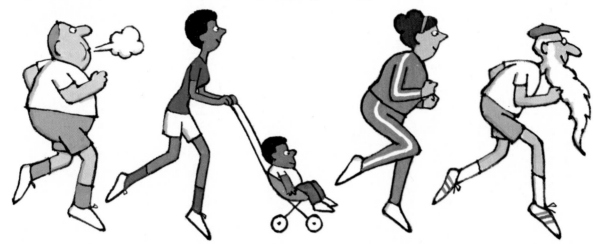

Suddenly it seems everyone is jogging. What is it with these people running in the parks and the streets at all hours? If you think you know, try answering these questions.

1. Most normal people are already in pretty good physical condition and don't need to make a point of exercising—true or false?

2. A regular program of weekend tennis or golf (no cart) can produce and maintain an adequate level of physical fitness—true or false?

3. Among the possible consequences of a long-term avoidance of conditioning exercise are (a) overweight, (b) atherosclerosis, (c) sluggishness and susceptibility to fatigue, (d) coronary heart disease, (e) loss of vital capacity in the lungs.

4. Jogging is just another exercise fad—true or false?

5. Adequate substitutes for jogging as conditioning exercise include (a) swimming, (b) calisthenics, (c) isometrics, (d) weight lifting, (e) bicycling.

6. Jogging on a regular basis can prevent heart attacks—true or false?

7. The essential quality of jogging that distinguishes it from calisthenics and other exercises is (a) the muscular effort required, (b) the equipment involved, (c) the rhythmic impact effect, (d) the demand for oxygen it generates.

8. Jogging can have damaging effects by loosening certain skeletal joints and displacing internal organs—true or false?

9. Jogging is equally beneficial to men and women—true or false?

10. Since women have far fewer heart attacks than men, they require less conditioning exercise—true or false?

11. On the average, jogging is an appropriate conditioning exercise up to the age of (a) 40, (b) 50, (c) 60, (d) 70.

12. No medical supervision is required for jogging—true or false?

13. Suppose that you, an experienced jogger weighing in at 160 lb, have just run two miles in the respectable time of 16 minutes, burning up a lot of energy. You can break even, calorie-wise, by allowing yourself (a) a cup of cottage cheese, (b) an eight-ounce sirloin steak, (c) a hot dog on a bun, (d) a piece of chocolate cake, (e) half a cheese pizza.

14. Now suppose that you run those two miles in 12 minutes, a very good pace indeed. How many more calories do you burn than at the slower pace? (a) 200, (b) 100, (c) 70, (d) 50, (e) 0.

15. A grassy area or cork track is better to jog on than a paved roadway—true or false?

16. Indoor jogging, with its more controlled conditions, is superior to outdoor—true or false?

17. The person who has already had a heart attack should avoid the stresses of jogging in favor of a regular program of light exercise—true or false?

18. Too much exercise can lead to an abnormally large "athletic heart"—true or false?

19. Children can safely take part in a regular jogging program—true or false?

20. In addition to conditioning the cardiovascular system, regular aerobic exercise like jogging can also (a) keep the muscular system toned, (b) reduce nervous tension and stress, (c) prevent arthritis, (d) cause new blood vessels to develop in muscles and heart, (e) increase the amount of blood in the body.

21. No special equipment is required for jogging—true or false?

Answers

1. False. For one example, Kenneth H. Cooper, Air Force surgeon and author of *Aerobics,* found that of a group of young recruits—all of whom had passed their induction physicals—65% rated from only fair to very poor on a simple test of physical endurance. The middle-aged population is even worse off.

2. False. Not even the most effective kind of exercise, which neither tennis nor golf is, can do much good if engaged in only once or twice a week.

3. All of them and more.

4. It does have its faddist aspects, but all we can hope is that, unlike other fads, it doesn't fade away in a matter of a few years, because this one is making us a healthier people.

5. (a) and (e). At best those others may build nice-looking muscles, but they won't do a thing for the cardiovascular system, which is what keeps us alive. Even walking would be better.

6. Evidence in medical questions involving cause and effect is usually more statistical than physical and almost always tentative to some degree, but the answer here is a cautious true: the achievement of a high level of fitness can prevent some, if not all, heart attacks.

7. (d). The prolonged controlled high demand for oxygen produced by "aerobic" exercises like jogging is the principal mechanism by which they produce improvement in fitness.

8. The claim has been made, but as yet no medical evidence has appeared in scientific literature. It may well be the inevitable reaction to the faddish aspects of jogging.

9. True. Were you expecting a trick question?

10. False. Beyond the other benefits to be derived from jogging, women ought to remember that their relative immunity against heart attack largely disappears after menopause.

11. No upper limit has been established. Experienced and fit joggers come in all ages, up to the redoubtable Larry Lewis of San Francisco, who ran six miles a day even after he was over 100 years of age. (He died at 106.)

12. The beginning jogger should assess his physical condition and, if 35 or older, should have a doctor do so as well. If all is well, no supervision should be necessary. A clinical history of heart disease, high blood pressure, diabetes, or certain other conditions calls for medical advice and consent before undertaking any program of exercise and probably continued monitoring thereafter.

13. (a) or (c), each at about 200 calories, which is what you burned up. (If you weigh 120, count only 165.) Those other temptations put you behind with 880 (steak), 445 (cake), and 740 (pizza) calories.

14. (e). Speed has very little effect on the rate of energy consumption. The principal determinant is weight.

15. False. You can jog safely on virtually any firm and reasonably smooth surface. The grass may even hide hazardous bumps and dips in the ground.

16. False. Mainly it's a matter of personal taste. Many prefer to jog in all weather and to be entertained by the passing scene; others do not. Some find an indoor track, often quite small, a boring place to spend an hour; others do not.

17. This used to be common advice, but evidence is rapidly accumulating that endurance training by jogging is highly beneficial to many heart patients. Strict medical supervision is required, of course. In 1973 seven heart attack victims, three of whom had had two attacks, finished the 26.2-mile Boston Marathon under the care of Terence Kavanagh of the Toronto Rehabilitation Centre.

18. True. However, there is no evidence that the larger than average hearts of many athletes are in any way unhealthy. The "enlarged heart" characteristic of some clinical conditions is entirely unrelated to the well-developed muscle that is the fit heart.

19. True. For most children, on the other hand, there is no particular reason that they should. If they have enough energy left over from their own normally vigorous activities to join in a family jog, fine. They shouldn't be pushed into training for the marathon, however.

20. (a), (b), (d), (e), and possibly (c).

21. Mainly true. But if you're going to do it regularly, proper shoes are a must. Striped shoes in primary colors may not be your idea of fashion, but why not look like an athlete two or three hours a week?

—Robert McHenry

The Importance of Fathering

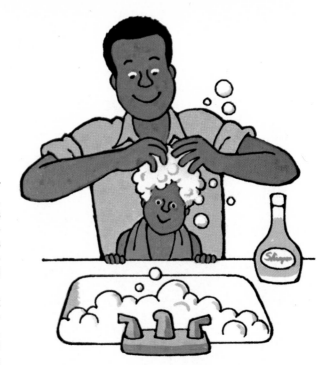

Until recently the importance of the role of the father in child development has been underestimated; rather, the focus has been on the mother-infant relationship as unique and vastly more important than any other relationship in the child's world. The mother typically takes on the role of primary caretaker, and so the first effective bond is presumed to develop from this continued association.

Recent studies, however, have demonstrated that the amount of time the infant and mother spend together is a poor predictor of the quality of their relationship. The best evidence for this is the fact that prolonged and extended daily separations from mothers such as by day-care attendance do not appear to disrupt the infant-mother attachment. It follows that there is no reason why the daily separations of the baby from a working father should be any more disruptive. The nature and quality of the interaction (whether with mother or father) are far more important. Just a few hours of happy interaction a day is much more conducive to the formation of strong, secure attachments than many, many hours of unstimulating interaction.

Many studies have shown that the interaction of infants with their fathers is mutually enjoyable and associated with highly positive emotions on both sides. The father's early involvement with his child is critical to the formation of a strong, lasting infant-father relationship. The concept that the father is outside the infant's social world must be put to rest.

Pregnancy and childbirth

Very often fathers-to-be feel left out during the mother's pregnancy. This factor sometimes sets in motion a pattern of noninvolvement. In our society a pregnant woman is a celebrity of sorts, and everybody fusses over her every twinge, ache, and pain. The mother-to-be proudly talks about "her" baby and probably unconsciously starts to believe that the new baby is her exclusive possession. Many a prospective father cannot help but resent the fuss and attention showered on his pregnant wife and "her" baby.

The fact is that we are all born with 46 chromosomes —23 from the mother and 23 from the father. The expectant father must remember that he is equally as important in the overall scheme of things. This approach will go a long way in minimizing the strain a pregnancy may place on the marriage. Further, parents adopting an "our" baby attitude will set the stage for

the father's positive, active participation in the upbringing of the child right from the start.

Pregnancy and childbirth should be important and exciting events for both parents. While society provides many supports for the mother as she adapts to her new role, as yet there are far too few such supports for the new father.

In recent years, however, more and more fathers have become active in the preparation for childbirth and now are even assisting in the birth itself. For example, many couples attend Lamaze classes together to prepare for the experience so that the father can encourage his wife throughout labor and delivery, which usually makes the process easier and less painful. This kind of participation means the father is not shut out, and there is immediate involvement of both parents with the newborn baby. The father is able to share the very special event with his wife, and fatherhood, appropriately, can begin at birth. Unfortunately, many hospitals still promote the belief that the father is superfluous and do not allow him to share in the birth or to interact with the baby during the first few days of life.

Sharing responsibility from the start

When the big day arrives and the new baby is brought home, many mothers feel that they are the only ones able to care for the infant. Again, much too often the new father is inadvertently left out. Too many of our children become overdependent on mother, and too many mothers become overprotective of their children.

Specialists in childhood development agree that the healthiest situation for the baby is to have the love and attention of both parents beginning on the first day of his or her life. The noted anthropologist Margaret Mead points out that infants naturally form attachments to

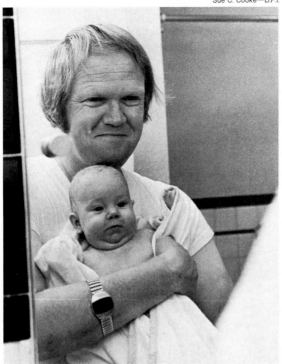

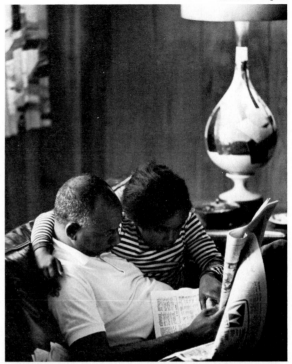

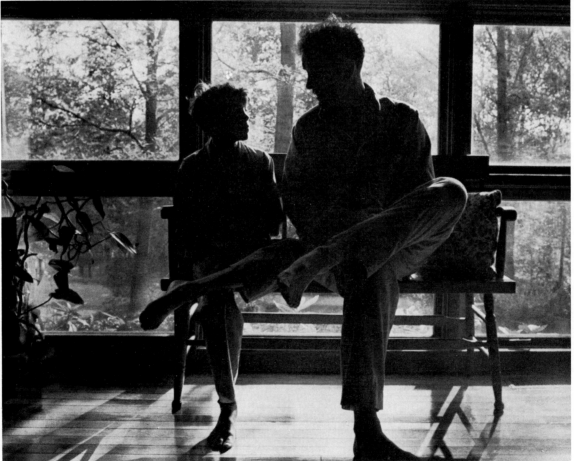

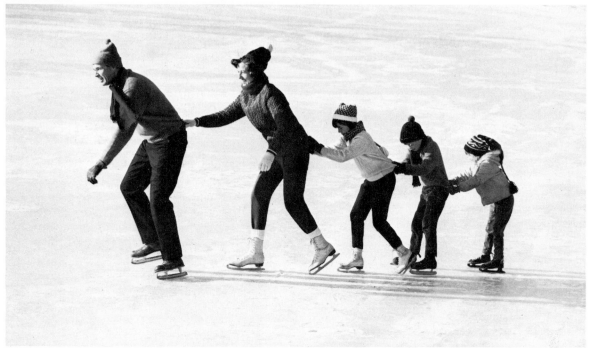

Every child needs the strength of a warm and nurturing relationship with both his parents. A father can participate in the preparations for childbirth, share in the care of the infant, and be a vital part of every aspect of his child's growing-up process. Strong father-child bonds are extremely important in the shaping of the child's personality and in his ability to form other healthy relationships.

more than one person—a phenomenon that has clear survival value since the child then has insurance against the loss of one parent. There is evidence that such babies grow up far more secure and self-reliant. Having both mother and father to relate to right from the beginning is unquestionably the ideal situation.

The arrival of the new baby drastically changes the ground rules at home. The baby's needs now come first. For the parents sleep is frequently interrupted, there is less privacy, and many more chores and tasks take away from their time together. Many mothers fall into the role of taking over the entire job. The result can be an overly tired and harried woman who devotes all her time to the new baby and who has no time or strength left for her husband—a situation that obviously can lead to marital stresses.

Many mothers complain that their husbands are no longer as attentive and loving as they were before the baby was born and that they are beginning to drift apart. Under the circumstances, this may be understandable. The father feels neglected and left out and unconsciously blames the new baby. Many a new father has confessed, "Had I known what our baby would do to our marriage, I would never have wanted to be a father." A marriage that was good before the pregnancy should not deteriorate because of the new baby. On the contrary, a new baby should further solidify and enhance the relationship. When the father feels

that he is as important as the mother in bringing up the infant and is very much needed for this purpose, all is well both for the marriage and for the child.

Given half a chance, most fathers will gladly involve themselves in the daily chores of infant rearing, feeding, bathing, changing diapers, and all the rest. And why not? There is nothing magical about handling a new baby. Nowhere has it been officially decreed that these tasks belong exclusively to the mother. The only clear exception, of course, is breast-feeding, but the father can certainly be involved in supplemental bottle feedings. Yet pediatricians frequently hear from anxious new fathers that they feel they are "in the way." On the contrary: their active involvement in all aspects of child care will help develop happy, secure, self-reliant children.

Unfortunate stereotypes

There is yet another factor that comes into play in determining what role the new father plays. Many among us have been indoctrinated to believe that it is somehow not manly for a father to feed or bathe his baby and, worse yet, to change the baby's diapers. This is utter nonsense. It is not manly for a father to abdicate his role and to just stand aside and watch. There is nothing unmasculine about loving and caring for and interacting with one's child. Indeed fathers should be partners, not spectators.

351

The importance of fathering

There is also nothing unmotherly about a woman wanting to pursue things other than raising her child. Even at the beginning caring for an infant can best be accomplished as a *cooperative* venture. For some couples detailed, well-planned schedules of assigned tasks work best. For others flexibility is the key. Obviously, sensible limits need to be set. For example, if the father comes home from work late at night and is exhausted and has to be up for an early morning appointment, he should not be expected to get up to take care of a 2 AM feeding. The important thing to strive for is active day-to-day involvement of both mother and father, in which the tasks are shared happily and equitably. This will pay large dividends as far as the emotional, moral, and intellectual development of the child is concerned.

An involved and competent father allows the mother to get out of the house and remain in touch with the outside world. While more mothers today are working, too many still spend month after month at home with their new baby. As a result the mother can completely lose touch with her other interests and activities, and this certainly is undesirable for all. Some fathers are even taking "paternity leaves" from their jobs to share infant care responsibilities.

The stereotyping of fathers solely as economic supporters of the family unit is far too common. This extraordinary prejudice can make it difficult for the young father to adjust to his new responsibility.

The "father figure"

Before a child reaches three years of age, the father typically acts as an occasional mother substitute and a source of emotional support for the mother. However, much recent evidence suggests that infants do form attachments to their fathers right from the start. It is gratifying to note that we are now starting to appreciate the importance of the father in terms of infant development. More and more fathers are making themselves accessible to their infants, enjoying interaction with them and becoming actively responsive to their signals. They, therefore, become important figures in the world of their babies—with their own special and distinct qualities—probably just as important as their wives, even though the father and infant may spend less time together. The infant who establishes close relationships with both parents has a tremendous advantage in the continuing process of socialization. A warm, caring, giving, involved man is the best kind of father figure a child can have.

There is no question that the warmth and quality of the father's relationship with his growing child, whether son or daughter, is crucial. The evidence is overwhelming that the establishment of satisfactory peer relationships is facilitated by the presence of an involved father. Nurturing and supportive fathers contribute greatly to the psychological adjustment of their children and improve the chances for the child to develop subsequent healthy relationships with other people.

There is a good deal of evidence suggesting that fathers exercise a strong influence—possibly more than the mother—over the child's intellectual development. Underachieving children often have inadequate relationships with their fathers, whom they regard as hostile or rejecting. Paternal encouragement is correlated with achievement. In general, a close father-child relationship in which the father is warm and democratic is associated with good performance in school and high academic achievement in both boys and girls. Studies have shown that "deprived" children with poor intellectual performance are often from homes where the father is absent.

Fathers also play an important role in the moral development of their children. In general, children who have the advantage of an involved and loving father (and mother) have a better chance of developing personalities that reflect generosity, altruism, and self-confidence. Children learn by example. "Delinquent" sons often come from homes where the father is antisocial. Statistics bear out the fact that a poor father-child relationship, even when there is an apparently normal mother-child relationship, is a common finding in the case histories of delinquents.

In recent years our family system has been subjected to great assault and strain. More and more marriages are ending in divorce, and so many children are being raised in single-parent families. There is good reason to believe that these children may be at greater risk of becoming poorly adjusted adults. Most studies suggest that father absence has its greatest impact on children when they are separated at a young age. Father absence can interfere with normal sex role development of the boy. In girls father absence has been reported to be associated with difficulties in relating to males later in life.

Within the family structure enduring relationships that are established very early are ideal. The father-child association is most successful when it is continuous rather than transient. Disruption, as in separation or divorce, may have adverse effects on the emotional development of the child. Nevertheless, many children are able to overcome the handicap of an absent father.

Though child raising is an imprecise art, all the evidence suggests that it is most successful and enjoyable when the job is shared by both mother and father within the context of a happy, secure marriage. There is no longer any question about the importance of the role of the father in infant and child development. However, thus far only a relatively small segment of our population perceives the father as playing as important a role as the mother. All children, including newborn infants, are entitled to the intimate loving care of *both* mother and father.

—*Alvin N. Eden, M.D.*

Fear

In a sense fear is a malignant disease. It is not caused by germs or viruses; yet it can be more destructive than physical illness itself. It is a disease transmitted from person to person, sometimes unwittingly, sometimes intentionally. It is one of the unfortunate side effects of the hectic, frenetic patterns of modern civilization.

There is no age, sex, or economic, cultural, or geographical group that is free from the emotional albatross of fear in this age of anxiety. Susceptibility to the disease is universal, and as yet there is no vaccine to immunize against it.

For many years doctors in all fields of medicine have been aware of and increasingly concerned with the number of patients who come to their offices overwhelmed by fears and anxiety. In most instances these patients' fears are disproportionate to the actual severity of the illnesses that brought them to their doctors. Yet so deeply ingrained are these fears that long after an illness is entirely cured, the patient still suffers the aftermaths of his or her unfounded anxiety. Doctors have noted that many people delay their intended visit by months, even years, for fear of substantiating their concern about an imagined, nonexistent disease.

The damaging effects of fear

Fear is everywhere. It is all-pervasive and flourishes with epidemic intensity. Slowly and insidiously it penetrates the physical, emotional, and spiritual fibers of man. Fear thrives on ignorance, weaving its snare gradually and subtly until one is caught in a web of confusion. To paraphrase Ralph Waldo Emerson, fear is a circle whose circumference is everywhere and whose center is nowhere. Fear can alter the destiny of people who allow themselves to be dominated by it. Fear plays havoc with professional and personal accomplishments.

Fear does not stand up to be counted. Rather its greatest potency lies in its being hidden. It therefore is not adequately charted in the diseases of man, although it ranks as one of the chief agents of demoralization and may often contribute to the onset and severity of disease.

Fear of all diseases as well as fear of cataclysmic destruction by atomic bomb and of economic upheaval all contribute to a never-ending bombardment against an individual and communal sense of inner security. This generation seems particularly plagued by anxiety and in fact seems to be tottering on the brink of destruction. Ironically, every generation has wanted to lay exclusive claim to this strange distinction, each insisting that theirs was the age of anxiety.

It is paradoxical that in this era of magnificent medi-

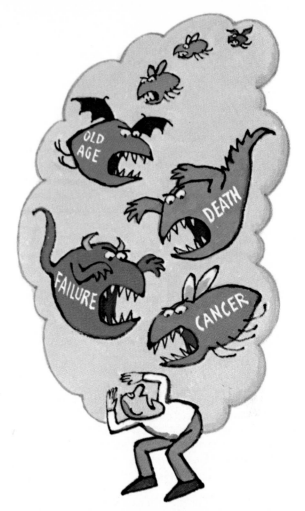

cal accomplishment so many people pass their lives in a slow and gradual death rather than living fully and with a sense of hope. That paradox is particularly poignant in light of these statistics: human life expectancy was 48 years at the turn of the century; by comparison, the male child born in 1980 will probably live to the age of 70, while the female child born in that year is expected to live to age 75.

Vaccination against poliomyelitis, tetanus, smallpox, whooping cough, diphtheria, measles, mumps, and rubella has saved the lives of many thousands of infants and children. Antibiotics have spared the lives of innumerable persons who might otherwise have succumbed to pneumonia, tuberculosis, mastoid disease, and other infections. The progress against some types of cancer and leukemia is encouraging. The strides in open-heart surgery, in dialysis for chronic kidney disorders, and in the control of diabetes and high blood pressure are all reasons for hope rather than fear.

In addition to being a disease, fear has also become big business. Medical publicity and propaganda—well-intentioned, but often ill-advised from a psychological point of view—have deluged the American people with statistics on death and devastation. Numerous health organizations, prompted by legitimate fund-raising needs, actually appeal to the public's fear with threatening exposés on the telltale symptoms of "their" particular disease. Widespread anxiety and fear should not be the aftermath of a fund-raising drive. Rather, health education for the public should be a carefully planned program, designed to teach but not frighten. Yet we are all familiar with the detailed catalog of symptoms and with the terrifying "one-out-of-five-will-get" warnings that dramatize our health drives. If we were to believe all the distorted, fear-provoking statistics with which we are assaulted, we might imagine our destiny in the following fashion:

By 1982 one out of 5 persons would be dying of cancer, while one out of 20 would be in a mental institution. These hospital patients would be visited from time to time by their children with cerebral palsy and rheumatic heart disease, their cousin with muscular dystrophy, their niece with multiple sclerosis, and their sister recovering from a stroke. This, of course, could occur only if they were fortunate enough to have escaped the combined effects of heart disease, tuberculosis, arthritis, and tobacco—*and* if they had not been previously killed in Fourth of July or Memorial Day accidents.

While this anxious vision of our individual fate in the very near future may seem ludicrous to many, there are nonetheless numerous people for whom this is a credible prediction. Therefore, it is not strange that doctors' patients reveal to them daily patterns of behavior directed by anxiety over physical ills. They follow a definite routine. They examine their tongues, check for redness in their eyes, and look for bleeding gums. The women feel for lumps in their breasts. The urine is intently inspected for cloudiness and unusual color, and excretions are carefully examined to be sure that they resemble "normal" feces. Some people even take their pulse rate, and finally at breakfast they turn to the obituary columns to check the ages of the recently deceased. This behavior sounds preposterous, yet there are thousands of people who follow similar routines with religious fervor, hoping that their existence can proceed uninterrupted for another day.

Fear versus anxiety

Although fear and anxiety seem to be identical, they are in reality significantly different. Fear is not always unfounded and irrational. Fear can be the body's reaction to anything threatening. It can in fact be an appropriate response to certain real-life situations, actually serving as a protective mechanism. When one is threatened by fire or by an oncoming automobile, fear physiologically triggers the mobilization of forces for self-protection. Motivated by fear, the body responds by pouring adrenaline into the bloodstream, rapidly increasing the heart rate, stimulating all the senses to become more acute, and causing the muscles to flex in anticipation of flight or self-defense.

Anxiety, however, is a vague, agonizing, diffused sense of apprehension. It is intangible and bewildering because it is unrelated to any specific threat and is characterized by an all-encompassing feeling of danger from an unknown source. So undefined is the threat that there is an inability to cope with it or run away from it. Anxiety has an ally in helplessness.

Each person must learn to function in his world despite the gnawings of fears and anxieties. Each age has held its terrors and uncertainties, which seem to be an inevitable part of the human condition.

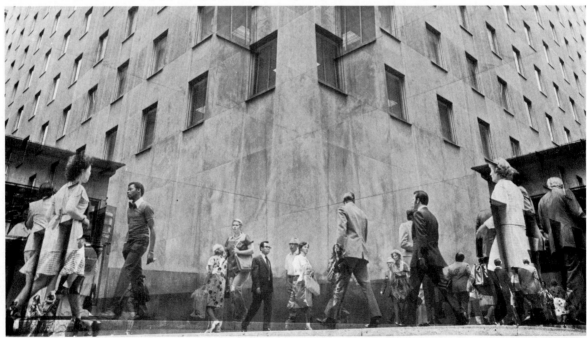

George Malave—Stock, Boston

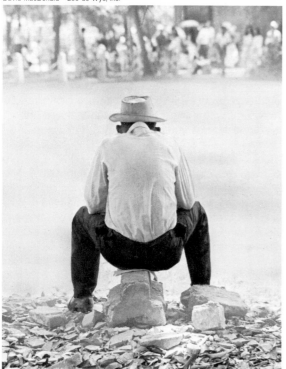

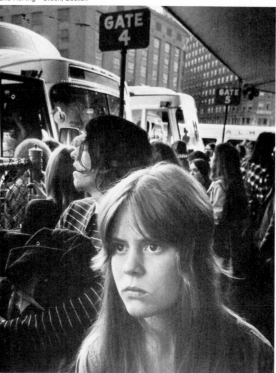

The fears plaguing the young may be different from those of the elderly, but they can be no less incapacitating. Anxiety becomes a danger rather than a valuable warning when it paralyzes the will and interferes with the ability to make decisions and to act.

Although distinct by strict definition, fear and anxiety both work their destruction by the incessant bombardment of the helpless. Fear and anxiety are interwoven into the entire fabric of life; no aspect of our daily existence is free from one or the other. To live is to have problems, and in turn to have problems means the need to make decisions. The ability to make decisions and to live with these decisions depends on freedom from fear and anxiety, particularly freedom from the powerfully destructive fear of the unknown.

Illness and fear

It is estimated that approximately one-third of all patients seen by doctors have no definite bodily, or somatic, disease to account for their ailments. Another third of all patients are estimated to have symptoms that are in part dependent upon emotional factors, which significantly add to the disability and prolongation of illness. The remaining third of all patients are those with diseases of a predominantly somatic nature that may or may not have an underlying basis in psychic disturbance. There is a general consensus among doctors that in each of the three classifications of disease, fear and anxiety play a significant role.

There is no longer any speculation regarding the relationship between emotional experiences and the functioning of the body (soma). It is now an accepted fact that the relationship between the psyche and the soma is a concrete factor in the understanding of all disease. The body and the mind are not two entirely separate, autonomous entities but are rather a closely intertwined unity. This psychosomatic relationship plays an important role in the understanding of all disease and markedly determines the effectiveness of treatment and the ultimate recovery from illness.

When a person has had a heart attack and has ostensibly recovered, the electrocardiogram is often used as an index of that recovery. For a person recovering from pneumonia, an X-ray of the chest is used as a criterion of recovery. Although the electrocardiogram and the X-ray indicate recovery from the *physical* aspect of disease, they are not necessarily a measure of *total* recovery. There is only one yardstick that is the true index of complete recovery: the patient's ability to resume his or her role in the home, at work, and in society as a functioning, productive human being.

Many patients who seem to have recovered from heart disease, for example, live in the constant fear of another heart attack. They may predicate their total behavior on the unfounded fear of an inevitable recurrence rather than accepting their real return to good health. Some persons who have recovered from a heart attack go back to work for only a few hours a day, returning home in the midafternoon. The rest of the day

355

and evening is spent pampering themselves, resting in bed, and in general playing the role of the chronic invalid. As the weeks go by, their unrealistic fears remain undiminished, and in essence they are still cardiac invalids despite normal electrocardiograms and physical evidence of complete recovery.

The real criterion of these patients' total recovery is their return to productivity. The continuing reassurance that chronic invalidism from heart disease is not inevitable provides the greatest possible contribution to their complete recovery. The alleviation of fear is the psychological antibiotic that determines their return to good health. Fortunately, heart patients are now also supported by psychological guidance and are induced to exercise and to return to all normal activities.

Nowhere is the grip of fear more evident than in people's desperate anxiety about cancer. These extreme fears are induced by the many reports of real or imagined causes of cancer. Food, water, canned foods, pesticides, smog, food additives, chemical pollution, contaminated streams, red dyes, plastic products, microwave oven radiation, and sugar substitutes are all alleged carcinogens, some or all of which most of us encounter on a regular basis. These contacts engender intense fear in many people despite the ironic fact that the average life span for Americans is today longer than ever before in the history of mankind. It is true that we must all eventually die and that the longer we live, the greater the chance of dying of cancer. One day the mysteries of cancer will be unlocked and the means of prevention found. Meanwhile, our cancer-phobic society will probably remain peopled with many helpless victims of irrational fear.

The elderly live in fear of imminently being incapacitated, chronically sick, and permanently dependent. Fear of the loss of personal dignity accounts for much of the unhappiness of the elderly. Fear of loneliness, of being unwanted, and of being dismissed from their jobs because of an arbitrary rule about retirement age upsets their emotional stability and complacency.

Along with the added years now granted the aging by the advances of medicine must also come a greater awareness of their needs, without which these added years may prove a burden rather than a gift. It is particularly sad when the elderly are relegated to inadequate nursing homes, being warehoused there until death releases them. On the other hand, if they can be made to feel wanted, loved, and accepted by society rather than discarded by it, the fears of growing older can be assuaged.

There is a delightful story told about a man, an accomplished musician, who at the age of 92 was still preparing for his annual concert for a small but enthusiastic audience. He had studied music with the great European masters and had taught music at an American university. He clearly demonstrated the sense of agelessness that the elderly ideally can enjoy.

He lived modestly through the years and had sustained pride in all of his past accomplishments. He had never competed with time, for each new year brought with it special and unique joys. When he was 76 years old and still actively engaged in teaching the piano, an elderly gentleman, a prospective pupil, called on him. "Are you still teaching?" he was asked. With a slight trace of irritation that he might be too old to teach at the age of 76, he said, "I most certainly am. Why do you ask? Surely, at your age you're not thinking of starting to study piano. How old are you?" The visitor answered, "I'm a little past 96, but I hear there's a great deal of music in heaven and I want to come prepared." For eight months the elderly pupil was taught the Bach two-part inventions and hymns, and then one day suddenly announced that he wanted to stop his studies. "But you're doing so well!" his teacher exclaimed. "Why stop now?" With introspective wisdom, the perquisite of the aged, he answered, "Because I think I now know enough to get by."

These two extraordinary people were fortunate because old age did not stop the flow of their creativity and enthusiasm. Neither one lived in the shadow of fear. Neither one would accept the stagnation that is thought to come with chronological age. Regrettably, they represent only a small portion of our aging population, who are too often sent out to pasture to wither and to wait.

Waging war on fear

How can fear be conquered? First of all, it must be faced frankly. Fear luxuriates in darkness and flourishes when it is hidden. Fear shrinks in daylight and can actually become a constructive force if it is brought out in the open and confronted.

The cure for the disease of fear does not lie in any of the new wonder drugs, but there is another kind of cure. It begins by recognizing that fear exists and by wanting to seek its cause and eradication. Confrontation with any problem brings it into focus. Too often a single, major problem becomes insidiously infused with small, insignificant problems, and it becomes very difficult to extricate oneself from the web of fear. This is the point at which help is needed. The family doctor, psychotherapist, counselor, or trained social worker can help one find relief from fear by gaining greater insight into its causes.

Fear is bondage. Emancipation and freedom from fear demand the courage to face fear. This is an era of hope, an era of unprecedented magnificent medical and scientific achievement. These advances, combined with ongoing developments in the social studies, augur well for the eventual uprooting of terror and anxiety. Fear is the single dominant disease that must be eradicated if we are to succeed in our rightful quest for peace of mind and inner security.

—Lester L. Coleman, M.D.

How Do You Rate as a Patient?

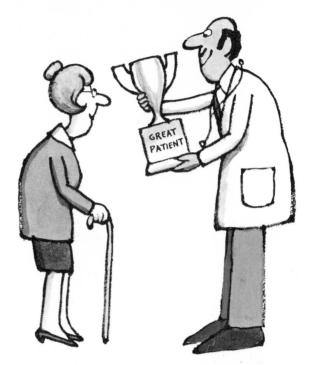

It has become increasingly useful to view the patient-doctor relationship as a mutual one, in which each partner has certain responsibilities to the other and to the process in which they are engaged. On the part of the patient, an intelligent, informed, and honest approach to health and medical care is becoming the expected norm. Your ability to answer such questions as the following will suggest how well you are prepared to be an equal partner in your own health maintenance.

1. The most common shortcoming in patients, as reported by doctors, is (a) unreliable memory of their medical history, (b) failure to follow instructions, (c) inability to understand simple medical terms, (d) hypochondria.

2. *Family practitioner* and *general practitioner* are essentially synonymous terms—true or false?

3. Osteopaths (doctors of osteopathy) and chiropractors receive similar training and provide similar services—true or false?

4. The normal adult resting pulse rate per minute is (a) 62–66, (b) 72–76, (c) 82–88, (d) 92–98, (e) 120–130.

5. In a physical examination the doctor uses his stethoscope to help assess the condition of the (a) heart, (b) lungs, (c) stomach and intestines, (d) abdominal blood circulation, (e) spleen.

6. Examination for possible symptoms of cancer should be performed only by a specialist known as an oncologist—true or false?

7. Polio immunization is no longer necessary in the United States since the disease has been eradicated—true or false?

8. No causal link between cigarette smoking and lung cancer, emphysema, and related conditions has been proved—true or false?

9. The normal adult respiration rate per minute is (a) 5–10, (b) 16–20, (c) 30–40, (d) 50–60, (e) 70–80.

10. Pains resulting from muscle strain or unusual or unaccustomed exertion are best treated by "working them out" with milder forms of the same movements—true or false?

11. When consulting a doctor about a particular problem or condition, it is best not to complicate or confuse the issue by offering extraneous facts of one's personal or family medical history—true or false?

12. It is wise practice to retain a moderate quantity of a prescription medication at the end of a course of treatment for use if the condition should recur in the future—true or false?

13. The normal adult blood pressure is approximately (a) 72, (b) 48/80, (c) 100, (d) 120/80, (e) 20/20.

14. Incidents of persistent abdominal pain can usually be treated at home with (a) heat packs, (b) mild laxatives, (c) aspirin, (d) rest, (e) massage.

15. The maintenance of good health requires, among other things, (a) competent primary medical care, (b) adequate secondary medical resources, (c) active participation by the individual, (d) an environment conducive to health.

16. Regular exercise, although currently fashionable and useful for maintaining muscular strength and appearance, has only marginal effect on total health—true or false?

17. There is no reliable way for the lay patient to judge a doctor's competence—true or false?

18. After surgical removal of the gallbladder, patients must follow a lifelong restricted diet—true or false?

19. Exposure to dampness and chills can cause colds—true or false?

20. Among the symptoms of a heart attack are (a) fever, (b) nausea, (c) shortness of breath, (d) chest pain, (e) shoulder, neck, or arm pain.

21. Diabetes is an essentially incurable disease—true or false?

22. Medication for hypertension is usually taken as needed, when the patient experiences symptoms—true or false?

357

Answers

1. (b). In particular, failure to take medication as often and for as long as instructed, to perform exercises, stick to diets, and generally endure inconveniences for the sake of their health.

2. False. The G.P., general practitioner, has no specialty license, such as for surgery, internal medicine, pediatrics, and so on. Family practice is one such specialty, emphasizing extra training in providing primary medical care.

3. False. Doctors of osteopathy are generally comparable to medical doctors in training and may prescribe drugs and perform surgery. Chiropractors may do neither; they generally limit themselves to physical manipulation, or "adjustment."

4. (b). The rate will be higher after even a slight exertion or after a meal and lower on waking, but this is a rough average.

5. (a), (b), (c), and (d). Handy, isn't it?

6. False. Examination for *symptoms* of most cancers is within the competence of most doctors. Certain symptoms, such as sores that fail to heal, warts or moles that undergo obvious changes, and the other warning signs well publicized by the American Cancer Society, should be watched for by every individual. Self-examination for signs of possible breast cancer is an easily learned technique every woman should master and practice monthly.

7. False. It has not been eradicated, nor have most other serious preventable diseases. There is fear that some of these diseases may again become potentially epidemic because of public apathy toward proper immunization.

8. True. The link that has been established is largely statistical; if you smoke, the findings say, your odds of developing one or more of the diseases are many times higher. It is an excellent bet that the causal link is there to be discovered, however, and won't you feel foolish then if you still haven't quit?

9. (b).

10. False. "Hair of the dog" will not impress sore muscles or joints, and it may turn soreness into full-blown injury. Rest, heat, appropriate dosage of aspirin, and massage may help.

11. Very false. Volunteer whatever information occurs to you. The doctor is the best judge of relevance.

Subtle clues from personal or family history may often speed the process of diagnosis.

12. False, twice. First, failure to complete the course of medication prescribed may hinder or even prevent full recovery. Second, many medications, including most antibiotics, become useless or even detrimental in a few weeks. They also pose a hazard in households with young and inquisitive children.

13. (d).

14. (d) only. The others are, as doctors say, contraindicated, meaning don't use them.

15. All are correct. This is less a question than a reminder.

16. False. Exercise can prevent many medical problems, can help speed recovery from others, and often adds a positive sense of well-being to a simple absence of physical disease. In other words, it can be the difference between "healthy" and merely "not sick."

17. As regards professional knowledge, diagnostic skill, and so on, this is largely true. The faith a patient necessarily invests in his doctor centers on these matters. On the other hand, as a partner engaged in a more or less formal relationship demanding certain social and psychological attributes, a doctor can and should be judged by the patient. That same faith depends upon the doctor's inspiring confidence, trust, and the desire to get well.

18. False. The gallbladder is essentially a storage organ, and many people can function quite well without it.

19. False. They may make you slightly more susceptible, but only direct exposure to the cold virus in one of its hundred varieties can bring on the disease.

20. All but (a).

21. True. It can be controlled by diet or medication but not cured. Therapy usually continues for life.

22. False. Hypertension is insidious precisely because it seldom exhibits symptoms. This makes it one of the commonest conditions in which patient noncompliance—failure to maintain the drug regimen—is a major complication.

—*Robert McHenry*

Health Education Unit 11

Measles and German Measles

Measles (rubeola)

Measles is a highly contagious viral disease that is characterized by fever, congested nose, inflamed eyes, and cough, followed by a typical generalized skin rash. It is predominantly a disease of infants and children. In developed countries serious complications now occur only rarely. The widespread use of measles vaccine in the U.S. beginning in the 1960s has led to a sharp decline in the incidence of the disease. However, in less developed areas of the world measles still presents very serious problems.

Measles was first described by the Persian physician known as Rhazes (AD 865–923). This disease is worldwide in its distribution and has played an interesting role in history. The parents and brother of Louis XV of France all died from measles and, as a result, Louis became king. About 20,000 Fiji Islanders died from measles in 1875, a total representing about one-fifth of the entire population. During the U.S. Civil War measles caused about 5,000 soldier deaths. In World War I reports showed that 90,000 soldiers contracted measles and over 2,000 of them died.

The course of the disease. After an incubation period of about ten days, the illness starts with fever and generalized weakness. Within 24 hours there is the beginning of coryza (running nose), conjunctivitis (eye inflammation), and cough. These symptoms gradually increase in severity and reach their peak about the same time the measles rash appears, which is usually on the fourth day of the illness. The rash usually begins at the hairline and forehead and behind the ear lobes. It then spreads downward to involve the face, neck, upper extremities, and trunk. By the seventh day it involves the entire body. It begins to fade after two or three days and fades as it appeared, one part of the body, then another—the face and upper body may be clear while the rash is still present on the legs.

During measles a child usually loses his appetite and looks ill. The glands in the neck may be enlarged. When the rash is at its peak, the child feels miserable. As the temperature starts to drop, the coryza and conjunctivitis clear, and the cough decreases in severity.

The typical case of measles is not difficult for the physician to diagnose. The combination of fever, cough, coryza, and conjunctivitis followed by the typical generalized rash is sufficient for a definitive diagnosis. Confirmatory laboratory examinations are usually not necessary. The diagnosis can be made with cer-

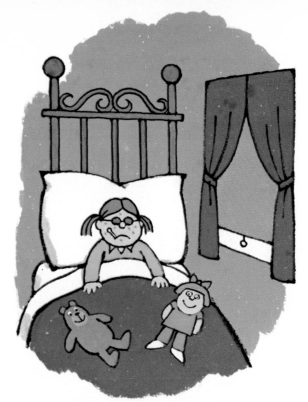

tainty if the child is found to have Koplik's spots on the mucous membranes inside the mouth. These characteristic spots are small and bright red, and in their centers are tiny white specks. They are seen before the child develops the generalized skin rash of measles.

The treatment of measles is largely supportive. Since it is a viral disease, antibiotics are ineffective. The child should be given plenty of fluids and a fever-reducing medication such as aspirin or acetaminophen. The family physician or pediatrician may wish to prescribe a cough preparation if the cough is severe. Bed rest is recommended and, because of the eye inflammation, the child should be protected from exposure to strong light.

Possible complications. The main complications are ear infections, pneumonia, and encephalitis.

Infection of the middle ear is one of the most common complications of measles. In such a case the child develops a severe earache. Occasionally the first sign of this infection will be a thick, purulent (pus-containing) discharge coming from the ear canal. Ear infection is usually accompanied by high fever that persists beyond the normal course of uncomplicated measles. Antibiotic treatment is necessary to clear up the infection, which is not caused by the measles virus itself but by bacteria.

Pneumonia is the next most common complication of measles and can be very severe and serious. A child with measles who remains feverish and continues to cough after the rash fades should be suspected of having pneumonia. The physician can make the diagnosis after examining the child's chest. He may require a chest X-ray to clarify the situation. Pneumonia secondary to measles is bacterial in origin and must be treated promptly with appropriate antibiotics.

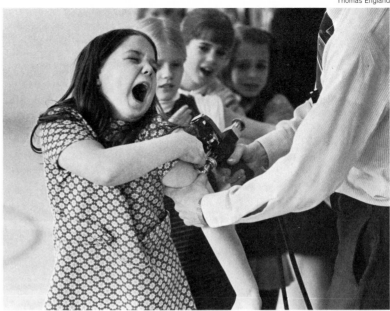

"Ouch!" The measles vaccine, licensed in 1963, has dramatically reduced the incidence of the disease, helping to protect children against potentially dangerous complications such as pneumonia and encephalitis.

Acute encephalitis (inflammation of the brain) is a serious, crippling, and sometimes fatal complication, occuring in approximately one out of every 1,000 cases of measles. Encephalitis causes headache, vomiting, convulsions, and coma. It most commonly develops three to six days after the start of the rash, and the course of the disease is extremely variable. It may be very mild, clearing completely in a few days, or it may be rapidly progressive and may terminate fatally within one or two days. Approximately 60% of the measles encephalitis patients recover completely; 25% recover but remain with signs of brain damage such as mental retardation, seizures, paralysis, or nerve deafness; and 15% die. There is no specific treatment for this most serious complication of measles. All that can be offered is supportive medical and nursing care, which, of course, must be carried out in the hospital.

The prognosis of measles has improved dramatically during the past 25 years. Many of the serious bacterial complications can be controlled with antibiotics. The majority of deaths due to measles are the result of severe pneumonia or measles encephalitis.

Controlling measles. One attack of measles usually confers permanent immunity. Most of the so-called second episodes of measles reflect mistakes in the original diagnosis. Mothers who have had the illness or have been vaccinated against it with the live measles vaccine pass on some passive immunity to their newborn babies. Newborns are protected against measles for the first six months and then rapidly lose immunity and become susceptible to the disease.

Measles is usually spread by direct contact via droplet spray, as from a cough or a sneeze. It is extremely contagious, and the period of contagion lasts for about a week after the beginning of the first symptoms. In general, measles is a disease of childhood. In crowded cities the highest incidence occurs in the infant and preschool age groups. In less crowded areas the highest incidence is in children from five to ten years of age. Measles is essentially a winter and spring disease, with the peak of the outbreaks occurring during March and April.

Measles can be modified or prevented by an injection of gamma globulin, an antibody-containing component of blood. Before the development of the live measles vaccine this was the usual method of attempting to reduce the severity of the illness in an infant or child exposed to the disease. The passive immunity developing from the gamma globulin lasts only about one month.

The licensing of a vaccine for the prevention of measles in 1963 was the big breakthrough in dramatically reducing the incidence of measles in the United States. During the five-year period before the vaccine, 1958–62, about 500,000 cases were reported each year. During 1972–76 an average of only about 28,000 cases were reported each year. The one injection of vaccine will produce lifelong immunity against this potentially fatal illness if given after the child is 15 months old. In high-risk countries and during some epidemic situations it may be necessary to immunize infants starting at six months of age, but under these circumstances a second measles vaccination is given after the infants are 15 months old in order to produce lifelong immunity. The vaccine is available as measles alone, measles-rubella, and measles-mumps-rubella vaccine.

Before the live measles vaccine was available, 300 to 400 cases of measles encephalitis were seen each year. The extensive use of the vaccine was followed by

360

a significant drop in the incidence of this deadly measles complication. This is the most important reason for immunizing every child. More than 90 million doses of measles vaccine have been given, and at present between 65 and 70% of infants and children in the U.S. have been immunized. However, the incidence of measles has been rising because of the substantial number of children who still have not been immunized. The 30 to 35% of unimmunized children of the 1960s have grown up without protection. During recent outbreaks a significant number of cases were seen in people over 15 years of age. If this susceptible group is not given the measles vaccination, more and more of them will grow into adulthood without protection and may contract this disease and its potentially life-threatening complications. Every effort should be made to identify and immunize this large unprotected segment of the population. Parents must make certain that their children receive the measles vaccine. It is safe, effective, and easily available from public health services. Immunizations are an essential aspect of every child's health care program.

German measles (rubella)

Rubella is an acute infectious viral disease that is characterized by mild systemic symptoms, a three-day rash, and generalized lymph-node enlargement, particularly of the nodes behind the ears. Before 1941 German measles was considered important mainly because it was responsible for epidemics in schools and because it was often confused with measles and scarlet fever. Since 1941 a great deal of interest has been focused on German measles because of its proven association with an increased incidence of severe birth defects when it has been contracted by women in the early months of pregnancy.

The course of the disease. German measles is caused by the rubella virus. The first symptoms occur after an incubation period of about 16 to 18 days. In children the first apparent sign of the illness is the appearance of the rash. In adolescents and adults, however, the rash is preceded by a one- to five-day period of a low-grade fever, headache, weakness, loss of appetite, sore throat, and cough. Rubella is characterized by lymph node enlargement, which may begin a few days before the rash appears; the most commonly affected lymph nodes are those behind the ear (post-occipital nodes). The swelling of these lymph nodes is usually greatest during the first day of the rash. The rash appears first on the face and then spreads downward rapidly to involve the neck, arms, trunk, and extremities. The rash appears, spreads, and disappears more quickly than does the rash of measles. By the end of the first day the entire body may be covered with the pink-red spots. By the end of the third day in a typical case the rash has entirely disappeared. In children the temperature may be either normal or slightly elevated. Fever rarely persists beyond the first day of the rash and is usually low grade.

Possible complications. Complications of childhood German measles are rare. Secondary bacterial infections, which are so commonly seen in measles, are generally not seen in German measles. However, the following complications have been observed, especially during epidemics.

Incidence of arthritic joint involvement in adolescents and adults with German measles is much more common than in children. It usually develops just as the

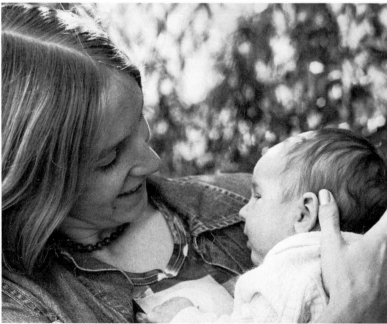

Erika Stone—Peter Arnold

While rubella, or German measles, is a mild and usually harmless disease, if it is contracted by a newly pregnant woman, the result may be a child born deaf, blind, retarded, or with a damaged heart. If all girls were protected by vaccination at an early age, their babies, like this one, could be protected from rubella's tragic consequences.

rash is fading on the second or third day of illness. Arthritic manifestations usually clear up completely within five to ten days.

Encephalitis or other complications of German measles involving the central nervous system are extremely rare. Encephalitis is less commonly seen after this disease than after measles or after chickenpox, occurring only about once in every 6,000 cases. Although electroencephalographic abnormalities are relatively common, the encephalitis itself is usually not severe and the child is very rarely left with any permanent damage.

The prognosis of German measles is almost always excellent, as rubella is one of the most benign of all infectious diseases in children. Many of the reported deaths attributed to German measles infection reflect errors in diagnosis.

Controlling German measles. One attack of German measles is usually followed by permanent immunity. Many of the so-called second or third attacks of German measles represent mistakes in diagnosis.

German measles is worldwide in distribution and is endemic in most large cities. In the temperate zones most cases occur during the spring months. This illness is rare in infants and is uncommon in preschool-age children. There is a higher incidence of the disease in older children, adolescents, and young adults.

German measles is spread by direct contact, usually via the respiratory tract. It is usually spread when a child who has the disease either coughs or sneezes on another child. A child with German measles is contagious a few days before the rash appears until the end of the first week of the rash.

There is no specific treatment for rubella. Since it is such a mild disease, nothing special need be done other than general supportive treatment.

If German measles is such a harmless and benign illness, why then is it necessary and so important to vaccinate against it? Rubella is very dangerous to the unborn child if the mother acquires this disease early in the pregnancy. In 1941 an Australian ophthalmologist named N. M. Gregg reported the occurrence of congenital abnormalities among 78 infants born after their mothers had acquired rubella infection during their pregnancies. More than half of those infants had severe congenital heart disease and many were blind from congenital cataracts. Since 1941 Gregg's report of the rubella syndrome has been confirmed by many others. All these studies demonstrate that the occurrence of German measles during the first three months of pregnancy is associated with a significantly in-

creased incidence of congenital malformations, stillbirths, and abortions. The congenital rubella syndrome is characterized by low birth weight, cataracts, microcephaly (small head), deafness, congenital heart disease, and mental retardation. The epidemic of rubella in the United States in 1964–65 had tragic consequences for about 50,000 pregnancies—30,000 of these were terminated before birth, and the remaining 20,000 infants were born with congenital abnormalities. Many of these youngsters suffered from multiple defects. The cost of hospitalization, medical care, rehabilitation, and special education of these handicapped survivors has been estimated to be over $1 billion. This devastating experience emphasizes the need for a safe and effective vaccine. Since a large percentage of babies born after their mothers are exposed to measles are adversely affected, it is very important that every effort be made to prevent this disease.

As of June 1969 a German measles vaccine was licensed for use in the United States. Mass immunization drives have been carried out for children under 12 years of age—the group most likely to spread the infection to pregnant women. The American Academy of Pediatrics now recommends that all children over the age of 15 months be vaccinated against German measles. One vaccination usually confers lifelong immunity. If all girls were protected before they reached childbearing age, the tragedy of the congenital rubella syndrome would be totally eliminated. Realistically, this goal cannot be achieved but, if a high enough percentage of all children are given the vaccine, the chances of an unprotected pregnant woman's contracting rubella will be greatly reduced. In 1977 an alarming upsurge of rubella cases was reported by the U.S. Center for Disease Control in Atlanta, Ga., posing a threat to the estimated 10–20% of women of childbearing age who have no immunity against rubella. Only by expanding immunization efforts can the needless tragedy of birth defects caused by rubella be avoided. Because the virus in the vaccine may damage the unborn child in the same way as the disease, women of childbearing age should never be immunized unless it is certain that they are not pregnant. Further, women must understand that they must not become pregnant within three months of the inoculation. Just as in the case of measles, prevention is the key to eliminating German measles.

—*Alvin N. Eden, M.D.*

Chickenpox, Shingles, and Smallpox

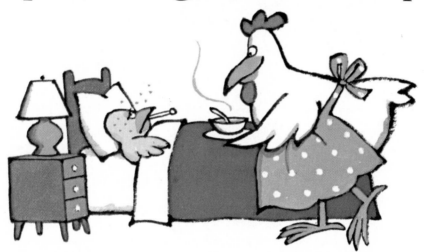

Chickenpox (varicella)

Chickenpox is a relatively harmless, highly contagious disease caused by the varicella-zoster (v-z) virus. The main manifestation of chickenpox is an itchy rash consisting of raised red spots, "water" blisters, and scabs. In children the effects of chickenpox are usually mild, and serious complications are very rare.

It is not certain how chickenpox came to receive its common English name. The disease varicella was referred to in print as "chicken pocks" as early as 1694, in Richard Morton's *Pyretologia*. According to the *Oxford English Dictionary* chicken connoted something that was "small, comparatively harmless," and varicella was "generally supposed to have been named from the mildness of the disease." In an agricultural society such analogies were easily and commonly made. However, a correspondent to the British medical journal *Lancet* suggests that the earliest common name might have been "itching-pox." Over the centuries the Old English word *gican*, "itch," may have been gradually replaced with *cicen* "chicken." The mildness connotation of chicken would have aided in the transformation. But certainly "itching-pox" would be an appropriate name for this mild but annoying disease.

The course of the disease. The incubation period of chickenpox is usually 14 to 16 days but can be as long as 21 days. The disease begins with low-grade fever, a generalized unwell feeling, and the appearance of the rash. The most striking characteristic of the chickenpox rash is the speed with which it progresses from flat red spots (macules) to raised red spots (papules) to so-called water blisters (vesicles) and then to the beginning of crusting—the changes may occur in less than one day. The diagnosis is made when the typical

crops of vesicles are seen. Before they rupture, the vesicles have a dewdrop appearance and are surrounded by a reddened area of skin. As these water blisters dry, they form small depressions and then a crust. After a two- to three-week period the scabs usually fall off, and eventually the skin looks perfectly normal, with no evidence of scar formation. The skin lesions of chickenpox that appear in crops are found mainly on the trunk and on the scalp, face, and arms and legs. The mucous membranes in the mouth can also be involved. A distinctive feature of the rash is the presence of lesions in all stages (macules, papules, vesicles, and crusts) in the same general area of the body at the same time.

The child with chickenpox is usually not very sick. The greater the severity of the rash, the higher the child's fever. When the rash is quite sparse, the temperature is usually only slightly elevated. Temperatures up to 105° F (40.6° C) are not unusual in severe cases of chickenpox, when almost the entire skin surface is covered with the rash. Along with the fever the child usually feels tired, loses his appetite, and may complain of a headache. In many cases, the most troublesome symptom is the severe itching of the skin.

The typical case of chickenpox can be recognized quite easily because of the rash. Certainty of exposure to the disease is also helpful in making the diagnosis, as other conditions involving the skin occasionally have to be taken into consideration in arriving at the correct diagnosis. When smallpox was widespread, this was sometimes a difficult task. Impetigo, an acute contagious skin disease, may also cause water blisters, but they differ from chickenpox lesions both in appearance and in distribution; they do not appear in

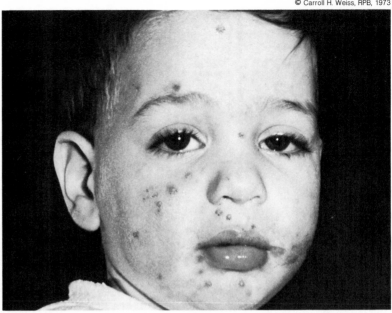

© Carroll H. Weiss, RPB, 1973

A young patient exhibits the characteristic rash of chickenpox. The rash usually clears without scarring the skin.

crops and do not involve the mucous membranes of the mouth. Multiple insect bites sometimes resemble the rash of chickenpox but do not have a water-blister appearance and do not have the typical distribution of the chickenpox rash.

Possible complications. The prognosis of chickenpox is excellent. Uneventful and complete recovery is the rule. Complications, rarely a problem, include secondary skin infection, encephalitis (inflammation of the brain), and pneumonia.

Secondary skin infections occur occasionally when bacteria gain entry into the skin lesions and produce an infected area (pyoderma). However, even before the use of antibiotics there was a very low incidence of this type of complication. If an infection of a local lesion does occur, it responds to simple measures such as warm compresses. If the infection is more severe, the physician may decide to prescribe an antibiotic.

Encephalitis occurs in less than one out of every 1,000 cases of chickenpox. The symptoms of this inflammation of the brain usually develop about a week after the rash. They are fever, headache, stiff neck, incoordination, and occasional convulsions and coma. If any of these symptoms occur, the physician must be notified immediately. Almost all cases of postchickenpox encephalitis make complete recoveries. It is a much milder form of encephalitis than the encephalitis seen following measles.

Chickenpox pneumonia rarely occurs in children but is seen more often in adults. It is characterized by severe cough, chest pain, and difficulty in breathing. If a child with chickenpox develops these symptoms, the doctor should be consulted. Severe varicella pneumonia in an adult may be potentially fatal, but in a child it is not as dangerous.

Chickenpox is almost always a benign disease of childhood—the typical case clears up completely without sequel and without skin scarring. Skin lesions that have become infected are more likely to leave permanent scars. Chickenpox in a newborn infant or in a child receiving corticosteroid therapy is more likely to be serious.

One attack of chickenpox usually confers lifelong immunity. Varicella is highly contagious and worldwide in distribution, being endemic in all large cities, where epidemics occur at regular intervals. It is predominantly a disease of childhood, with the highest incidence between ages two and eight, and is rarely seen in adults. Unlike measles, it may occur in early infancy in spite of a history of previous chickenpox in the mother. The infection is spread chiefly by direct contact with someone who has the disease. A patient with chickenpox can spread the disease to other susceptible people from about one day before the beginning of the rash until all the water blisters have become dry.

Treating chickenpox. Chickenpox is a self-limited disease, and so treatment is entirely for symptoms. Antipyretic (fever-reducing) drugs such as aspirin or acetaminophen are indicated for high fever. Local application of a lotion or an antipruritic (anti-itching) ointment may help in relieving the itching caused by the rash, and severe itching occasionally requires the use of an oral antihistamine. Fingernails should be kept short and clean in order to help prevent secondary skin infections caused by scratching. No preventive measures are recommended for a normal child who has been exposed to varicella. Since chickenpox is more serious in an adult, it is safer for a child to acquire the disease so that he is protected for life. A patient with chickenpox should be kept at home until the water blisters have dried. Contacts need not be quarantined but merely observed. Special isolation precautions within the home to protect brothers and sisters are useless and should not be attempted. At the present time there is no vaccine available against chickenpox, but since this is such a mild disease with so few serious complications, there is no urgency in developing such a vaccine. Zoster immune globulin, prepared from the plasma of convalescing chickenpox patients, is high in antibodies and confers immunity when administered within three days after exposure to the disease. It is prescribed for debilitated or severely ill patients only, and sometimes for newborn infants.

Herpes zoster (shingles)

The same varicella-zoster virus that causes chickenpox also causes herpes zoster. This is a unique biological phenomenon in that the identical virus is responsible for two separate, distinct diseases. The present-day consensus is that zoster is probably caused by the reactivation of latent v-z virus: a person who previously had chickenpox carries the latent v-z virus in his body for many years without any trouble and, for some as yet unknown reason, in a small percentage of cases the dormant v-z virus is activated, and shingles, or herpes zoster, develops. It is known that the v-z virus can be activated in patients with Hodgkin's disease or in those receiving immunosuppressive therapy. Herpes zoster manifests itself by the breaking out of localized crops of skin vesicles, which follow along the course of a nerve. This disease is more common and more painful in adults than in children.

The course of the disease. The incubation period of zoster is unknown. For a few days before the characteristic signs of the disease develop, the patient may have a generalized unwell feeling, with slight fever or gastrointestinal upsets. The area of the body that is served by the affected nerve may be painful. The classic case of shingles is characterized by the rash, which progresses through the same stages as the chickenpox rash. The rash may appear on the trunk, shoulders, arms, or neck or may involve the lower extremities. The common name for the disease, shingles, is derived from the Latin word for belt, or girdle, indicating that the disease frequently appears in the waist area. The lesions are almost always located on one side of the body only, appearing on the skin over the nerve, which is located deep in body tissue. If one of the cranial nerves is involved, the lesions can appear on the face. The skin of the eyelids may carry lesions, and in ophthalmic herpes zoster the cornea can be damaged by ulcerations and opaque areas. Zoster affecting the eyes must be carefully monitored by an ophthalmologist.

Pain at the site of the rash is not much of a problem in a child with zoster—itching is a more common problem. By contrast, zoster in an adult can often cause excruciating pain, which sometimes lasts for weeks. Some patients' skin becomes so sensitive that even the touch of clothing is intolerable. Adults are also

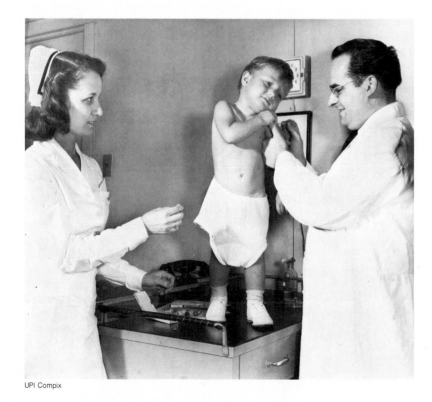

UPI Compix

In 1944, when this photograph was taken, smallpox immunization was a part of the ordinary regimen of vaccination for every child. In 1971 this practice was finally discontinued; the last case of smallpox was recorded in the United States in 1949.

more likely than children to develop eye involvement.

Although herpes zoster is chiefly an adult disease—it most commonly affects people over 50—it is not unusual for infants and children to be affected. In the reported cases of childhood shingles, there is almost always a previous history of chickenpox. The v-z virus can be isolated and identified by withdrawing some fluid from one of the vesicles of the rash and examining it microscopically.

Treating herpes zoster. In children the clinical course of zoster is usually mild, and the prognosis is excellent. There are very few complications, and no specific treatment is indicated. If the rash is severe, soaks or drying lotions may be helpful. The rash clears in one to two weeks in most children. The pain that some children with zoster experience can be controlled readily with aspirin.

The more pronounced symptoms in adults require somewhat more rigorous supportive care. Analgesics may be prescribed to control pain and barbiturates to control the tension and nervousness associated with neuralgia. In severe cases of zoster hospitalization may be necessary. The skin vesicles should be protected from infection to minimize scarring.

The usual course of the disease is only a few weeks. With rare exceptions, one attack of zoster confers lifelong immunity. Postherpetic neuralgia may persist for months or even years, a result most common in the elderly.

The possibility that herpes zoster may follow exposure to chickenpox should be kept in mind when the exposed person previously has had chickenpox. The antibodies produced in the blood by the past chickenpox infection will not protect against herpes zoster. Conversely, chickenpox can follow exposure to herpes zoster if the exposed person never had chickenpox as a child.

Smallpox (variola)

Today smallpox has just about been eradicated from the face of the Earth. Throughout the ages smallpox epidemics have resulted in the deaths of millions of people—some epidemics resulted in a death rate of up to 50% of entire populations. As of 1978 smallpox has become a disease of the past. This remarkable accomplishment has been primarily due to the widespread use of the smallpox vaccine. In 1796 Edward Jenner proved that the inoculation of humans with a vaccine against an animal and human disease, cowpox, led to complete immunity and protection against the human disease smallpox. Cowpox and smallpox belong to the same "pox" group of viruses, which cause diseases characterized by pustules, or skin eruptions; cowpox is sufficiently related to smallpox that acquiring a case of cowpox by vaccination results in the development of immunity against the dangerous and potentially lethal disease smallpox.

Smallpox eradication. Until recent years vaccination against smallpox was considered a routine procedure in the United States, part of the regular series of childhood immunizations. However, in 1971 this policy was radically changed when the U.S. Public Health Service and the American Academy of Pediatrics announced that routine smallpox vaccination was no longer necessary. Because the last case of smallpox in the United States was recorded in 1949, and since the dangers of complications following smallpox vaccination were greater than the possibility of acquiring the disease, routine smallpox immunization ceased.

In 1966 the World Health Organization (WHO) announced an all-out attack against smallpox, and now this killer of millions has been virtually eradicated from the Earth. The history of smallpox is a most dramatic example of the conquering and elimination of one of the most dangerous diseases known to man by the use of a vaccine and by proper public health surveillance. The head of the World Health Organization has said, "To do what has been done is nothing short of a public health miracle."

—*Alvin N. Eden, M.D.*

Health Education Unit 13
Peptic Ulcers

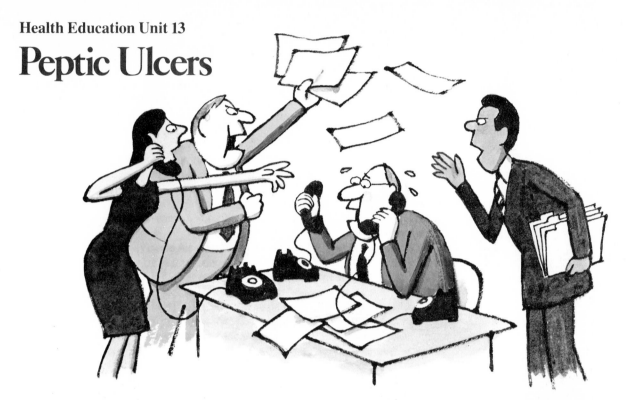

Peptic ulcers of the stomach (gastric ulcers) and of the small intestine (duodenal ulcers) were once considered a disease of the tycoons of industry. But such a select group are not the only victims of this disease. Ulcers are a complaint of advertising executives, bank managers, doctors, lawyers, college professors, shoe salesmen, taxi drivers, sanitation workers, and many others. There is evidence, however, that in recent years fewer people in the United States and in Scandinavian countries have been developing ulcers. But everyone likes to attribute his ulcer to the unique tensions of his particular job and to the seemingly limitless pressures made on him by his family and friends and by society.

The fact of the matter is that no one in any occupation at any economic or social level is free of the possibility of developing an ulcer. Both men and women in every geographical area can be burdened with this distressing condition. And contrary to general belief, children, too, can develop ulcers. It has been estimated that 5% of the adult population in the United States suffer from peptic ulcer disease, men being affected three times as often as women.

It is commonly thought that there is a typical profile or portrait of the ulcer-prone personality. A person who is tense, high-strung, hard driving, conscientious, ambitious, and aggressive is considered to be susceptible to ulcers. The calm, tranquil, and passive individual, it is supposed, is less frequently affected. But this assumption is not necessarily true. Sometimes, apparently tranquil, easy-going people may not be expressing

their real feelings. In fact, suppressing the emotions can create conflicts that add stress to a person's life and upset the little understood and delicate balance between the body and the mind.

This general description of the ulcer-prone person is reflected in the medical cliché that a stomach ulcer is not necessarily caused by what you eat but rather by what's eating you. But the mind and the body can both be intricately involved in every aspect of the development of, treatment of, and recovery from a peptic ulcer. However, many widespread beliefs about ulcers, including the role of stress as a cause, are being questioned. Some researchers have come to doubt that stress is as important a factor as it has long been thought to be.

Causes of ulcers

Peptic ulcers are small breaks in the delicate mucous membrane that lines the stomach and the upper small intestine. When the protective layer has been broken, a small crater forms, usually 1 to 2.5 cm in diameter. It has been definitely established that such ulcers are related to the pepsin and hydrochloric acid that are secreted in the stomach for the digestion of food. Pepsin is an enzyme produced in the stomach that breaks down proteins into simpler components. The acid content of gastric juices helps liquefy food and prepare it for further breakdown. Since everybody secretes acid, why do some people develop ulcers and others not? The answer is not known. It is known that persons with peptic ulcer disease have acid secretion rates no

367

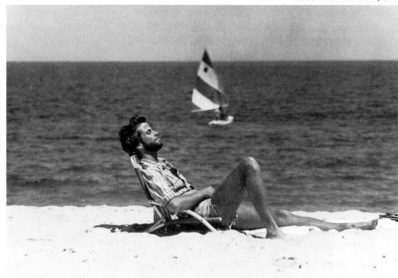

The seemingly placid, relaxed, and easy-going person may not conform to our ideas of the typical ulcer sufferer, but ulcers afflict many types of people of all ages, even children. The conditions leading to the formation of ulcers may be more complex than was once thought.

greater than normal, while persons with duodenal ulcers may secrete two to three times more acid than normal.

There are many other factors that may be involved in ulcer formation, not all of them well understood. One assumption is that the mucous membrane lining of the stomach and intestine may, for some unknown reason, lose its own protective capacity. Alcohol and tobacco are thought to compound the damage and cause additional weakening of the mucosa.

Studies show that ulcers do not occur in any fixed or well-established geographical or occupational pattern. Gastric ulcers tend to develop later in life than do duodenal ulcers. Men are affected far more frequently than women. Heredity is not of particular significance, although sometimes several members of a family do develop ulcers. It is generally believed that psychological stress and the inability to cope with social or financial problems may be partly responsible for the development of peptic ulcers. It is known that ulcers can be brought on as a result of injury to the central nervous system, even by brain surgery. Ulcers sometimes form in burn or shock victims or during the course of some drug therapies.

Symptoms of ulcers

The symptoms of peptic ulcers show definite patterns. There are variations, of course, but almost always pain is the predominant complaint. The pain is frequently described as being constant or gnawing, typical of a so-called hunger pang. There may also be an aching soreness and an empty feeling in the upper abdomen just below the breastbone.

A person with a duodenal ulcer has a distinctive pattern of pain. The symptoms are so typical, in fact, that many doctors make an initial diagnosis based on the patient's description of the pain alone. Pain is rarely present when the person first awakens. Occasionally, the pain begins in midmorning. It is almost always relieved by eating but may return an hour or so later. The pain may awaken a person from sleep.

The symptoms of a gastric ulcer do not always follow this pattern. Eating may, in fact, cause pain rather than relieve it. In both types of peptic ulcer the dull, aching, or burning sensation may be rhythmic or steady, depending on the depth of the ulcer and its size, severity, and possible complications.

Bleeding from ulcers of the stomach and the duodenum may first evidence itself in black, tarry stools. This symptom can cause alarm in persons taking iron compounds, which also can produce such stools. Bleeding is caused when the ulcer erodes into an artery or vein, or when the granulation tissue on the ulcer begins to hemorrhage. Surgery may be indicated if the bleeding recurs or is severe.

Diagnosis of ulcers

The diagnosis of peptic ulcer is not determined, of course, by the patient's description of the pain alone. If an ulcer is suspected, the doctor inquires into the patient's eating habits and use of tobacco and alcohol. The doctor has tests performed by which a definite diagnosis can be made. Ulcers must be distinguished from gallbladder and liver disease and from disorders of the pancreas. Hiatal hernia and ulcers of the lower end of the esophagus must be ruled out. Secretions taken from the stomach are studied to determine if there is an absence or excess of hydrochloric acid. X-rays are an important diagnostic tool. When a patient is given a small amount of barium, the crater formation of an ulcer can readily be seen by X-ray.

A new important diagnostic instrument is the fiber-optic gastroduodenoscope. The instrument is passed through the mouth into the stomach and duodenum.

Almost every area of the stomach and duodenum can be carefully visualized through the scope. It is possible to take photographs of the entire inner lining of the wall of this area in order to find the exact position of a peptic ulcer. Smears, secretions, and biopsy material can be removed through the fiberoptic instrument and evaluated by chemical and microscopic examinations. Because cancer of the stomach in its early stages may mimic the symptoms usually ascribed to peptic ulcers, a direct view of the inside of the stomach through a scope is of tremendous value.

Treatment of ulcers

When a diagnosis of peptic ulcer is definitely established, treatment tries to neutralize or decrease the acidity in the stomach. Every substance that can create acidity—this includes many kinds of foods and many varieties of medication, both prescription and nonprescription—is eliminated.

There has been a marked change in the attitude toward diet in the treatment of ulcers. Until a few years ago a bland diet that included regular hourly feedings of milk and cream was considered essential for the control of ulcers in their acute stages. Fatty foods, spices, fruit juices, tea, coffee, cocoa, and cola drinks —all of which stimulate acid and pepsin secretions— were prohibited.

In recent years there has been a tendency to liberalize some of these restrictions. A patient is now permitted to eat a sensible, more normal diet with fewer limitations. The use of milk and cream to neutralize excess stomach acid has been abandoned. It is now recognized, in fact, that the protein in milk actually stimulates, rather than depresses, peptic activity and causes increased acidity.

Some fruit juices and spicy foods are still not generally permitted. Some physicians, however, do permit patients to season foods delicately unless spices provoke ulcer pain. There is less emphasis today on the need for frequent feedings. Ulcer patients are encouraged to eat three meals a day. Food before bedtime is not recommended because it tends to stimulate acid secretion and induce pain during the night. Today there is also far less emphasis than there used to be on eating pureed or chopped foods.

There has been, however, absolutely no change in the rule that alcohol and smoking should be eliminated. Both alcohol and tobacco may be factors in the production of peptic ulcers and may delay healing. It is believed that both have adverse effects on the intrinsic capacity of the lining of the stomach to heal itself. Coffee, tea, and cola drinks are also still generally forbidden. Even decaffeinated coffee is considered an irritant that should be avoided.

It has been established that aspirin and compounds containing aspirin are related to the production of gas-

The diagram shows ulcers in the stomach itself and in the duodenum just beyond the stomach, another common site. The cross sectional close-up shows the craterlike nature of the lesion.

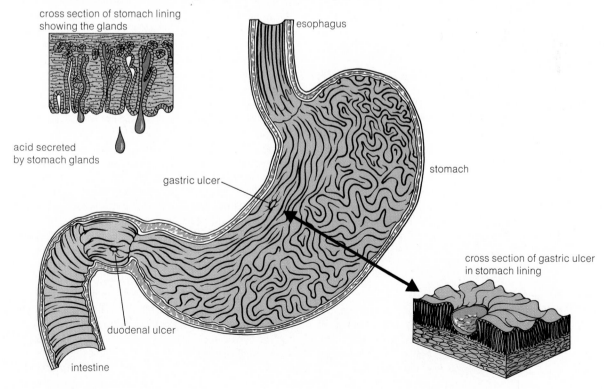

cross section of stomach lining
showing the glands

acid secreted
by stomach glands

esophagus

stomach

gastric ulcer

cross section of gastric ulcer
in stomach lining

duodenal ulcer

intestine

tric ulcers. Although aspirin's effect on duodenal ulcers has not been clearly determined, all ulcer patients should avoid aspirin in any form. In addition, because aspirin has a "blood-thinning" property, it may stimulate bleeding from ulcers. Cortisone and a number of other drugs that can cause peptic ulcers and their complications should also be avoided.

Antacid therapy

The treatment of ulcers tries to eliminate or reduce those factors that stimulate the production of hydrochloric acid and pepsin. Consequently, the use of antacid drugs can be of enormous benefit. Antacids neutralize stomach acids, control pain, and can even promote the healing of uncomplicated ulcers.

To be effective antacids cannot be used haphazardly. They must be taken in sufficient quantity and at times when they will remain active in the stomach for a number of hours. If a person has very little or no food in the stomach, antacids can leave the stomach within half an hour, which is not enough time for them to neutralize the acid.

If antacids are taken about an hour after a meal, they remain in the stomach for about three hours. This practice gives antacids a great deal more time to work. The ideal time to take an antacid is generally considered to be 45 minutes to an hour after eating. The dose is repeated in about three hours.

Not all antacids are equally beneficial. Antacids that contain calcium may have undesirable side effects. Sodium bicarbonate should not be taken over long periods of time. Doctors should carefully evaluate the antacids that they prescribe in order to be certain that the drugs do not contain excessive salt for patients with high blood pressure or heart disorders. Patients with kidney disease should not take antacids that contain magnesium. In fact, before embarking on antacid therapy, a patient should specifically discuss such problems with the doctor. Only in this way can the maximum benefit from antacids be achieved.

A special group of drugs known as anticholinergics have been used for years to delay the emptying of the stomach. By doing so, they also diminish acid secretion and help to reduce the frequency and severity of ulcer pain. These drugs should also be carefully evaluated before they are prescribed. Patients who have a tendency to develop glaucoma, who are markedly debilitated, who have an enlargement of the prostate gland, or who have difficulty urinating should not take anticholinergics.

New drugs

In recent years there have been many new drugs developed for the treatment of peptic ulcers. The drugs produce their beneficial effects in different ways. Although it is not fully understood how these substances work, they relieve ulcer pain dramatically.

Probably the most dramatic new drug is a chemical compound known as cimetidine. Ulcers respond to its use in a short time. The drug works most effectively in the reduction of the acid in the stomach that is normally produced by food, tobacco, coffee, and drugs. Cimetidine seems to promote rapid healing of ulcers and to bring relief from their distressing symptoms.

Studies with the new drugs are continuing in order to determine which are the most promising. Both their value and their possible toxic side effects are being considered. Even though new drugs are on the horizon for the treatment of peptic ulcers, patients must not believe that they may be careless or neglectful of early symptoms. To delay treatment of a gastric or duodenal ulcer is to allow a simple problem to develop into a complicated one.

Surgery

Medical treatment for patients with peptic ulcers is effective in a large majority of cases. To the extent that stress may be involved, psychological help may also be effective. Consequently, today less and less surgery is being performed. With a better understanding of the causes and effective treatment of ulcers, and with the new drugs being developed, the necessity for surgery has been greatly reduced. Today approximately 15% of patients with duodenal ulcers will ultimately require surgery. Surgery is now used when bleeding cannot be controlled, when scar tissue has formed an obstruction in the digestive tract, when there is a suspicion of cancer, or when there is a possibility that the ulcer is becoming deeper and is about to perforate the wall of the stomach or intestine. When acute perforation does occur, immediate surgery is required. The longer the time between perforation and surgery, the poorer the prognosis. An ulcer that perforates into the peritoneal cavity must be regarded as an acute emergency. Peritonitis can result quickly, a life-threatening complication.

Surgery for ulcers is of several types and has several purposes. Overstimulation of acid-secreting tissue may be corrected by a vagotomy, in which various portions of the vagus nerve are severed. In addition, passage of stomach contents may be facilitated by several procedures that refashion the connection of the stomach to the small intestine. The ulcerated tissue itself can be excised. The lower portion of the stomach, in which acid-secreting cells are located, is frequently removed in a gastric resection, or gastrectomy. Ulcers that are not actually removed in surgery still benefit from the environment of reduced acidity, which allows natural healing to take place more successfully.

The total picture of peptic ulcers of the stomach and the duodenum is not as bleak as it once was. The outlook for the successful cure can usually be determined by a person's own respect for the delicacy of these vital organs.

— Lester L. Coleman, M.D.

Alcoholism

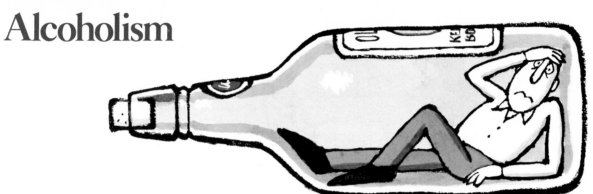

Alcoholism is the term used to identify excessive and compulsive drinking that results in the destruction of mind and body. It is not known with accuracy how many people in the world live with this problem; for the U.S. alone estimates range from 10 million to 20 million. The alcoholic is believed to suffer from a disease, a very special disease that is both chronic and incurable. Once a person is afflicted with alcoholism, he or she must accept the undeniable truth that it will always persist.

Because alcoholism is incurable, does this mean that it cannot be controlled? Many alcoholics whose handicap no longer prevents them from being normal, productive human beings say emphatically no. Experience has shown that, once this complicated disorder has been understood by the alcoholic and by friends and family, all of these forces can join in returning him or her to health and happiness.

Who is an alcoholic?

As recently as a generation ago this devastating problem was considered only in moral or legal terms. Alcoholism was a character weakness, and the alcoholic was rejected by society as a worthless, hopeless drunkard. No other illness ever provoked such a totally unsympathetic response. It was not until alcoholism was approached scientifically like a disease in terms of diagnosis, treatment, and prevention that society was able to accept the alcoholic as a victim rather than an offender. Currently even the disease concept is sometimes regarded as too simplistic. The causes of alcoholism are multiple and appear to involve both genetic and environmental factors whose interactions are yet poorly understood.

The nature of alcoholism is further complicated by subtle shades of difference between the heavy social drinker and the alcoholic. At times the heavy social drinker may drink without restraint and appear to have the "alcoholic personality." Usually the alcoholic, once drinking has begun, continues without interruption, sometimes to the point of unconsciousness. Yet there are some alcoholics who, by choice or under pressure of family, friends, or physician, are able to go weeks or months with only moderate drinking until a stressful situation arises. Then follows an uncontrollable drive to seek oblivion with total intoxication. With this pattern of drinking, a cycle of controlled and uncontrolled drinking is established—a cycle that is in some ways contrary to the assumption that continual craving is the rule in all alcoholics.

Why does a person become an alcoholic?

Drinking is part of a social pastime that seems to offer some escape from the inner tensions of modern living. Most people are able to maintain a pattern of social drinking without any significant alteration of personality and without loss of social responsibility. Those afflicted with alcoholism, however, may drink the same amount as others and yet be affected in an entirely different way. For them a small quantity of liquor is not usually adequate. Ever larger quantities at more frequent intervals are needed to relieve their real or fanciful burdens of anxiety.

A purely psychological approach to the problem of alcoholism, however, is insufficient. Alcohol or ethanol, the intoxicating constituent of all alcoholic beverages, is a drug and as such must be considered in terms of its effects on the body. Unfortunately, despite its potential danger, alcohol is the drug that for the alcoholic alleviates the very misery associated with drinking. With it the confirmed drinker feels better, for it blocks out many of the unpleasant symptoms commonly associated with withdrawal of the drug.

Uncontrolled craving for alcohol may well be, at least in part, the result of a metabolic or chemical disorder in the body. Scientific investigators have variously suggested nutritional deficiencies, allergies, disorders of the endocrine (hormone) system, and even neurologic or brain dysfunctions. There may even be some hereditary pattern similar to the predispositions that occur in families for other diseases. These abnormal physiological requirements of the body, coupled with the effects of psychological stress, may work to convert a stable human being into an uncontrolled alcoholic.

371

How does alcoholism show itself?

Even though its cause is not yet known, alcoholism can be identified and treated. Like other diseases it has symptoms, some obvious and others difficult to detect because they can be so cleverly masked. Pain, fever, and swelling directly pinpoint an infectious disease; attacking it, therefore, becomes relatively simple. Unfortunately, alcoholism does not present outward evidence that makes it readily visible in its earliest stages. By the time it is recognized, its severity and complications make treatment more difficult.

The early phases of alcoholism present symptoms so subtle that only the suspicion itself can reinforce the diagnosis. The gentle, considerate person may become angry, hostile, and aggressive with alcohol. The dependable worker may grow progressively unstable and undependable. Changes in attitude toward spouse, children, or friends are at first barely perceptible. The suggestion or accusation that the person is drinking too much is denied or resented. There may be a loss of appetite, a loss of weight, irritability, slurring of speech, or explosions of anger without provocation. During an evening of social drinking such changes

Most people are lucky: they can participate in the social aspects of drinking without suffering damage or alteration of personality.

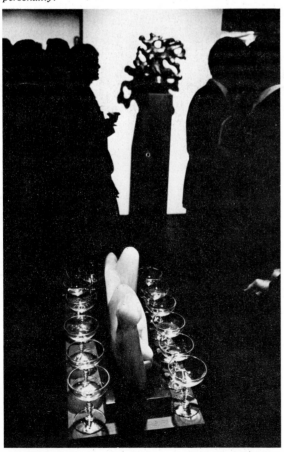

Dan Budnik—Woodfin Camp

become more apparent. When challenged, the drinker may not yet be ready to face the reality that these unpleasant changes of behavior are an important clue to early alcoholism.

The drinker may ingeniously create endless excuses to cover the awareness that a problem exists. The pressures of work, conflicts within the home, and financial difficulties often appear among the rationalizations. If unchecked, the alcoholic soon finds these "straw men" materializing into very real threats. Reflexes are so diminished that normal activity on the job is impossible and automobile driving becomes hazardous. A carelessly handled cigarette may threaten the lives of loved ones or destroy valuable property. Belligerency, so often stimulated by alcohol, frequently erupts into chronic abuse and physical violence.

In the middle phases of alcoholism the victim may become deceptive and try to conceal drinking. Telltale alcoholic breath is sometimes overtly avoided by drinking nearly odorless vodka. When confronted, many alcoholics will concede that some small problem exists but are deluded into believing that they can correct it whenever they want. But personal dignity soon fades, and the alcoholic departs from social grace, caring less and less about the reaction of others. Any offers of help from family or friends become intrusions on privacy. What was before an occasional flare-up of temper becomes flamboyant behavior, full of anger, guilt, self-pity, and despair. It commonly becomes necessary to be thoroughly intoxicated early in the morning in order to face the rigors of the day.

The late phases of alcoholism are characterized by limitless, mostly solitary alcohol intake, which occurs without shame or disguise. The urge to drink is uncontrollable. Deterioration within the heart, the brain, the liver, and other body organs finally reduces the alcoholic to the point of physical incapacitation. Malnutrition, changes in the circulatory system, inflammation of the nerves, and impaired kidney function, coupled with successive drunken binges, eventually result in the need for hospitalization or treatment in a psychiatric institution or a special alcoholism center. Persistent remorse and indefinable anxieties make return to any semblance of normal life impossible.

What can be done to help the alcoholic?

Before there can be any hope of recovery, the alcoholic must take one crucial step: he or she must admit the need for help. It is estimated, however, that only one of every ten alcoholics eventually does so. It is extremely difficult for a person to accept the realization that the problem is alcoholism. All alibis must be exhausted before the inevitable confrontation. When the reality of alcoholism finally is accepted, it usually takes the coordinated drive of family and friends to convince the alcoholic of the need for medical and psychological guidance.

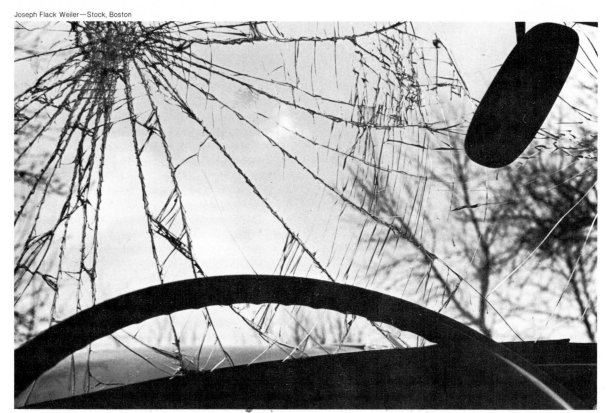

Alcohol and drugs are a dangerous combination. The impairment of coordination and slowing of reflex time that result create a tremendous hazard on the highways.

Alcoholism is not a sign of inadequacy, frailty, or incompetence. When the alcoholic recognizes that addiction to alcohol is not a personal weakness, the feelings of guilt and the attempt to deny the existence of an overwhelming problem disappear. Then, with the knowledge that one's own body defenses are powerless against this affliction comes admission that outside support is essential.

Alcoholism can be treated and controlled, but only by the most persistent and intensive efforts. Once the alcoholic and his family have ceased to pretend that a drinking problem does not exist, consultation with a doctor and with a psychiatrist is the next most important step toward recovery. From then on, management or treatment can be outlined and begun, either in a hospital or at home.

As with any illness, complete understanding by the patient ensures the greatest possibility that the suggested medical treatment will be followed. Unless one has a complete comprehension of heart disease, high blood pressure, or stomach ulcers, one cannot fully appreciate the need for restricted activities, special diets, or the constant use of drugs. Without such understanding, patients often rebel against the limitations imposed on them. When the nature of a problem is completely explained to the patient, however, treatment becomes purposeful rather than punishing.

There was a time when it was believed that all alcoholics needed at least a month of hospitalization to be "dried out," or detoxified. This period has been shortened and, in fact, it is now accepted that not more than 10% of all severe alcoholics need prolonged hospitalization. Nevertheless, a thorough physical examination, including blood studies, urinalysis, and complete profiles of the heart, lungs, liver, and brain, is imperative. The liver undoubtedly reflects to the greatest degree the destructive effect of chronic alcoholism.

During treatment the alcoholic and his family may look for a miracle drug that will totally eradicate the disorder. Although no such drug exists, there is a drug called Antabuse or disulfiram, which works in a strange way. It is not a cure but a substance that causes unpleasant reactions in people who drink alcoholic beverages. Consequently, the person who is given Antabuse is warned that taking even the slightest amount of alcohol while the drug is still in the body can cause violently distressing symptoms of severe nausea, vomiting, and dehydration and even death. Used properly, Antabuse can deter the alcoholic from embarking on a period of drinking.

When intensive treatment is begun, craving for alcohol can sometimes be reduced by the use of tranquilizing drugs. Psychotherapy is extremely supportive to the alcoholic and can offer insight into some of the ramifications of the disease. Assurance, reassurance, and intense interest in the patient establish a firm bond between therapist and patient and offer the greatest chance for recovery.

In recent years the spread of government-sponsored alcoholism centers, the growth of behavioral and family therapy programs directed against alcoholism, and the establishment of halfway houses and rehabilitation techniques have eased the task of the physician and family in helping the alcoholic. Yet despite these developments Alcoholics Anonymous, founded in 1935, remains the cornerstone of efforts in the U.S. to rehabilitate the drinker. With some 200,000 members this dedicated organization is a constant persuasive force generated by people who tirelessly devote themselves to the painful struggle of the alcoholic to regain health, emotional strength, and personal dignity. At AA the family is also indoctrinated. Since alcoholism affects each member of the family, every element in the foundation and total structure of that family must be considered, evaluated, and incorporated into the alcoholic's recovery.

Recently many industrial alcoholism programs have begun to treat alcoholic employees rather than fire them. An alcoholic worker can endanger his own health and safety. Moreover, employee alcoholism is prevalent at all levels. Major industrial firms have estimated that the alcoholic employee loses approximately 22 more working days per year and suffers twice as many accidents as the nonalcoholic. The National Council on Alcoholism (NCA) and the National Institute for Alcohol Abuse and Alcoholism (NIAAA) estimate that 7–10% of the work force are alcoholic. Fortunately, the employer is particularly well suited to intervene. As many as two-thirds of those who undergo treatment are restored to normal job performance.

Can alcoholism be prevented?

Alcoholism can be stamped out or modified in its frequency and destructiveness if its source is assiduously attacked. When does alcoholism begin? Many children today have already started to drink by age 12. The high incidence of alcoholism in high schools and colleges is convincing proof that young people are becoming more and more susceptible.

The child born to a family in which at least one member is an alcoholic has a far greater chance of developing alcoholism than does the child born to a nonalcoholic family. In the light of this finding, the drinking patterns of teenagers and young adults whose families have drinking problems need to be meticulously monitored before the signs of alcohol dependency become evident.

Even those children from nonalcoholic backgrounds present alarming statistics relating to alcoholism. One high school student, in reaching out for help, told the following story of the slow transition from "just tasting" to confirmed dependency on alcohol. "I first tasted beer when I was 12 years old. I hated it. By 13 I loved it. I drank it a lot. I couldn't get enough of it. My parents didn't know why all the beer in the refrigerator disappeared so quickly. I did. They themselves drank so much beer it was hard for them to keep track of it. By the time I was 15 they began to wonder why the vodka bottle always seemed to be empty. They didn't know but I did. Now I'm hooked on alcohol."

So are almost one million other high school and college students in the U.S. who are considered hard-core alcoholics, a number that is rapidly rising. During the past 25 years use of alcohol by college students has increased substantially. Most of these had established their drinking habits in high school.

To compound the problem, it has been noted that the drinking of alcohol is definitely associated with the smoking of cigarettes and marijuana. In a study of more than 8,000 high school students 94% of all illicit drug users were found to have been beer, wine, and hard liquor drinkers. It was shown, too, that students who admitted having been intoxicated during the school year were much more likely to have used marijuana, amphetamines, barbiturates, and LSD.

The interaction between alcohol and other drugs is particularly dangerous. Impairment of coordination by alcohol alone, and especially in combination with other drugs, makes the automobile a lethal weapon. More and more evidence is also coming to light that the pregnant woman who drinks as little as two alcoholic drinks per day may be risking damage to her developing fetus. A large number of serious birth defects, including mental retardation, have been definitely linked to excessive consumption of alcohol during pregnancy.

Of course, little needs to be said about the destructive effects of alcohol even in the nonalcoholic. At the very least, moderate drinking results in impaired thought and judgment. Increasingly heavy consumption disturbs motor coordination, makes clear speech difficult, and greatly increases the risk of accidental injury to the drinker and others. A severe drunken binge can have effects equivalent to surgical anesthesia, including unconsciousness, coma, and even death.

The most successful treatment of alcoholism depends on its recognition and verified diagnosis. Once that diagnosis has been established, it must be communicated to the patient and to his family. Since alcoholism is a family problem, communication with all members of the family is essential. Drugs are available to make the withdrawal period from alcohol less terrifying and less difficult. It is during a period free from alcohol intoxication that psychotherapy and guidance can be most effective. Support by Alcoholics Anonymous and other community-sponsored groups can provide the alcoholic with insight into the magnitude of the problem and the hope for rehabilitation.

— Lester L. Coleman, M.D.

Health Education Unit 15

Cosmetic Surgery

There was a time, not too long ago, when cosmetic surgery was usually reserved for people in the theater and in films and for those prominent people whose features were constantly under scrutiny by the general public. Slowly a transition was made to include among the candidates for such surgery virtually anyone who wanted to improve his or her physical image.

Liking one's self is an important part of personal happiness. For this reason one chooses clothes carefully, maintains a hairstyle meticulously, and artistically applies cosmetics to enhance beauty. It is not surprising, therefore, that cosmetic, or aesthetic, surgery has blossomed into a significant surgical specialty. The secrecy that used to surround a cosmetic operation is more and more being replaced by a casual attitude of frankness and a general acceptance that having cosmetic surgery is just another way of improving one's appearance.

Psychological aspects

An important extension of cosmetic surgery is the better understanding of the psychological needs of the people who seek it. Psychological "reconstruction" is intimately involved in every aspect of this type of plastic surgery.

Initially, the reconstruction of the nose dominated this specialized form of surgery. Later, large and asymmetrical ears became the target. Now aesthetic surgery brings gratifying results in the removal of sagging eyelids, wrinkled cheeks, hanging neck and face tissue, pendulous breasts, and even "saddlebag" thighs. "Stretch marks"—striations of abdominal skin after multiple pregnancies or following marked loss of weight—may be corrected by plastic surgery. Enlargement of the breasts for women can enhance both appearance and state of mind.

All surgery carries with it some risk. Fortunately, cosmetic surgery is usually desired by healthy people who have no special medical problems to contraindicate it. As with all surgery, the choice of the surgeon must never be a haphazard one. The family doctor is usually a primary source of referral. Since the doctor is conversant with the physical and emotional needs of the patient, he is the ideal person to direct his patient to the "ideal" plastic surgeon. Plastic surgeons, after a long period of surgical training, offer their credentials to hospitals, colleagues, and other doctors in the community. A patient choosing a plastic surgeon should consider the doctor's training and hospital affiliations as important criteria.

Unfortunately, their surgical training, elaborate as it

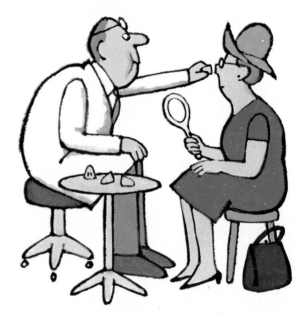

is, is not always commensurate with their understanding of the patient's psychological motivations. Unless the objectives and hopes of the patient are completely evaluated, there is always the danger that the end result of cosmetic surgery will be disappointing.

A hypothetical case illustrates this point. An attractive young woman may have a minor nasal deformity—a crooked nose, with a wide bridge—that induces her to seek surgical reconstruction. However, the crooked nose may not be the only reason for her inner dissatisfaction. There may be an underlying feeling of insecurity or social inadequacy. Her hope is that successful cosmetic surgery will help her make a new social adjustment—that a "perfect nose" will make others like her more and will ultimately bring her happiness. Unless the patient and the doctor frankly and openly examine every detail of the motive for the surgery, the psychological aftermath may be painful. A fine, anatomically correct, well-shaped nose is the surgeon's contribution to her appearance. But when the patient does not find the psychological rebirth and social fulfillment she had expected, a precarious emotional state may result. For years this person may have attributed her failures to the nasal distortion. Now, with a highly improved physical appearance, she may be deprived of the excuse that she had used in the past to account for other deficiencies.

It is becoming more and more obvious to plastic surgeons that the body and mind cannot be separated. No operation can provide the complete solution for emotional turbulence, psychological inadequacy, and lack of social attainment. Some patients whose hopes have not been realized after cosmetic surgery may, in fact, find themselves in a state of severe depression. Some will conclude that the surgery was not adequate; the nose is still not beautiful. All plastic surgeons have

375

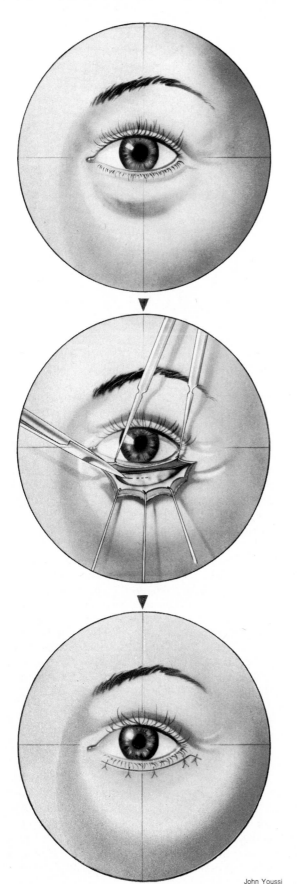

John Youssi

had the experience of a patient begging to have an additional change, perhaps the slightest, barely perceptible elevation of the tip of the nose. The patient is convinced that this might be the answer to his or her frustrations. When a surgeon says he cannot fulfill such expectations, the patient may take the request from doctor to doctor, hoping to find one who will perform the miracle. Others may undergo surgery and never be satisfied, seeking a new surgeon to repair the mistake of the previous one.

Happily, for both surgeons and patients, this experience is the exception rather than the rule. Many patients are delighted with their new, improved appearance, and they flourish socially and in business. The ultimate satisfaction from plastic surgery depends on open discussion of all the physical and emotional ramifications of the operation *before* surgery is undertaken. Sometimes the simple question "Why do you want the operation?" is all that is needed to uncover the feelings that indicate to the surgeon who will be a good candidate for surgery and who will be a risky one. Cases where disfigurement is barely visible must be particularly carefully evaluated.

Who should have cosmetic surgery?

Few areas of surgery have developed so many remarkable, intricate, and ingenious techniques as has the field of cosmetic surgery. The dualities of artistic endeavor and surgical skill are nowhere more important than in the aesthetic remodeling of facial deformities. Some bony structures of the face and some skin textures of the neck lend themselves more than others to successful cosmetic surgery. Patients between the ages of 40 and 60 are usually the most favorable candidates for complete facial repair. But age itself is not the only criterion. Many people over 70 achieve dramatic results, both physical and psychological.

Adolescents seem to have the best prognosis for the total benefits of cosmetic surgery. They are still in a formative stage, and their body image is constantly changing. The outlook is especially good when an adolescent patient has the long-standing feeling that a physical defect has interfered with development of self-esteem, maturity, and body image. Adults tend to have more complicated reasons for cosmetic surgery. Men especially, who comprise about 10% of such patients, may have more deep-seated and more psychologically significant motivations.

Just as there are ideal candidates for surgery, so there are individuals with specific contraindications to

Blepharoplasty corrects the bags under the eyes that give a sleepy expression. An incision is made just under the lower eyelashes through the skin and facial muscle, forming a flap. Excess fat is removed through a series of stab wounds in the orbital septum. The incision is closed with sutures, leaving a smoother contour under the eye and an improved appearance.

it. One problem, for example, that will dissuade a surgeon from operating is the genetic tendency of some people to form thick, unattractive scars known as keloids. Although keloid formation may be minimized by X-ray radiation at the time of surgery, plastic surgeons are hesitant to undertake extensive surgical procedures on those who have a known history of keloids.

Even those who do not have this characteristic cannot always be expected to heal with minimal scarring. There are numerous genetic and metabolic factors that determine how quickly and how perfectly a scar will form. One person may heal with a delicate, barely noticeable scar. Another may heal with a widened scar. Some may bleed more than others, thus delaying the absorption of blood and the ultimate recovery from surgery. Surgeons use similar techniques for most of their patients; yet fine shades of healing differences occur from one patient to another. In all cosmetic surgery the initial incision is made in the natural creases of the skin to make scarring as unnoticeable as possible. But "scarless" surgery simply does not exist.

Common cosmetic operations

Several kinds of cosmetic operations are performed to improve facial features, skin, and body contours. Some of the more common ones are discussed here.

Rhinoplasty, or nasal reconstruction, is probably the most common operation for the repair of facial disfigurement. It is also one of the most surgically demanding procedures. The artistic talent of the surgeon combines with surgical skill to remove a bony hump on the nose, to shorten the nose, or to narrow a thickened, bulbous tip. In addition to effecting fine structural change, the surgeon must attempt to fashion a nose that is in harmony with the rest of the face. Another major objective is to ensure that the nasal reconstruction will not be obvious and thus easily identified as "another nose job." It is also imperative that cosmetic surgery should not interfere with normal breathing through the nose or alter the sense of smell. Frequently, along with rhinoplasty—that is, the external surgery of the nose—a repair is made to the nasal septum, the cartilage that divides one side of the nose from the other. Rhinoplasty is almost always performed under local anesthesia. It is painless and usually can be completed in less than an hour.

Rhytidoplasty, or "face lift," is a technique to remove the wrinkles, furrows, creases, and sagging of the skin that inevitably come with age. The face lift was originally used to correct sagging jowls and the stretching of the skin of the neck. With the realization that such remedies as expensive creams and hormones were totally ineffective came the birth of the idea of surgical intervention.

The operation, which must be performed by a highly skilled surgeon, can produce dramatic results distinctly apparent after a few days. As with all surgery there is

a moderate risk, but advances in modern anesthesiology have reduced such risks to a minimum. Nevertheless, the surgeon and the anesthesiologist make extensive preoperative studies of the total general condition of the patient in order to further reduce the possibility of operative and postoperative complications. The operation almost always is performed under general anesthesia and lasts about two or three hours, depending on the extent of the surgery. Because the incisions are not made in exposed areas, scarring is barely visible. Delicate nerves, tiny blood vessels, and the muscles of the face are handled with exquisite gentleness in order to avoid injury to them. Excess skin on the face and neck is removed with great care so that the postoperative result will not be a too tight, masklike appearance.

Once the operation is performed, there is always the possibility that the continued aging process may make reoperation necessary at a later time. Not to understand this is to mistakenly identify the progressive changes of aging with inadequate or improperly performed surgery.

Blepharoplasty, or repair of eyelids, is an operation that may or may not be done at the same time as the face lift. The blepharoplasty operation is aimed at removing excess skin of the upper and lower eyelids. "Hanging bags" under the eyes, a source of great annoyance to cosmetically conscious people, are removed as part of this procedure.

Mammaplasty, or cosmetic surgery of the breast, is done to enlarge the breasts, to minimize them, and to make them symmetrical. In some instances, as following the removal of a breast for cancer, special operations have been developed to restore the normal contour, obviating the need for artificial padding. Studies have shown that cosmetic operations on the breasts do not increase the possibility of developing breast cancer at a later date.

The reduction of the size of the breasts is particularly important when large, pendulous breasts, besides being disfiguring, cause strain on the muscles of the chest and pain at the back of the neck and shoulders. Such surgery is rarely performed on people who are markedly overweight. Plastic surgeons prefer that the operation be done only after a period of arduous dieting and the attainment of the ideal weight.

Liquid silicone was one of the first substances used for breast enlargement in flat-chested women. The technique was greeted with a great deal of enthusiasm and was thought to be the panacea for a variety of plastic surgical procedures. Unfortunately, liquid silicone proved to be hazardous and caused many severe reactions. It has, therefore, been entirely discontinued for this purpose. Instead, a soft silicone gel is now used, enveloped in a plastic bag so that the silicone itself is not in contact with any of the breast and muscle tissue. Liquid silicone, however, is still used in very small amounts to eradicate tiny facial lines and wrinkles.

The incisions for mammaplasty, both for the reduction and the augmentation of the breast, are made in the crevice beneath the breast. When healing is uncomplicated, the scar is barely visible, and the results are enthusiastically welcomed.

Enlargement of the breast in boys sometimes occurs during puberty and adolescence. The condition, known as *gynecomastia*, is attributed to a hormone imbalance. Usually, with normal growth, gynecomastia is a temporary condition. However, it may be the cause of embarrassment and may produce deep psychological problems. If the enlarged breasts do not return to normal size within a reasonable period of time, a relatively simple surgical procedure can correct the gynecomastia.

Lipectomy, or the repair of double chins, can be easily accomplished by the removal of the fat pad. Lipectomy is usually done at the same time that the total face lift is performed. Receding chins can be built up with bone, cartilage, or synthetic material to offer a fine profile as an end result. As in all cosmetic surgery, the initial incision is made in the natural creases of the skin to make scarring as invisible as possible.

Otoplasty, or correction of the ears, is a simple operation for the reduction and reshaping of floppy or protruding ears. The operation is a safe and painless one. Young boys, in particular, pay a penalty for this anatomical deformity by being teased and unkindly nicknamed. The long hairstyles were a boon to those with this problem, but since hairstyles tend to change, young people may once again find it a source of distress. The operation should be performed before embarrassment leaves its psychological impact. The scars behind the ears are not detectable, and the end result is exceptionally gratifying.

Hair tranplants are a surgical technique for restoration of hair. Baldness, or *alopecia*, is sufficiently distressing that it drives many men in any direction that offers hope. Salves, ointments, hormones, diets, and electric and manual massages have all been tried for male "pattern baldness." There now seems to be acceptance of the concept that this type of baldness has some hereditary factor. The failure of other remedies has led scientists, dermatologists, and plastic surgeons to seek surgical means of solving this problem.

There are several variations in technique by which small plugs of hair, taken from another part of the skull, are implanted into the bald and balding areas. Results are gratifying in some cases, not so in all. The operation is time-consuming because it is done in stages. The transplants are painlessly inserted, usually in the doctor's office, under local anesthesia.

Dermabrasion, or skin planing, is a technique by which the outer layers of the skin are removed. Pitted scars that follow chickenpox, smallpox, or acne are in this way markedly reduced. Electrically driven fine sandpaper or metal brushes smooth out the skin surface and help to obliterate indentations. Scars following injury or surgery can often be improved by this method. Skin specialists as well as plastic surgeons effectively use dermabrasion.

Gnathoplasty, or reduction of the jaw, is another frequently performed cosmetic procedure. The markedly projecting jaw, known as *prognathism*, can now be repaired by removing a segment of jawbone. Lips that are thickened and heavy can be reduced in size by another specialized technique known as *cheiloplasty*.

Operations for recontouring the body—including the correction of sagging abdomen and thick, heavy thighs and buttocks, and the removal of rolls of skin made apparent after marked loss of weight—are now performed with regularity.

Cosmetic surgery must be differentiated from other reconstructive operations in plastic surgery. Burns, birth defects, gunshot wounds, and facial deformities of genetic origin are some of the problems corrected by this extensive specialty. Nowhere in the field of surgery are more intricate and dramatic results attained than in the correction of birth defects and severe injuries.

As in all forms of medicine, plastic surgery must approach the patient as a total human being if the operation is to fulfill its ultimate objective. The plastic surgeon must identify the emotional needs of his patients in order to best help them to realize their aspirations. In this sense cosmetic plastic surgery is rehabilitative surgery.

— Lester L. Coleman, M.D.

What Do You Know About Sex?

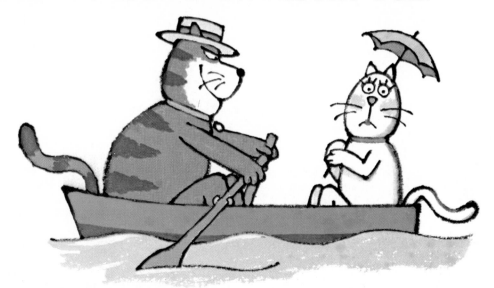

That slightly impertinent question worries a great many people these days. Some of them are perhaps discovering a nostalgic feeling for the days of their great-grandparents, when sexual misinformation commonly prevailed and many happily proclaimed their entire ignorance of the topic. As in most things, however, the only cure for the problems of a little knowledge is more knowledge. And who knows? We may yet all end up peacefully at ease with our own disturbing selves.

1. Sexual problems or difficulties affect about (a) 10, (b) 25, (c) 50, (d) 75% of Americans.

2. A principal cause of sexual difficulty is (a) organic disease, (b) unrealistic expectations, (c) ignorance, (d) overexposure to sexually oriented films, literature, etc.

3. The most common sexual problem for married couples today is (a) satyriasis, (b) impotence, (c) frigidity, (d) lack of sexual desire.

4. The normal frequency of intercourse for women between 30 and 35 years of age is (a) 2 times, (b) 4 times, (c) 12 times, (d) 20 times per month.

5. Homosexuality is almost always a treatable mental aberration—true or false?

6. Confirmed homosexuality usually results from one or two homosexual experiences in childhood or adolescence—true or false?

7. Sexual desire in women usually fades after menopause—true or false?

8. In the average man sexual potency disappears at age (a) 65, (b) 70, (c) 75, (d) 80.

9. Alfred C. Kinsey, the famous sex researcher, was by profession a (a) zoologist, (b) sexologist, (c) psychologist, (d) psychiatrist.

10. Simultaneous orgasm is (a) the ultimate test of compatibility, (b) more likely to result in pregnancy, (c) inconsequential, (d) the result of much practice.

11. The likelihood of any given act of intercourse resulting in pregnancy is about (a) 84, (b) 56, (c) 24, (d) 6%.

12. The mechanism by which the IUD (intrauterine device) prevents conception is unknown—true or false?

13. "Tubal ligation" is (a) the implantation of a fertilized ovum in the fallopian tube, (b) a form of gynecological examination, (c) a method of sterilization, (d) a procedure used to hasten a difficult labor.

14. The consensus among sex researchers now holds that the vaginal orgasm is more fundamentally satisfying than the clitoral—true or false?

15. The percentage of women who regularly achieve orgasm during intercourse is about (a) 30, (b) 50, (c) 70, (d) 90.

16. Impotence in men is usually traceable to physical causes such as disease, alcohol, or medication—true or false?

17. The "double standard" of allowing or condoning premarital or extramarital sexual relations on the part of males but not females is peculiar to Western societies—true or false?

18. Alcohol is a sexual stimulant—true or false?

19. Intercourse is safe during the first trimester of pregnancy, allowable with proper precautions during the second, and hazardous during the third—true or false?

20. Males do not undergo menopause—true or false?

21. Sexual fantasies, especially during sexual activity, are indicative of sexual immaturity or pathology—true or false?

22. The human female is not unique among species in having a menstrual cycle—true or false?

379

Answers

1. (c). Half of us, in some degree.

2. (b). Pressure to perform in certain ways and to measure up to certain unfounded standards derived from popular myth is one of the most common causes of sexual problems.

3. (d). According to psychiatrist Helen Singer Kaplan of the New York Hospital at Cornell University, this problem is complicated by the reluctance of people to admit it.

4. None of the above. There is no "normal" figure for either sex or any age. The range of actual frequencies is very wide and varies greatly with changing circumstances even for single individuals. If you missed this one, go back to question 2.

5. False. Certain forms of therapy, such as psychotherapy, hypnosis, and aversion training, have succeeded in changing homosexual behavior in a small number of cases only. It is not clear that homosexuality is a condition to be "cured" in any case, nor that most homosexuals would wish to be cured.

6. False. A great many, perhaps a majority of persons, have such experiences. Genuine homosexuality stems from much deeper roots.

7. False. It remains relatively constant.

8. None of the above. With good health it need not disappear.

9. (a). His main subject of study before coming to human sexual behavior was the gall wasp.

10. (c). The idea seems to have arisen among writers of prurient fiction and been accepted by uncounted and otherwise content victims.

11. (d). However, the likelihood does exist for even a single act.

12. True. It may in some way prevent a fertilized ovum from implanting in the uterine wall.

13. (c). It refers to the tying closed of the ducts by which ova descend from the ovaries.

14. False. The consensus is now that the distinction between them has no basis in fact.

15. (a). This is not to say that the other 70% don't at all, but that additional clitoral stimulation before, during, or after intercourse may be necessary.

16. False. Each of these may be the cause in any given case, but their incidence is small compared with the major cause, anxiety in one form or another.

17. False. It is very common throughout the world and is characteristic of perhaps a majority of societies.

18. False. Alcohol is a depressant and even in moderate quantities can inhibit sexual responsiveness. It is a common cause of temporary male impotence. Its undue reputation doubtless stems from its supposed utility in seduction.

19. False. Intercourse and other sexual activities (not unduly strenuous) are safe throughout pregnancy.

20. True. In the literal sense there is no "male menopause." But the male can experience a variety of symptoms that have been recognized as the *male climacteric.* These include fatigue, depression, impotence, asocial behavior, and even hot flashes, and in general they appear over a much longer span of years than in women. Studies have shown a gradual decline in the production of testosterone in men starting in the fifth decade of life; this is accompanied by a gradual rise in the pituitary hormone FSH. Many men, however, experience no symptoms and, as a rule, fewer consequences—psychological and physical—occur in men than in women.

21. False. In fact, they are virtually universal.

22. True. The great apes, the Old World monkeys, and possibly the elephant shrew also discharge blood from the uterus at regular intervals.

—Robert McHenry

Hyperactive Children

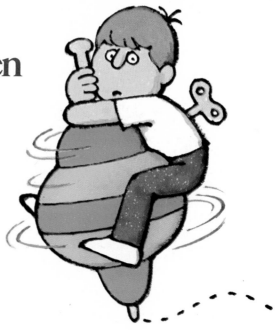

It is estimated that 5% of all schoolchildren suffer from hyperactivity, or hyperkinesis, and from learning disabilities. Three-fourths of this total are boys. The hyperactive child is usually of average intelligence but has learning or behavioral difficulties that range from mild to severe. In addition, various combinations of defects in perception, conceptualization, language, memory, control, attention, and impulse may be present. And, finally, there usually are defects in the child's motor function.

The entire subject of hyperactivity is complicated and confusing. Over 40 different terms have been used to describe this group of children, including hyperkinetic child, hyperactive child, minimal brain injury, dyslexia, and maturation lag. This behavioral-learning defect syndrome is now gradually becoming known as minimal brain dysfunction (MBD), a term first used by neuropsychiatrist Alfred Strauss in 1940. The apparent recent increase in the frequency of this condition is probably due to the increased sophistication of physicians, educators, and parents in suspecting the diagnosis rather than an actual increase in the numbers of cases.

Diagnosing MBD

How can one recognize a child with MBD? Hyperactivity may be the first symptom noticed—it is the most readily recognized symptom of MBD. The child often is so hyperactive that it is virtually impossible for him to maintain any semblance of control over his behavior. This continuous nonstop motor activity is usually impulsive and purposeless. An MBD child often has poor muscle coordination and is described as being clumsy. He may have trouble tying his shoelaces, throwing a ball, or buttoning his shirt. Still other MBD children have a great deal of trouble learning to read or write. Their very short attention spans make it difficult to communicate with them. The MBD youngster may be prone to temper tantrums and emotional lability, being calm and happy one minute and violent and angry the next. The problem in diagnosis is that each MBD child is different from the next. Unfortunately, there is no one sure sign or symptom that can be used to make a definite diagnosis. As a result, many children are not diagnosed soon enough, while many others are incorrectly labeled as having MBD. A child may be active, mischievous, curious, and continually looking for new adventures. If this is the only "problem" he has, he obviously does not have MBD. Parents may suspect trouble, but they should never attempt to make the actual diagnosis, which is always best left to the experts. It should be emphasized that most children with learning disabilities do not have MBD, nor do most very active children.

Since the proper diagnosis and subsequent treatment of MBD is so important for the well-being of the child, it is important that the correct diagnosis be made as early as possible. An untreated MBD child rapidly becomes severely handicapped in both his educational and social development. If a parent suspects that a child may have this syndrome, a doctor should be consulted and allowed to proceed from there. The diagnosis may require not only the physician but also the help of teachers, learning disability specialists, neurologists, and psychologists. This multidisciplinary approach may be necessary not only to establish the diagnosis but to plan proper treatment as well.

Although there are many theories as to its origins, the cause or causes of MBD are not known. There is frequently a history of a difficult labor or delivery, and many MBD children are born prematurely, but most MBD children with this diagnosis are full-term and delivered normally. A genetic factor has been implicated, since learning disabilities occasionally appear to run in families. However, identical twin studies do not bear out this theory, since there are many reported cases of one identical twin having MBD while the other is unaffected. Low blood sugar or a biochemical abnormality have both been blamed, but these charges are also unsubstantiated. In recent years there has been much publicity about a non-food-additive diet that is said to cure many hyperactive children. Proponents of this special diet believe that the various additives in many foods are the cause of MBD symptoms.

It is important to emphasize that the MBD child is *not* mentally retarded, nor does he have cerebral palsy or epilepsy. Put in the simplest terms, MBD should be considered a disorder of the central nervous system that in some as yet unknown way adversely affects the child and does not allow him to function and learn at the usual rate and manner. There is a delay in the mental maturation process.

In the toddler one of the first signs of MBD is excessive motor activity. Mothers report that these children always are in "trouble," "getting into things," having accidents, and they often wander away from home. They are always on the move and just don't seem to understand the meaning of the word *no*. Many preschool age children who later are diagnosed as definitely having MBD have a history of impulsiveness, temper tantrums, and short attention span. They often are poorly coordinated and nonathletic, and many also have sleep problems. Another early feature is that they start talking later than the average child. If a toddler or preschooler appears to fit this type of behavior pattern, it would be wise to consult a pediatrician or family practitioner about it.

Most MBD children are diagnosed after they have started school. The usual story is that of a child who

Liveliness should not be confused with hyperactivity, or minimal brain dysfunction. This complex problem can be diagnosed only by careful analysis by a trained specialist.

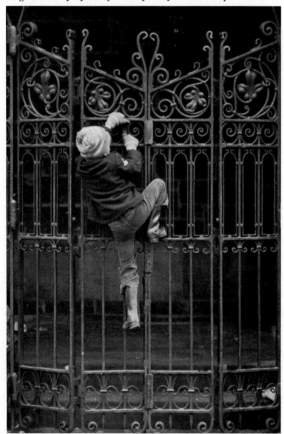

Mike Mazzaschi—Stock, Boston

cannot learn to read or to solve conceptual or abstract problems. The school-age child with MBD usually does better in memory work such as spelling and multiplication but has trouble understanding and following instructions. All these difficulties contribute to his school failure. Since he is continually at odds with his teachers, he remains under increasing emotional stress and tension. His classmates often ridicule him, and this, of course, aggravates his emotional problems. In addition to difficulty in school work, the MBD child is also often hyperactive and erratic in his behavior. This combination of traits causes chaos in the classroom and presents the teacher with a number of frustrations and problems.

Treating the hyperactive child

Once the diagnosis of MBD is established, treatment should be started as soon as possible. The management of this condition is complex and requires a multifaceted approach. There are three proven methods of treatment: family counseling, remedial education, and the use of drugs. All cases of MBD require both family counseling and remedial education programs, and many of the children with MBD also require some form of drug therapy.

Family counseling. Too often parents faced with coping with a child with MBD respond with guilt and anxiety and wrongly assume that they are at fault and the cause of the problem. This erroneous belief must be completely dispelled before any effective management can be started. The cause of this syndrome remains unknown. The delay in the maturation of the child's central nervous system is unrelated to the parents. Unfortunately, the child with MBD often begins to see himself as unworthy, unloved, and inadequate. Since he is continually in trouble at home, in school, and with his friends, his self-esteem is steadily and continually being eroded. Parents must be counseled to keep this in mind and must be advised to use praise whenever possible and emphasize successful activities rather than constantly criticizing and finding fault. This advice is not easy to follow, but it is vital in order to help build up the self-confidence of the MBD child. Parents should try to take short periodic vacations away from the child if at all possible. These breaks in the daily routine can help to reduce the many anxieties and frustrations that can be involved in the struggle to effectively treat children who have MBD.

Parents should make every attempt to establish a structured, calm routine in the home. Both parents must be consistent in their approach to the child. Tasks should be presented only one at a time in order to reduce the tension on the child, who, although he is trying so hard to please, cannot overcome his handicaps overnight. It is important for parents to provide him with a quiet room, free from distractions, for his homework. Most authorities in this field agree that tu-

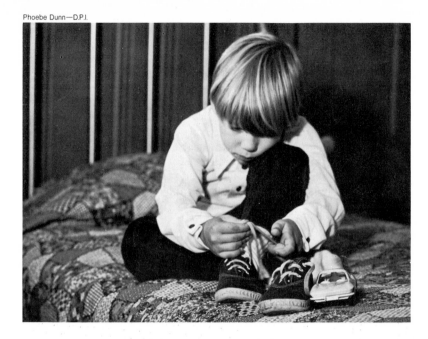

Phoebe Dunn—D.P.I.

In addition to his ceaseless, uncontrolled activity, the hyperactive child may have learning disabilities and be poorly coordinated.

toring should be left to the professionals rather than to the parents.

During the past few years great strides have been made in helping parents improve the behavior of MBD children. Much of this success is due to the use of a set of basic learning principles called behavior modification. The basic concept of this approach is a system of rewards and punishments—good behavior is rewarded and undesirable behavior punished. To this is added the principle of imitative learning, with the underlying rationale that an individual can learn by observing others. The behavior modification technique is very effective in helping the MBD child learn socially acceptable behavior.

A discussion of proper family counseling techniques would not be complete without stating that, although the ideal is difficult to achieve, it is extremely important for the parents to do everything they can to provide a warm, affectionate, loving, and accepting environment for their child.

Remedial education. Persistent failure in school is one of the most damaging situations that the MBD child faces. Special education that is begun early goes a long way toward improving the ultimate outcome. The quality of the special remedial education program is most important.

It is not within the scope of this article to discuss in detail all the special educational program possibilities and the wide variety of techniques involving motor, sensory, and visual training programs that may be available in each community or school system. There is no question that remedial education is the cornerstone for proper treatment of MBD. Specific class placement should be determined by the teachers and educational consultants according to the type and se-

verity of the disorder and the available educational resources in the community. Many schools have established special learning disability classes. Others have part-time tutorial programs, and still others have so-called resource rooms, which are separate classrooms set aside for special teaching. The MBD child needs all the remedial education he can get, and it is mandatory for the parents to find out exactly what resources are available in their community. The goal of any education program is to help guide the child in acquiring the knowledge, skills, and emotional adjustment he needs to relate successfully to himself and to the world and to allow him to reach his optimum in becoming a self-sufficient, functioning adult.

Drug therapy. The use of drugs is not indicated for all children with MBD. However, if family counseling, behavior modification techniques, and remedial education programs are found to be insufficient in managing the child, medication may well be indicated. A number of drugs have been found to be useful in reducing the hyperactivity and in prolonging the attention span of the MBD child. The physician may decide to give the child a therapeutic trial with one of these medications, which very often is found to be effective and becomes an integral part of the overall treatment. Some of the commonly prescribed drugs are Ritalin, Dexedrine, Benzedrine, and Cylert, which are stimulants. Paradoxically, the administration of a stimulant to an already overstimulated child somehow calms and slows down the child. It is interesting to note that giving a sedative to an MBD child acts just in the opposite way and stimulates and excites him. There are some complicated neurophysiologic theories that attempt to explain this peculiar paradoxical response. While some children tend to show dramatic improvement after the administration of such medications, some pediatricians are becoming concerned about the possible unwanted side effects. It must always be remembered that these are potent drugs with possible toxic effects, and they must always be carefully administered under the strict supervision of a physician. Stimulant drugs generally should not be used in children under six years old. Many MBD children are maintained on drug treatment for long periods of time, often for many years. It has been recommended that a child receiving drugs for hyperactive symptoms be taken off the medication periodically in order to assess the condition.

There has been much recent publicity about a dramatic new method of treating MBD. The food-additive-free diet developed by Benjamin Feingold of Kaiser-Permanente Medical Center (San Francisco) is claimed to markedly improve the functioning of 40 to 50% of the children with MBD. The proponents of this diet, which eliminates all artificial flavors, colorings, and other food additives, are most enthusiastic and vocal about its effectiveness. However, to date controlled studies have largely failed to substantiate these claims, and additional investigations are in progress. Basically this diet, called the K-P diet (Kaiser-Permanente), eliminates most fruits, luncheon meats, hot dogs, sausage, jams, chewing gum, candies, oleomargarine, ice creams containing artificial flavors and coloring agents, and soft drinks. Since this diet is basically nutritious, there appears to be no objection to trying it out for a week or two in order to see whether or not it calms the youngster down. It requires a great deal of time and trouble for the parents to keep their MBD child on this diet, so the question yet to be answered is whether the improvement noted in some of these children is due to the extra attention they are given in the monitoring of each and every mouthful of food they consume or actually is due to the elimination of the additives.

There is little reliable information about the long-term prognosis of MBD. The variability of the handicaps complicates the problem of predicting the outcome. Everybody agrees that early recognition and treatment improve the outlook. A poor parent-child relationship in a disrupted or chaotic family structure usually will result in a less favorable outcome. A normal intelligence quotient is a good prognostic sign. Successfully controlling the hyperkinetic behavior that impairs the child's ability to interact successfully with his peers and to function well in school certainly will improve the overall prognosis. Most children with MBD learn to read and to master basic mathematics, although they remain relatively weak in these areas. On the other hand, the majority of these children complete high school and many go on to college. While it is true that their learning disabilities tend to damage their self-esteem, as adults they tend to compensate and even overcompensate and often become hard and effective workers. Most MBD children experience substantial improvement by 12 years of age. The adolescent MBD child still may be restless and impulsive and have difficulty in concentrating, but he usually has fewer problems in school and in his peer relationships. With adequate family counseling, remedial education programs, and the use of medication, these children can be helped dramatically. The overall prognosis is good. It takes a great deal of patience, understanding, and hard work, but the stakes are so high that it is well worth the effort.

The following is a selection of books available on the subject of hyperactive children:

Alabiso, Frank P., and Hansen, James C. *The Hyperactive Child in the Classroom*. Springfield, Ill.: Charles C. Thomas, 1977.

Bittinger, Marvin L., ed. *Living with Our Hyperactive Children*. New York: BPS Books, 1977.

Bosco, James J., and Robin, Stanley S., eds. *The Hyperactive Child and Stimulant Drugs*. Chicago: University of Chicago Press, 1977.

Feingold, Benjamin F. *Why Your Child Is Hyperactive*. New York: Random House, 1975.

Millichap, J. Gordon. *The Hyperactive Child with Minimal Brain Dysfunction*. Chicago: Year Book Medical Publishers, 1975.

Minde, K. A. *A Parent's Guide to Hyperactivity*. New York: J. Norton, 1972.

Ross, Dorothea M., and Ross, Sheila A. *Hyperactivity: Research, Theory, and Action*. New York: John Wiley & Sons, 1976.

Stewart, Mark A., and Olds, Sally W. *Raising a Hyperactive Child*. New York: Harper and Row, 1973.

Sugarman, Gerald I., and Stone, Margaret N. *Your Hyperactive Child*. Chicago: Henry Regnery Co., 1974.

—Alvin N. Eden, M.D.

Living Wills and Organ Donation

The growing focus on death and dying in medical and psychiatric research has yielded fresh and valuable information. Widespread publication of these findings has in turn initiated a gradual change in our attitudes about death.

Until this recent change, we had shunned the direct mention and contemplation of death, as if by mentally and verbally avoiding it, we might ignore it. A measure of the change is reflected in the current addenda of courses on death to many elementary and high school curricula. Medical schools, which for years approached death from a purely physiological standpoint, are becoming increasingly concerned with the social and psychological problems of the terminally ill. It seems that we are finally laying to rest our squeamishness about death. In short, we are finally learning to live with death.

Living Wills

Ironically, just as we are coming to terms with our own mortality, the definition of death has, for technological reasons, become more elusive. Those who in earlier eras of medical science would have succumbed naturally and rapidly to disease or accident can now be kept alive, often indefinitely and in a coma, with drugs and mechanical life-support systems. For some these medical advances represent a welcome extension of life. For others the artificial maintenance of life is a cruel and unwelcome invasion of individual privacy. The growing community of those who insist upon the right to die naturally and with dignity is now voicing its wishes in a document called a Living Will. This document requests, in the event that illness or accident leaves the signer without reasonable hope of physical or mental recovery and without a mode of self-expression, that no "artificial means or 'heroic measures'" be used to keep the individual alive.

Although not legally binding, the Living Will is nonetheless widely recognized throughout the United States. To ensure the effectiveness of the will, it is recommended that you sign and date it before two witnesses and that copies of the document be given to your personal physician and to your family, who should be fully informed of your wishes concerning your own death. Further information and a copy of the Living Will, as well as a condensed, wallet-sized version, can be obtained by writing to:

Euthanasia Educational Council
250 W. 57th Street
New York, N.Y. 10019

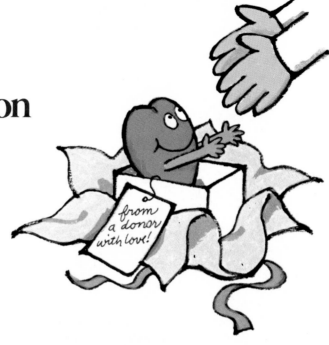

Organ donation: living legacies

For those who confront it squarely, death can afford a final moment in which to reaffirm life. The body that we now inhabit becomes in death an ephemeral vessel storing a host of vital organs and tissues that can literally restore another to life and health or enable invaluable advances in medical research.

Under the Uniform Anatomical Gift Act, now effective in every state, the donation after death of all or parts of one's body can readily be made by an individual or by his or her family. Such generous anatomical gifts are fundamental to medical research and an essential tool in the training of new physicians and dentists. Their value to individual transplant recipients is incalculable. Cornea transplants, for example, can restore sight to the blind. Healthy kidneys offer new hope to renal dialysis patients. Hormonal extracts from the pituitary gland yield the necessary stimulus for growth to thousands of hormonally deficient children. Skin can be used for dressing or grafting in severe burn cases, and blood can provide life-saving transfusions. Bone, tendons, fascia (tissue covering the muscles), heart valves, dura (the membrane covering the brain), and cartilage are also transplantable; and the heart, lung, liver, pancreas, and bone marrow are now being experimentally transplanted.

Although the number of organ transplants is increasing each year, there are still far more patients awaiting organs than there are organs available. This situation results in part from the fact that many people simply do not make known their willingness to donate. Unlike in some European countries, U.S. physicians are unable to routinely remove for transplant healthy, vitally needed organs from patients who have died. In the European countries in point, one is considered a donor un-

385

TO MY FAMILY, MY PHYSICIAN, MY LAWYER, MY CLERGYMAN
TO ANY MEDICAL FACILITY IN WHOSE CARE I HAPPEN TO BE
TO ANY INDIVIDUAL WHO MAY BECOME RESPONSIBLE FOR MY HEALTH, WELFARE OR
AFFAIRS

Death is as much a reality as birth, growth, maturity and old age—it is the one certainty of life. If the time comes when I, _____ can no longer take part in decisions for my own future, let this statement stand as an expression of my wishes, while I am still of sound mind.

If the situation should arise in which there is no reasonable expectation of my recovery from physical or mental disability, I request that I be allowed to die and not be kept alive by artificial means or "heroic measures". I do not fear death itself as much as the indignities of deterioration, dependence and hopeless pain. I, therefore, ask that medication be mercifully administered to me to alleviate suffering even though this may hasten the moment of death.

This request is made after careful consideration. I hope you who care for me will feel morally bound to follow its mandate. I recognize that this appears to place a heavy responsibility upon you, but it is with the intention of relieving you of such responsibility and of placing it upon myself in accordance with my strong convictions, that this statement is made.

Signed _____

Date _____

Witness _____

Witness _____

Copies of this request have been given to _____

_____

_____

_____

This is a sample of a Living Will, a document that directs the decisions of persons who might be called on when an individual is no longer able to make his own decisions. In the event of irreversible illness or injury from which there is no hope of recovery, the signer requests that he or she will not be kept alive through artificial, mechanical means. Copies of this will are available from the Euthanasia Educational Council, whose address is given on the previous page.

less he or she, or the family, has expressly stipulated otherwise. In the U.S. just the opposite is true: the individual or his or her family must give prior permission for organ donation. Hence, if you wish to bequeath anatomical gifts, it is important to make provisions to do so. Whatever the specific arrangements, you should fully inform your family and close friends of your wishes. You should additionally inform your physician of your plans in writing and, if you have made a will, specify these intentions therein.

If you wish to donate your body for medical research, you should contact the anatomy department of the medical school nearest you for further information. Note that medical schools will not accept bodies that have been embalmed, autopsied, or from which organs, other than the eyes, have been removed for donation. Hence, a funeral with a display of the embalmed body precludes donation of the body for research. Similarly, if you wish to bequeath individual organs or tissues, you will be unable to donate your body for research. It should also be noted that bodies, organs, and tissues may only be given, not sold, and that medical schools are under no obligation to accept anatomical gifts. Rather medical schools take bodies only as they are needed, and thus a generously offered anatomical gift may be refused if there is no need.

Arrangements for transportation of the body and related expenses vary from school to school. In general medical schools dispose of the remains of bodies given for research by cremation and, if requested, will return the ashes to the family; the bodies of organ donors are usually returned to the family for burial or cremation.

Removal of an organ or tissue for donation is a simple medical procedure that does no more harm to the body than the process of embalming. Funeral display of the body, if desired, is in no way affected by organ or tissue removal. If you wish to bequeath individual organs or tissues (though you cannot specify the recipient), you may contact either the national headquarters or local branches of specialized organ banks, one of the growing number of multiorgan banks, or one of the clearing house organizations that coordinate the bequeathal of a variety of anatomical gifts.

Specialized Organ Banks

Ear: The Deafness Research Foundation
366 Madison Avenue
New York, N.Y. 10017

National Temporal Bone Banks Center
Johns Hopkins University
Baltimore, Md. 21205

Eye: Eye-Bank Association of America*
3195 Maplewood Avenue
Winston-Salem, N.C. 27103

TO MY FAMILY, MY PHYSICIAN AND ANY HOSPITAL

If there is no reasonable expectation of my recovery from physical or mental disability . . .

I request that I be allowed to die and not be kept alive by artificial means and heroic measures. I ask that medication be mercifully administered to me for terminal suffering even if it hastens the moment of death.

I hope that you who care for me will feel morally bound to act in accordance with this urgent request.

_____
SIGNATURE

This condensed, wallet-sized version of the Living Will on the preceding page can be easily carried and will be discovered in case of accident.

Kidney: National Kidney Foundation*
116 E. 27th Street
New York, N.Y. 10016

Pituitary: National Pituitary Agency*
Suite 503–7
210 W. Fayette Street
Baltimore, Md. 21201

Multiorgan Banks and Donor Clearing Houses

Northern California Transplant Bank
751 S. Bascom Avenue
San Jose, Calif. 95128   (408) 998-4550
   (408) 289-8200 (24-hour emergency)

Living Bank*
P.O. Box 6725
Houston, Texas 77005   (713) 528-2971

Medic-Alert*
1000 N. Palm Street
Turlock, Calif. 95380   (209) 632-2371

The Tissue Bank
Naval Medical Research Institute
NNMC
Bethesda, Md. 20014   (202) 295-1121

Contact one of the organizations listed above, your physician, or a medical school or hospital near you to inquire about donor organizations in your area.

UNIFORM DONOR CARD

OF _____

Print or Type name of donor

In the hope that I may help others, I hereby make this anatomical gift, if medically acceptable, to take effect upon my death. The words and marks below indicate my desires.

I give: (a) _____ any needed organs or parts

(b) _____ only the following organs or parts

_____

Specify the organ(s) or part(s)

for the purposes of transplantation, therapy, medical research or education;

(c) _____ my body for anatomical study if needed.

Limitations or
special wishes, if any: _____

Signed by the donor and the following two witnesses in the presence of each other:

_____ _____
Signature of Donor   Date of Birth of Donor

_____ _____
Date Signed   City & State

_____ _____
Witness   Witness

This is a legal document under the Uniform Anatomical Gift Act or similar laws.

For further information consult your physician or

American Medical Association
535 N. Dearborn, Chicago, Ill. 60610

This is a sample of a Uniform Donor Card, directing the prompt and efficient utilization of organs for transplant. It is simply carried by the signer. Copies are available by writing to the addresses on this page and the preceding page.

Uniform Donor Card

The Uniform Donor Card represents another effort to coordinate and facilitate the collection of anatomical gifts. The card, when signed, is a legally binding document throughout the U.S. under the Uniform Anatomical Gift Act. The card permits the donor to specify whether the entire body or just certain organs and tissues are to be donated and whether they are to be used for medical research or for transplant. The donor may also indicate any special wishes or stipulations regarding the donation.

The card should be filled out, and signed and dated in the presence of two witnesses. Family, friends, and your physician should be notified of your wishes, but the card should not be sent to anyone. Instead, the card should be carried in your wallet as it must be available at the time of death. In the event that, after signing the card, you later decide against being a donor, you need only destroy the card. Acceptance of the anatomical gifts offered through the Uniform Donor Card is similarly dependent upon the circumstances and locale of the donor's death.

* The Uniform Donor Card may be obtained, free of charge, from the above-listed organizations and additionally from:

American Medical Association
535 N. Dearborn Street
Chicago, Ill. 60610

— *Christine Timmons*

Glaucoma and Cataracts

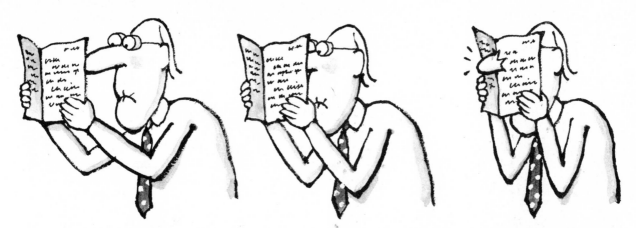

The ability to see is often taken for granted. Only when some threat to vision occurs does panic erupt and persist during the anxious attempts to save sight. The key to the preservation of vision lies in the early detection of visual disturbances and in the determination of their causes. Once the underlying reason for impaired sight is found, intensive treatment can almost always prevent its progression.

There is cause for hope for victims of eye disease within the framework of modern medicine and surgery. Far too often a person delays by months his visit to the ophthalmologist or eye specialist for fear of learning that he may be losing his sight. It is just such procrastination that perpetuates unnecessary anxiety and allows eye diseases to do irreparable damage.

When a person finally decides to go to the "eye doctor," he should know what kind of practitioner to contact. An *ophthalmologist* (or *oculist*) is a physician who has taken a full program of medical studies along with specialized study of eye diseases and visual disorders; he may diagnose a condition and treat it medically or surgically. An *optometrist* is licensed to examine the eyes and prescribe corrective eyeglasses and exercises. An *optician* fills prescriptions for visual aids such as eyeglasses. For serious conditions such as glaucoma and cataracts and for complete treatment of the eyes one should contact an ophthalmologist.

Glaucoma and cataracts are two of the most common maladies of the eye and the most frequent causes of blindness. It has been estimated that nearly two million people in the U.S. 35 years of age and older have glaucoma to some degree and that nearly three million people of all ages experience some form of vision impairment from cataracts. Of Americans living in 1976, 66,000 had lost their sight to glaucoma and more than 78,000 to age-related, or senile, cataracts. These two diseases are not infections, contagious diseases, or cancers. Most cases of blindness due to glaucoma and cataracts are preventable. Glaucoma can be treated medically and surgically; cataracts can be removed by surgery. There is no relationship between the two conditions. Should these both be present in one person, it must be considered coincidental.

When these axioms are understood, distressing fears can be eliminated. A person who understands the true nature of an illness or a physical disorder such as glaucoma or cataracts is more likely to cooperate with his physician or surgeon and to adhere to planned programs of treatment. Conversely, when a person is confused about his illness, he tends to depart from fixed regimens of treatment.

How the eye functions

The normal human eyeball is a nearly spherical, fluid-filled sac with opaque walls and a transparent window called the cornea. Behind the cornea is an inner space called the aqueous chamber, which is divided into a larger, anterior portion and a smaller, posterior portion by the iris, the colored part of the eye. In the middle of the iris is a hole called the pupil, which can expand and contract to let in varying amounts of light. The aqueous chamber is separated from yet another compartment, a large rear cavity called the vitreous chamber, by a clear lens that lies a little behind the iris. Lining the inside back of this rear chamber is the retina, an arrangement of light-sensitive nerve cells.

When light from an object enters the eye, it is focused by the lens (and to some degree by the cornea) into an inverted image of the object on the retina. Almost instantly the retinal cells convert this image into electrical impulses that are carried by the optic nerve to a small region of the brain associated with vision. The brain then decodes these impulses to form a mental image of the object that later can be recalled and

389

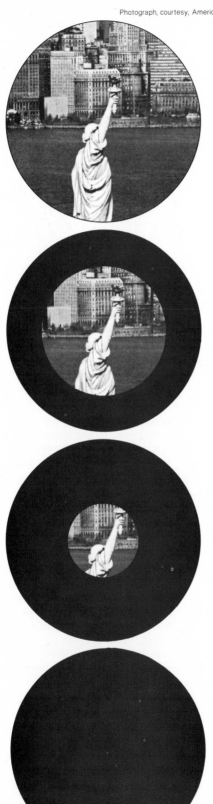

Photograph, courtesy, American Airlines

distinguished from millions of other complex images.

The crystal clear lens, a tiny oval body about one-eighth of an inch thick and convex on both surfaces, can adjust for near and far vision. Tiny muscles (called ciliary muscles) and ligaments attached to the edges of the lens gently but efficiently stretch or relax it in order to bring objects into sharp focus. In the elderly both the muscles and the lens lose some of their flexibility and elasticity and cause a farsighted condition known as presbyopia. Presbyopia is not responsible for blindness and can be corrected easily with ordinary or bifocal glasses. The same holds true for nearsightedness, or myopia.

Glaucoma

Just as the outer surface of the eye is cleansed by tears, so must the inside of the eye be cleansed and nourished by fluid. In particular, the cornea and lens, which have no blood supply of their own, need this regenerative fluid action. The aqueous chamber, with one portion adjacent to the cornea and the other adjacent to the lens, contains a clear watery fluid that is constantly being manufactured by membranous tissue associated with the ciliary muscles. At regular intervals this fluid empties through a tiny tube, the canal of Schlemm. It is by this process that the pressure of fluid within the eye is maintained at a constant level. When something interrupts this circulation so that fluid within the eye begins to increase, tension mounts and early evidence of the condition known as glaucoma appears.

The large vitreous chamber of the eye contains the vitreous body, another kind of fluid, which is thick and has the consistency of gelatin. In the healthy eye both fluids remain at normal pressure. When glaucoma occurs and goes untreated, however, excess pressure in the aqueous chamber is transmitted to the vitreous body and then to the retina at the back of the eyeball. The pressure compresses blood vessels that supply the retinal nerves, causing some nerve fibers to die from deficient blood supply, and part of the retina becomes useless, resulting in permanent blindness in that segment of the eye.

There is a mistaken notion that the increased pressure of glaucoma is related to high blood pressure, or hypertension. No such relationship exists. Many people with a family history of glaucoma live in terror that they are also inevitable candidates for the same disorder. Although this is not necessarily so, it is recommended that those people have regular checkups to ensure early recognition of glaucoma.

Untreated glaucoma may lead to blindness. This series of photographs illustrates the diminished field of vision as glaucoma progresses. The first photograph is the field of vision of a person with normal eyesight. The final stage of the progress of glaucoma is a total loss of sight.

Fortunately there are highly sophisticated instruments, called tonometers, by which the slightest elevation of pressure within the eyeball can be immediately recognized. One touch to the eyeball by a tonometer probe during an office visit to the ophthalmologist or optometrist is all that is needed for a measurement. Once the presence of glaucoma is established, examinations at regular intervals can follow any increases in pressure that may affect vision.

It is difficult to diagnose glaucoma solely on the basis of subjective early symptoms. Definitive signs may be absent entirely until the advanced stages of the disease. When symptoms are present they are often confusing and may induce anxieties about a problem that really does not exist. Therefore, when there are intermittent periods of blurred or oddly colored vision or pains in and behind the eye, or when prescribed eyeglasses are no longer satisfactory, a visit to the ophthalmologist is essential. By bringing unusual experiences to the attention of the eye specialist, a patient guards against delayed recognition of the existence of glaucoma or any other eye condition.

Treatment of glaucoma depends on its exact nature and the particular type of glaucoma that is present. Not all cases of glaucoma demand surgery for control. In some instances special eye drops are remarkably effective in reducing increased pressure. Other drugs produce the same effect when taken by mouth. Since glaucoma does not improve spontaneously, use of drops and drugs may be necessary for months or years. During this time it is imperative that there be no interruption of regular visits to the eye doctor.

When despite the use of eye drops excess pressure within the eyeball persists, and when there is any evidence of sudden or prolonged loss of vision, surgery is considered. In many cases the increased pressure is due to a condition in which the outer rim of the iris has moved too close to the wall of the eyeball, so as to cover the outlet to the canal of Schlemm. To correct this problem a simple, safe, and painless operation called an iridectomy is often performed. A small piece of the colored portion of the eye, the iris, is removed near its outer margin. As a result the accumulated fluid can reach the canal of Schlemm more readily, lessening the chance of compression damage to the nervous structures responsible for normal vision. Other, less common causes of fluid blockage can also be treated surgically.

The essence of preservation of sight in glaucoma is prevention of the progress of the disease. Many patients with early glaucoma carry with them identification cards that indicate the nature of the condition and the drops that are being used. In any emergency this information is of great importance to the examining doctor. Pilocarpine is one of the basic ingredients of some of the eye drops used for glaucoma. Because it makes the pupil of the eye contract, it is essential that medical

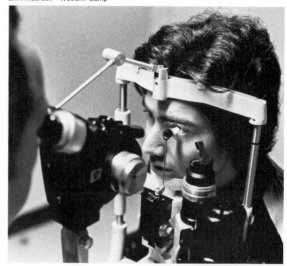

A tonometer, which measures the pressure within the eyeball, is used to diagnose the presence of glaucoma and to trace its progress.

personnel do not mistakenly attribute this effect to some other condition that also might produce it.

Damage to the retina from glaucoma is presently considered irreversible, but other maladies involving the retina that were once thought hopeless can now be corrected. For example, detachment of the retina from the inner wall of the eye was formerly synonymous with blindness. The delicate retinal structure can sometimes be torn or separated from its fixed position by an injury to the eye or by some severe disease. With surgery, however, almost 90% of all such tears and detachments can now be repaired with almost total preservation of sight. Surgical techniques for repair of the retina include spot welding using intense light from a laser, high-frequency electric current passing through miniature electrodes, and deep-freezing probes. If future research efforts discover the secrets of successful tissue transplantation, surgical techniques like those just mentioned may be used to replace damaged retinal nerves in the eye blinded by glaucoma.

Cataracts

A cataract is a dulling or clouding of the lens as a result of chemical changes in its structure. When cataracts occur, vision becomes blurred and outlines of images grow indistinct. The degree of impaired vision depends on how cloudy the lens becomes. Seeing through a healthy lens is comparable to looking outside through a clear, clean window. If this window suddenly steams up, distinctness of the images seen through the window is reduced. This situation might be compared to an early cataract. Should a freezing rain or snow completely cover the window, the scene outside, except for color and shadow, would be almost featureless. This last case is comparable to an advanced cataract.

Most cataracts occur in the elderly and are referred to as senile cataracts. This is a misleading term that should no longer be used, for senility has nothing to do with the onset or character of cataracts. The years added to the average human life-span during the 20th century are accompanied by degenerative changes in all the organs of the body. Advanced years are not senile years; advanced cataracts are not cataracts of the senile.

There are a number of different kinds of cataracts, the distinctions being technical ones. Overexposure to radiation, injury in which the eye is penetrated, diabetes, and certain eye diseases are some of the known causes. Cataracts can also appear as birth defects, brought on either by some prenatal event such as a disease contracted by the mother during pregnancy or as the result of a genetic disorder of the fetus.

There is no way to predict the speed with which a cataract will develop. Often there is no progression, and any mild interference with vision, if present at all, needs no special care. For Americans aged 65 and older about 75% will have some degree of lens cloudiness upon examination, but in only 15% will consequent vision loss be a handicap. Sometimes the condition worsens, however, until there is almost total obliteration of vision. Once a cataract in the eye is recognized by the eye specialist, it is kept under observation at repeated intervals. Only in this way can a progression of cloudiness be noted.

As cataracts progress, they are said to "ripen." The victim of ripening cataracts often will need brighter lights for reading and may tend to hold printed matter closer to the eyes. Night driving is affected because the light from such bright sources as headlights and street lamps scatters from the cloudy lens, making vision even more hazy. Changes in eyeglass prescriptions may help for a time, but eventually the the economic and social handicap of failing vision may force the victim to seek a permanent solution.

There are no drops or medications that can reverse clouding of the lens and return clarity of vision. Some people fall prey to mail-order advertising persuasion that glaucoma and cataracts can be prevented by expensive miracle drugs. Such quackery flourishes and extracts hundreds of thousands of dollars from those who sidetrack the confrontation with the truth, the need for an operation. It is hoped that real advances in medicine and surgery eventually will be able to prevent the onset and reverse the progression of cataracts. Currently this is not possible, and there is danger that an unusual delay when surgery is needed may convert a relatively simple operation into a complex one.

Highly refined techniques make cataract surgery painless, rapid, successful, and remarkably safe. It is estimated that normal vision returns in more than 95% of all cases following all types of cataract surgery. Only rarely do troublesome problems arise during or after the operation. Results are gratifying and, within a few weeks at most, vision is restored.

The most radical departure from the preferred surgical procedure was made about 15 years ago. The older yet highly successful traditional method involved making incisions in the cornea and iris, through which the lens was removed with suitable instruments. Although this method is still in wide use, a new method called phacoemulsification has been substituted in some cases. In this procedure the lens is fragmented with a beam of very-high-frequency sound from an instrument similar to the dentist's ultrasonic dental cleaner. The tiny pieces of lens that remain are then sucked up through a hollow needle. Phacoemulsification has reduced the length of time required for cataract removal and has brought to a minimum the incapacitation and hospitalization following cataract operations. Not all people of all ages who have cataracts are candidates for this highly individualized type of surgery. And not all surgeons have the specialized skills for performing phacoemulsification.

Because the lens is essential for clear vision, there must be a substitute for a lens that has been surgically removed. At one time thick, heavy, vision-distorting eyeglasses were necessary for the restoration of useful eyesight. Today skillful advances in the manufacture and shaping of hard and soft contact lenses make it possible to substitute these convenient devices for spectacles. After wearers learn to insert, remove, and clean their contact lenses without difficulty, they find their vision remarkably enhanced. Unfortunately the mechanical agility required to manipulate these tiny objects makes them unsuitable for some persons, particularly many of the elderly.

In the past few years another alternative to eyeglasses has been used successfully in specially selected cases. A substitute plastic lens is implanted at the time of cataract surgery to replace the clouded lens just removed. The major advantage of this approach is that contact lenses or eyeglasses are not needed except for reading. A great many surgeons, however, are still skeptical about the value of lens implants. When the success of this kind of operation has been more firmly established, it may look less attractive in the long run, since surgeons may not be as discriminating in choosing ideal cases for it.

It is hoped that within a few years a new type of contact lens will become available, one that can be worn continuously without fear of irritation or infection. This, of course, would be a boon to the elderly and feeble as well as all wearers of contact lenses and eyeglasses. Currently, however, the best hope for victims of severe cataracts lies with corrective eyeglasses and conventional contact lenses.

—*Lester L. Coleman, M.D.*

Beware
of Mixing Drugs

"Do not mix with household ammonia," cautions the label on a bottle of chlorine bleach, "or poisonous fumes will result." This warning and others like it on dozens of household products are welcome reminders of the potentially dangerous reactions that can result when the wrong chemicals are combined. If such a reaction occurs in a scrub bucket or washing machine, one can escape the danger by leaving the vicinity. But what if a similar situation were to happen within one's own body—say, severe depression of the central nervous system as the result of mixing alcoholic beverages with sleeping pills or tranquilizers? There might be no way to escape the consequences, which can range from extreme drowsiness to unconsciousness and even death. Moreover, there might not be a precautionary warning on the bottle of medicine—a warning that could serve to head off the disaster.

The human body is a likely caldron for the interaction of all kinds of chemicals: prescription drugs; over-the-counter items such as cold remedies, vitamins, and antacids; alcohol; and even common foods such as milk or bananas. In the daily process of eating, working, keeping calm, fighting off illness, and trying to get to sleep, a person can easily consume a half dozen substances that have the potential to rendezvous unexpectedly in the bloodstream, stomach, liver, or other body organs. The effect can be merely mildly unpleasant or, in rare cases, it can threaten life.

Chemical substances can interact in the body in several ways. Some drugs intensify the expected effects of other drugs. For example, aspirin can combine with anticoagulants, or anticlotting agents (e.g., Coumadin, dicumarol, and Panwarfin), to promote minor bleeding and possible hemorrhage. Other chemicals reduce or block the therapeutic effects of some medicines. A common case of this type is the inhibitory effect of the calcium in milk, yogurt, and other dairy products on the antibiotic action of tetracycline. Again, one chemical substance may aggravate the very condition a second substance is being taken to correct. Eating large amounts of natural licorice, for instance, puts a chemical into the body that can elevate blood pressure and thus counteract the benefits of taking medicine for hypertension.

Some combinations of substances may have rather unique effects. One of the most hazardous is the interaction between monoamine oxidase (MAO) inhibitors, which are drugs sometimes prescribed for depression or hypertension, and a food substance called

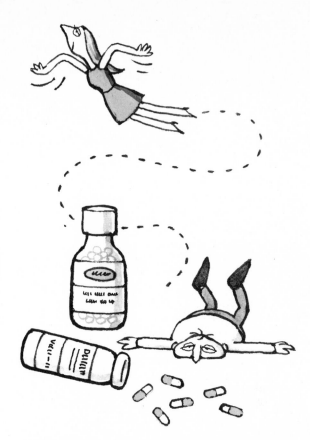

tyramine. Such foods as pickled herring, aged cheese, chicken livers, ripe bananas, Chianti wine, beer, yogurt, and sour cream contain high concentrations of tyramine, which reacts with MAO inhibitors to cause a rapid, dangerous rise in blood pressure. Antidepressant drugs like Tofranil, Elavil, and Norpramin also do not fare well with MAO inhibitors; their combination can result in blood pressure fluctuations, hyperexcitability, and fever.

Some common problems

Alcohol is a much-abused drug that interacts in the body with a large number of chemical substances. As mentioned above, mixing tranquilizers and alcohol sometimes results in deep sedation and has been a well-publicized cause of many deaths. Alcohol can diminish or exaggerate the major effects or side effects of many drugs including anticonvulsants, anticoagulants, antihistamines, and analgesics. Taken orally by itself, aspirin normally causes a small amount of bleeding in the stomach; combined with alcohol, however, it can induce considerable irritation of the stomach lining and substantial gastrointestinal bleeding. Alcohol and antidepressants are known to produce deep sedation and a drop in body temperature.

Oral contraceptives are a class of drugs in very common use. When they are taken regularly over long periods of time, their continual presence in the body is likely to be forgotten. Birth control pills often have an inhibitory effect on other drugs, particularly oral an-

Common Food-Drug Interactions

Food	Incompatible Drug	Possible Effect of Combining
dairy products	tetracycline antibiotics	reduces therapeutic effects of antibiotic
foods containing sugar	antidiabetics	increases requirement for drug
foods rich in vitamin B_6 (beef, liver, pork, wheat germ)	levodopa (Larodopa), used to treat parkinsonism	blocks drug effects
fruit juices	penicillin G	decreases drug action
goitrogen-containing vegetables (soybeans, turnips, cabbage, rutabagas, brussels sprouts)	thyroid medication	opposes drug action
green leafy vegetables (high in vitamin K)	anticoagulants (Coumadin, dicumarol, phenindione, warfarin)	reduces blood-thinning effects
licorice (excessive)	heart or blood pressure medication	may cause headache, high blood pressure, heart failure
tyramine-containing foods (pickled herring, ripened or aged cheese, Chianti wine, beer, fermented sausages, chicken liver, excessive chocolate, and others)	monoamine oxidase inhibitors (Marplan, Nardil, Parnate for depression; Eutonyl, Eutron for blood pressure control)	causes rapid rise in blood pressure (hypertensive crisis), severe headaches, vomiting, even death

Alcohol and Drugs That Do Not Mix

Drug	Possible Effect of Combining with Alcohol
anticoagulants	increases or decreases anticoagulant effect
anticonvulsants (Dilantin, Mesantoin, phenytoin)	diminishes or enhances drug effect
antidepressants	causes increased sedation; has led to several deaths
antidiabetics insulin oral (Diabinese, Orinase, Tolinase)	produces mild to serious symptoms of low blood sugar causes severe nausea and vomiting
antihistamines	may cause drowsiness and respiratory depression
antihypertensives (guanethidine for blood pressure control)	causes dizziness and fainting spells
aspirin	increases gastrointestinal bleeding induced by aspirin
codeine	causes respiratory depression, dizziness, and drowsiness
propoxyphene hydrochloride (Darvon)	causes dizziness and drowsiness; excessive amounts may be fatal
sedatives, sleeping pills, and minor tranquilizers (barbiturates, Librium, Miltown, Valium)	produces severe effects on central nervous system; excessive amounts may cause death

Common Drug-Drug Interactions

Drug	Incompatible Drug	Possible Effect of Combining
antibiotics lincomycin hydrochloride (Lincocin)	products containing kaolin (Donnagel, Kaopectate)	reduces antibiotic activity
tetracyclines	antacids	decreases antibiotic absorption
	iron compounds	decreases drug effect
anticoagulants, oral (Coumadin, dicumarol, phenindione, warfarin)	aspirin and analgesic pain relievers, barbiturates, chloramphenicol (Chloromycetin), clofibrate, phenylbutazone (Butazolidin), quinidine (Quinaglute), thyroid hormone preparations	increases bleeding, possible hemorrhage
	birth control pills, glutethimide (Doriden), griseofulvin (Grifulvin V)	decreases drug effect
	corticosteroids	increases or decreases anticoagulant activity
anticonvulsants (Dilantin, Mesantoin, phenytoin)	chloramphenicol, dicumarol, isoniazid (INH), phenylbutazone, some sulfonamide antibacterials (Orisul, Sulfabid, Thiosulfil)	causes side effects by raising phenytoin blood levels too high
antidepressants (Aventyl, Elavil, Norpramin, Tofranil)	anticoagulants	causes internal bleeding
	guanethidine (Ismelin)	blocks antihypertensive drug effect
	minor tranquilizers	may result in additional sedation
	monoamine oxidase inhibitors (Marplan, Nardil, Parnate for depression; Eutonyl, Eutron for blood pressure control)	may cause hyperexcitability, fever, muscular rigidity, wide blood pressure fluctuations
antifungals griseofulvin (Grifulvin V)	barbiturates	decreases antifungal effect
aspirin and aspirin-containing products	anticoagulants	increases bleeding, possible hemorrhage
	arthritis medications (indomethacin)	decreases drug effect
	oral antidiabetic drugs	causes increased effect of antidiabetic drugs
birth control pills	antihistamines, barbiturates, phenylbutazone, major tranquilizers, antituberculosis drugs	may decrease contraceptive effect
	oral anticoagulants	may decrease blood-thinning effect
	antidiabetics	may decrease effect of antidiabetic
cardiac glycosides (digitalis, digoxin)	antacids	decreases drug effect
cold and cough preparations antihistamines	codeine	results in extreme drowsiness, dizziness
	sedatives, sleeping pills, and minor tranquilizers	causes dizziness, drowsiness, and respiratory depression from excessive doses
sedatives, sleeping pills, and minor tranquilizers (barbiturates, Equanil, Librium, Miltown, Quaalude, Valium)	antidepressant drugs	enhances sedative effect
	antihistamines	exaggerates sedative effect

ticoagulants and antidiabetic drugs (*e.g.,* Diabinese and Orinase). They can also deplete the body of vitamin C, folic acid, and vitamins B_6 and B_{12}, which then may need to be replenished with vitamin supplements. On the other hand, certain antihistamines, barbiturates, arthritis medications, tranquilizers, and tuberculosis drugs are thought by some medical researchers to speed up the metabolism of contraceptive drugs in the body, thus decreasing their effectiveness and raising the chances for pregnancy.

The relationship between oral contraceptives and vitamins is part of a larger class of food-drug interactions that can influence how the body absorbs nourishment. Laxatives, for instance, may speed up movement of food through the gastrointestinal tract and thus reduce the time the intestines have to absorb nutrients. Some substances such as mineral oil and the antigout drug colchicine affect the bowel wall and also prevent nutrient absorption. Used repeatedly as a laxative, mineral oil can hinder absorption of vitamins D and K and of carotene, which the body converts to vitamin A. The antituberculosis drug isoniazid and a drug for hypertension called hydralazine upset the body's ability to process or absorb vitamin B_6; similarly the antibiotic neomycin can inhibit absorption of vitamin B_{12}. Taking certain of these and other drugs over long periods of time can cause specific nutrition deficiencies, particularly in the old, the young, the malnourished, and the chronically ill, unless dietary habits are improved or nutrition supplements are taken.

Preventing unwanted interactions

At present few labels on prescription or over-the-counter drug packages provide comprehensive information about possible reactions with food or other drugs. When they do, it cannot be stressed enough that these labels should be read and the warnings heeded. Under guidelines of the U.S. Food and Drug Administration—regulations effective in 1979—drug manufacturers must specify known adverse reactions with foods or drugs on the package inserts accompanying certain prescription medicines. Product labeling intended for the physician must also carry more information on such interactions.

Correcting labeling deficiencies, however, is not the only way to reduce the number of drug-related accidents. Consumers can do much to protect themselves by taking a few simple precautions:

1. Always tell the doctor about all drugs presently being taken—including easily overlooked items such as aspirin and birth-control pills—and ask about their possible interactions with any new drug being prescribed. In this era of medical specialization a patient may be consulting several doctors, each of whom may know nothing of the others' therapy. Also inform the doctor of any habit of consuming large amounts of certain foods or beverages.

2. Follow the doctor's instructions carefully, particularly concerning when prescribed drugs should be taken and what foods and other drugs should be avoided.

3. Double-check the doctor's instructions with the pharmacist. Sometimes this procedure can uncover a fact that the doctor forgot to mention or was not aware of.

4. Avoid taking any new medicines without checking with the doctor or, at least, with the pharmacist.

5. Make it a rule to avoid swallowing pills or capsules with liquids other than water—particularly milk, fruit juices, coffee, or soft drinks—unless the doctor specifies otherwise.

The tables accompanying this article constitute a selective list of some of the more common food-drug and drug-drug interactions. However, it should be noted that the consequences of the combined effects of two drugs are not limited to those given and may vary widely from person to person.

—*Charles M. Cegielski*

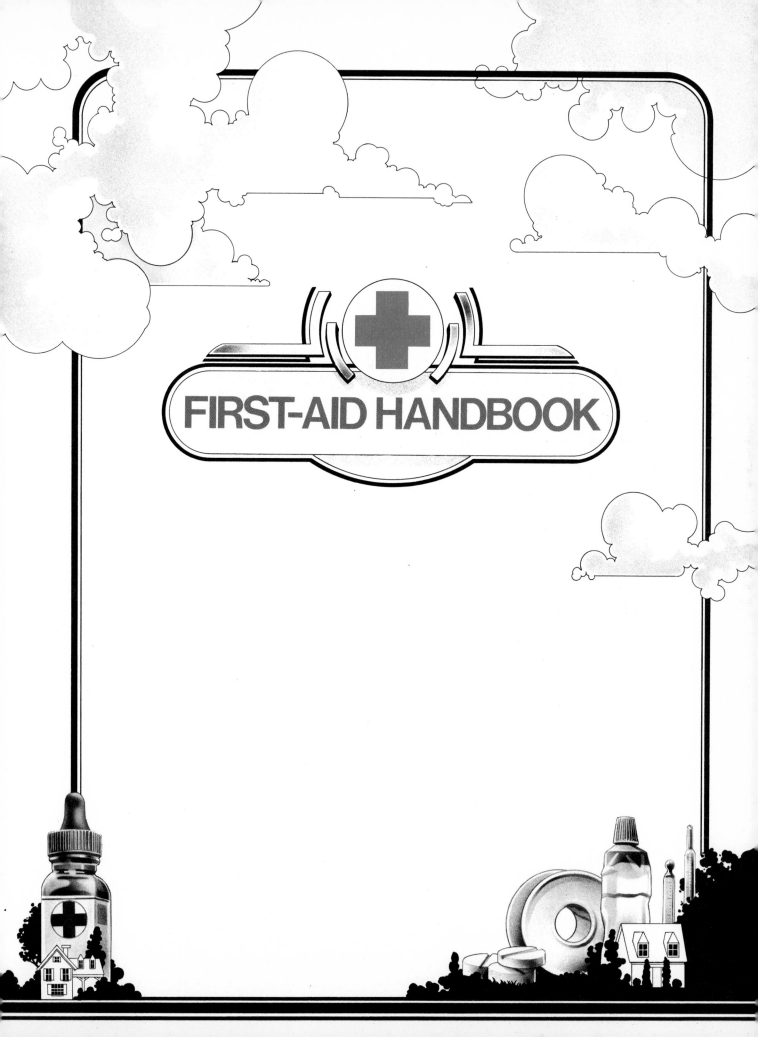

FIRST-AID HANDBOOK

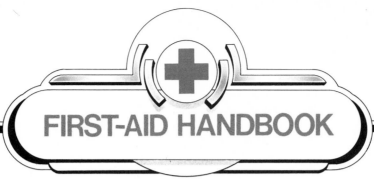

FIRST-AID HANDBOOK

Produced in cooperation with the Educational Materials Committee
of the American College of Emergency Physicians,
B. Ken Gray, M.D., Chairman.

Authors

Roy D. Beebe, M.D., and G. Richard Braen, M.D.

ACEP Educational Materials Committee

G. Richard Braen, M.D.
Philip M. Buttaravoli, M.D.
Desmond P. Colohan, M.D.
B. Ken Gray, M.D.
Robert M. Stryker, M.D.
Roger S. Taylor, M.D.

Contents

Illustrations by John Youssi

Emergency Care and First Aid

Properly administered first aid can make the difference between life and death, between temporary and permanent disability, or between rapid recovery and long hospitalization. First aid is most frequently employed to help a family member, a close friend, or an associate, and everyone should be familiar with first aid techniques and should know how best to use the emergency care system.

Public education and public awareness of potential roles in first aid have lagged behind the development of the emergency care system, which includes emergency medicine as a special area of medicine, better equipped and better staffed emergency facilities, paramedical care, communications, and transportation. The concept of first aid as simply the immediate care of the injured person is obsolete. Today a person administering first aid must be able to establish priorities in care and must understand and implement *basic life support* in an attempt to maintain vital functions. Education will reduce the chances of error and the possibly harmful results of well-meant but misdirected efforts.

Accidents are the leading cause of death among persons one to 38 years of age. In addition, over 800,000 Americans die annually of heart attacks, and a great majority of these die before they reach a hospital. The annual cost of medical attention and loss of earning ability amounts to billions of dollars, not to mention the toll in pain, suffering, disability, and personal tragedy. Thus, the delivery of quality emergency care and public education in basic life support and first aid must be accorded a high priority.

Use of This Handbook

The purpose of this handbook is both to educate and to serve as resource material for commonly encountered emergencies. It is arranged in three sections. The first deals with basic life support and the treatment of immediately life-threatening emergencies. One must understand these concepts *before* an emergency arises, since the necessary techniques must be employed immediately, almost by reflex, if the victim is to be saved.

The second section deals with emergencies that are not immediately life-threatening. It covers the common emergencies in alphabetical order.

The final section covers prevention, preparation, and use of the emergency care system. Prevention is still the least expensive medicine, and several of its most important principles will be discussed. Each home should be prepared for an emergency by having a readily accessible first aid kit, appropriate telephone numbers, etc. This section also discusses what to do and what to expect at the emergency department.

Section One:
Basic Life Support—Treatment of Immediately Life-Threatening Emergencies

Cardiopulmonary Arrest (Heart and Respiratory Failure)

Cardiac arrest is the most life-threatening of all emergencies. If circulation and breathing are not reestablished within minutes, the brain will suffer irreparable damage. Cardiopulmonary resuscitation (CPR), or basic life support, can be begun by *any person* who has taken time to learn the technique, and there is no need for special equipment. (In addition to reading the description of CPR technique that follows, one would be well advised to undertake formal training in the procedure, available through either the Red Cross or the American Heart Association.)

What Is Cardiopulmonary Arrest?

There are two absolutely vital systems in the body that must function if life is to continue: the *respiratory* system (lungs and respiratory tree) and the *circulatory* system (heart and blood vessels). The overall function of these two systems is to get oxygen from the air into the blood and then to all parts of the body. If either of these systems fails, or "arrests," death occurs very quickly unless the function is restored by CPR.

0-4 MIN.	CLINICAL DEATH	BRAIN DAMAGE not likely
4-6 MIN.		BRAIN DAMAGE probable
6-10 MIN.	BIOLOGICAL DEATH	BRAIN DAMAGE probable
OVER 10 MIN.		BRAIN DAMAGE almost certain

Phases of brain damage and death following cardiac arrest.

Respiratory or breathing failure has two basic causes: 1) obstruction of the intake of air or of the exchange of oxygen into the blood, and 2) impairment of the part of the brain that controls the rate and depth of breathing. Obstruction can result from several factors, including the presence of large pieces of foreign material (such as food) in the upper airway, swelling and closure of the airway (as in severe acute allergic reactions), and damage to the oxygen-exchanging membranes in the lung (from drowning and smoke inhalation). The most common sources of interference with the brain's ability to control breathing are drugs (narcotics, sedatives, alcohol), and carbon monoxide, electric shock, and an interrupted supply of oxygen to the brain, as when the heart has stopped.

If the heart stops pumping, or arrests, the tissues of the body do not receive the blood and oxygen they need. When this happens to the brain, there is an almost immediate loss of consciousness and breathing stops.

What To Look For

If a cardiopulmonary arrest has occurred, the victim *always:* is unconscious; has no pulse in the neck (carotid pulse); is not breathing. The carotid pulse can be checked by feeling with the thumb and index finger on either side of the windpipe (trachea). If a pulse is present, it will be felt here.

What To Consider

Any person who suddenly collapses (becomes unconscious), has no detectable pulse in the neck, and is not breathing has suffered a cardiopulmonary arrest. (A person who collapses while eating and is unable to breathe may well have a large piece of food caught in his windpipe. This is not purely a cardiac arrest, but has been called a "café coronary" and will be discussed below.)

What To Do: The ABCs of CPR

If a person suddenly collapses and loses consciousness, it must be decided immediately whether a cardiopulmonary arrest has occurred. Any delay can result in permanent brain damage or death. Try to arouse the victim. If he cannot be awakened, begin the ABCs of cardiopulmonary resuscitation.

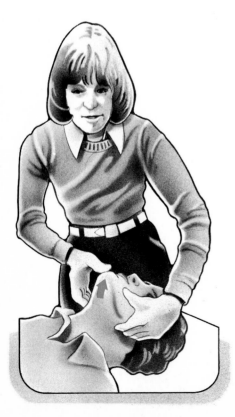

Lifting the jaw forward will help to open the airway.

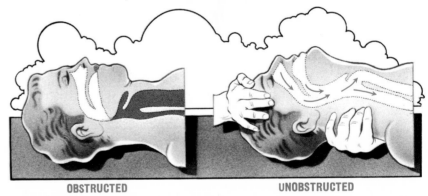

OBSTRUCTED **UNOBSTRUCTED**

The back of the tongue may obstruct the airway. Lifting the victim's neck and tilting the head backward will open the airway.

(A) Airway. **The first requirement is to assure a clear, unobstructed airway.**
1. Place the victim on his back.
2. Hyperextend the neck (lift the victim's neck and tilt his head backward); this lifts the tongue away from the back of the throat and helps to enlarge the airway.
3. Listen for breathing by placing your ear near the victim's mouth, and watch the victim's chest for signs of breathing.
4. If there is no evidence of breathing, open the victim's mouth and remove any obvious foreign materials—false teeth, food, vomitus.

(B) Breathing (Mouth-to-Mouth Resuscitation). **If opening and clearing the airway do not produce spontaneous breathing, it will be necessary to breathe for the victim.**
1. With the victim's head in the hyperextended position, pinch his nostrils closed, take a deep breath, and place your mouth tightly over his mouth.

2. Exhale quickly and deeply, four times in rapid succession, each time removing your mouth and letting air escape passively from the victim's mouth.

3. If there is great resistance to your breath, no rise in the victim's chest, and no escape of air from his mouth, the airway may still be obstructed.
   a) Further hyperextend the victim's neck and lift his jaw.
   b) Look again for foreign objects in the mouth and throat.
   c) If none are found, you will have to try a different approach. Roll the victim on his side and deliver four firm slaps between the shoulder blades. With the victim on his back, place your fist just above his navel and forcefully push once. Combined, these may force air out of his lungs and dislodge any foreign body that is trapped deeper in the airway; if so, the material should be removed from the victim's mouth.

4. If the mouth cannot be opened or is severely damaged, mouth-to-nose resuscitation may be used.

(C) Chest Compression. After assuring an open airway and delivering four breaths, check for carotid pulse in the neck, on either side of the windpipe. If there is no pulse, perform chest compression, or external cardiac massage.

1. Kneel beside the victim.
2. Place the heel of your hand just below the middle of the victim's breastbone and your other hand on top of the first. Do not let your fingers touch the victim's ribs; you may compress the wrong part of the chest.
3. Leaning directly over the patient, give a firm thrust straight downward. Let the weight of your shoulders do the work.
4. The breastbone should be pushed downward about two inches in the adult, and the compressions should be repeated 60 to 80 times each minute. (Note: Use of this procedure may crack some of the victim's ribs; proceed carefully, but do not stop CPR, since the alternative is death.
5. CHEST COMPRESSION OR EXTERNAL CARDIAC MASSAGE SHOULD ALWAYS BE ACCOMPANIED BY ARTIFICIAL RESPIRATION!
   a) If there are *two rescuers:* one ventilation should be interposed between every five compressions at a compression rate of 60 per minute.
   b) If there is only *one rescuer:* one ventilation should be interposed between every 15 compressions at a compression rate of 80 per minute.
6. If the victim is a child, the ABCs of CPR are the same except:
   a) Foreign bodies are more common in the airway.
   b) The person administering CPR puts his mouth over both the mouth and the nose of the victim.
   c) If an infant's head is flexed back too much, further obstruction of the airway can occur.

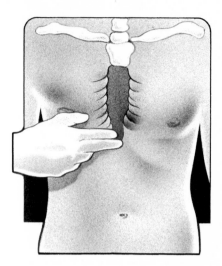

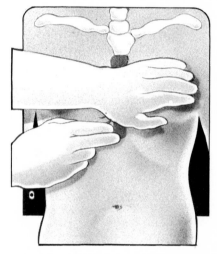

Find the tip of the sternum. The correct hand position for cardiac compression is two finger breadths above the tip of the sternum.

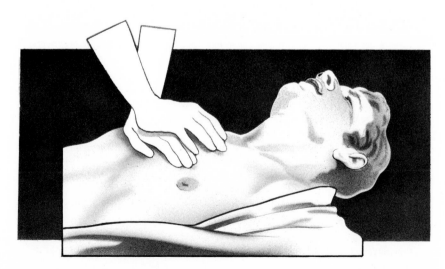

Place the heel of one hand on the sternum, and the heel of the other hand on the back of the first. Compressions of the chest should be done without placing the fingers on the chest wall.

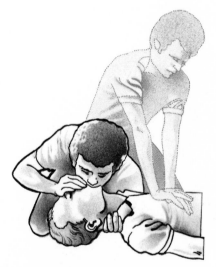

In "two-man" resuscitation, give one breath between compressions at the ratio of one breath for every five compressions.

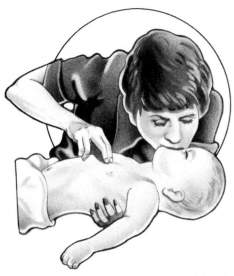

One person can resuscitate an infant by giving quick breaths while compressing the chest with the fingers of one hand.

d) Shallower breaths (puffs) should be used at a rate of 25 to 30 per minute.

e) Exert pressure over the center of the breastbone, as the heart chambers (ventricles) to be compressed are higher in a child's body.

f) Using only your fingertips, compress the chest ¾ to 1½ inches at a rate of 100 to 125 compressions each minute.

What Not To Do

1. Do not try to use CPR on any person who is alert and awake, or on any person who is unconscious but is breathing and has pulses.
2. Never compress the upper or lower ends of the breastbone; CPR is effective only when the flexible part of the breastbone that lies directly over the heart is compressed.
3. Do not interrupt CPR for more than 15 seconds, even to transport the victim.
4. Unless completely exhausted, do not stop CPR either until the victim is breathing adequately on his own and has a pulse, or until the care of the victim is taken over by more experienced medical personnel.
5. If the victim is revived, do not leave him unattended, because he may arrest again and require further CPR.

"Café Coronary" or Severe Choking While Eating

Anyone who collapses while eating may well have had a heart attack, but he may be choking on a large piece of food (usually meat). This most frequently occurs in older people, usually those who have poor teeth or false teeth, and frequently it is associated with some alcohol intake.

What To Look For

1. Before collapsing and losing consciousness, a victim who has been eating, possibly while also talking or laughing, may suddenly stand up and walk from the table, clutch his throat, or exhibit violent motions.
2. *He will not be able to talk*.
3. He may become blue.

What To Consider

The victim may be having a heart attack, but heart attack victims usually are able to talk prior to collapsing; they usually do not display quick violent motions, but collapse suddenly.

What To Do

The person will soon become unconscious and die if the obstructed airway is not cleared.

If the person is still standing:

1. Ask the victim to nod if he has food stuck in his throat.
2. Stand behind him and place one clenched fist in the middle, upper abdomen just below the ribs. Place your other hand on top of the first hand.
3. Give a very forceful pull of the clenched fist directly backward and upward under the rib cage (a bear hug from behind).
4. This will, ideally, act like a plunger and force the diaphragm upward, pushing any air left in the lungs out the windpipe and expelling or loosening the trapped object. The procedure may be repeated several times.
5. Once loosened, the foreign object can be pulled out.

If the victim has already collapsed:

1. Place him on his back, open his mouth and look for and remove any visible foreign material.
2. If none is seen, place the heel of your hand on the victim's mid-upper abdomen and give a forceful push.
3. This should dislodge the foreign material into the mouth, from which it can be removed. Repeat the procedure as often as necessary.
4. If, after the object has been cleared, the victim still is not breathing, is unconscious, and is without a pulse, begin CPR.

What Not To Do

Do not stop CPR efforts until the victim revives or more experienced personnel arrive.

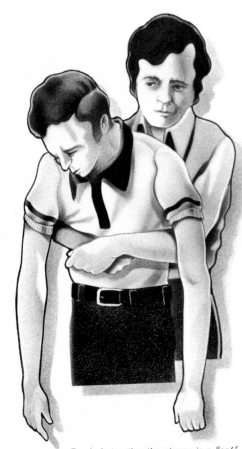

Food obstructing the airway in a "café coronary" may be loosened or expelled by an upper abdominal thrust or hug; using the fist of one hand placed in the abdomen just below the rib cage, give a forceful jerk upward.

What To Expect

If the problem is noted early and foreign material is removed, the chances for the victim's survival are excellent.

Drowning

Drowning and near drowning are common occurrences. Like cardiac arrest and "café coronary," drowning requires immediate action and basic life support.

What Is It?

Many more people nearly drown than actually drown (suffer cardiac arrest). The near drowning victim may have no symptoms or he may need help because of severe respiratory distress and confusion. The drowned victim will be unconscious, will have no pulse, and will not be breathing.

What To Consider

1. The water may damage the lining of the lungs, resulting in a decreased ability to exchange oxygen from the air into the blood. Following a near drowning the victim may suffer a cardiac arrest.
2. Always consider the possibility of an associated injury—for example, a broken neck, which is likely if the victim has dived into the water.

What To Do

1. Begin mouth-to-mouth resuscitation if the victim is unconscious, is not breathing, and is without pulse, even while he is still in the water.

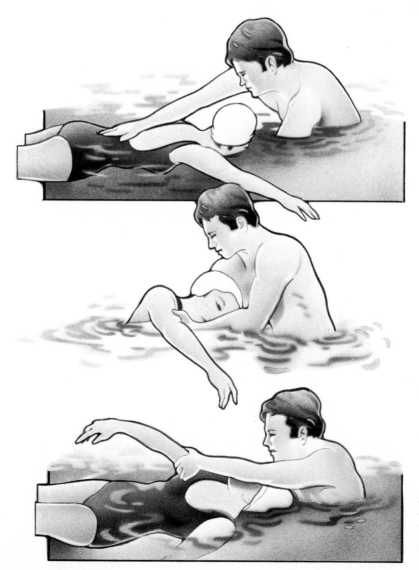

If there is a chance that a drowning victim has also injured his neck, particular care should be taken to protect the neck from further injury. The victim may be floated onto a board for removal from the water (see following page).

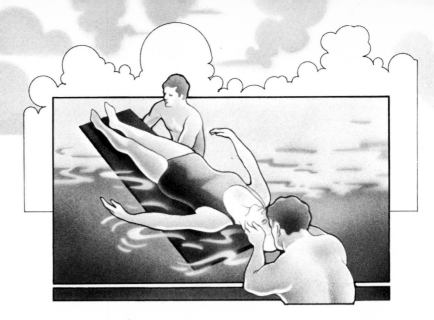

2. Give four quick breaths, followed by one breath every five to ten seconds.
3. Remove the victim from the water without interrupting artificial respiration except for a few seconds (one minute at most). Once he is out of the water begin CPR.
4. If the victim has a suspected spinal injury, he should be placed on his back on a flat board for removal.
5. The victim of near drowning should be taken to the hospital *immediately*. If oxygen is available it should be used, and the victim should be watched closely for the possibility of cardiac arrest.
6. The distressed victim who has difficulty breathing, has blue color, and is semiconscious may require only artificial respiration, but be sure.

What Not To Do

1. Do not use the manual (arm lift) method of artificial respiration; it doesn't work.
2. Do not try to drain water from the victim's lungs.
3. Do not fail to take near drowning victims to the hospital immediately; such victims may quickly develop respiratory difficulty.
4. Do not stop CPR until more experienced medical personnel take over, or until you are completely exhausted.

Electric Shock

What Is It?

Even the relatively low voltages of electrical appliances that are used around the home can cause fatal electrocution. Death results from paralysis of the breathing center in the brain, from paralysis of the heart, or from uncontrolled, extremely rapid twitching (fibrillation) of the heart muscle.

What To Look For

1. The possibility of electrocution should be considered whenever an unconscious victim is found near an electric wire, a socket, or an appliance.
2. Electrical burns may or may not be apparent.

What To Consider

1. There are other possible reasons for unconsciousness, such as a head injury, a cardiac arrest, or a seizure.
2. Think of possible associated injuries (head injury, neck injury) before moving the victim.

What To Do

1. Disconnect the victim from the electrical source as quickly and safely as possible. This can be done by disconnecting the plug or appliance or by shutting off the main switch in the fuse box.
2. Alternately, use a dry, nonconductive, nonmetallic stick or pole to move the wire or victim. DO NOT TOUCH THE VICTIM UNTIL HE IS DISCONNECTED OR YOU MAY BECOME ANOTHER VICTIM.

3. If the victim remains unconscious and shows no pulse or respiration, begin CPR immediately. Continue until the victim revives or until more experienced medical personnel take over.
4. If there is an associated head, neck, or back injury, let trained medical personnel transport the victim.
5. Upon awakening, victims of electric shock often are confused and agitated, and, for a short time, they may need protection from falls and additional injuries.

What Not To Do

1. DO NOT TOUCH THE VICTIM UNTIL HE IS DISCONNECTED.
2. DO NOT MOVE THE VICTIM IF THERE IS A HEAD, NECK, OR BACK INJURY, EXCEPT TO REMOVE HIM FROM DANGER.

What To Expect

Even with adequate CPR the victim may need more advanced life support such as electric heart shock. However, he generally can be managed with basic CPR until more advanced life support becomes available.

Drug Overdose and Carbon Monoxide Poisoning

What Is It?

Although deaths from drug overdose and carbon monoxide poisoning may be associated with suicide attempts, such deaths do occur in other settings. An unsuspecting heroin addict may inject an exceptionally pure cut of the narcotic. A child may explore the medicine cabinet and ingest some sleeping pills, pain pills, or even antidiarrheal pills. Carbon monoxide poisoning occurs frequently in automobiles with faulty exhaust systems, in industry, and in burning buildings. These poisons all suppress the breathing center in the brain.

What To Do

1. If the person who has ingested pills is unconscious and without pulse or breathing, begin CPR.
2. If the victim is unconscious and is not breathing, but *has* pulses, perform mouth-to-mouth resuscitation only. Respiratory arrest is common in drug overdoses.
3. When transferring the victim to the hospital, take along any bottles and pills that may be associated with the poisoning.
4. Remove the victim from the carbon monoxide exposure and begin CPR.

What To Expect

Following a large drug overdose, even with adequate CPR the victim may not begin to breathe on his own or may not wake up for many hours, and he may need extended life support at the hospital in an intensive care unit.

Massive Hemorrhage (Bleeding)

Following the control of a victim's cardiorespiratory function, the next most urgent priority for the person giving first aid is to control hemorrhaging.

What Is It?

If major bleeding occurs, a large vessel (artery or vein) may be involved. Lacerated arteries tend to produce a pulsating stream of blood, signifying an injury that needs immediate first aid.

What To Consider

If the victim is bleeding massively, shock or inadequate blood circulation may develop and the victim may become unconscious or may have a cardiopulmonary arrest.

What To Do

1. Have the victim lie down to prevent fainting.
2. If he already has fainted, raise his feet higher than his head.
3. If the victim is unconscious, and there are no pulses or breathing, begin CPR.
4. With a clean cloth or sterile dressing, apply *direct pressure* over the wound to halt the bleeding. Most major bleeding (even arterial) will stop in a few

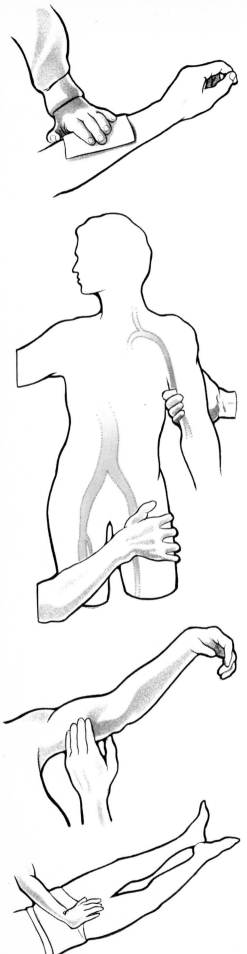

minutes if this method is used.

5. Maintain the pressure until better trained medical personnel take over.
6. If severe bleeding of an arm or leg does not stop after several minutes of direct pressure, try to stop the circulation in the artery supplying the blood by pressing firmly against it with your hand or fingers. There are three points on each side of the body where arterial pressure can be used to stop bleeding. (There are also pressure points in the head and neck, but they should *not* be used because of the danger of interrupting the supply of blood to the brain or the intake of air.)
7. Tourniquets are used only as a last resort, when all else has failed and the victim continues to hemorrhage profusely. Once a tourniquet has been applied, note the exact time and transport the victim to a hospital immediately.
8. When the bleeding stops, tie the dressing firmly in place.

What Not To Do

1. Do Not Try To Use Arterial Pressure Points In The Head Or Neck.
2. Do Not Use A Tourniquet Until You Are Absolutely Certain That Nothing Else Will Work. If the limb around which a tourniquet is applied is deprived of oxygen long enough, it may have to be amputated.
3. If the injury has been caused by a large foreign object that is protruding from the victim's body, do not remove it, or you may further aggravate the injury.

What To Expect

1. Most bleeding can be controlled by direct pressure.
2. Lacerations of the scalp bleed profusely but are rarely associated with massive blood loss.
3. Lacerations of the torso may have penetrated into the chest or abdomen and must be evaluated by a physician.

Section Two:
Common, Not Immediately Life-Threatening Emergencies

Animal Bites

All animal bites (dog, cat, and wild animal, as well as human) are dangerous and need medical attention. In addition to the injury itself, there is a chance of infection, including tetanus and rabies.

Bites from wild animals, particularly skunks, foxes, raccoons, and bats, always should be evaluated by a physician.

What To Do

1. Thoroughly scrub the wound with soap and water to flush out the animal saliva. This should be done for at least ten minutes.
2. Cover the wound with a dry, clean cloth or dressing.
3. Consult a physician immediately for further cleansing, infection control, repair, and possibly for tetanus and rabies prevention.
4. If possible the animal should be caught or identified and reported to the local authorities for observation.

What Not To Do

Do not mutilate the animal, particularly its head. (If it is a wild animal and is killed, tests can be run by the local authorities to determine if it was rabid.)

Automobile Accidents

Even with the slower, safer speeds on U.S. highways, automobile accidents still account for the largest number of the nation's accidental deaths, as well as for numerous fatalities elsewhere. Automobile accidents may cause complex or multiple injuries, and priorities must be considered for the care of the injured.

What To Do

1. Turn the car's engine off if it is still running.
2. Do as much first aid as possible *in* the car.
3. Move the victim only under the following circumstances.

a) The car is on fire.

b) Gasoline has spilled and there is a *danger* of fire.

c) The area is congested, unsafe, and presents the danger of a second accident.

4. Check the patient for breathing and pulses.

5. Control any hemorrhaging.

6. If there is a head and neck injury or fracture of an extremity, wait for medical help before moving the victim, except to insure breathing or to stop significant bleeding.

7. If the victim must be moved to a medical facility, splint any fractures and support his head and neck on a board.

What Not To Do

Do not move unnecessarily a victim who is unconscious or who has a head or neck injury. It may be necessary to move a victim who has no pulse and is not breathing, or who is bleeding severely.

Backache, Acute

Most frequently, back pain is of recent onset and follows some type of acute exertion or unusual activity, such as the lifting of a heavy object. The pain usually results from muscular strain and is not of great significance. However, back pain that is associated with acute injury or with pain radiating down the legs may be important and demands immediate medical evaluation. In addition backache accompanied by blood in the urine might indicate injury to the kidney or the presence of a kidney stone, while backache with fever or urinary pain might signify a urinary tract infection.

What To Do

1. If a backache is nagging, mild, of recent onset, and is associated with recent activity, and if there is no pain radiating into the hip or leg, and if there is no bowel or urinary problem, it may be treated with:

   a) Absolute bed rest for 24–72 hours.

   b) A firm, nonsagging bed—a bed board might be used.

   c) Local heat or warm tub baths.

   d) Two aspirin every four hours.

2. If the back pain is severe, with pain radiating into the hip or legs, or if it is associated with bowel or urinary problems, the victim should see a physician as soon as possible.

3. If the back pain follows an accident, it should be evaluated by a physician.

4. Back pain that does not improve within 48 hours should be evaluated by a physician.

Bleeding from the Rectum

The acute onset of bright red bleeding from the rectum may be caused by bleeding *hemorrhoidal* veins. The usual history includes constipation and straining to defecate, leading to bright red blood dripping into the toilet bowl and onto the toilet paper, frequently with associated rectal pain. The problem is common among pregnant women.

If rectal bleeding is not due to hemorrhoids, it needs medical evaluation. If the stools are black and tarry, it is imperative to get a medical evaluation as soon as possible. The possibility that the bleeding originates higher in the intestinal tract must be considered, since rectal bleeding may be a sign of an ulcer, tumor, or inflammation.

What To Do

1. If the bleeding is due to hemorrhoids:

   a) Warm tub baths three or four times daily may promote healing.

   b) Lubricating ointment such as petrolatum may decrease irritation to the hemorrhoids during bowel movements.

   c) Drinking plenty of fluids will soften the stool, as will bran cereals or stool softeners available from drug stores.

2. If bleeding persists, see a physician.

Direct, firm pressure is frequently the best way to stop bleeding. If bleeding is too extensive to stop with direct pressure, locate the brachial or femoral arteries and apply pressure to stop bleeding distal to those points.

3. Get a physician's evaluation for black, tarry stools or for bright red rectal bleeding that is not known to be from hemorrhoids.

Blisters

Blisters are generally caused either by burns or by friction on the skin. Burn-related blisters can result from contact with flame or hot objects or with certain chemicals, and from severe sunburn or scalds. Blisters represent injuries to only a partial thickness of the skin. When a blister breaks, there is a loss of the natural protective insulation of the skin. Open, broken blisters are vulnerable to infection and tend to promote the loss of body fluids by evaporation. If blisters are very large, evaporation may be severe and may result in dehydration.

What To Do

1. Small blisters should not be opened. They should be protected with dry, soft dressings to prevent rupture.
2. Blisters resulting from contact with chemicals should be immediately and copiously washed with tap water to dilute the offending agent.
3. If a blister ruptures, the area should be washed gently but thoroughly with mild soap and water. The skin that covered the blister should be carefully removed, and the wound should be covered with a dry, sterile dressing.
4. Blisters of large areas of the body should be treated by a physician.

What To Expect

1. The pain from blisters usually subsides after one to two days.
2. Almost all blisters break and slough after four or five days, and the wound heals in about two weeks.
3. Ruptured blisters often become infected. Note any increased redness, pain, swelling, or heat about the wound, and be particularly aware of any red streaking up the extremity, pus from the wound, or fever.

Boils, Pimples, and Styes

When sweat glands of the skin become plugged, there may be bacterial growth and an accumulation of infected material (pus) inside the gland. Frequently, the accumulation of pus is absorbed by the body's natural defense processes. Occasionally, the area of infection expands, forming an abscess or boil (called a stye when on the eyelid). These are painful swellings that are red, warm, and can vary from less than a half inch to several inches in size. When these infections have reached this stage, the only way that the body can heal itself is to let the pus out through the skin.

What To Do

1. Apply warm, moist compresses as often as possible throughout the day (for 15 minutes every four hours).
2. When the boil or stye "points" and then ruptures, wipe the pus away gently with a dry, sterile cloth and cover it with a dressing. Continue to use warm, moist compresses.
3. If there are multiple boils or if the infection seems to be large, contact a physician.

What Not To Do

Do not attempt to squeeze or puncture boils, pimples, or styes. If hot compresses are used, early boils and styes may resolve. Most will "point" and rupture in two or three days and will then rapidly heal.

Broken Bones (Fractures)

A broken bone should be suspected whenever a person complains of pain with the loss of the normal use of an extremity. Fractures are seldom in and of themselves life-threatening emergencies, and one must make sure that the victim is safe from further harm and has good respiration and pulses before making any attempt to immobilize or move an injured person. Any victim suspected of having a broken neck or broken back should be handled in a special manner. (*See* Broken Neck or Back, below.)

There are two types of fractures that are important to recognize. Most frac-

Simple fracture.

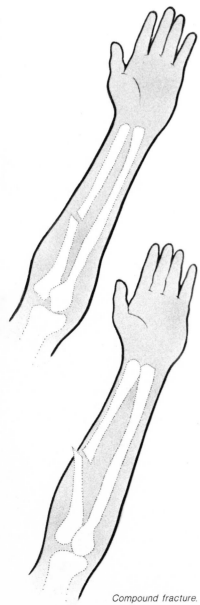

Compound fracture.

tures are "simple" or "closed," and the broken bone does not protrude through the skin. There are times, however, when the broken bone does pierce the skin; such breaks are known as "compound" or "open" fractures.

A word about sprains is in order here. Sprains may be managed at home if they are very mild. Aspirin, rest, elevation of the affected extremity, and local ice packs are the best treatment. If a sprain is severe, however, it should be treated like a fracture, and medical attention should be sought.

What To Do

1. Make certain that the victim is breathing adequately and has pulses before even considering first aid for the fracture.
2. When there is reason to suspect multiple broken bones, or when the neck, back, pelvis, or thigh might be broken, it would be best to let trained emergency personnel transport the victim to the hospital.
3. If the broken bone protrudes through the skin, cover it with a dry sterile dressing, but do not try to push it back in. If there is excessive bleeding, use direct pressure to stop it. (*See* Massive Hemorrhage, above.)

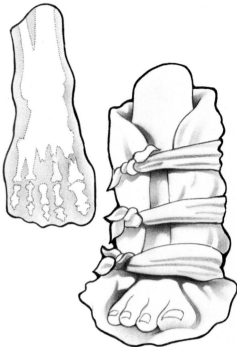

A simple splint for a broken ankle or foot may be made with a pillow or folded blanket or jacket and secured with roller bandages, tape, and so forth.

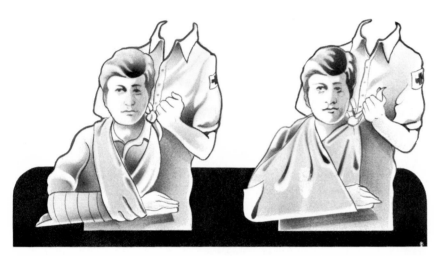

A broken forearm bone should be splinted, and a sling should be applied. If a splint is not available, the sling itself will reduce the pain.

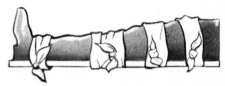

A broken bone in the lower leg should be splinted before transporting the victim.

4. If the victim must be moved, the fracture should be immobilized with splints to prevent further damage and to make the victim more comfortable (the pain of a fracture is caused by the two ends of the broken bone rubbing together.) The basic principle of splinting is to immobilize the broken bone by securing the affected limb to some firm object (a piece of wood, broom handle, ski pole, several newspapers or magazines, or even an injured leg to the uninjured leg). Both ends of the splint must extend beyond the area of suspected fracture; the splint may be secured with bandages, belts, sheets, or neckties. Most injuries of the arm, wrist, or hand can be stabilized simply with a sling.

What Not To Do

1. Do not try to transport any accident victim who has an obviously unstable (floppy) extremity without stabilizing or splinting it first. Even though fractures can be disturbingly displaced, deformed, and very painful in themselves, they rarely represent life-threatening emergencies. If fractures are immobilized adequately, there frequently is a marked reduction in pain.
2. Do not attempt to move a victim with a suspected broken neck or back without trained medical personnel, unless it is absolutely necessary to do so.

Broken Neck or Back

The possibility of injury to the spine (neck and back) must be considered whenever a person is:

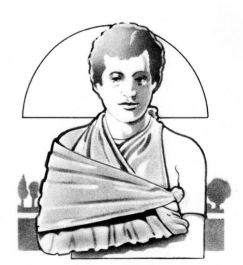

A broken collarbone can be splinted by first applying a sling to the arm, and then applying a wrap around the arm and chest, to reduce movement of the arm.

1. Involved in an accident of any type and subsequently complains of back or neck pain, has any degree of paralysis or weakness of an extremity, or has numbness or tingling of an extremity or part of his body.
2. Injured about the face or head in an accident, or is rendered unconscious.

What To Do
1. Make certain the victim is breathing and has pulses.
2. Unless it is absolutely necessary, do not move the victim, but let trained medical personnel do it.
3. Unless he is unconscious, the victim is safest on his back; avoid attempts to pick up his head or to move his neck.
4. If the victim is unconscious, convulsive, or vomiting, he should be rolled—carefully, and preferably by two people—onto his side, and his head should be supported very carefully on a pillow or coat.
5. If it is absolutely necessary to move the victim, he should be placed on a firm board. This should be done cautiously, with several people supporting the whole spine and the head. The neck or back should not be flexed (chin moved toward the chest or head dropped back).

What Not To Do
1. Do not allow any accident victim who complains of neck or back pain to sit or stand.
2. Do not give the victim anything to eat or drink.

Bruises and Black Eyes

Any direct trauma to the soft tissues (skin, muscles, etc.) of the body may injure the blood vessels as well. The damaged blood vessels then leak blood which, when it accumulates under the skin, at first looks black, in a few days looks yellow-brown, and then is reabsorbed. Also, direct trauma may cause swelling or fluid collection under the skin. The area about the eye, because of the loose tissue present, is particularly prone to this swelling, and when blood collects the result is a "black eye".

Bruises are frequent problems and are usually benign in that they represent minimal injury and get better by themselves. However, if the force is adequate, associated injuries can occur, including fractures, ruptured abdominal organs, collapsed lungs, and injuries to the eyeball. If there is an obvious deformity, severe pain, or impaired motion of an extremity, or if there is impaired vision, blindness, severe pain in the eye itself, or double vision, a physician should evaluate the injury.

What To Do
1. As soon as possible, place a cold compress or an ice bag (a towel soaked in ice water or a towel-covered plastic bag of ice) on the bruise. This will reduce the pain and swelling and should be continued for several hours.
2. Restrict any movement of the injured part, because the less it is used during the first few hours, the less it will swell. Elevation of the bruised part above the level of the heart also decreases swelling.

If the injury is only a bruise, the victim should be able to use the extremity. Most bruises and black eyes will enlarge and worsen in appearance for up to 48 hours after the injury, after which they will gradually shrink. The blue-black color becomes yellow-brown and then disappears in 10–14 days. If multiple bruises that are not associated with trauma appear over the body, a physician should be contacted, because this may indicate a blood clotting disorder.

Burns

The skin can be burned by flames, hot objects, hot liquids (scalds), excessive sun exposure, chemicals, and contact with electricity. There are three degrees or depths of burns:
First degree—reddened, hot, very painful, no blisters. Heals spontaneously.
Second degree—painful, red, blistered. Usually heals spontaneously.
Third degree—deep burns can be white or black and are always painless. These may require skin grafts.

Many burns that appear to be first degree may later develop blisters and may actually be second degree. Second-degree and third-degree burns frequently become infected and need more attention and care than do first-degree burns. Electrical burns frequently look small but may be much deeper than suspected. Burns in children and older people are more serious.

What To Do

1. For sunburn see below.
2. For flash burns, scalds, and small burns, towels or sheets soaked in cool water should be applied immediately for comfort.
3. If it is a chemical burn, the area should be washed copiously and continuously (under a running faucet if possible) for 15–30 minutes.
4. The burn should be dressed with sterile, dry, soft dressings.
5. If burns involve large areas of the hands or face, they should be examined by a physician.
6. Electrical burns should be treated by a physician.
7. Burns, like cuts, require tetanus prevention.

What Not To Do

1. Do not apply ointments, sprays, or greases to large wounds.
2. Never use butter on any burn.
3. Do not break blisters.
4. Do not pull off any clothing that adheres to the burn.

If a small burn becomes encrusted, has pus, or shows red streaking, it may be infected and should be seen by a physician. If large areas of the body have second- or third-degree burns, there may be an excessive water loss from the body with consequent shock. People with extensive burns, especially young children and old people, are very likely to go into shock, and they should be transported to a hospital emergency department as soon as possible. "Shock," in this case, refers to a low level of circulating bodily fluids, not to a psychological state.

Chest Pain

It is well established now that most heart attack deaths result from *treatable* disturbances of the heartbeat. The overall emphasis must be to get the person with a heart attack into an intensive care unit as soon as possible. To accomplish this there must be:

1. Equipped and staffed emergency departments.
2. Better prehospital care and transportation.
3. Public education on the signs and symptoms of a heart attack.
4. Public education on the techniques of basic life support—CPR. (*See* Cardiopulmonary Arrest, above.)

Denial of the pain and its significance, ascribing it to other causes (heartburn, gas, or pulled muscles), and trying different remedies (antacids or antiflatulence medications) often lead to fatal delays in proper medical treatment. Everyone must be aware of the significance of chest pain and heart attack.

Severe chest pain must always be considered a medical emergency. A correct diagnosis can only be made by a *physician*, using an appropriate medical history, an examination, and sometimes several laboratory tests—an electrocardiogram, chest X-ray, and blood tests.

There are several aspects of chest pain that are important. Heart attack pain is often described as a *dull* ache, tightness, squeezing, or as a heavy feeling that is usually diffusely located over the front of the chest. It is often associated with aching in the shoulders, neck, arms, or jaw. Many people become short of breath, sweaty, nauseated, and may vomit. If any of these symptoms occurs in an adult, he must be transported immediately to the nearest physician or emergency department.

What To Do

1. Chest pain, especially with the symptoms listed above, demands *immediate* medical attention. An ambulance should be called immediately.
2. While waiting, make the person comfortable and reassure him.

3. Do not give him anything by mouth except what a physician has prescribed.
4. Do not make him lie down if he is more comfortable sitting.
5. Do not leave him unattended. He may suffer a cardiac arrest and may require basic life support (CPR).

There are many other causes of chest pain that may need medical attention. Chest pain associated with fever and cough could be a symptom of pneumonia. Chest pain associated with coughing up blood or associated with thrombo-phlebitis (pain in the calf or thigh) might represent a blood clot in the lungs. A collapsed lung might cause chest pain and sudden shortness of breath.

There are numerous causes of chest pain, such as severe heartburn, viral pneumonia, inflammation of the cartilages of the ribs, and pulled muscles, that are not life-threatening, but a physician must make these diagnoses.

Childbirth, Emergency

Childbirth is a natural and normal phenomenon, and it rarely requires advanced medical training to carry out a safe delivery. For a variety of reasons (inadequate transportation, very short labor, etc.) many babies are born unexpectedly, outside of the hospital.

Labor is the cyclical contraction of the uterus (womb) which helps to open up the end of the uterus (cervix) to allow passage of the baby. These contractions usually are painful and occur with increasing frequency and duration until the delivery. The overall duration of labor is different for every woman. Frequently labor lasts for 12 or more hours for a woman's first baby, but the time may be reduced to a few hours or less for the woman who has borne several children.

Delivery is the passage of the baby through the birth canal and the vagina. The mother will usually experience *rectal* pressure and will know that the child is being born. The reflex action is to push or "bear down." The child's head and hair will be visible at the opening of the vagina. If the woman is "pushing" and the infant is visible, the birth is imminent. If a foot, an arm, the buttocks, or the umbilical cord is first to appear, take the mother to a hospital immediately.

What To Do

1. Let nature take its course. Do not try to hurry the birth or interfere with it.
2. Wash your hands and keep the surroundings (sheets, etc.) as clean as possible. (Fresh newspaper is often sterile, if sheets or blankets are unavailable.)
3. Support the emerging baby and let it slide out.
4. Once the baby is delivered, support him with both hands, keeping his head lower than the rest of his body. This will allow the fluid to drain from his mouth.
5. Place the infant on a dry towel or sheet and cover him immediately. Heat loss is a problem for newborn babies.
6. Aluminum foil wrapped around the baby will retard heat loss.
7. If the baby is not breathing begin mouth-to-mouth resuscitation, very gently, using puffs of air from your cheeks.
8. It is not necessary to cut the umbilical cord, and one may choose to have this done at the hospital. If medical care will be significantly delayed, however, use the following procedure to cut the cord: using a clean (boiled) ribbon, cord, or string, tie the cord tightly at two points, one that is four inches from the baby and the other at least eight inches from the baby. Cut the cord with clean, boiled scissors between the two ties.
9. Do not wash the white material from the baby (this is protective).
10. Warmly wrap the infant and transport it to the hospital.
11. Knead the womb after the child has been delivered.
12. The mother should remain supine until the bleeding stops and the placenta has been expelled.
13. When the placenta is expelled, minutes after the birth of the child, it should be retained and taken to the hospital for examination.

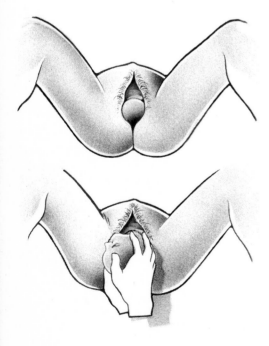

If childbirth is imminent, the top of the baby's head will begin to bulge through the mother's labia. Support the head with one hand on each side (not over the baby's face), and ease the shoulders out. The baby will be quite slippery, so be careful not to drop it.

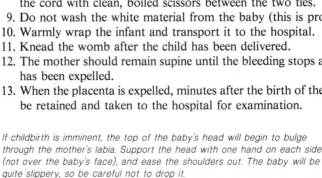

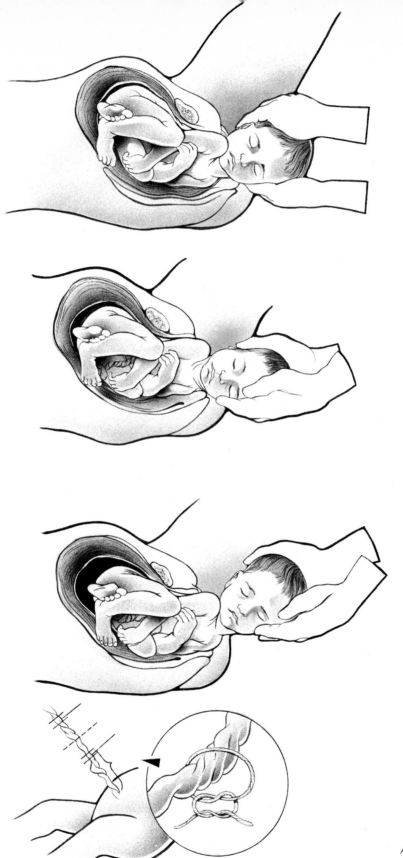

After delivery, the umbilical cord may be tied using a sterilized cord. Tie the cords at four and eight inches from the baby.

Cold, Overexposure, and Frostbite

Overexposure. Each year many people die from cold exposure resulting in *hypothermia*. The people who are particularly at risk include elderly persons with poor circulation, individuals who unpreparedly become exposed to low temperatures and high winds, and people who are intoxicated with alcohol.

CORE TEMPERATURE	SYMPTOMS
94°	CONFUSION
90°	HEARTBEAT BECOMES IRREGULAR
86°	LOSS OF MUSCLE STRENGTH DROWSINESS AND UNCONSCIOUSNESS
77°	CARDIAC ARREST AND DEATH

As the body's core (central) temperature drops, the victim becomes confused and ultimately may die.

Poor circulation, poor protection from the elements, and alcohol dilate blood vessels in the skin and allow heat loss that lowers the body core (central) temperature. Malfunction of the brain, heart, and lungs may then occur.

What To Do

1. Remove the person from cold exposure and place him in the warmest place possible.
2. Use hot water bottles or warm blankets to warm the victim as quickly as possible.
3. If the victim is awake and able to swallow, give him *warm, nonalcoholic* drinks.
4. Watch for a cardiac arrest and be prepared to carry out CPR.

What Not To Do

1. Do not give alcoholic beverages.
2. Do not leave the person unattended.
3. Do not place a hot water bottle directly against the victim's skin; wrap it in a sheet or towel.

Frostbite. Frostbite is a common injury in winter weather, particularly when low temperatures are combined with wind. Exposed, small parts of the body are the most susceptible (nose, ears, fingers, toes, and face). Again, the elderly and the intoxicated are the most susceptible. Initially, the involved part begins to tingle and then becomes numb. Frozen tissue usually is dead white in color.

What To Do

1. Remove the person from the cold as soon as possible.
2. Every effort should be made to protect the frozen part. If there is a chance that the part might refreeze before reaching medical care, it may be more harmful to thaw it and let it refreeze than to await arrival at the treatment area for thawing.
3. Rapid rewarming is essential. Use lukewarm (not hot) water between 100° and 110° F (37–43° C) or use warmed blankets. Within about 30 minutes, sensation may return to the part, which may become red and swollen. At first the rewarmed part will tingle, but it will begin to be painful and tender to the touch.
4. When the part is warm, keep it *dry* and clean. If blisters appear, use sterile dressings.
5. See a physician as soon as possible.

What Not To Do

1. Do not give alcoholic beverages.
2. Take care not to burn the person by using water that is too hot.
3. Do not let the part refreeze.
4. Do not rub the injured part; friction may cause further damage.

Convulsions

Convulsions and epileptic attacks are frightening to watch. The victim's lips may become blue, he may make a crying noise, his eyes may roll back, and his body may be jerked by uncontrollable spasms. Many seizures occur in people with known seizure disorders who have forgotten their medications, in alcohol abusers who have recently stopped drinking, and in children with an acute febrile illness (febrile seizures). *Febrile convulsions* are quite common among children aged six months to three years. They result from an abrupt rise in the child's temperature and are generally of short duration (usually ending by the time the victim arrives at the emergency department). The victim usually awakens soon after the seizure.

What To Do

1. Turn the victim onto his side so that saliva is able to drain out without being inhaled into the victim's lungs.
2. If it can be done safely, place a rolled handkerchief in the victim's mouth between his teeth to prevent him from biting his tongue. Do not force a spoon or other object into the victim's mouth.

414

3. Most people who have had a seizure need prompt medical attention at the nearest emergency department.
4. The child with febrile convulsions is treated by reducing the fever. Cool towels or sponge baths may help to lower the child's temperature.
5. If the victim has fallen or shows evidence of head trauma, he should be assumed to have a broken neck and should be treated accordingly. (*See* Broken Neck or Back, above.)

What Not To Do

1. Do not force objects into the mouth of the convulsing person.
2. Do not get bitten by the convulsing person.
3. Do not try to restrain the convulsive movements. Protect the victim from further injury.

Following the seizure (most last less than ten minutes) the person will usually fall asleep or will be confused.

Do not assume that the seizure is "just a seizure" in either a child or an adult, since seizures may be signs of other problems such as head injury, meningitis, or tumor.

Croup

What Is It?

In the fall and winter months, when houses are dry and warm, young children (usually younger than three years) may develop a "croupy," barking cough. This condition usually is caused by a viral inflammation of the trachea (windpipe) and of the larger airways, and the infection may cause severe respiratory distress.

What To Do

1. For mild cases (most cases), lowering the temperature in the room and using a humidifier will quickly help the croupy breathing. A bathroom filled with steam from a running shower may be helpful.
2. Aspirin and liquids may be used to combat low-grade fever.
3. If there is a high fever, difficulty in swallowing or talking, or respiratory distress, the child should be seen by a physician as soon as possible.

Most cases of croup are mild, and they will usually clear up after two or three days if corrective measures are taken.

Cuts, Scratches, Abrasions

Small cuts, abrasions, and scratches are common occurrences and generally require only thorough cleansing and bandaging for protection. Some cuts are larger and may require stitches for closure to minimize scarring, to reduce the chance of infection, and to restore function. Deeper cuts may involve blood vessels, and they may cause extensive bleeding or may damage muscles, tendons, or nerves.

What To Do

1. All minor wounds and abrasions should be *thoroughly* washed. There should be no dirt, glass, or foreign material left in the wound. Mild soap and water are all that are necessary.
2. Bleeding can be stopped by direct pressure that is applied over the wound with a sterile, dry dressing, and by elevating the injured part.
3. Most wounds should be covered with a dressing to protect them from further harm and contamination.
4. All bites (human or animal) should be treated by a physician because of the likelihood of infection. (*See* Animal Bites, above.)
5. If there is any question about the need for sutures, the wound should be examined by a physician.
6. If the wound is dirty or extensive, or if the victim's tetanus immunization is not up to date, there may be the need for a booster immunization.
7. Watch carefully for signs of infection (usually they do not appear for several days). The signs are:
   a) a reddened, hot, painful area surrounding the wound,
   b) red streaks radiating from the wound,

c) swelling around the wound, with fever and chills.

If an infection appears, see a doctor at once.

Diabetic Coma and Insulin Reaction

Diabetics have difficulty using the sugar in their blood. *Insulin* lowers the blood sugar level. As would be expected, it may be difficult to adjust the daily insulin requirement to the intake of sugar-containing foods and to the individual's activity level. Because of this, some diabetics occasionally suffer either from *insulin reaction* (which is a blood sugar level that is too low) or from *diabetic coma* (which can be thought of as a blood sugar level that is too high).

Insulin reaction, or acute hypoglycemia, may cause the person to become acutely confused, incoherent, sweaty, or shaky. Eventually, the person may lose consciousness.

What To Do

1. Determine if the victim is a diabetic.
2. If he is *conscious*, give him some form of sugar (a lump of sugar, candy, sweets, or soft drinks that are not artificially sweetened).
3. If recovery is prompt, take the victim to the nearest physician.

What Not To Do

Do not try to give sugar to someone who is unconscious.

Diabetic coma with hyperglycemia (a high blood sugar level) is quite different. The onset is more gradual, taking several hours or longer. The victim may have warm, flushed skin, with a very dry mouth and tongue. He frequently may be drowsy but rarely is unconscious. His breath may smell fruity (like nail polish remover), and he may be dehydrated.

What To Do

A person in a diabetic coma needs prompt treatment by a physician.

Diarrhea (in a small child)

Diarrhea may be caused by many factors, ranging from simple nondigestion of eaten foods to such conditions as bacterial or viral infections of the intestinal tract. In a small child, acute prolonged diarrhea may rapidly cause dehydration and death. The younger the child and the more prolonged the diarrhea, the more dangerous is the threat to health. Maintenance of adequate hydration is the main goal of therapy.

The signs of dehydration are: lethargy, dryness of the mouth and armpits, sunken eyes, weight loss, and the absence of urination. A child who continues regularly to wet his diapers generally is not dehydrated.

What To Do

1. Small children with acute diarrhea should be given water, liquid Jell-O, or pediatric salt solutions. Milk and whole foods should be withheld for the first 24–48 hours of the diarrhea. In acute diarrhea, the bowel is unable to digest and absorb some of the sugars in milk, which worsens the diarrhea.
2. If the diarrhea persists for more than 48 hours, a physician should be contacted.
3. If the diarrhea causes signs of dehydration, or if the child stops taking in fluids, a physician should be contacted immediately.
4. Almost all diarrheal states in children are well on the road to recovery within 48 hours. For the bottle-fed child, half-strength formula can be substituted for regular formula for one or two days before resuming full-strength formula. If the diarrhea persists, a physician should be consulted.

What Not To Do

1. Do not continue milk and whole food during an acute diarrheal state.
2. Do not use adult antidiarrheal medications for children.

Dislocated Joints

It is frequently impossible to tell the difference between dislocated joints and broken bones until X-rays have been taken.

416

What To Do

1. Probable dislocations in the hand, arm, shoulder, or jaw usually do not require an ambulance for transportation to the hospital. Victims should, however, be transported safely and comfortably.
2. If there is a dislocation of the hip or knee, ambulance transportation will be needed.
3. Slings or splints may be helpful. (*See* Broken Bones, above.)

What Not To Do

Do not attempt to move or manipulate the joint, or to set a dislocation yourself; the bone may be broken if these procedures are done improperly.

Eye Pain (something in the eye)

Even a small speck of dirt in the eye can cause intense pain. The covering of the eye is quite sensitive and, even after the foreign material is removed, there may be a feeling of irritation. Redness and tears are frequently present.

What To Do

1. Examine the eye by pulling the lower lid down while lifting the upper lid off the eyeball. Most specks will be visible.
2. Gently attempt to wipe the speck off with a moistened corner of a clean cloth, handkerchief, or cotton swab.
3. If the speck does not come off *easily*, or if there is persistent discomfort, a physician should be seen as soon as possible.
4. If irritating liquids are splashed into the eye, irrigate the eye with cool tap water for 30 minutes.

Fainting—Dizziness

Fainting is a sudden but momentary loss of consciousness. There are a variety of causes for it, including fatigue, hunger, sudden emotional upset, poor ventilation, etc. The person who has fainted looks pale and limp but is breathing and has a normal pulse. Simple fainting is not associated with chest pain or seizures, and the unconsciousness does not last for more than one or two minutes.

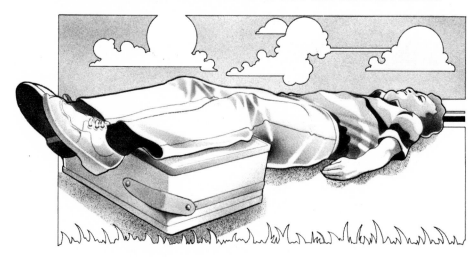

If a person faints, place him on his back or side and elevate the legs above the head.

What To Do

1. Place the victim on his back or side, with his legs higher than his head.
2. Check his airway, breathing, and pulses.
3. Apply cold compresses to the victim's forehead, and have him inhale aromatic spirits of ammonia.
4. If fainting is associated with chest pains, seizures, or severe headache, or if it lasts more than one or two minutes, the victim should be transported by ambulance to a physician.
5. If a person reports that he feels faint, have him sit with his face in his lap or stretch out on his back until he feels better.

Fainting is a relatively common problem and almost always quickly resolves in one or two minutes. Nevertheless, other causes should be considered—heart attack, stroke, internal bleeding, and insulin reaction.

Fever

Fever is an elevated oral temperature above 98.6° Fahrenheit or above 37° Celsius. Fever is a manifestation of the body's response to infection (viral or bacterial) or to foreign substances that the body is attempting to reject. People with fever frequently report muscle and bone pains, headaches, chills, and a hot feeling. Viral infections (colds, influenza, and even viral gastroenteritis) almost invariably are associated with low-grade fevers and are the most common causes of such fevers.

In susceptible children younger than three years of age, a *rapidly* rising fever may induce febrile seizures.

What To Do—Adults

1. Aspirin and acetaminophen (aspirin substitute) are the two most effective antifever medicines available. If used appropriately, they not only effectively lower the temperature but also will provide some relief for the bone and muscle aches.
2. The person with fever should take a lot of fluids, as higher temperatures increase evaporation of water and thus accelerate dehydration.
3. Bed rest helps.
4. If the fever is very high (102° or more) and persistent (most fevers last less than 24 hours), a physician should be consulted.
5. Fever associated with chest pains, shortness of breath, cough, or with the production of sputum, or with confusion, headache, a stiff neck, abdominal pain, or earache should be evaluated by a physician as soon as possible.

What To Do—Children

1. Fever of 100° or more in an infant (less than 30 days old) is always an emergency, and the child should be seen immediately by a physician. Every household should have a thermometer for taking children's temperatures.
2. In addition to fluids and bed rest, children with temperatures over 100° may be given aspirin or acetaminophen (aspirin substitute) every four hours in doses of not more than 60 mg for each year of life.
3. The child *should not be* overly dressed but should be dressed lightly (T-shirt and diapers are enough).
4. If a child develops a temperature of 103° or more, and the fever does not respond to aspirin or acetaminophen, the child should be placed in a tub of lukewarm water (not cold) and should be sponged for at least 30 minutes.
5. If the fever still does not respond, a physician should be contacted.
6. Any child with a febrile seizure, lethargy, signs of dehydration, or excess irritability should be seen by a physician.

What Not To Do

Do not sponge a child with alcohol; it is potentially toxic and is flammable. The sudden cold is often frightening to a child.

Food Poisoning

Food poisoning is a term applied to the combination of nausea, vomiting, or diarrhea that is attributed to contaminated food. The symptoms may be identical to those of viral gastroenteritis (stomach flu), but with the lack of an associated fever. Some other causes of the same symptoms include emotional stress, viral infections, inorganic or organic poisons, or food intolerance. Food poisoning itself is caused by toxins produced by bacteria growing in the food. The most common organism causing food poisoning is the *Staphylococcus*. In *Staphylococcus* food poisoning, vomiting and diarrhea generally develop within one to 18 hours following ingestion of the contaminated food.

What To Do

1. Generally, food poisoning resolves spontaneously within a few hours. Clear liquids should be offered as tolerated.

418

2. If vomiting or diarrhea is prolonged, dehydration may develop. In some cases, medical attention should be sought.

What Not To Do

1. Do not take antibiotics. They are useless in this type of poisoning.
2. Do not force the victim of food poisoning to drink fluids if he has any respiratory difficulty. Victims who develop respiratory difficulty should be seen immediately by a physician.

Foreign Objects in the Nose, Ear, Throat

Nose

1. If the object cannot be withdrawn or teased out easily, consult a physician at once.
2. Do not allow violent nose-blowing.
3. Do not deeply probe the nose yourself. You may push the object deeper into the nostril or you may cause harm to the nasal tissues.

Ear

1. If the object cannot be withdrawn easily, consult a physician.
2. The tissues of the ear are very delicate and can easily be damaged. Pushing the object in further may even rupture the eardrum.

Throat

1. Large objects caught in the throat can cause severe difficulty in breathing (*see* Café Coronary, above). This requires immediate care.
2. Small objects can be swallowed—coins, fishbones, etc. Such smaller objects that get caught or that irritate the throat and that cause no difficulty in swallowing or breathing should be given a chance to pass. Drinks of water followed by eating soft foods—such as bread—may help. If the object remains caught or if irritation persists for more than two or three hours a physician should be notified.
3. Someone who has an irregular object—such as a pull tab from a beverage can, a piece of wire, or glass—caught in his throat needs immediate medical attention.

Head Injury

Injuries to the head may include lacerations and contusions of the scalp, fractures of the skull, or brain injuries. Whenever someone has suffered a serious injury to his head, one must always consider whether there might have been an associated injury to the neck. If there is a possibility of an associated neck injury, the victim should not be moved except by skilled personnel unless there is a chance that he might inhale secretions or vomitus. In that case, the victim may be very carefully rolled onto his side.

What To Do

1. Severe, deep lacerations should not be cleansed or irrigated. Instead, sterile dressings should be placed over the wound and should be secured snugly with a roller bandage. Heavy pressure should not be applied to severe lacerations because there may be an associated fracture of the skull and too much pressure may drive a fragment of bone into the brain.
2. Note any loss of consciousness or altered mental status. An examining physician will need this information.
3. Make sure that the victim's pulse and respiration are normal. If the victim might inhale his secretions or stomach contents, very carefully turn him onto his side. Note the size of the victim's pupils. If the victim is unconscious or confused and his pupils become unequally dilated, this is a medical emergency and he should be seen immediately by a physician.
4. Keep the victim lying down, but do not place a pillow under his head since doing so may cause further damage to the neck if it also has been injured.
5. Make sure that the victim's airway remains open. At times, CPR or artificial respiration (see above) may be needed.

Any head injury accompanied by a loss of consciousness should be evaluated

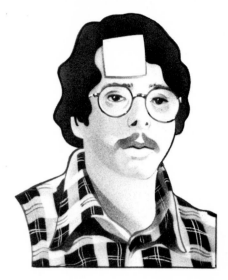

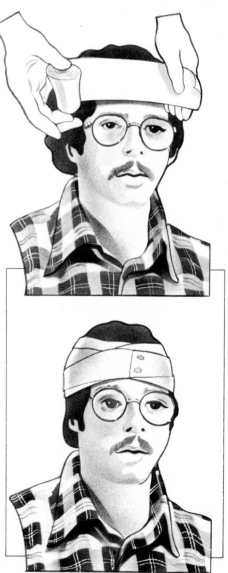

If there is an open head injury, apply a sterile dressing and secure it with a roller bandage. If there is significant bleeding, apply the roller bandage firmly.

by a physician. This evaluation should be done as soon as possible after the injury. Even though the victim may regain consciousness, further brain damage may develop.

Heatstroke (sunstroke), Heat Exhaustion (heat prostration), and Heat Cramps

Heat exhaustion and heat cramps result from salt depletion generally in association with dehydration. Heat cramps are characterized by muscle spasms in the extremities and in the abdomen. Heat exhaustion is manifested by shock (low blood pressure), mental confusion, and muscular incoordination. Other symptoms may include weakness, dizziness, or headaches.

Heatstroke is rare and generally affects the elderly, persons with heart disease, persons who are physically exhausted, or persons who have been consuming alcohol to excess. In this condition and in sunstroke there is a failure of the heat-regulating mechanisms in the body. The victim has a high fever and dry skin. The pulse generally is rapid and irregular and the blood pressure is low. The victim's temperature may reach 107° to 111° F (41.7° to 44° C). First aid is the same for heatstroke and sunstroke.

What To Do

1. For heat exhaustion, move the victim to a cool place and elevate his legs. If he can take fluids by mouth, give him salt water (½ teaspoon of salt in a glass of water).
2. Heat cramps may also be treated with salt solutions taken orally.
3. Heatstroke, manifested primarily by a very high temperature, should be treated by placing the patient in a cool place, by removing his clothing, and by applying cool water or ice packs to his body. The victim's extremities should be massaged vigorously to aid circulation.
4. If the victim has suffered from heatstroke, heat exhaustion, or prolonged heat cramps, medical attention should be sought.

What Not To Do

1. Avoid giving water without added salt, because this may further deplete the body's salt concentration.
2. Avoid the immediate reexposure of the victim to the heat, because he may be very sensitive to high temperatures for a time.

Nosebleeds

Nosebleeds are generally caused by trauma to the nose, which can result from nose-picking, from colds when there is hard nose-blowing, or from drying of the nasal mucosa. Most commonly, nosebleeds originate from the area of the nasal septum. Nosebleeds may also be associated with hypertension, bleeding disorders, or nasal tumors.

What To Do

1. To prevent the inhalation or swallowing of blood, have the person sit up and lean forward.
2. Gently squeeze the affected side of the nose closed for 10 to 15 minutes.
3. If the bleeding stops have the victim rest quietly for a few hours. During this time there should be no stooping, lifting, or vigorous nose blowing. Seek medical attention if the nosebleed is profuse or prolonged. The blood loss from a nosebleed can be considerable, and some people even go into hemorrhagic shock following a nosebleed.

What Not To Do

Do not allow the victim to resume normal activities for a few hours after the nosebleed has subsided.

Poisoning

Poisoning is a common occurrence, particularly in households in which there are children. For the most part poisoning is accidental, but occasionally someone will ingest a poison during a suicide attempt. Households should be equipped to handle poisoning, and syrup of ipecac should be available.

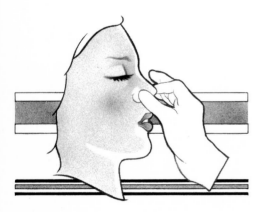

A nosebleed frequently can be stopped by firmly pinching the nose closed.

Generally there are five kinds of poisons that might be ingested: a) pesticides, b) drugs, c) strong alkalies and acids, d) petroleum products, e) poisonous plants.

Two of these, petroleum products and strong alkalies and acids, are worthy of special note, because vomiting should *never* be induced if they have been ingested. Examples of petroleum products include turpentine, paint thinner, furniture polish, gasoline, and liquid shoe polish. Examples of strong alkalies include drain cleaner, lye, and some bleaches. In the case of strong alkalies or other strong substances that may cause chemical burns, the mouth and esophagus are burned when the poison is swallowed. If the person is made to vomit, he will be burned a second time as the chemical is passed up the esophagus and out the mouth again. In the case of petroleum products, vomiting may lead to inhalation of the poison, with a resulting chemical pneumonia.

The best way to handle poisons is to take precautions against their ingestion, particularly when small children are present. Medicines, detergents, and cleaning products should all be placed on a high shelf, not under the sink where children can easily find them. In addition, poisons should be kept in appropriate containers. It is dangerous to keep gasoline or furniture polish in a soft drink bottle because a child may drink from that bottle, thinking that it contains a soft drink.

What To Do

1. Initially, give ½ glass of water or milk to anyone who has ingested a poison, unless the victim is *unconscious* or is having convulsions.
2. Decide whether or not to induce vomiting. Look in the victim's mouth for burns that might indicate the ingestion of an acid or alkali. Also, smell the victim's breath to see if it smells like a petroleum product. If either sign is present, do not induce vomiting. If the poisoning has been caused by pesticides, drugs, or poisonous plants, vomiting may be induced by putting one's fingers into the back of the victim's throat to induce gagging and vomiting, or by using syrup of ipecac. Children should be given approximately one teaspoon to one tablespoon of syrup of ipecac, and adults should be given two tablespoons. Vomiting should occur within 20 to 30 minutes.
3. Contact your local physician or emergency department for further instructions. A Poison Control Center may recommend specific antidotes. Antidotes that are listed on the packaging of poisonous products may not be correct or the procedure for their administration may be faulty. It may be better to contact a Poison Control Center for specific, step-by-step instructions.
4. If respiratory difficulty or shock develop, they should be treated appropriately.

What Not To Do

1. Do not allow poisons to be within the reach of children.
2. Do not induce vomiting if alkalies, acids, or petroleum products have been ingested.
3. If the victim is unconscious or is having convulsions, do not give him water, and do not induce vomiting.
4. Do not store poisonous materials in food bottles or jars.

Poison Ivy, Poison Oak, and Poison Sumac

Contact with poisonous plants such as poison ivy, oak, or sumac frequently produces local itching and redness in allergic individuals. In some people the rash that develops is characterized by vesicles (small blisters). More severe reactions include headache, fever, and malaise.

What To Do

1. Contaminated clothing should be removed and all exposed areas of the body should be washed with soap and water.
2. Once the rash has developed, soothing lotions may be applied to the skin. Many of these lotions are available without prescription at a pharmacy. Cool, moist compresses also are valuable for relieving itching.
3. If blisters appear and begin to ooze, they may be treated with wet dressings —sterile gauze pads saturated with a solution of baking soda and water

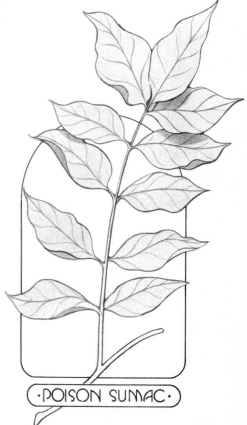

·POISON SUMAC·

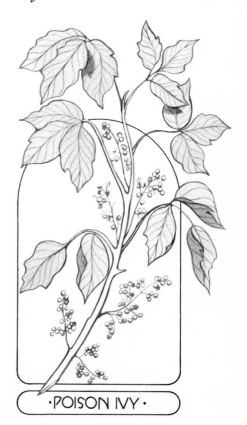

·POISON IVY·

421

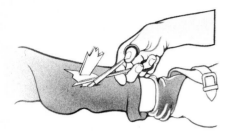

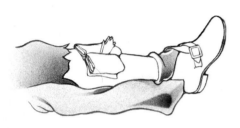

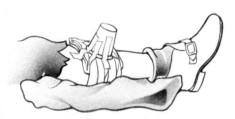

Objects stuck deep through the skin (or into the eye) should not be removed. If the object is too large to be secured in place by simply using a dressing, a paper cup taped over it may reduce further injury.

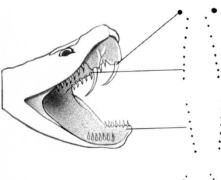

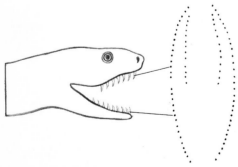

Pit vipers generally produce conspicuous fang marks. Nonpoisonous snakes and coral snakes will not leave fang marks.

(one tablespoon of baking soda to one pint of water).

4. If a severe reaction occurs, if there is a fever, or if a large area of the body is involved, seek medical advice.

Puncture Wounds

Puncture wounds are created by penetrating objects such as nails, knives, sticks, and needles. Puncture wounds do not bleed as readily as lacerations and thus there is less natural cleansing of the wound and a higher rate of infection.

What To Do

1. The site of the puncture wound should be cleansed with soap and water, after which a clean dressing should be applied.
2. For severe puncture wounds, seek medical attention for tetanus prophylaxis and for consideration of antibiotic therapy.

What Not To Do

Do not remove any foreign object that is protruding from the wound. As moving the object may cause further damage, the physician should attend to such wounds.

Rape

Rape is the unlawful carnal knowledge of a woman by a man, forcibly and against the woman's will. In the United States, rape is common, and friends or relatives are frequently called on to render assistance to rape victims.

What To Do

1. The rape victim should be protected from further harm and should be assured that she is safe.
2. If she is injured and is bleeding, direct pressure should be applied to the bleeding points. Never, however, apply hard pressure to the rectal or vaginal areas.
3. If she has a broken extremity, it should be treated appropriately.
4. Always remember that a rape victim has an absolute right to refuse medical, legal, or psychological help; however, she should be encouraged to see a physician as soon as possible.

What Not To Do

1. Even though the victim may feel unclean, she should be advised not to bathe, douche, or urinate, because doing so may destroy some evidence needed by the medical examiner.
2. The scene of the crime should not be touched, because this may invalidate existing evidence that would lead to the conviction of the attacker.
3. The victim should be advised not to change her clothing until she has been examined medically, because some evidence may be lost.

The trauma of the rape victim does not end with the rape itself. She may develop psychological problems or have marital difficulties for days or even years following the incident. In many communities, counseling services have been established specifically for the benefit of these victims.

Snakebite

In the United States there are two groups of poisonous snakes: the coral snakes and the pit vipers. The coral snake is found from North Carolina to Florida, through Louisiana to central Texas. The Sonoran coral snake is found in Arizona and southwestern New Mexico. The pit vipers include the copperhead, water moccasin, and rattlesnake. Rattlesnakes and other pit vipers account for the greatest number of the venomous snakebites in the United States, while coral snakes account for a very small number. Coral snakes produce relatively inconspicuous fang marks. Pit vipers produce a more conspicuous injury, with fang marks surrounded by swelling and blood-filled blisters.

The effect of a poisonous snake's bite depends on the size of the victim, the location of the bite, the amount of venom injected, the speed of absorption of the venom into the victim's circulation, and the amount of time between the bite and the application of specific antivenom therapy.

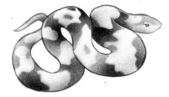
copperhead

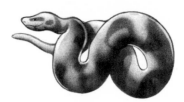
water moccasin

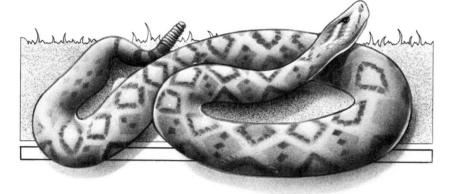
diamondback rattler

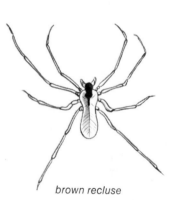
coral snake

What To Do

1. First aid begins with reassuring and calming the victim.
2. The victim should be transferred to a physician as soon as possible. Even if the bite was inflicted by a nonpoisonous snake, a physician may want to give tetanus prophylaxis and antibiotic therapy.
3. Immobilization of the bitten extremity will help retard absorption of the toxin.
4. Application of an ice pack at the site of the fang mark may also slow absorption.

What Not To Do

1. Incisions over the fang marks are not recommended, nor are constricting tourniquets.
2. Do not give the victim alcohol in any form.

Spider Bites and Scorpion Stings

The reaction to the toxins of spiders and scorpions varies from mild, with resulting local pain, redness, and swelling, to severe, with convulsion, nausea, vomiting, muscular pain, and even shock. In the United States the two spiders that are generally the most harmful are the black widow spider (*Latrodectus mactans*) and the brown recluse (*Loxosceles reclusa*).

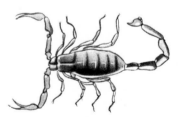
brown recluse

What To Do

1. The two best first aid measures for spider bites and scorpion stings are the immobilization of the affected part and the application of ice packs to the site of the bite or sting.
2. A medication like aspirin may help relieve the pain.
3. For brown recluse bites, black widow bites, and some scorpion bites, a physician's attention should be sought.
4. If the spider or scorpion has been killed, don't discard it. A physician may be able to further identify the species if he sees it.

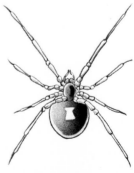
scorpion

Stings (Wasp, Bee, Yellow Jacket, and Hornet)

The stings from these insects are relatively common, and they rarely cause death except in highly sensitive individuals. The sting may be painful, but the symptoms are usually mild and are of short duration.

black widow

423

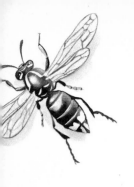

Some people are highly sensitive to insect stings and may develop an allergic reaction, possibly with anaphylaxis (a massive allergic reaction) and subsequent death.

What To Do

1. Most people have no problem from an insect sting if they apply local cool compresses or a solution of water and baking soda.
2. Aspirin sometimes helps.
3. If the person is highly sensitive to insect bites and has developed allergic reactions in the past, seek immediate medical attention. If medical attention will be delayed more than a few minutes, attempt to remove and discard the stinger and attached venom sac if present, being careful not to squeeze it.

wasp

yellow jacket

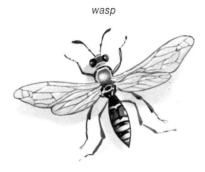

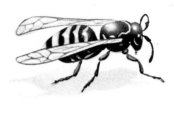

honeybee

bumblebee

hornet

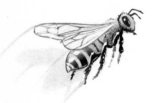

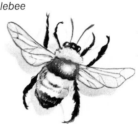

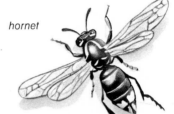

Stroke

Strokes are often referred to as cerebral vascular accidents. "Cerebral vascular" refers to the blood vessels in the brain, which are affected either by a clot or by rupture with subsequent hemorrhage. Major strokes may be accompanied by facial weakness, an inability to talk, the slurring of speech, loss of bladder and bowel control, unconsciousness, paralysis or weakness (particularly on one side of the body), or difficulty in breathing and swallowing. Sometimes strokes are associated with vomiting, convulsions, or headaches.

The most important things to watch are breathing and vomiting. Recovery from strokes is quite variable.

What To Do

1. If the victim is having difficulty breathing, his airway should be opened. (*See* Cardiopulmonary Arrest, above.)
2. The victim should be positioned on his side so that his secretions will drain out of his mouth and not into his airway.
3. If vomiting occurs, the victim should be kept on his side and his mouth should be wiped clean of vomitus.
4. Get prompt medical attention for all stroke victims.

What Not To Do

1. Fluids should never be administered by mouth unless the victim is fully conscious.
2. The victim should not be left alone for any length of time because of the chance of his vomiting and then inhaling the vomitus.

Sunburn

Ordinary sunburn is caused by overexposure to the sun's ultraviolet rays. The initial symptoms may begin as early as one hour after exposure and are manifested in painful redness and swelling of the area, and, in more severe cases, in the formation of blisters over the sun-exposed areas. When very large areas of skin are involved, fever, gastrointestinal upset, and weakness may occur.

Fair-skinned people and people taking certain medications should avoid exposure to the sun. Even dark-skinned people should initially avoid being in the bright midday sun for longer than 30 minutes. For added protection there are many good sun-screening ointments, creams, and lotions available. The most common and most effective ingredient in these is para-aminobenzoic acid (PABA), which screens out the ultraviolet rays that cause sunburn.

What To Do

1. Mild sunburn can be treated at home with cool compresses.
2. If there is an accompanying fever, aspirin may help.
3. Commercially available lotions often have a soothing effect on the skin.
4. For more severe cases, it may be necessary to consult a physician.

What Not To Do

1. Avoid further exposure to the sun until the acute reactions have subsided.
2. Avoid greasy preparations.

Sunburns usually resolve themselves, but occasionally the blisters become infected. If much of the skin has peeled off, the underlying skin will be quite sensitive to reexposure to the sun for several days or weeks.

Unconsciousness

Unconsciousness is a sleeplike state from which one may or may not be arousable. A person in "stupor" may be aroused with stimulation and only then with difficulty, while a person in coma cannot be aroused even by the most powerful stimuli.

The most common causes of unconsciousness are fainting, intoxication with alcohol, head trauma, strokes, poisoning or drug overdoses, seizures, diabetic acidosis, hypoglycemia, various types of shock, and hypoxia. Elderly, poorly nourished, or otherwise debilitated people are more prone to unconsciousness regardless of the nature of their illness.

The cause of unconsciousness is often difficult for even a physician to diagnose, and laymen should be careful not to ascribe a patient's unconscious state to something like intoxication. Alcoholics are of course not immune to other more serious causes of unconsciousness.

What To Do

1. Any unconscious person should be checked for an open airway and for palpable carotid pulses (*see* Cardiopulmonary Arrest, above).
2. If the person is not arousable but is breathing well and has good carotid pulses, he should be placed on his side so that he will not inhale any stomach contents if he vomits.
3. Anyone who is comatose should be evaluated by a physician. If drug ingestion or poison is suspected, the containers from the suspected toxin should be brought to the emergency department. Observations made about the person before his lapse into unconsciousness also will be of great help to the examining physician.

What Not To Do

1. Unconscious persons should not be left alone for any length of time, except for summoning help.
2. Fluids should never be administered by mouth and vomiting should never be induced.
3. Do not unnecessarily move an unconscious person unless you are certain he does not have a neck injury.

If unconsciousness resulted from a fainting attack, the victim may awaken within a few minutes. If unconsciousness recurs or if the person remains unconscious for several minutes, an evaluation by a physician should be sought.

Vomiting

Vomiting is the action by which the stomach rids itself of its contents. Vomiting can be caused by disturbances in either the abdomen or the head.

Causes of vomiting arising in the abdomen include: irritation or mechanical obstruction at any level of the intestinal tract, or irritation of abdominal organs like the gallbladder.

Causes of vomiting that originates in the vomiting centers in the head include: emetics (drugs), various toxins (poisons), increased pressure inside the head, decreased oxygen content of the blood in the head, disturbances of the semicircular canals of the ear (as occurs with seasickness), and, occasionally, psychological factors.

Severe or prolonged vomiting may lead to dehydration. When vomiting is associated with respiratory difficulty it may indicate that some of the vomitus was inhaled, and this is a medical emergency.

Simple acute vomiting may be caused by the effects of alcohol on the stomach lining, by dietary indiscretions, by viral gastroenteritis, or by the morning sickness of pregnancy. Severe or prolonged vomiting may reflect more severe gastrointestinal or systemic disease.

What To Do

1. Care should be taken to turn bedridden people onto their sides, so that they do not inhale any vomited stomach contents.
2. If a comatose person vomits, he should be turned onto his side and the vomitus should be cleared from his mouth.
3. After the initial episode of vomiting, solid food should be withheld temporarily and clear liquids should be given. (A clear liquid is one through which it is possible to read a newspaper.)
4. If the person goes twelve hours without vomiting, solid foods may be resumed, beginning with dry foods such as crackers.
5. If vomiting is prolonged or associated with severe abdominal pain, seek medical attention.

What Not To Do

1. Milk or formula should not be given to infants until the vomiting has subsided.
2. Solid foods should not be given to adults and children until the vomiting has subsided.

Section Three:

The Emergency Care System

To be most effective, emergency care must begin as soon as possible at the scene of an accident. In the home—one of the most common accident sites—there are two important steps that should be taken *before* an accident occurs: prevention and preparation.

The cheapest and most effective medicine is prevention. Every attempt to make the home as safe as possible is mandatory. Accidents in the home may be prevented by keeping stairways well lit and entryways unobstructed, by the careful placement of loose rugs, by proper care and maintenance of electrical appliances and cords, and by the proper shielding and use of power tools.

Particular care should be taken in the home to prevent poisoning. All prescription and over-the-counter drugs (including aspirin, cold remedies, and vitamins) should be stored in "child-proof" containers. In addition, old medications should be flushed down the toilet. The passage of time may cause drugs either to lose their potency or, through evaporation, to increase in potency. All medicine should be stored out of the sight and reach of children.

All cleaning solutions, drain and oven cleaners, solvents, and petroleum products (kerosene, gasoline, turpentine, charcoal lighter), insect spray, roach tablets and roach powder should be stored on high or locked shelves where children can't get at them. Never put any of these substances in a beverage or food container. Beverage bottles look particularly inviting to toddlers.

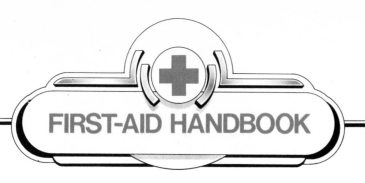

FIRST-AID HANDBOOK

Every home should have a separate box (not just the medicine cabinet)
containing at least the following supplies

First Aid Tools

Thermometer, oral
Thermometer, rectal
Flashlight
Hot water bag
Pair of scissors
Pair of tweezers
Packet of needles
Safety matches
Ice bag

First Aid Material

Aspirin, adult
Aspirin, children's, or aspirin substitute
Bottle of ipecac syrup (2 to 3 oz)
Bottle of aromatic spirits of ammonia
Antiseptic cream for burns
Sunscreen medication (para-aminobenzoic acid)

First Aid Dressings

Sterile 4″ × 4″ dressings
Gauze (2″ wide) for bandaging
Box of assorted adhesive dressings
1″ adhesive tape

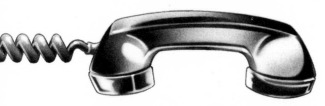

Appropriate List of Telephone Numbers

911 (the universal emergency call number in some communities)
Local hospital emergency department
Ambulance or rescue squad
Police department
Family physician
Poison Control Center (if one is available in the area)
Fire department

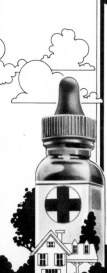

Prehospital Care

Wherever there is a serious accident, or when there is any question of serious injury, it is best to call an experienced ambulance or rescue squad. Many services are upgrading their capabilities with better equipment and training. Most ambulance drivers and attendants are at least basic Emergency Medical Technicians (EMTs). The EMTs have received 81 hours of intensive first aid training, have passed a minimal proficiency test, and are certified by a state health agency. Many communities also have advanced EMTs (paramedics) available for emergency care. These individuals are basic EMTs but have had an additional 500 to 1,000 hours of intensive training in advanced life support (defibrillation, use of intravenous medications, advanced airway management, etc.). They generally function through radiocommunications with a hospital-based physician.

To Summon Emergency Aid

Have the telephone numbers of an ambulance service or, if none is available, the local police or fire department readily accessible. When you call, be as calm as possible. *Do not* hang up until all of the following information has been given: a) your name; b) your location (how to get there); c) your telephone number; d) the type of emergency (number of people involved, etc.).

The Emergency Department

The emergency department of the local hospital is the best facility to evaluate and treat true emergencies. Because many people may be seeking emergency care at the same time for different degrees of emergencies, the emergency department might seem to be a very confusing place. Most emergency departments, however, are organized to quickly establish priorities for care, and to provide appropriate treatment for each individual as soon as possible within the limits of those priorities.

The system starts with the nurse, who usually sees the victim first and, by means of a few basic medical questions or tests (temperature, blood pressure, pulse, etc.), attempts to determine the nature of the victim's problem. This nurse is trained to recognize life-threatening problems and to assure that they are seen and evaluated first. In an emergency department patients are not seen on a first-come, first-served basis. For example, a person with a sprained ankle would have to wait to be seen until a man with severe chest pains had been treated.

Better hospital emergency departments have physicians present around the clock to see and treat emergencies. These physicians are specialists in the treatment of emergency problems. Their availability in the hospital and their special training make them the physicians best suited to initially evaluate and stabilize any true emergency. The emergency physician's practice frequently is confined to the emergency department, and he should not be assumed to be in competition with one's regular physician.

Index

d

e

diabetes **77**–265
  juvenile diabetes cause and treatment **79**–337
  first aid for insulin reaction **78**–420; **77**–422
  guidelines for use **78**–382
  hormonal mechanisms **78**–242, il. 243; **77**–264
  obesity effect on production **77**–398
  Yalow's research **79**–224
insulin reaction
  first aid **79**–416
insurance
  Australia **78**–321; **77**–335
  Canada **78**–323; **77**–337
  cancer screening coverage **78**–191
  health care **79**–227, il. 228; **78**–132
    care systems **77**–112, 341
    cost increases **78**–231; **77**–257
    technology **77**–222
  occupational safety policies **77**–304
  outpatient care coverage **78**–233, 304
  patients' rights **77**–281
  malpractice premiums rise **79**–234
  sports safety coverage **79**–292
  see also national health insurance
intensive care
  anesthesiology **78**–184; **77**–200
  emergency care coordination **78**–226
  premature infant care **77**–223, il. 224
interferon (IF) **78**–256; **77**–197
  antiviral drug research **79**–248
  viral disease treatment **79**–112
intermittent hydroarthrosis of the knee **77**–150
internal medicine **77**–287, 306, 349
International Chiropractors Association **77**–84
internship **77**–26, 306
interstitial brachytherapy **78**–298
intestine
  abdominal pain causes **78**–377
  bypass surgery for weight loss **79**–205
  digestive system diseases **78**–217
  fiber deficiency complications **79**–241
  radiation injuries **77**–322
  ulcers **79**–367
  see also colon
intima **78**–197, 374
intoxication **77**–193
intracellular infections **77**–274, il. 275
intralipid **77**–325
intraocular lens **77**–254
intrauterine device (IUD) **79**–344; **77**–204
  patient package inserts **79**–181
intravenous anesthetic **78**–35, 183
intravenous feeding **77**–325
iodine
  cancer link to deficiency **78**–390
  diagnostic uses **77**–237
ionizing radiation **77**–322
Iowa
  pseudorabies epidemic **78**–319
ipecac
  vomiting induction **77**–427
Iran
  ancient sexual taboos **78**–248
  digestive system cancer **77**–246
  zinc deficiency in diet **77**–246
Iraq
  smallpox **79**–127
Ireland
  heart attack incidence **77**–391
Ir (immune response) gene **77**–198
iridectomy **79**–391
iris **79**–389
iritis **77**–154
I-RNA (immune-RNA) **77**–277
iron **78**–215
  breast-feeding effect on absorption **79**–291
iron lung il. **79**–115
irregular heartbeat: *see* arrhythmia
isatin (thiosemicarbazone) **79**–248
Islam
  sexual taboos **78**–248
Islamic medicine **77**–11
Islets of Langerhans **77**–265
isoniazid **79**–261; **77**–276
  vitamin absorption efffect **79**–396
isoprinosine **79**–248
Israel
  aging studies **78**–117
  cholera epidemic **79**–322
  Dead Sea spa **77**–324
  diabetes study **78**–214; **77**–267
  hypochondria incidence study **79**–16

Italy
  cancer treatment study **78**–192
  health care system **77**–344
  medical education history **77**–12
  Seveso incident **78**–309, il. 308
  world medical news **79**–322
IUD: *see* intrauterine device
Ivy, Andrew
  Krebiozen controversy **77**–91

j

Jackson, Charles T.
  anesthesia history **78**–23
Jacob, François **77**–294
Jamaica
  marijuana effect study **77**–250
Janet, Pierre **78**–293
Japan
  aging studies **78**–117
  antismoking campaign **79**–324
  cancer **77**–211
    diet relation **78**–212; **77**–242
    stomach cancer **77**–246
  health care system **77**–343
  Minamata incident **78**–308
jaundice **77**–246
jaw
  dentistry advances **78**–210
  facial surgery **79**–312, 378
    reconstructive surgery il. **78**–287
  first aid for dislocation **77**–422
  wiring for weight loss **79**–206
JCAH (Joint Commission on Accreditation of Hospitals) **79**–233
Jefferson, Thomas **79**–332
jejunum
  bypass surgery for weight loss **79**–205
Jenner, Edward
  smallpox control history **79**–129
jet injector
  smallpox vaccination **79**–133
jet lag
  travelers' maladies **78**–371
Jews
  breast cancer incidence **78**–212
  culture and health **78**–111; **77**–127
  hypochondria incidence study **79**–17
  jogging **79**–293; **78**–399
  health quiz **79**–347
John of Arderne **77**–48
Johns Hopkins Hospital **79**–67, il. 68
Johns Hopkins University **77**–23, il. 25
Johnson, Samuel
  hypochondria **79**–9
Johnson, Timothy **79**–318
Johnson, Virginia **77**–271, 377, il. 378
Joint Commission on Accreditation of Hospitals (JCAH) **79**–233
Joints and Muscles 79–251. **See Connective Tissue Diseases 78**–204; **77**–226. **See Muscle Diseases 78**–265; **77**–295
  diseases
    arthritic symptoms **78**–361; **77**–145
    immunology research **77**–291
    rubella hazards **79**–361
    vitamin E therapy risks **77**–240
  first aid **79**–416; **78**–422; **77**–422
  jogging and running risks **79**–294
  osteopathic emphasis **78**–270; **77**–306
  physical therapy **78**–285; **77**–310
  prosthetic joints **77**–314
  sports medicine research **78**–54
  sprain cause and treatment **78**–360
Jordan
  cholera epidemic **79**–322
Journal of the American Medical Association **77**–240
Jung, Carl Gustav **78**–170, il. 171
Jungle, The (Sinclair) **79**–24
junk food
  child obesity causes **79**–335
juvenile delinquency: *see* delinquency
juvenile diabetes **79**–337, **77**–265
  viral causation theory **79**–109
juvenile rheumatoid arthritis: *see* Still's disease

k

Kaiser, Edgar F. **78**–125
Kaiser-Permanente Medical Care Program **78**–124
kallikrein **78**–200
Katz, Bernard **77**–292
Kawasaki disease (mucocutaneous lymph node syndrome) **79**–288
Kawasaki, Tomisaku il. **79**–288
Kefauver-Harris Drug Amendments **77**–92
Kell blood group system **77**–207
Kelly, Howard A. il. **77**–23
keloids
  cosmetic surgery risk **79**–377
Kelsey, Frances O. **79**–30
Kennedy-Corman plan **79**–231
Kennedy-Griffith proposal **77**–281
Kenya
  smallpox eradication program **79**–140
  world medical news **79**–322
kepone **79**–279; **78**–308; **77**–320
Kernaghan, Salvinija G. **78**–305
Kessling pressure appliance **78**–283
keto acids **77**–265
ketone **77**–265, 353
ketonemia **77**–353
ketonuria **77**–353
ketosis **79**–203; **77**–265
kidney
  blood filtration **78**–350
  blood pressure regulation **78**–200
  body water conservation **77**–264
  cell loss in aging process **77**–190
  jogging and running risks **79**–296
Kidney Diseases 79–255
  abdominal pain causes **78**–377
  amphotericin side effects **77**–276
  anesthetic risks **78**–33
  bench surgery **79**–320
  cancer **78**–185
  gout complications **77**–152
  hemodialysis **78**–260, 314, il. 261
  hypertension damage **77**–395
  infection risk **79**–311
  myoglobinuria complications **78**–267
  pregnancy risk increase **77**–313
  transplantation **78**–314; **77**–328, il. 329
    immunology research **77**–196
    immunosuppression **77**–291
    surgical advances **79**–309; **77**–326, il. 327
    wart occurrence **78**–300
  urology **77**–330
kidney stone **78**–379
kinins **78**–200
Kinsey, Alfred C. **77**–271, 380
Kitasato, Shibasaburo **79**–116
knee
  arthritic symptoms and treatment **78**–361
  jogging and running risks **79**–295
  osteoarthrosis results **77**–147, ils. 146, 150
  prosthetic joints **77**–314
kneecap (patella)
  jogging and running risks **79**–295
Koch, Robert **77**–17
Kokich, Vincent G. **78**–211
Kolff, Willem J. **77**–315
Koplik's spots **79**–359
Kornberg, Arthur **77**–295
Korsakoff's psychosis **77**–194
Kosterlitz, Hans W. **78**–277
K-P diet **79**–384
Krebiozen **77**–91
Krebs, Ernst T., Jr. **78**–237
Kuan Kung **78**–155, il. 153
kuru **79**–277; **77**–299

l

LAAM: *see* levo-alpha-acetyl-methadol
labeling **79**–25

drug interaction warnings **79**–396
saccharin and sugar labeling **79**–199
labile hypertensives **77**–394
labor unions **79**–234
  workers' health action **79**–279
laceration
  first aid **79**–405; **78**–359, 409
lactate **77**–216
lactic acidosis **79**–34
lactogen **77**–263
Ladee, G. A. **79**–16
Laënnec, R. T. H. **77**–17
laetrile **79**–186; **78**–237, il. 238; **77**–92
Lain Entralgo, P. **77**–38
Lakes Region General Hospital (Laconia, New Hampshire) **79**–71
Lalonde, Marc **78**–87, 324; **77**–339
laminar flow rooms **79**–154; il. **78**–259
language **77**–367
laparoscopy
  diagnostic use **77**–303
  sterilization use **79**–178, 343, il. 179; **77**–205
laparotomy **79**–343
Laragh, John **78**–200
Larrey, Dominique-Jean **78**–17
laryngitis **77**–401
larynx
  artificial replacement design **77**–315
  cancer
    alcoholism link **78**–111
    environmental carcinogens il. **77**–211
    smoking link **78**–390
  upper respiratory infections **77**–401
laser
  cauterization use **77**–246
  photocoagulation use **79**–216, 218
Latham, Michael **79**–200
Latrodectus mactans: see black widow spider
law: *see* Health Care Law
Law, The (Hippocrates) **77**–176, il. 175
laxative
  appendicitis causes **78**–380
  muscle disease causes **78**–267
  nutrient absorption effect **79**–396
lead poisoning **78**–309; **77**–231
  occupational risks **79**–281
Leaf, Alexander **78**–81
learning
  aging process **77**–191
  depression susceptibility **77**–233
  hospital care stress **77**–360
  Importance of Play, The **77**–367
learning disabilities **79**–381
  osteopathic study **78**–271
Lebanon
  cholera epidemic **79**–322
LE cell **79**–253; **77**–155
lecithin **77**–248, 302
leg
  first aid **79**–406, il. 409; **78**–410; il. 413
  jogging and running risks **79**–295
  physical examination **78**–346
  restless-legs syndrome **78**–265
Legionnaires' disease **79**–262; **78**–256
leishmaniasis **77**–60, il. 61
lens **79**–389; **77**–254, 315
leprosy **79**–95, il. 94; **77**–275
  ancient care il. **77**–35
  pre-Columbian incidence **77**–62
  South African research **78**–328
  thalidomide benefits **78**–219
less developed countries **79**–321
  immunization problems **79**–121
leukapheresis **77**–207
leukemia **78**–188, 257
  Acute Leukemias, The **79**–142
  animals as carriers **78**–319
  BCG use **77**–215
  cancer **79**–185
  childhood illnesses **77**–224
  incidence **78**–389
  Living with Leukemia **79**–158
  occupational risks **79**–280
  radiation hazards **77**–320
  veterinary medicine research **77**–335
  viral organ theory **77**–278
leukocyte
  Acute Leukemias, The **79**–142
  blood separation methods **77**–206
  connective tissue diseases **78**–204
  interferon preparation **79**–249
  leukemia **78**–188, 257
  life span **77**–190
  radiation injury treament **77**–322
levamisole **79**–252; **77**–215